3

Health Psychology
An Introduction to Behavior and Health

3

Health Psychology
An Introduction to Behavior and Health

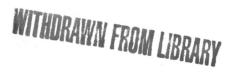
Linda Brannon
Jess Feist

McNeese State University

Brooks/Cole Publishing Company

I(T)P® An International Thomson Publishing Company

Pacific Grove • Albany • Bonn • Boston • Cincinnati • Detroit • London • Madrid • Melbourne
Mexico City • New York • Paris • San Francisco • Singapore • Tokyo • Toronto • Washington

295943   NOV 1 0 2004

Sponsoring Editor: *Marianne Taflinger*
Marketing Representative: *Carolyn Crockett*
Editorial Assistant: *Laura Donahue/Scott Brearton*
Production Editor: *Tessa A. McGlasson*
Manuscript Editor: *Patterson Lamb*
Design Coordination: *E. Kelly Shoemaker*
Interior and Cover Design: *Laurie Albrecht*
Cover Photo: *The Image Bank/Wy*

Permissions Editor: *Catherine Gingras*
Art Editor: *Lisa Torri*
Interior Illustration: *John and Judy Waller*
Photo Editor: *Robert Western*
Marketing Team: *Gay Meixel and Romy Taormina*
Typesetting: *Colortype, San Diego*
Cover Printing: *Phoenix Color Corporation*
Printing and Binding: *Quebecor/Fairfield*

BROOKS/COLE PUBLISHING COMPANY
511 Forest Lodge Road
Pacific Grove, CA 93950
USA

International Thomson Publishing Europe
Berkshire House 168-173
High Holborn
London WC1V 7AA
England

Thomas Nelson Australia
102 Dodds Street
South Melbourne, 3205
Victoria, Australia

Nelson Canada
1120 Birchmount Road
Scarborough, Ontario
Canada M1K 5G4

International Thomson Editores
Campos Eliseos 385, Piso 7
Col. Polanco
11560 México D. F. México

International Thomson Publishing GmbH
Königswinterer Strasse 418
53227 Bonn
Germany

International Thomson Publishing Asia
221 Henderson Road
#05-10 Henderson Building
Singapore 0315

International Thomson Publishing Japan
Hirakawacho Kyowa Building, 3F
2-2-1 Hirakawacho
Chiyoda-ku, Tokyo 102
Japan

Printed in the United States of America

10   9   8   7   6   5   4   3   2   1

Library of Congress Cataloging-in-Publication Data
Brannon, Linda, [date]–
    Health psychology : an introduction to behavior and health / Linda Brannon, Jess Feist.—3rd ed.
        p.   cm.
    Includes bibliographical references and index.
    ISBN 0-534-34306-6
    1. Medicine and psychology.   2. Sick—Psychology.   3. Health behavior.   I. Feist, Jess.   II. Title.
R726.5.B72   1996
616'.001'9—dc20   96-2626
                                                                    CIP

Brief Contents

Contents

Preface

At the beginning of the 20th century, most serious illnesses were caused by contact with viruses and bacteria. People had little individual responsibility for preventing diseases because these microorganisms were nearly impossible to avoid. Today, most serious diseases occur partly as the result of individual behaviors — or failures to behave. As health and illness became more closely linked to behavior, psychology — the science of behavior — became involved with many health-related issues. This involvement led to the birth and development of *health psychology,* the scientific study of behaviors that relate to health enhancement, disease prevention, and rehabilitation.

At about the same time, two other disciplines began to emerge — behavioral medicine and behavioral health. *Behavioral medicine,* an interdisciplinary field oriented toward treatment, has grown rapidly as a result of the recognition that behavior is an important and controllable contributor to the development of illness. *Behavioral health* includes the wide variety of research and interventions that explore ways to keep healthy people from becoming sick.

The field of health psychology has continued to grow and progress since the publication of the first and second editions of *Health Psychology: An Introduction to Behavior and Health*. The first edition of the book, for example, contained a rationale for the existence of a textbook for health psychology at the undergraduate level, but now no such rationale is necessary: Undergraduate health psychology courses have appeared at many universities, colleges, and community colleges. The field is no longer fighting for acceptance as a teaching area in undergraduate curricula.

Our purpose in writing a third edition was to reflect the changes in the field of health psychology, to update the material in the book by including some of the voluminous research on behavior and health, and to give students a balanced view of health psychology — one that includes both behavioral medicine and behavioral health.

THE THIRD EDITION

We have organized the third edition of *Health Psychology: An Introduction to Behavior and Health* into four areas. In addition to an introductory section, we include two major sections that correspond to the fields of behavioral medicine and behavioral health. The final section highlights the growth of health psychology and looks to future challenges. In addition, the third edition expands the coverage of many topics and adds several new topics.

Expanded Coverage

The volume of health-related research that appears daily was a primary motivation to write a new edition of *Health Psychology*. We have added over 900 references, updating the existing topics and adding new ones.

We have streamlined Chapter 1, emphasizing the different models available to explain the involvement of health and psychology in health. Additions include information on leading causes of death for young adults, the age of most students, and expanded information on *gender* and *ethnic factors* in health.

Chapter 2 reviews research methodology in psychology and epidemiology. One major section of Chapter 2 covers research methods in psychology, and the section on *research methods in epidemiology* represents almost half this chapter. We believe that students who take a course in health psychology benefit from a discussion of how psychology research is done and require an introduction to the research methods in epidemiology. Our organization of this material aims for easy comparisons of methodology in psychology and in epidemiology. A comparison of these research approaches allows students to appreciate and understand the research presented in later chapters. To facilitate comparisons, we have chosen to present example studies oriented around one topic — cardiovascular disease — to allow students to see how each of the many research methods in both psychology and epidemiology can be used to investigate a single topic.

After the introductory chapters, students are introduced to Part 2, "Behavior and Illness," which includes topics within behavioral medicine and begins with two chapters on stress. Chapter 3 covers the theories, sources, and measurement of stress and new information on the relationship between sleep and the immune system. Chapter 4 examines the relationship between stress and illness, updating the review of psychoneuroimmunology and cardiac reactivity. Chapter 5 discusses the topic of pain, including the physiology of the somatosensory system, pain syndromes, theories, and measurement. Because of the similarities in their techniques, stress management and pain management both appear in Chapter 6 along with an evaluation of the effectiveness of each technique.

Chapter 7 presents information on seeking health care. We have added a review and critique of several theories that attempt to explain why people seek health care. In addition, this chapter includes the review of factors involved in seeking medical care and being hospitalized. Chapter 8 reviews patients' compliance with medical advice, presenting not only research evidence but also theories that are relevant to adherence.

Chapter 9 identifies factors involved in cardiovascular disease, updating the extensive research on this topic. We have expanded the coverage of cholesterol as a factor in cardiovascular disease and have traced the evolution of the Type A behavior pattern. Chapter 10 reviews behavioral factors in cancer, with expanded discussion on the value of psychosocial support for cancer patients. The expanded coverage in Chapter 11 includes new information on the causes of Alzheimer's disease and up-

dated coverage of the human immunodeficiency virus (HIV) and acquired immune deficiency syndrome (AIDS).

Chapters 13 through 16 examine the health consequences of smoking, drinking and drug use, eating and efforts toward weight control, and exercising. All these chapters contain updated information about these health-related behaviors. In addition, Chapter 15 contains reorganized information on dieting and asks questions about the value and success of dieting to control weight.

Chapter 17 offers predictions about the role of health psychology in the future, oriented around health goals for the United States.

New Topics

In addition to this expanded coverage, we have included several new topics and a new chapter.

In the second edition, Chapter 2 contained a review of theories, but the third edition separates these theories into various chapters where students can see the practical application of theoretical models to a variety of issues. The *diathesis-stress model* is an addition to Chapter 4. Chapter 5 now poses a contrast between the *specificity theory* and the *gate control theory* of pain and integrates Melzack's neuromatrix concept of pain into the gate control theory. The *theory of reasoned action, theory of planned behavior, self-regulation theory, stages of change theory,* and the *precaution adoption process* all appear in Chapter 7 in the context of seeking health care. Theories of compliance appear in Chapter 8.

Other chapters have new sections and new information. New sections in Chapter 3 reorganize the information on sources of stress, with sections on *personal relationships* and *urban press* as sources of stress as well as several of the new measuring instruments to assess stress. Included in the updated version of Chapter 4 is a new section on *stress and negative mood,* which presents information on negative affect and illness as well as new information on posttraumatic stress disorder.

Chapter 5 now contains new sections on *preventing pain* and the *limitations of medical treatments.* Chapter 6 now includes a section of the value of *expressing emotion.*

Chapter 7 has a new title, "Seeking Health Care," and the chapter concentrates on factors relating to the decision about consulting health care professionals and being in the hospital. The third edition includes an added section to Chapter 8 on adherence called "Does Adherence Pay Off?"

Chapter 9 now includes new sections on *types of cholesterol* and *cholesterol and the elderly,* which allows a more thorough exploration of this important and often misunderstood risk factor for cardiovascular disease. In addition, the expanded coverage of diet as a risk factor includes sections on *fat, fiber,* and *vitamins* as important dietary components. Additions to the coverage of the Type A behavior pattern include the recent research on anger as the toxic component. Chapter 10 has an added section on *perceived dangers of smoking.*

Chapter 12, "Staying Healthy," is a new chapter, which begins the section on "Behavioral Health." This chapter examines issues of injury prevention and control of violence. These factors are related to accidental and violent deaths, the leading cause of deaths for people in the United States under age 45. This chapter also includes information on mass media campaigns, workplace wellness programs, and communitywide health campaigns.

Chapter 13 contains a new section on *smoking and weight control.* Chapter 14 has a new section on *cognitive-behavioral theories* of drinking, which includes two theories that appeared in the second edition, the tension reduction model and the self-awareness model, plus a new model called *alcohol myopia.* The section of this chapter that deals with other drugs includes new material on *drug use and abuse, treatment for drug abuse,* and *preventing and controlling drug use.* Chapter 16 has expanded coverage of the cardiovascular benefits of exercise, which includes added sections on *exercise and stroke* and exercise as a *protection against diabetes.*

Chapter 17, the final chapter, has a new subtitle, "Growth and Future Challenges," which summarizes our view of the future of health psychology. This chapter contains a great deal of new material, organized around the goals in *Healthy People 2000* (U.S. Department of Health and Human Services, 1990c) and added challenges for controlling health care costs.

WRITING STYLE

Although *Health Psychology: An Introduction to Behavior and Health* (3rd ed.) frequently explores complex issues and difficult topics, we use clear, concise, and comprehensible language as well as an informal writing style. The book is designed for upper-division undergraduate students and should be easily understood by those with a minimal background in psychology. Health psychology courses typically draw students from a variety of college majors, necessitating the inclusion of some elementary material that may be repetitive to some students. For other students, this material will fill in the background they need to comprehend the material unique to health psychology.

Technical terms first appear in **boldface type**, and a definition usually appears at that point in the text. These terms also appear in the glossary at the end of the book.

INSTRUCTIONAL AIDS

Besides a glossary, we have supplied several other features to help both students and instructors. These include "Would You Believe . . . ?" boxes, annotated reading lists, and case studies.

"Would You Believe . . . ?" Boxes

The boxes throughout the book all take the form of "Would You Believe . . . ?" We asked this question repeatedly to highlight particularly intriguing findings in health psychology, and we chose material we thought might be provocative for inclusion in the boxes.

Annotated Suggested Readings

At the end of each chapter we have included four or five suggested readings along with a short description of each. These readings have been carefully chosen for their recency, their readability, and their importance to the chapter subject. They will direct students to further study.

Case Studies

We begin every chapter except the final one with a case study. Some of these case studies are new to the third edition, and others have appeared in the previous editions; all illustrate the topics for each chapter. The cases are never perfect examples, and we have received many comments about them, asking why we included specific features or behavior in a certain case. The case studies fail to be perfect examples because they are real people. We have never invented any specific characteristics for these people but have chosen cases we believe will help students relate the chapter's scientific information to real people. Each case matches research findings only imperfectly, but we hope this imperfection will illustrate to students that real people do not fit the statistical profiles in every way.

We would like to thank the people who shared their stories with us so that we could write these case studies. We have changed some details of their lives to protect their privacy, but we have preserved the details of their cases that relate to their health and behavior.

Chapter Outlines and Chapter Summaries

The chapter outlines orient students to chapter content by previewing major topics to be covered in each chapter. Chapter summaries contain enough detail to provide a quick review of important concepts.

STUDY GUIDE

We have authored the study guide for the third edition of *Health Psychology: An Introduction to Behavior and Health* because we feel that a study guide written by the textbook's authors provides students with a more accurate and meaningful account of the contents of the text. Like the textbook, the study guide is divided into 17 chapters, and each chapter contains a detailed summary outline and a variety of test questions. We believe the study guide will help students organize their study methods and will also enhance their chances of achieving their best scores on class quizzes.

INSTRUCTOR'S MANUAL

This edition of *Health Psychology: An Introduction to Behavior and Health* is accompanied by a comprehensive instructor's manual. Each chapter begins with a lecture outline, a summary in outline form of the headings from the chapter. This outline should assist instructors in preparing lecture material from the text.

Multiple-choice test items make up a large section of each chapter of the instructor's manual. These test items were written by the authors and will reduce the instructor's work in preparing tests. Each item lists the page in the text on which the material appears, and each is marked with the correct answer.

Essay questions are included for each chapter, along with an outline answer of the critical points that should appear in answers to these questions.

Also included for each chapter are suggested activities. These activities vary widely — from video recommendations to student research to classroom debates. We have tried to include more activities than any instructor can feasibly assign during a semester so as to give instructors a choice for activities.

ACKNOWLEDGMENTS

Many people have contributed to the completion of this book, and we wish to express our gratitude. First, we thank Patrick Moreno, who has acted as adviser, librarian, reviewer, and proofreader. His untiring efforts to make the book better have made the book better.

Next we acknowledge the considerable assistance of all the staff at the McNeese library, whose help has been essential for the completion of this project. Joanne Durand and Brantley Cagle have been especially helpful — both have exhibited outstanding skill and constant good humor in acquiring material for our use. We also thank Imogene Park, Medical Librarian at St. Patrick Hospital in Lake Charles, Louisiana, for her help.

In addition, we would like to thank the people at Brooks/Cole for their assistance. Marianne Taflinger supervised this edition, and we are grateful for her interest and assistance. Ken King, who was our original editor at Wadsworth, did a great deal to shape the book. Although he is no longer our editor, his influence is still apparent in this edition. We express our gratitude to Tessa McGlasson, production editor, whose expert skill greatly enhanced this book. Copyeditor Patterson Lamb's impressive knowledge of the English language helped improve our writing style. Thanks also go to Kelly Shoemaker and Laurie

Albrecht, designers; Lisa Torri, art editor; and Bob Western, photo editor.

We are also indebted to a number of reviewers who read all or parts of the manuscript for either the first or second edition and made valuable comments, for which we are grateful: Mary Arbogast; Cole Barton, Davidson College; Jim Blascovich, University of California, Santa Barbara; Bernard L. Bloom, University of Colorado, Boulder; Sandra A. Brown, University of California, San Diego; William E. Bruce, University of North Carolina, Asheville; Kenneth D. Craig, University of British Columbia; Tom DiLorenzo, University of Missouri; Leonard Doerfler, Auburn University; Carol-Ann Emmons, University of Michigan; Anita Fields, McNeese State University; Arthur J. Gonchar, University of La Verne; Sergio Guglielmi, University of Virginia; David Hanson, James Madison University; David Hines, Ball State University; John Jung, California State University, Long Beach; Elizabeth Klonoff, California State University, San Bernardino; Richard Lazarus, University of California, Berkeley; David I. Mostofsky, Boston University; Susan G. Nash, University of Houston; Mary K. O'Keeffe, Providence College; Ralph Paffenbarger, Jr., Stanford School of Medicine; Paul B. Paulus, University of Texas, Arlington; R. Douglas Peters, Jacksonville State University; Antonio C. Puente, University of North Carolina, Wilmington; Thomas Reischl, Michigan State University; Frederic Shaffer, Northeast Missouri State University; Margaret K. Snooks, University of Houston, Clear Lake; Cecie Starr; Robert M. Stern, Pennsylvania State University; and Diane C. Tucker, University of Alabama at Birmingham.

Authors typically thank their spouses for being understanding, supportive, and sacrificing. We thank our spouses, Barry Humphus and Mary Jo Feist, because they were understanding, supportive, and sacrificing. But they have also provided more than the traditional emotional support. Both have made contributions that have helped to shape the book. In addition to his creative contributions to the book, Barry provided generous, patient, live-in, expert computer consultation that proved essential in the preparation of the manuscript, and Mary Jo has made suggestions on style and content.

Linda Brannon
Jess Feist

1

Foundations of Health Psychology

Introducing Health Psychology

Dwayne, a 21-year-old college junior, seldom thinks about his health—either his present or his future health. In fact, Dwayne seems to believe that he is invincible. He sees his present lack of illness as a sign of good health and assumes that he will always be free of disease and disability.

Perhaps Dwayne should be more concerned because many of his present habits may have some effect on his future health. Probably his most damaging health practice is his diet, which consists mostly of fast-food hamburgers, with an occasional fried fish sandwich for variety. However, variety is a very low priority for Dwayne, who eats three meals a day, six days a week at the same fast-food restaurant. For breakfast he almost always eats a biscuit, scrambled eggs, sausage, and a soft drink (because he doesn't like coffee). Lunch invariably consists of French fries, a hamburger, and another soft drink. Dwayne's evening meal is usually a repeat of lunch, except occasionally he will have a fried fish sandwich in place of the hamburger. In addition to these meals, he eats lots of sweets between meals; he is especially fond of ice cream, candy bars, and doughnuts.

Dwayne's diet is not his only health risk. He seldom exercises, never uses seatbelts, and has few close friends. Also, he tends to believe that his future health is beyond his personal control. He believes that heart disease, cancer, and accidents are matters of genetics, chance, or fate rather than his behavior. Thus, he has thought little about ways of enhancing his future health or decreasing his chances of developing a debilitating illness or avoiding premature death. When he becomes sick he adopts a passive attitude toward his own cure, hoping that the over-the-counter medication he takes will help him feel better.

On the other hand, Dwayne does some things right. He does not smoke cigarettes or drink alcohol, and he has very little stress in his life. When he filled out the popular Social Readjustment Rating Scale (Holmes & Rahe, 1967; see Chapter 3 for a discussion of this scale), he reported only one stressful life event—Christmas. Although Dwayne does not smoke, his reasons for refraining have nothing to do with health. When he smoked a cigarette as a young adolescent, he became sick and lost any motivation to try again. He avoids alcohol for religious reasons and not because he thinks it is harmful to his health.

Robyn is also a 21-year-old college junior, but her attitude toward health is quite different from Dwayne's. She believes that she has primary responsibility for her own health, and she has adopted a lifestyle that she believes will keep her healthy. Like Dwayne, she does not smoke. She tried to take a puff from a cigarette when she was in the fourth grade, but after coughing for awhile, she decided that smoking wasn't for her. She never tried again. Her father is a smoker, but several years ago she and her mother convinced him not to smoke in their house. Robyn is acutely aware of the potential dangers of passive smoking, and when possible, she avoids all enclosed places where people are allowed to smoke.

She has confidence that she will never smoke, and she believes that smoking contributes to both heart disease and cancer. Unlike Dwayne, Robyn drinks in moderation. Her parents are also moderate drinkers, and Robyn has lived all her life with a variety of alcoholic beverages in her home. She feels confident that her drinking will not escalate and has no fear of becoming a problem drinker.

Robyn's diet is quite different from Dwayne's. She seldom eats eggs, whole milk products, beef, or pork; she concentrates on eating lots of fruits and vegetables. She occasionally allows herself a dessert, such as a small piece of cake, pie, or pudding. In selecting her meals, she chooses food that is low in fat, calories, sodium, and cholesterol. Her grandfather died of heart disease at 63, and Robyn is convinced that his smoking and high-fat, high-cholesterol diet hastened his death.

Robyn has also begun a regular exercise routine. She is currently enrolled in an aerobic dancing class that meets three times a week. On three of the other days she walks briskly for 30 minutes a day. When not enrolled in an aerobics class, she walks six days a week. She seldom allows weather, class work, job, or social engagements to interfere with exercising.

Unlike Dwayne, who thinks that illness is caused by agents beyond his control, Robyn believes that disease results from a combination of biological, psychological, and social causes and that a person has considerable control over the psychological and social forces. This chapter, and the rest of the book, examines these psychological and social factors as they apply to health and illness.

THE CHANGING FIELD OF HEALTH

At the beginning of the 20th century, most people in the United States had views of illness and health similar to Dwayne's. People's illnesses were largely the result of contact with impure drinking water, contaminated foods, or sick people. Once they were ill, people were expected to seek medical care to be cured, but medicine had few cures to offer. The duration of most illnesses—such as typhoid fever, pneumonia, and diphtheria—was relatively short; a person either died or got well in a matter of weeks. People felt very limited responsibility for contracting an illness because they believed it was impos-

sible to avoid contagious disease. At that time, Dwayne's view of illness would have been considered accurate. But during the last years of the 20th century, such a view is becoming obsolete.

During the 20th century, health in the United States changed in several important ways. First, the leading causes of death have changed from infectious diseases to those that relate to unhealthy behavior and lifestyle. Second, the escalating cost of medical care has spotlighted the importance of educating people about how health-related practices can lower their risk of becoming ill. Third, a new definition of health has emerged, so that health is now seen as the presence of positive well-being, not merely the absence of disease. Fourth, some in the health care field have advocated a broader perspective of health and disease, questioning the usefulness of the traditional biomedical model.

PATTERNS OF ILLNESS AND DEATH

Today the major health problems in the United States no longer come from infectious diseases but from **chronic diseases**, illnesses that develop, persist, or recur over a long period of time. Chronic disorders include heart disease, cancer, chronic obstructive pulmonary disease, and stroke—the four major causes of death in the United States. These diseases are not new, of course, but the proportion of people who die of them has changed dramatically since 1900. Table 1.1 reveals important differences in the leading causes of death in the United States as recorded in 1900 and 1993. Although cardiovascular diseases (including both heart disease and stroke) head both lists, there are few other similarities. In 1900, the majority of deaths were from diseases that were rooted in public or community health problems, such as influenza, pneumonia, tuberculosis, diphtheria, and typhoid fever. By 1993, most deaths were attributable to diseases associated with individual behavior and lifestyle. Cardiovascular disease (including stroke), cancer, chronic obstructive pulmonary disease (including both emphysema and chronic bronchitis), accidental death, diabetes, suicide, and cirrhosis of the liver have been linked to stress, cigarette smoking, alcohol abuse, unwise eating, and sedentary lifestyle. In addition, the rapid rise of infectious and parasitic diseases is linked to the human immunodeficiency virus (HIV) which is largely the result of unsafe behaviors.

Table 1.1 **The ten leading causes of death in the United States, 1900 and 1993 (rates per 100,000 population)**

1900	Rate	1993	Rate
1. Cardiovascular diseases (heart disease, stroke)	345	1. Cardiovascular diseases (heart disease, stroke)	366
2. Influenza and pneumonia	202	2. Cancer	206
3. Tuberculosis	194	3. Chronic obstructive pulmonary diseases	39
4. Gastritis, duodenitis, enteritis, and colitis	143	4. Accidents	34
5. Accidents	72	5. Influenza and pneumonia	32
6. Cancer	64	6. Diabetes	21
7. Diphtheria	40	7. Other infectious and parasitic diseases	18
8. Typhoid fever	31	8. Suicide	12
9. Measles	13	9. Homicide and legal intervention	9.9
10. Chronic liver diseases and cirrhosis	*	10. Chronic liver diseases and cirrhosis	9.6

*data unavailable
SOURCE: Figures for 1900 from *Historical Statistics of the United States: Colonial Times to 1970, Pt. 1* by U.S. Bureau of the Census, 1975, Washington, DC: U.S. Government Printing Office. Figures for 1993 from *Statistical Abstracts of the United States* by U.S. Bureau of the Census, 1995, Washington, DC: U.S. Government Printing Office.

McGinnis and Foege (1993) estimated that in 1990 more than one million deaths in the United States, or about half the total deaths, had preventable causes. These authors calculated that tobacco accounted for about 400,000 deaths, or 19% of all deaths. In addition, diet and physical inactivity were responsible for about 300,000 (14%) deaths, and alcohol, firearms, sexual behaviors, motor vehicles, and illicit drug use killed about 200,000 more (9%).

These causes of death apply to the population as a whole but differ for various age and ethnic groups. The chronic diseases that are the leading causes of death are more likely to affect the middle-aged and elderly, but as Figure 1.1 shows, young people between 15 and 24 years old die from accidents or unintentional injuries more often than from any other cause. In 1993, accidents were responsible for about 40% of the deaths in this age group; homicides accounted for 23%; suicide, 13%; cancer, 5%; heart disease, 2%; and HIV infection, less than 2%. In 1993, HIV infection replaced unintentional injuries as the primary killer of adults between 25 and 44 years of age (Centers for Disease Control and Pre-

vention [CDC], 1995b). In this age group, these two causes of death are followed by cancer, heart disease, suicide, and homicide (United States Bureau of the Census [USBC], 1995).

Ethnic background is also a factor in life expectancy and cause of death. If African Americans and European Americans in the United States were considered to be different nations, White America would rank 12th in the world in mortality rate whereas Black America would rank 33rd (Dwyer, 1995). Despite these dramatic differences, it is not clear what component or components connected to ethnicity raise the risks. Some researchers (Centerwall, 1984, 1985; Navarro, 1990; Pappas, 1994) have contended that social class is the underlying factor, saying that socioeconomic status is associated with mortality more strongly than is ethnicity. In addition, the factors of income, occupation, and education all relate to ethnicity.

Poverty is a factor in illness and decreased life expectancy. Separating ethnic background and socioeconomic status is very difficult in the United States because a disproportionate number of African Americans, Hispanic Americans, and Native Americans

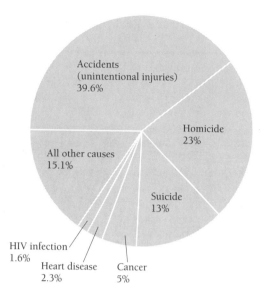

Figure 1.1 Leading causes of death among young adults, 15 to 24, United States, 1993.
SOURCE: Data from *Statistical Abstracts of the United States, 1995* (115th ed.). by U. S. Bureau of the Census, 1995, Washington, DC, U.S. Government Printing Office, p. 94.

are poor and unable to afford adequate medical care. Fisher (1995) found that ethnic minority Americans were less likely than European Americans to have insurance coverage, an important factor in access to medical care. Poverty is also associated with poorer health habits (Gibbons, 1991) and thus is related to increased risks for disease as well as difficulties in accessing medical care.

About one-third of African Americans live below the poverty line, but only about 12% of European Americans are poor (Gorman, 1991). The risks of living in poverty have substantial health implications, beginning before birth. With no prenatal care, poor women are more likely to deliver low-birth-weight infants, who are more likely to die than infants with normal birth weight. Cutbacks in federal immunization programs during the 1980s resulted in an increasing percentage of poor children without protection against measles and other childhood diseases. Children and adolescents living in urban poverty are vulnerable to neighborhood violence and are less likely than wealthier children and adolescents to have regular health care. Poor adults also have limited access to regular health care, with local

hospital emergency rooms providing the only accessible care for many (Gorman, 1991). Poverty is a serious health risk.

Educational level is another factor that is related to ethnic background as well as to life expectancy, occupation, income, and social class (Navarro, 1990; Rogers, 1992). In addition, lower educational level is related to behaviors that increase health risks such as smoking, eating a high-fat diet, and maintaining a sedentary lifestyle (Pappas, 1994; Winkleby, Jatulis, Frank, & Fortmann, 1992).

Therefore, the variable of ethnicity is associated with other factors that relate to health status and mortality, complicating the interpretation of studies on this topic. Only studies that control for socioeconomic factors and then compare ethnic groups can show ethnic differences, and many such studies fail to find differences. For example, Keil, Sutherland, Knapp, and Tyroler (1992) followed African American and European American men for 28 years and found that when socioeconomic status (defined by educational level and occupational status) was held constant, mortality rate differences between the two groups disappeared.

Although the majority of deaths in all ethnic groups, as well as deaths among young adults, can be attributed to lifestyle and unhealthy behaviors, Americans have started doing some things right, and deaths related to behavior and lifestyle are decreasing. For example, deaths from cardiovascular disease peaked in 1960 and have declined by almost 30% since 1970 (USBC, 1995).

Partially as a consequence of the movement toward healthier lifestyles, the life expectancy of people in the United States continues to increase. In 1900, life expectancy was 47.3 years (USBC, 1975) whereas today it is nearly 76 years (USBC, 1995). In other words, infants born today can, on average, expect to live more than a generation longer than their great-great-grandparents born at the beginning of the 20th century.

What factors have accounted for the nearly 30-year increase in life expectancy during the 20th century? A more health-conscious lifestyle is a factor, but the control of many infectious diseases and the reduction of infant mortality rates have been more important. Widespread vaccination, safer drinking water and milk supplies, and more effi-

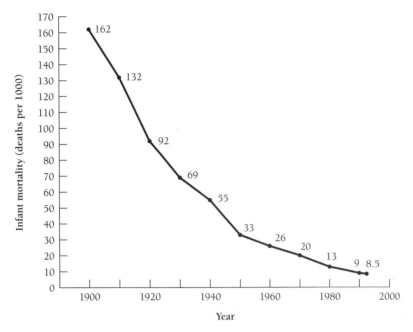

Figure 1.2 Decline in infant mortality in the United States, 1900 to 1992. SOURCE: Data from *Statistical Abstracts of the United States,* by U.S. Bureau of the Census, 1995, Washington, DC: U.S. Government Printing Office, pp. 90–91 and from *Historical Statistics of the United States: Colonial Times to 1970* by U.S. Bureau of the Census, 1975, Washington, DC: U.S. Government Printing Office, p. 60.

cient disposal of sewage have helped contain infectious diseases. In addition, improved nutrition has increased people's resistance to infection, and antibiotics have provided a cure for many infectious diseases. Improved medical care, such as surgical technology, improved paramedic teams, and better intensive care units also have made some contribution to longevity.

Although these advances have helped extend lives, the lowering of infant mortality has contributed even more to average increased life expectancy. When infants die before their first birthday, these deaths greatly lower the population's average life expectancy. Thus, decreasing deaths at a young age can have a substantial statistical impact. As Figure 1.2 shows, a dramatic decline in infant death rates occurred between 1900 and 1992. The total death rates have also decreased, but not as rapidly as for infants. Indeed, life expectancy at age 65 has increased little, indicating that the lifestyle changes, public health measures, and improvements in medical care have not had as great an impact on life expectancy for the elderly (USBC, 1995).

In summary, four important patterns of illness and death have emerged in the United States during the 20th century. First, chronic illnesses have replaced infectious diseases as the leading causes of death; second, accidents, homicide, and suicide account for more than three-fourths of all deaths among young adults; third, disparities exist in the health and life expectancy among ethnic groups, but the underlying reasons for these differences may be more a result of socioeconomic and educational levels than ethnic background; fourth, life expectancy has increased by about 30 years, but most of this improvement has been the result of reduced infant mortality rates.

ESCALATING COST OF MEDICAL CARE

The second major change within the field of health has been the escalating cost of medical care, and these costs are related to the increase in life expectancy. As people live to middle and old age, they tend to develop chronic illnesses, which require extended (and often expensive) medical treatment.

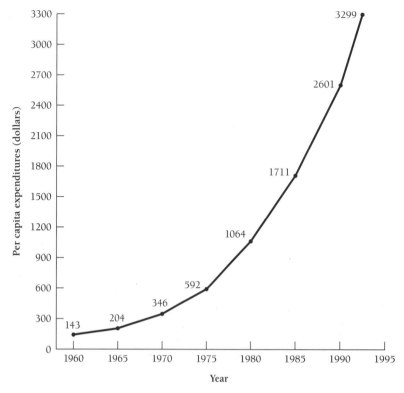

Figure 1.3   Per capita health expenditures, United States, 1960 to 1993.   SOURCE: Data from *Statistical Abstracts of the United States, 1995* by U.S. Bureau of the Census, 1995, Washington, DC: U.S. Government Printing Office, p. 109.

Medical costs, however, are increasing at a much faster rate than inflation, and year to year they represent a larger and larger proportion of the gross domestic product. In 1977, a concerned physician, John Knowles, warned that if this trend in the cost of medical care continued, it would "loom as large and pregnant to the American people in the future as the mushrooming atomic cloud does today" (Knowles, 1977, p. 58). Unfortunately, the trend has not only continued but, like the atomic cloud, has begun to mushroom. Figure 1.3 shows that from 1975 to 1993, the total yearly cost of health care increased from $592 per person to $3,299, a jump of more than 500% and a much faster annual increase than that reported for the years 1960 to 1975. By 1993, Americans were spending more than $884 billion a year on health care. This figure represented 13.9% of the gross domestic product, nearly triple the 5.3% spent in 1960 (USBC, 1995).

Although medical treatment during the 20th century has performed nearly miraculous cures for some individuals, the mounting monetary costs of medical miracles militate against the traditional philosophy of health, which has emphasized diagnosis, treatment, and cure. Expensive medical procedures such as heart surgery, hemodialysis, and high-technology imaging techniques have contributed substantially to the rising cost of health care in the United States, even though they are used with only a relatively small proportion of the population.

Mounting medical costs require a greater emphasis on the early detection of disease and on changes to a healthier lifestyle and to behaviors that help prevent illness. For example, early detection of high blood pressure, high serum cholesterol, and other precursors of heart disease allows these conditions to be controlled, thereby decreasing the risk of serious illness or death. Screening people for risk is preferable to remedial treatment because chronic diseases are quite difficult to cure and living with chronic illness decreases quality of life. Even more preferable to treating illnesses or screening for risks is maintaining health through a healthy lifestyle. Staying healthy is typically easier and less costly than getting well. Thus, prevention of disease through a healthy lifestyle, early detection of symptoms, and reduction of health risks have all become part of the changing philosophy within the health care field.

WHAT IS HEALTH?

What does it mean to be healthy? Is health an absence of disease, or is it the presence of some positive condition? How do people know they are healthy? Is health a single condition or is it multidimensional?

According to George Stone (1987), definitions of health fall into two categories: those that portray health as an ideal state and those that portray health as movement in a positive direction. The first definition implies that any disease or injury is a deviation from good health and that the ideal state can be restored by removing the disease or disability. With this limited definition of health, a blind concert violinist would not be healthy, despite his or her accomplishments, productivity, and contribution to society. The second definition avoids this problem by considering health as a direction on a continuum. This

definition implies that movement toward greater health is better than movement in the opposite direction. But because health is multidimensional, all aspects of living—biological, psychological, and social—must be considered. By this definition, a scientist who disregards personal safety or physical health to search for a cure for contagious disease would be moving away from biological health but toward social and perhaps psychological health.

One part of good health, in Stone's view, is improved biological functioning, such as normal blood pressure, superior cardiac output, a high level of respiratory volume, and the ability to withstand stress, infection, and physical injury. Stone proposes that the psychological manifestation of health is a subjective feeling of well-being. Social manifestations of health include the capacity for high levels of social productivity and low demands on the health care system.

Is health merely the absence of illness or are some additional elements necessary for health? Does health result from the removal of a negative state or must some positive state be attained? As Table 1.2 summarizes, people in various cultures during different times have held varying views of health. In 1946,

Table 1.2 Definitions of health held by various cultures

Culture	Time Period	Health Is . . .
Prehistoric	10,000 B.C.	endangered by spirits that enter the body from outside
Babylonians and Assyrians	1800–700 B.C.	endangered by the gods, who send illness as a punishment
Ancient Hebrews	1000–300 B.C.	a gift from God, but illness is a punishment from God
Ancient Greeks	500 B.C.	a wholistic unity of body and spirit
Ancient China	1100–200 B.C.	a balance of the forces of nature
Galen in Ancient Rome	200 A.D.	the absence of pathogens, such as bad air or body fluids, that cause disease
Early Christians	to 600 A.D.	not as important as illness, which is a sign that one is chosen by God
Descartes in Renaissance	1600	a condition of the mechanical body, which is separate from the mind
Vichow in Germany	late 1800s	endangered by microscopic organisms that invade cells, producing disease
Freud in Vienna	late 1800s	influenced by emotions and the mind

the United Nations established the World Health Organization (WHO) and wrote into the preamble of its constitution a modern, Western definition: "Health is a state of complete physical, mental and social well-being, and not merely the absence of disease or infirmity." This definition clearly affirms that health is a positive state.

How do people view health and illness? Millstein and Irwin (1987) attempted to answer this question by interviewing adolescents about their conceptions of health, and they found that only 28% of the young people defined health as an absence of illness. Instead, these adolescents tended to include both physical and psychosocial factors, such as the ability to perform certain activities and the presence of positive emotional states. Thus, the young people in this study defined both health and illness in multidimensional terms and saw health and lack of illness as being related but not identical. Not being sick was part of their definition of health, but it was not the whole picture.

To Dwayne, health is an absence of disease. Because he does not feel sick most of the time, he believes he is healthy. However, his lifestyle includes few behaviors that might increase his chances for a healthy future. Dwayne's diet of fatty foods and his lack of exercise make him a candidate for elevated cholesterol, which has been linked to early heart disease. In addition, his diet of fried food with few fruits and vegetables elevates his chances of developing cancer. Yet Dwayne believes that he has good health—at least when he is not sick.

In contrast, Robyn sees health as a positive condition, not merely freedom from disease. As a consequence, she works hard to achieve an enhanced sense of total well-being. Her reasons for eating a healthy diet, exercising, not smoking, and drinking alcohol moderately have little to do with avoiding illness. She engages in healthy behavior not to guard against disease but to achieve a positive state of health. And her lifestyle is paying off. She is able to study for long hours without becoming bored or lethargic; she enjoys being with other people but also likes solitude; she is able to exercise for 30 minutes a day without undue fatigue; and she very seldom suffers from headaches, depression, or general malaise. In short, she has approached the level of complete health described by the World Health Organization.

Dwayne and Robyn personify the two separate definitions of health. To Dwayne, health is a condition of not being sick whereas Robyn regards health as a positive state of physical, mental, and social well-being that can be achieved through healthy behavior and lifestyle.

CHANGING MODELS OF HEALTH

Throughout the 20th century, the biomedical model has allowed medicine to conquer or control many of the diseases that once ravaged humanity. The notion that illnesses are caused by a specific **pathogen**, a disease-causing organism, spurred the development of synthetic drugs and medical technology, which in turn engendered optimism that many diseases could be cured. However, the belief that a disease is traceable to a specific agent places more focus on disease than on health. In addition, this biomedical model defines health exclusively in terms of the absence of disease.

Although the biomedical model of disease has been the predominant view in medicine, a few physicians have begun to advocate a holistic approach to medicine—that is, one that considers social, psychological, physiological, and even spiritual aspects of a person. During the last quarter of the 20th century, more physicians, many psychologists, and some sociologists have even begun to question the usefulness of the biomedical model. Although they concede that the model has stimulated much progress in disease treatment, they question its limited definition of health.

Currently, people in the health care field are debating which model researchers and practitioners should use. Some have become dissatisfied with the traditional biomedical model and have challenged its adequacy. Dissatisfaction, however, is not sufficient grounds to prompt a change. An alternative model must be available, and this alternative must have the power of the old model plus the ability to solve problems that the old model failed to solve. Recently, an alternative model has begun to emerge, one that incorporates not only biological but also psychological and social factors. In this *biopsychosocial* model, health is once again seen as a positive condition. Advocates of the biopsychosocial model believe it has both these advantages.

The biopsychosocial model of illness incorporates not only physical factors but also psychological and social factors:

> To provide a basis for understanding the determinants of disease and arriving at rational treatments and patterns of health care, a medical model must also take into account the patient, the social context in which he lives and the complementary system devised by society to deal with the disruptive effects of illness, that is, the physician role and the health care system. This requires a biopsychosocial model. (Engel, 1977, p. 132)

How crucial is the acceptance of the biopsychosocial model of illness? In 1977, Engel warned of an impending crisis in medicine resulting from adherence to the outdated biomedical model. He described this crisis as coming from the frustration of those seeking medical care and the discrepancy between their needs and the care that the biomedical establishment provides. Not only are patients in need of a different philosophy of medical care, Engel stated, but many young medical students are eager to learn about the psychosocial dimensions of illness. The changing patterns of illness and the escalating cost of medical care may make acceptance of the biopsychosocial model more urgent.

Although the biomedical model has been the dominant view of medicine in the 20th century, before 1900 most physicians held a view of illness that emphasized the patient more than the symptoms. Joseph Matarazzo (1994), a pioneer in the development of health psychology, argued that before the widespread use of drugs, a compassionate, empathic bedside manner was about all that a physician had to offer patients. He also contended that the relatively recent explosion of scientific knowledge in such areas as biology, physiology, chemistry, and microbiology has produced several generations of physicians who know little about that type of bedside manner.

Nevertheless, some research has suggested that today's physicians may also conceptualize disease in ways that include psychological and social factors. Schmelkin, Wachtel, Schneiderman, and Hecht (1988) investigated medical students' concepts of disease and found that these students do distinguish between physiologically based diseases and those that appear to have heavy psychological involvement. This analysis demonstrates that even those who should be most indoctrinated in the biomedical approach still tend to include psychological factors in their thinking, a finding that supports the biopsychosocial model.

PSYCHOLOGY'S INVOLVEMENT IN HEALTH

Although chronic diseases have many causes, no one seriously disputes the evidence that individual behavior and lifestyle are strongly implicated in their development. Because most chronic diseases stem at least partly from individual behavior, psychology — the science of behavior — has become involved in health. One psychologist summarized the rationale for this involvement as follows:

> In short, the most serious medical problems that today plague the majority of Americans are not ultimately medical problems at all; they are behavior problems, requiring the alteration of characteristic response patterns, and thus fall squarely within the province of psychology. (Stachnik, 1980, p. 8)

According to Taylor (1990), a large part of psychology's involvement in health is a commitment to keeping people healthy rather than waiting to treat them after they become ill. Psychology shares this role with medicine and other health care disciplines, but unlike medicine (which tends to study specific diseases), psychology contributes certain broad principles of behavior that cut across specific diseases and specific issues of health. Among psychology's contributions to health are techniques for changing behaviors that have been implicated in chronic diseases. In addition to changing unhealthy behaviors, psychologists have also used their skills to relieve pain and reduce stress, improve compliance with medical advice, and help patients and family members live with chronic illnesses.

PSYCHOLOGY IN MEDICAL SETTINGS

Psychology has been involved with people's physical health almost from the beginning of the 20th century. In 1911, the American Psychological Association (APA) convened a panel to discuss the role of psychology in medical education (Rodin & Stone, 1987). In 1912, psychologist John B. Watson (1878–1958) proposed a course in psychology for medical students. He believed that regardless of medical specialty, physicians needed training in psychology to deal with patients as human beings. As reasonable as this proposal now seems, most medical schools failed to pursue the recommendation. The APA again broached the topic in 1928 and once more in 1950, but medical schools implemented few changes during this time. According to a 1913 survey of medical schools, only 27% of those with academic affiliations collaborated with psychology departments (Franz, 1913).

During the 1940s, medical training typically incorporated the study of psychological factors as they relate to illness, but this training was usually conducted by physicians and was limited to the medical specialty of psychiatry. Before 1950, only a handful of psychologists were employed in medical schools (Matarazzo, 1994), and the duties of most of those were limited largely to teaching. A few of these clinical psychologists provided psychological services, such as testing and psychotherapy for patients with emotional problems, but few were involved in research. Also, psychologists seldom collaborated with medical specialists other than psychiatrists. Pattishall (1989, p. 45) summarized the relationship between psychology and psychiatry by saying, "Behavioral science and psychiatry was a good marriage . . . until the behavioral scientists were sought out by other medical departments such as family medicine, pediatrics, internal medicine, and preventive medicine for clinical and research collaboration." As psychology became more widespread in medical training and as the research base increased to give behavioral science academic credibility, psychology's involvement in medical settings began to expand.

Behavioral science became part of the curriculum in most medical schools in the 1960s, when many new medical schools were established and new curricula for these schools were developed (Pattishall, 1989). By the 1970s, all except two medical schools in the United States had psychologists on staff. Matarazzo (1994) estimated that the number of psychologists who held academic appointments on

medical school faculties nearly tripled from 1969 to 1993. At this latter time, 3,500 psychologists were employed in medical settings, a number greater than the total membership of Division 38 (Health Psychology) of the American Psychological Association. By the 1990s, health psychologists were no longer considered by physicians as merely statistical consultants, test administrators, or therapists with skills largely limited to psychosomatic illness. They, along with neuropsychologists and rehabilitation psychologists, had become accepted members of most major hospital staffs (Sweet, Rozensky, & Tovian, 1991).

PSYCHOSOMATIC MEDICINE

Psychosomatic medicine encompasses the view that physical illnesses have emotional and psychological components and that psychological and somatic (or physical) factors interact to produce disease. The notion that psychological and emotional factors can contribute to physical ailments is older than history (Kaplan, 1985). Prehistoric humans saw disease as spiritual as well as physical, and many cultures in ancient history included psychological and social factors in their views of disease. The more modern concept of psychosomatic medicine received some impetus from Freud, who emphasized the importance of unconscious psychological factors in the development of physical symptoms. But Freud's methods relied on clinical experience and intuitive hunches that were unverified by laboratory research.

The research base for psychosomatic medicine began with Walter Cannon's observation in 1932 that physiological changes accompany emotion (Kimball, 1981). Cannon's research demonstrated that emotion could cause physiological changes that might be related to the development of physical disease; that is, emotion can cause changes, which in turn could cause disease. From this finding, Helen Flanders Dunbar (1943) developed the notion that habitual responses, which people exhibit as part of their personalities, are related to specific diseases. In other words, Dunbar hypothesized a relationship between personality and disease.

Franz Alexander (1950), a one-time follower of Freud, saw psychosomatic disorders as resting on a link between personal conflicts and specific diseases. During Alexander's time, such diseases as peptic ulcer, rheumatoid arthritis, hypertension, asthma, hyperthyroidism, neurodermatitis, and ulcerative colitis were believed to be psychosomatic. Alexander believed that certain people were more vulnerable than others to the effects of stress on their organ systems and that when organ vulnerability and stress coincided, these susceptible people would develop the disease to which they were vulnerable.

Although stress and its effects on physiology and the development of disease has remained a prominent part of psychosomatic medicine, by the 1970s the emphasis had shifted away from specific diseases, and the term *psychosomatic* was no longer applied to diseases but to an approach to the study and treatment of disease. Kimball (1981, p. 132) summarized this newer pychosomatic approach, referring to physicians who express in their practice the belief that "human illness cannot be conceptualized or treated by a single factor–single disease approach, but that all illness depends on a multiplicity of factors involving the somatic and psychological processes of the individual in relationship to environment."

Thus those physicians who believed in psychosomatic illness were the first in modern medicine to accept a biopsychosocial model for disease and to call for an enlargement of the prevailing biomedical model. Oken (1987) contended that under the new definition of psychosomatic illness, all illnesses are psychosomatic because all illnesses include psychological and social components.

McHugh and Vallis (1986) described psychosomatic medicine as a reformist movement within medicine, but they declared that it has not lived up to its objectives of emphasizing the psychological and social components of somatic illness. These authors contended that psychosomatic medicine is the domain of psychiatry, a branch of medicine. They also suggested that the collaborative goals of the psychosomatic movement have not been attained; that is, the psychological and physiological aspects of disease have not yet been totally integrated. They claimed, instead, that the objectives of the psychosomatic movement have been subsumed under the area of *behavioral medicine.*

BEHAVIORAL MEDICINE

Although some psychologists have worked in medical settings since the beginning of the 20th century, only during the past two decades have their contributions begun to be recognized by the medical establishment. Until the 1970s, the role of psychologists in medicine was mostly restricted to medical education, psychological testing, psychosomatic medicine, and psychotherapy. Psychologists rarely participated in the psychological aspects of medical treatment, and their expertise was generally thought to be limited to mental health problems. Although psychologists considered their discipline the science of behavior, their skills were rarely called on to help people stop smoking, eat a healthy diet, exercise wisely, reduce stress, or control pain.

A growing knowledge of the link between behavior and illness and psychology's development of effective techniques to change problem behaviors led to an increased role for psychology in health care. A 1977 conference at Yale University led to the definition of a new field, **behavioral medicine**, defined as "the interdisciplinary field concerned with the development and integration of behavioral and biomedical science knowledge and techniques relevant to health and illness and the application of this knowledge and these techniques to prevention, diagnosis, treatment and rehabilitation" (Schwartz & Weiss, 1978, p. 250).

This definition indicates that behavioral medicine is designed to integrate medicine and the various behavioral sciences, especially psychology (Pomerleau, 1982). The goals of behavioral medicine are similar to those in other areas of health care: improved prevention, diagnosis, treatment, and rehabilitation. Behavioral medicine, then, attempts to use psychology and the behavioral sciences in conjunction with medicine to promote health and treat illness. Chapters 3 through 11 cover topics in behavioral medicine.

BEHAVIORAL HEALTH

A new discipline called **behavioral health** began to emerge at about the same time behavioral medicine was establishing its identity. Behavioral health emphasizes the enhancement of health and the prevention of illness in healthy people rather than the diagnosis and treatment of disorders in sick people. Furthermore, it is an "interdisciplinary subspecialty within behavioral medicine specifically concerned with the maintenance of health and the prevention of illness and dysfunction in currently healthy persons" (Matarazzo, 1980, p. 807). Behavioral health includes such concerns as preventing illness, cigarette smoking, alcohol use, diet, and exercise, topics discussed in Chapters 12 through 16.

The focus of behavioral health is on individual responsibility for health and wellness rather than on physician-based diagnosis, treatment, or rehabilitation (Matarazzo, 1984a, 1994). All those behaviors and lifestyles that maintain or enhance health fall within the purview of behavioral health. Although people are generally accepting more responsibility for their health, the formal discipline of behavioral health has not emerged as a rival to the fields of behavioral medicine or health psychology (Matarazzo, 1994).

HEALTH PSYCHOLOGY

Related to both behavioral medicine and behavioral health is a relatively new discipline within the field of psychology called **health psychology**, that branch of psychology that relates to individual behaviors and lifestyles that affect a person's physical health. Health psychology includes psychology's contributions to the enhancement of health, the prevention and treatment of illness, the identification of health risk factors, the improvement of the health care system, and the shaping of public opinion with regard to health. More specifically, it involves the application of psychological principles to such physical health areas as lowering high blood pressure, controlling cholesterol, managing stress, alleviating pain, stopping smoking, moderating other risky behaviors, and encouraging regular exercise, medical and dental checkups, and safer behaviors. In addition, health psychology contributes to identifying the correlates of health, diagnosing and treating certain chronic diseases, and modifying the behavioral factors involved in physiological and psychological rehabilitation. As such, health psychology contributes to and overlaps with both behavioral medicine and behavioral health (see Figure 1.4).

The Development of Health Psychology

As an identifiable area, health psychology received its first important impetus in 1973, when the Board of Scientific Affairs of the American Psychological Association (APA) appointed a task force to study the potential for psychology's role in health research. That task force reported in 1976 that few psychologists were involved in health research and that research conducted by psychologists in the area of health was not often reported in the psychology journals. However, the report envisioned a future in which health psychology might contribute to the enhancement of health and the prevention of disease. The task force stated that

> there is probably no specialty field within psychology that cannot contribute to the discovery of behavioral variables crucial to a full understanding of susceptibility to physical illness, adaptation to such illness, and prophylactically motivated behaviors. (American Psychological Association, 1976, p. 272)

This directive led to the establishment of the Section of Health Research within APA's Division of Psychologists in the Public Service. In 1978, the American Psychological Association established Division 38, Health Psychology, as "a scientific, educational, and professional organization for psychologists interested in (or working in) areas at one or another of the interfaces of medicine and psychology" (Matarazzo, 1994, p. 31). Four years later, in 1982, the journal *Health Psychology* began publication as the official journal of Division 38.

Health Psychology's Position within Psychology

How does health psychology fit within the field of psychology? Matarazzo (1987b) addressed this question nearly a decade after health psychology was established as Division 38 within the APA. He insisted that health psychology was still an emerging field and would continue as such for at least another decade. In a thoughtfully prepared position paper, Matarazzo reviewed the history of psychology since the Boulder Conference in 1949, which established psychology as both a scientific discipline and a practicing profession. From that time, every doctoral program within a department of psychology

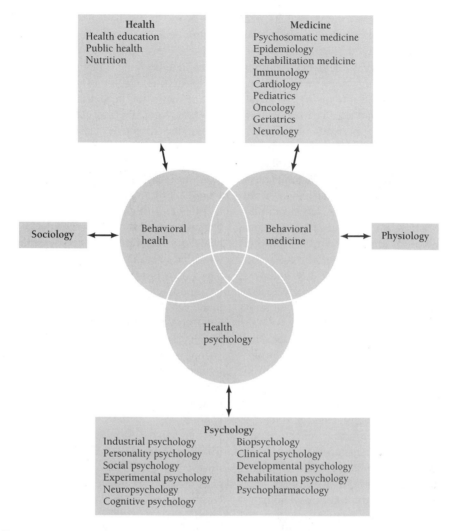

Figure 1.4 *Relationship of health psychology to other health-related fields.*

has offered nearly the same core of generic course work for psychologists.

Along with the core courses required of all psychologists, health psychologists take courses in such fields as biostatistics, epidemiology, physiology, biochemistry, and cardiology. In other words, health psychologists are psychologists first and specialists in health second. According to Matarazzo, "psychology" is the *noun* that identifies the subject matter; and "health" is the *adjective* that describes the client, problem, or setting to which psychology is applied. Like other fields of psychology, health psychology applies the principles of generic psychology to a

particular area. Health psychology does not exist as a profession separate from generic psychology; rather, "health psychology is today nothing more than the application of the accumulated knowledge from the science and profession of generic psychology to the area of health" (Matarazzo, 1987b, p. 55).

Matarazzo believes that health psychology will not emerge as a clearly unique profession until it has proceeded through at least eight steps, stages through which even clinical psychology has not yet passed. At this time, health psychology has successfully passed through the first three. It has (1) founded its own national and international associations; (2) established a number of its own journals in addition to *Health Psychology;* and (3) received acknowledgment from professionals in other fields of psychology that its subject matter, methods, and applications are different from theirs. The remaining five obstacles have yet to be hurdled. They include (4) postdoctoral training that is specific to health psychology and distinct from clinical and other fields of psychology; (5) recognition from the National Institutes of Health and other federal agencies that health psychology exists as a separate discipline; (6) establishment of departments of health psychology within medical schools, schools of public health, universities, and hospitals; (7) acceptance by other psychologists and by the legal profession that health psychologists are experts who can be differentiated from clinical and other psychologists; and (8) designation by the American Board of Professional Psychology and state licensing boards that health psychology is a separate profession.

Matarazzo forecasts that health psychology will continue to be regarded as the science and profession of psychology applied to the field of health for several years. It will not become a separate entity until it passes through the eight stages listed above and establishes "nationally designated and accredited postdoctoral training programs which are publicly identified as offering preparation for work as a specialist" (Matarazzo, 1987b, p. 59). Like other fields within psychology, health psychology relies on and contributes to the basic core of psychological research and then applies this knowledge to a particular field of specialization.

CHAPTER SUMMARY

Psychology began making significant contributions to health as a result of several important changes within the field of health. One such event was the changing pattern of illness and death in the United States. Chronic illnesses such as heart disease, cancer, emphysema, acquired immune deficiency syndrome (AIDS), and adult-onset diabetes are now among the leading causes of death. In large measure, these and other chronic illnesses are a result of individual or societal behaviors or "misbehaviors." Psychology, as the science of behavior, clearly has a

role in modifying behaviors implicated in chronic illness.

The increase in chronic illness has contributed to a second important trend: the escalating cost of medical care. Total health costs, which showed a significant increase in the decades prior to 1980, have shown no signs of decreasing. These escalating costs are not due solely to increases in population or to the rising rate of inflation but represent a greater and greater percentage of the gross domestic product.

A third major change is the gradual acceptance of a new definition of health. Although some people still view health as the absence of disease, others are beginning to view it as the presence of positive well-being, a definition that encourages health enhancement and not simply disease prevention. The acceptance of this new definition of health sparked a fourth trend: the emergence of a biopsychosocial model of health. The biopsychosocial model is a departure from the traditional biomedical model, which views illness as the result of a specific biochemical abnormality with the person. This newer model emphasizes positive health and sees illness, particularly chronic illness, as resulting from the interaction of biological, psychological, and social conditions.

Psychology has been involved in health almost from the beginning of the 20th century. During those early years, however, only a few psychologists worked in medical settings and most were considered adjuncts rather than full partners with physicians. Psychosomatic medicine emphasized psychological explanations of somatic illnesses and increased the need for psychologists in the health field. By the 1960s and early 1970s, psychology and other behavioral sciences were beginning to make a contribution to the prevention and treatment of chronic diseases and to the promotion of positive health. These contributions led to the development of two new fields: behavioral medicine and behavioral health.

Behavioral medicine is an interdisciplinary field concerned with applying the knowledge and techniques of behavioral science to the maintenance of physical health and to prevention, diagnosis, treatment, and rehabilitation. *Behavioral health* is a subspecialty within behavioral medicine concerned with health maintenance and disease prevention in currently healthy individuals. Although both behavioral medicine and behavioral health are related to psychology, both are disciplines outside the field of psychology. In 1978, the American Psychological Association established Division 38, *Health Psychology*, a specialty within psychology that contributes to both behavioral medicine and behavioral health and uses the science of psychology to enhance health, prevent and treat illness, identify risk factors, improve the health care system, and shape public opinion with regard to health.

SUGGESTED READINGS

Matarazzo, J. D. (1994). Health and behavior: The coming together of science and practice in psychology and medicine after a century of benign neglect. *Journal of Clinical Psychology in Medical Settings, 1,* 7–39. Matarazzo covers many of the same issues discussed in this chapter; in addition, he briefly discusses some examples of misbehaviors, such as smoking, overeating, and living a hostile lifestyle.

Rodin, J., & Salovey, P. (1989). Health psychology. *Annual Review of Psychology, 40,* 533–579. This article is an excellent overview of the status of health psychology 20 years into its history. Rodin and Salovey summarize the literature dealing with factors related to health and illness. They also suggest a broader definition of health, one of positive well-being, instead of simply the absence of disease.

Stone, G. C. (1982). Health Psychology: A new journal for a new field. *Health Psychology, 1,* 1–6. This editorial appeared in the first issue of *Health Psychology* and helped to define the field by outlining the types of articles considered appropriate for publication.

2 Conducting Health Research

Diane was a 22-year-old college senior who wanted to quit smoking. Her roommate was taking a health psychology course and told Diane that smoking was one of the topics included in the course. They had not yet covered the chapter on smoking, so her roommate could not tell Diane about quitting, but she advised Diane to talk to the professor who taught health psychology. Diane visited the professor in her office and asked her to recommend a hypnotherapist to hypnotize her so she could quit smoking.

The professor asked Diane why she wanted to use hypnosis rather than some other smoking cessation program, and Diane replied that she had en-

rolled in a group class in hypnosis two years earlier and had quit smoking for almost a year. The professor explained that hypnosis has a number of uses and can be effective for some problems but that hypnosis is not very useful in helping people quit smoking. Diane believed that if hypnosis had been successful for her once, it would be successful a second time. She did not see her resumption of smoking as a failure of the hypnotherapy; instead, she blamed herself and the stresses in her life for her resuming her smoking habit. Despite the professor's explanation, Diane believed that hypnosis was an effective smoking cessation treatment.

Furthermore, Diane was adamant that hypnosis was the technique she wanted despite the professor's contention that research on smoking and hypnosis had shown that it was ineffective. Evidence from research was not important to Diane because her personal experience was the evidence that she believed. She was convinced that hypnosis worked for her, even if it does not work for other people.

Diane is similar to many people in her reliance on personal experience rather than research evidence. She believed that her own observations were more valid (especially for her) than research conducted on large groups of people. She did not see that her own biases were interfering with her judgment of the value of hypnosis—that is, Diane had trouble accepting the value of scientific research on a personal level.

She had, however, accepted the idea that smoking was dangerous to her health, and she acknowledged that the evidence for this belief also had come from research. Diane is also like many people in her choosing what research to accept and what to ignore. Although some of the information on health-related behaviors is biased and comes from individuals and organizations trying to sell a product, a vast body of scientific evidence exists that is relatively objective and free from self-serving claims. This evidence is produced by researchers trained in the behavioral and biomedical sciences who typically are associated with universities and hospitals. Because these men and women use the methods of science in their work, evidence usually accumulates gradually over an extended period of time. Dramatic breakthroughs are rare.

When scientists are familiar with one another's work, use controlled methods, keep personal biases from contaminating results, make claims cautiously, and are able to replicate their studies, evidence is more likely to be evolutionary than revolutionary. Claims to the contrary are most often motivated by financial or other personal interests. News reports must get readers' attention, so the headlines often misrepresent scientific findings. (see box, Would You Believe . . . ?). And, of course, commercial advertisements that champion their product as a revolutionary new cure for insomnia, an effortless way to eat all you desire and still lose weight, a simple way to stop smoking, or a food that protects you against cancer or heart disease either are not using or are distorting scientific evidence when they make their claims.

This chapter looks at the way scientists work, emphasizing the behavioral and biomedical sciences—that is, psychology and epidemiology. These two disciplines share some methods for investigating health-related behaviors, but the two areas also have their own unique contributions to scientific methodology. Before we begin to examine the methods that psychologists and epidemiologists use in their research, we need to consider what the professor was trying to explain to Diane—that her success with hypnosis might have been due to the **placebo effect**, an effect of treatment that is due to expectation rather than to effectiveness of the treatment.

THE PLACEBO IN RESEARCH AND TREATMENT

The problem that Diane found so difficult to accept—how an ineffective treatment can be effective through expectation alone—can be an advantage for people like Diane, who actually benefit from their expectation. For researchers, however, the placebo effect makes the evaluation of effective treatment difficult.

Placebo is a Latin word that translates into English as "I shall please," but the term now refers to those effects caused by people's beliefs or expectations. In other words, a placebo is an inactive substance or condition that has the appearance of an active treatment and may cause participants in an experiment to improve or change their behavior as a result of their belief in the placebo's efficacy. When a treatment is presented, either in research or in clinical practice, people like Diane tend to expect that the treatment will produce an effect.

This expectation is capable of causing effects separate from any influence of the treatment itself. The literal translation of placebo is not exactly an accurate description of the effect. People do not act to please, but rather they act in the ways that they *think* they should, and their actions are based more on their expectations than on any effects of the experiment. In other words, people's actions tend to be consistent with their expectations.

The effects of "sugar pills" have long been known (Wolf, 1950). Indeed, the ability of inert substances to mimic drug effects are the best known of all placebo effects. A slightly cynical view suggests, in fact, that the history of pharmacology is a study of the placebo effect (Evans, 1985). Placebos have been found to cure a remarkable range of disorders, including insomnia, headache, fever, the common cold, and warts. Placebos have also caused side effects, just as drugs do. They have been shown to produce dependence, and their removal may prompt withdrawal symptoms.

The form of the placebo also affects its potency (Shapiro, 1970). Injections are more powerful than pills. Very large and very small pills are perceived as stronger than medium-sized ones. Colored pills are more effective than plain white pills; capsules produce stronger effects than tablets; brand-name drugs are believed to be better than generics. Drug companies take advantage of all these perceptions in creating and marketing their products.

The placebo effect is capable of more than merely alleviating the imaginary illnesses of hypochondriacs

WOULD YOU BELIEVE . . . ?

Misleading Media Messages

Would you believe that you can't believe all the health reports you read? Health research has become a common topic in the media, with reports appearing daily in newspapers, magazines, and television. But one day the reports seem to say one thing, and a few months later, just the opposite. First we hear that a study has found that coffee is related to pancreatic cancer, then another study has failed to find any risk. Next comes a report that coffee is not related to cancer but to raised cholesterol levels. One study says that alcohol seems to raise the risk of breast cancer whereas another, larger study finds no increased risk. Which studies are correct, and how do we know what to believe? Even more important, how do we decide which results should prompt changes in our behavior?

Part of the problem with understanding research results is the medium through which most people obtain health information. Newspaper, magazine, and television reports omit technical details and tend to simplify research designs and conclusions so that everyone can understand the study. In this process, simplification can become oversimplification. In addition, journalists who prepare stories are interested in a piece that will catch people's attention, a tendency that may result in sensationalism.

Anthony Schmitz (1991) explored some of the reasons for problems in science reporting. He found that even without intending to distort findings, science reporters often do. These reporters may not have the training in science to completely understand the research, and their reports may reflect their lack of understanding. In addition, the stories that they write may be cut to

fit the space available, omitting the limitations and qualifying information at the end of the stories.

Schmitz offered several suggestions to guide people in getting information from media reports, saying "you can defend yourself against half-baked findings and wild advice — if you read carefully" (p. 45). Schmitz advised people to be wary of the headline, which was probably constructed by someone other than the person who prepared the story. Headlines are designed to catch attention and may suggest findings that are more dramatic or important than the research warranted.

Schmitz advised people to "count the legs" of the subjects in the study and to be cautious if the number of legs differs from their own. That is, if the study used nonhuman animals, the results are not as clearly applicable to people as studies that use human participants. He also pointed out that the number of participants is important, with more participant and more representative samples providing more persuasive results.

A related concern comes from the characteristics of participants, which may differ from those of the general population. For example, a great deal of biomedical research has used only White, middle-class men as participants, and they have become the standard for comparison (Tavris, 1992). The results of studies with European-American participants do not necessarily apply to other ethnic groups, and generalizing results from men to women can lead to unsound conclusions. In addition to knowing the number of legs of participants, it is important to know the characteristics of the sample and to be cautious in

accepting results from participants who differ from you.

Schmitz also recommended that people find out the source of the story, and he made a distinction in credibility between studies that had appeared in reputable scientific journals and those presented at conferences. The latter studies are not subjected to intense review whereas the former are. The source of funding for a study can also make a difference in credibility, with some sources of research funding leading to obvious potential for bias. For example, if a study on smoking has been funded by a tobacco company or a study on the cholesterol-lowering properties of oat bran have been funded by a cereal manufacturer, skepticism is in order. Funding by government grants does not guarantee a lack of bias, but corporate funding can lead to an obvious conflict of interest for researchers.

"Don't let one study change your life" was the advice given by Jane Brody, *New York Times* health writer (in Schmitz, 1991, p. 47). Even if a study appeared in a prestigious journal and had thousands of participants, one study is usually not sufficient evidence to prompt lifestyle changes. The results from such a study may or may not be confirmed by other studies. Disconfirming studies rarely get the publicity that positive results do. On the other hand, a body of research that has yielded consistent results warrants more serious consideration. If the lifestyle changes are unlikely to do harm (even if they don't do any good) and if the changes are relatively easy to make, consider changing your life.

and those who exaggerate their symptoms. The medical effects of placebos are complex and physiologically real, and placebo treatments are capable of curing physical symptoms in a variety of medical disorders. The improvements are sometimes the same as those caused by physiologically active drugs and other specific medical treatments (Levine, Gordon, & Fields, 1978). Indeed, in most situations involving medical treatment, the improvements shown by patients may be a combination of the specific effects of the treatment plus the placebo effect (Evans, 1985). Unless patients are treated without their knowledge, the placebo effect is a factor.

The placebo effect presents a problem in evaluating drug effectiveness because a physiologically inactive substance may sometimes produce improvements and even side effects. Therefore, to demonstrate that a drug has unique effects, the effects of that drug must be compared with the effects of a placebo. The comparison must be made using at least two groups: one that has received the drug and another that has received the placebo. Both groups must have equal expectations concerning the effectiveness of the treatment. In order to create equal expectancy, not only must the participants receiving each substance be ignorant of who is getting a placebo and who is getting a drug, but the experimenters who dispense both substances must also be unaware of or "blind" as to which group is which. The arrangement in which neither participants nor experimenters know about treatment conditions, called a **double blind** design, is common in drug research.

Does the placebo effect also apply to psychological treatments? Because psychological treatments also create expectancy, the placebo effect would seem to be a likely factor in changing behavior. The power of the placebo appeared in a 1962 study by Stanley Schachter and Jerome Singer. In an attempt to understand the components of emotional reactions, Schachter and Singer administered the drug epinephrine to one group of participants and a placebo injection, a saline solution, to another group. Half the members of the group injected with epinephrine were told that they might feel a bit jittery, notice an elevated heart rate, and experience sweaty palms. The other half of the participants who received epinephrine were not informed of its effects, leaving them without a way to interpret the biological effects of epinephrine. The group that received the placebo injection was also divided, with half not being told about side effects of the injection and half being told to expect the same effects that epinephrine produces.

The results of Schachter and Singer's experiment demonstrated a strong expectancy effect. Participants who were injected with the placebo and led to expect physiological effects exhibited the high degree of arousal typically produced by epinephrine. Their reactions were not quite as strong as those of participants who had actually received epinephrine but who were uninformed of its effect. However, the misinformed placebo group reacted more strongly than those who received epinephrine and were correctly informed of its effects. The diminished effect of epinephrine in this group was also a type of expectancy effect: When a label is available for their physiological reactions, people tend to explain their reactions according to the labeled expectation. The placebo group that had not been led to expect effects should not have felt any, and this prediction held true. Schachter and Singer's study demonstrated that placebos are potent factors in psychological research and treatment.

Improvement rates due simply to the placebo effect are frequently reported to be about one-third. However, Turner, Deyo, Loeser, Von Korff, and Fordyce (1994) reviewed more than 200 articles dealing with the placebo effect on pain and found that improvement rates are often much higher than 33% and that most physicians greatly underestimate the power of the placebo effect. Turner et al. found that both physician and patient expectations can produce reductions in pain, as can the reputation of the physician, the expense of treatment, the physical setting, and the attention, interest, and concern shown by the physician. These authors also reported that placebos often produce adverse effects, a condition called the **nocebo effect**. In their review, Turner et al. found that nearly 20% of healthy volunteers given a placebo in a double-blind study experienced some negative effect as a result of the nocebo effect.

Because health psychologists use behavioral interventions and because the patients they work with often receive drug or other medical treatment, the placebo effect is an ever-present factor in psychological research and practice. Researchers in the health care fields, including health psychology, must assess the effectiveness of therapy cautiously, because expectancy is a factor in both medical and behavioral therapies. Without careful research design, the effectiveness of therapies can be overestimated. It is interesting that psychological placebos have been found about as effective as medical placebos (Blanchard & Andrasik, 1982). Both types of placebos have been shown to provide about a 35% rate of improvement for a wide variety of conditions (Evans, 1985).

Although the placebo effect is a complication for research, it may be used advantageously by practitioners. The association of the placebo effect with "sugar pills" has led many people to believe that placebo cures are not "real" and that they cure only psychological conditions that have no physical basis. This belief is not founded on research. Placebos yield improvements in a substantial percentage of cases for a wide variety of conditions and frequently bring about physiological changes as well.

Practitioners may increase patients' expectations about the effectiveness of therapy, thus prompting improvements due to expectancy. Because improvement is the goal of therapy, *any* factor that enhances treatment effectiveness is a bonus. The underlying causes for improvement are the concern of researchers more than practitioners. Therefore, the placebo effect may be considered a positive factor in medical and behavioral therapies, as it was for Diane. Indeed, Diane's belief in the effectiveness of this therapy might lead her to change her behavior, even if hypnosis were ineffective as a therapy for smoking.

Ornstein and Sobel (1987) emphasized the advantages to practitioners who accept and maximize placebo effects rather than belittle them. They pointed out that placebo-induced cures are indistinguishable from improvements that occur as a result of other treatments. A cure is a cure, and the method of cure makes no difference to the well-being of patients. Ornstein and Sobel argued that placebo effects are a tribute to the ability of humans to heal themselves, and they advised practitioners to enlist this ability to a greater extent.

RESEARCH METHODS IN PSYCHOLOGY

Like many people, Diane is concerned about her health. She not only wants to quit smoking, but she tries to exercise regularly, watch her diet, and avoid too much stress. But how do people, such as Diane, know that these health practices will, indeed, contribute to better health? What is the source of health information? Who conducts the basic research that suggests which behaviors are healthy and which are harmful?

Much health-related information comes from studies conducted by behavioral and biomedical scientists using a variety of research methods. The methods chosen depend in large part on what questions the scientists are trying to answer. Questions regarding heart disease, for example, may require different research methods to lead to a comprehensive understanding of this illness. This chapter looks at different methods, both within psychology and epidemiology, that health researchers have used to increase their understanding of behavioral factors in heart disease as well as other topics pertinent to their discipline.

When scientists wish to learn as much as possible about a single individual, they usually employ a *case study;* when they are interested in what factors predict or are related to either an illness or healthy functioning, they use *correlational techniques;* when they want to compare people across different ages or ethnic groups, they rely on *cross-sectional studies;* when they desire information on stability or instability of health status over a period of time, they use *longitudinal studies;* and when they wish to compare one groups of participants with another, they can use either an *experimental study* or an *ex post facto design.* Case studies, correlational techniques, cross-sectional studies, longitudinal investigations, experimental studies, and ex post facto designs, then, are all methods from the discipline of psychology that have application to the field of health.

CASE STUDIES

Although most psychological investigations employ many participants, studies using only one person have a legitimate role in science. **Case studies** provide an in-depth analysis of only one individual and are one type of the single-subject design.

In a case study, a researcher extensively studies one subject, usually because that person presents a particularly interesting or unusual case. The advantage of the case study is that it ordinarily provides a more complete analysis of an individual than can be obtained by investigations of large numbers of participants. The principal disadvantage is that it magnifies sampling errors. One purpose of any scientific investigation is to allow generalization to other participants or even to an entire population. Although all studies on population samples suffer from problems of generalization, case studies are more limited than multiple-subject studies in their ability to permit general inferences.

Many areas of health psychology can be examined from a variety of views, and case studies offer one such view. For example, cardiovascular disease (CVD) can be studied using several different methods, including the case study. One such study was described by Gore and Fallon (1994) who presented the case study of a 25-year-old man with congestive heart failure and a recent diagnosis of diabetes. The vast number of measures gathered from this single case yields information that is not ordinarily available in studies with many participants. From the description given by Gore and Fallon, we know that this man was an only child, living at home with both parents, and working in a clerical job when he developed an irregular heart beat and a severe upper respiratory tract infection. After a week of bed rest, the infection subsided, but continual heart palpitations led him to seek the care of a **cardiologist** — that is, a medical doctor who specialized in heart disease. Gore and Fallon described the man as weak, fatigued, and having symptoms of diabetes. Their description also included dozens of other pieces of information on such heart-related measures as blood glucose concentration, **electrocardiogram (ECG)** signals, cholesterol levels, pulse, blood pressure, jugular vein pressure, and white-cell count. One year after treatment for both heart disease and liver ailment, the patient had no symptoms of heart disease, was working full time, and had become engaged to be married. Such detailed reports allow health psychologists and physicians to learn about

heart disease in a relatively young patient and to see how this disease may, in some cases, be related to diabetes.

CORRELATIONAL STUDIES

Correlational studies yield information about the degree of relationship between two variables, such as personality factors and heart disease. Correlational studies *describe* this relationship and are, therefore, a type of **descriptive research** design. Although scientists cannot determine causal relationships through descriptive research, the degree of relationship is valuable information that can be used as an exploratory tool before an experimental study is designed. On the other hand, information about the degree of relationship may be exactly what a researcher wants to know and may thus be the preferred method of investigation.

To assess the degree of relationship between two variables, the researcher measures each variable in a group of participants and then computes a correlation coefficient. Many types of correlation coefficients exist, but the one most commonly used in psychology is the *Pearson product-moment correlation coefficient*. This **correlation coefficient** is described by a formula, and the correlation is computed by applying the formula to the data that the researcher has gathered. The computation yields a number that varies between -1.00 and $+1.00$. Correlations that are closer to 1.00 (either positive or negative) indicate stronger relationships than do correlations that are closer to 0. Small correlations — those less than 0.10 — can be *statistically significant* if they are based on a very large number of scores. However, such small correlations, though not random, offer the researcher very little ability to predict scores on one variable from knowledge of scores on the other variable.

Positive correlations occur when the two variables increase or decrease together. Negative correlations occur when one of the variables increases as the other decreases. For example, a researcher might wish to study the relationship between psychological factors, such as stress, and a variety of factors known to relate to heart disease. This was one of the purposes of a study by Hollis, Connett, Stevens, and Greenlick (1990), who wished to learn whether stressful life events were correlated with other risks for coronary heart disease. They gathered information from nearly 13,000 men with multiple risks for heart disease and correlated stressful experiences with such coronary *risk factors* as age, education, income, diastolic blood pressure, serum cholesterol level, and cigarette smoking. (A **risk factor** is any characteristic or condition that occurs with greater frequency in people with a disease than in people free from that disease.) All resulting correlations, though statistically significant, were quite small, with negative correlations ranging from −0.03 for diastolic blood pressure to −0.10 for age, and positive correlations ranging from 0.03 for education to 0.10 for number of cigarettes smoked per day. In other words, this study found that stressful life events were somewhat positively related to such coronary risk factors as cigarette smoking and somewhat negatively associated with other risks, such as age.

Compared with the case study, correlational studies are rather impersonal, but they offer much more information concerning the factors that are associated with or predict a particular risk factor, disorder, or other event.

CROSS-SECTIONAL AND LONGITUDINAL STUDIES

In addition to decisions about the number of participants in a study, researchers have choices to make about the time span of their studies. **Cross-sectional studies** are those conducted during only one point in time, whereas **longitudinal studies** follow participants over an extended period.

In a cross-sectional design, the investigator studies a representative sample of people from at least two different age groups or developmental periods or from two different ethnic groups to determine the possible effects of age or ethnicity on a particular variable. For example, a researcher may want to know whether total cholesterol levels are related to heart disease for people at different ages. Kronmal, Cain, Ye, and Omenn (1993) conducted such a study, and the results showed that cholesterol was not positively related to heart disease among people over the age of 50. This finding, however, cannot suggest that older people somehow outgrow their

need to maintain moderate cholesterol levels. Because people 70 or 80 years old were born at an earlier time than 40- to 50-year-old participants and thus had different experiences that might relate to heart disease, we cannot conclude that younger people with high cholesterol levels can avoid heart problems if they can only survive into their 70s or 80s. Older people with high cholesterol may have simply outlived their age-mates with high cholesterol because they were blessed with better genes for coronary health.

Longitudinal studies can yield more useful results than cross-sectional studies because they assess the same people over time. However, longitudinal studies have one obvious drawback: They take time. In addition, longitudinal studies are usually more costly than cross-sectional studies, and they frequently require a large team of researchers.

Although cross-sectional studies have the advantage of speed, they have a disadvantage as well. Whereas longitudinal studies compare individuals to themselves, cross-sectional studies compare two separate groups of individuals. Cross-sectional studies can show differences, but they cannot yield information about changes in people over a period of time. For example, a cross-sectional study may find that a group of 20- to 30-year-olds have lower cholesterol levels than a group of 50- to 60-year-olds, but such information does not demonstrate that cholesterol levels go up as people become older. Only a longitudinal study, looking at the same people over a long period of time, can show that cholesterol increases with age. Thus, longitudinal studies allow researchers to assess developmental trends and draw conclusions concerning the course of a particular condition. The choice between a longitudinal method and a cross-sectional method depends partly on which questions the researcher is asking and partly on the amount of time and resources available.

Cross-sectional and longitudinal studies can be combined, allowing researchers to examine differences among people at different ages and then to follow them over time to measure developmental differences. Such a design was conducted by Keltikangas-Järvinen and Räikkönen (1990a, 1990b). These investigators selected a large group of healthy adolescents and young adults, ages 12, 15, and 18, and assessed their coronary risk factors three times over a 6-year period. The cross-sectional phase of the study allowed the researchers to compare coronary risk factors among three different age groups whereas the longitudinal aspect of the study permitted an examination of risk factor changes. Keltikangas-Järvinen and Räikkönen found that participants with high risk factors—that is, those with high blood pressure, high cholesterol, and a high body-mass index—were more likely than those with low risk factors to be aggressive-competitive but less likely to be closely involved with other people. They also found that male and female participants were quite similar in risk factors, a finding that suggests that early risk factors do not explain the later higher death rates from heart disease experienced by men.

Case studies, correlational studies, cross-sectional designs, and longitudinal studies all have important uses in psychology, but none of them is able to suggest causality. Sometimes psychologists desire information on the ability of one variable to cause or influence another, requiring an experimental design.

EXPERIMENTAL DESIGNS

Health psychologists sometimes use experimental studies to learn the effects of a health-related behavior (such as eating a low-fat diet) on an illness (such as heart disease). Experimental designs are valuable because they generally yield information about cause-and-effect relationships that no other method can reveal.

In an experimental study, the experimenter begins with a sample of participants, divides them randomly into two or more groups, administers the condition of interest to one group, and administers a different condition to the other group or groups. The group receiving the condition of particular interest is called the *experimental group;* the participants receiving the comparison condition make up the *control group.* Often the experimental condition consists of administering a treatment whereas the control condition consists of withholding that treatment, but other combinations of treatment and control conditions are possible.

In an experimental design, the participants in the experimental group must receive treatment identical

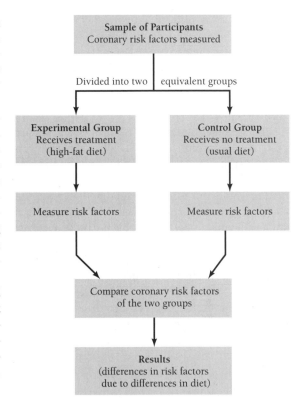

Figure 2.1 Example of the experimental method.

to that of participants in the control group except for one factor. The only difference between the two groups must be that they differ in their exposure to the **independent variable**. The experimental group receives one level of the independent variable, and the control group receives a different level. The independent variable is systematically manipulated to observe its influence on behavior—that is, on the **dependent variable**. If manipulation of the independent variable causes a change in the dependent variable, which can be evaluated by contrasting the experimental and control groups, the independent variable has a cause-and-effect relationship with the dependent variable.

In the example of the low-fat diet and heart disease, the experimental group would be placed on a low-fat diet and the control group would eat a regular diet (see Figure 2.1). If the two groups are equal in all other important respects—such as baseline levels of diastolic and systolic blood pressure, age, gender, weight, and other dietary factors—and if the two groups differed only in diet during the course of the experiment, then any posttest differences between the two groups in cardiovascular disease could be attributed to differences in diet. Such an experimental design allows the investigator to speak of causation or at least of probable causes of a particular disorder.

Experimental designs with health outcomes are problematic for ethical reasons. Participants who might be put in the control group could not be prevented, for example, from eating a low-fat diet, and neither could those in the experimental group be compelled to each such a diet. Two experimental studies illustrate how this problem can be avoided. In one experiment, Kramsch, Aspen, Abramowitz, Kreimendahl, and Hood (1981) used nonhuman subjects to investigate the effects of a high-fat diet on serum cholesterol levels, **atherosclerosis** (narrowing of the arteries), and sudden death from heart failure. The researchers randomly divided 27 monkeys into three groups. All animals were fed a very high-fat diet, but those in the two control groups were permitted little exercise whereas those in the experimental group were forced to run on a treadmill for 1 hour, three times a week. After 3 1/2 years, monkeys in the exercise group had the same total cholesterol levels as the sedentary monkeys, but they had higher levels of "good" cholesterol, lower levels of "bad" cholesterol, and less atherosclerosis. In addition, the only monkeys to die suddenly were the sedentary ones. This study demonstrated that exercise can protect against coronary risk factors in monkeys; it suggested similar result for humans, if one is willing to generalize from monkeys to humans.

Another experimental study, the Multiple Risk Factor Intervention Trial (MRFIT), used humans as participants, but researchers did not force some people to eat a high-fat diet or prevent others from doing so. The study was a large-scale investigation of more than 12,000 men between 35 and 57 years of age at the start of the study (Caggiula et al., 1981; Dolecek et al., 1986). At the beginning of this study, all the men were at risk for heart disease by virtue of being cigarette smokers with elevated blood pressure and high serum cholesterol levels. The participants were randomly assigned to either an intervention group or a control group. The intervention was

not a low-fat diet; rather, it consisted of a program of counseling and advice about the benefits of a low-fat diet. Men in the control group were referred to their physicians for "usual care." Although participants in both groups reduced their daily intake of dietary cholesterol to some extent, those in the experimental group changed their diets and lowered their serum cholesterol levels much more than did men in the control group.

Achieving equivalence between the two groups is often a challenging problem in experimental studies. If one group receives a special type of intervention, that group differs in two ways from the control group that does not receive the intervention: (1) the presence of the intervention and (2) the knowledge that they are in a group getting special attention. This knowledge may lead to expectancies about the treatment that interfere with assessment of the treatment's effectiveness. To deal with this problem, researchers may give the control group a *placebo,* as discussed earlier.

Although a well-designed experiment can yield information about causal relationships, not all variables of interest in psychology can be manipulated. If the independent variable is not or cannot be manipulated, the study does not meet the requirements of the experimental method. When researchers are prevented by either ethical or practical restrictions from manipulating variables in a systematic manner, they sometimes rely on ex post facto designs.

EX POST FACTO DESIGNS

Ex post facto designs, which are one of several types of quasi-experimental studies, resemble experiments in some ways but differ in others. Both types of studies involve contrasting groups to determine differences, but ex post facto designs do not involve the manipulation of independent variables. Instead, researchers choose a variable of interest and select participants who differ on this variable, called a **subject variable.** By placing participants in groups according to different values of the subject variable, researchers can contrast these groups according to responses in a dependent variable. The most common reasons for this research strategy are practical and ethical limitations on the manipulations that an experimenter can perform.

Ex post facto designs are very common in health psychology because researchers are interested in investigating variables they cannot manipulate. For example, researchers interested in investigating the effect of a high-fat diet on the development of atherosclerosis have used nonhuman animal subjects rather than humans. An alternative approach would be to select a group of participants who already eat a high-fat diet and also select a comparison group of those who eat a diet lower in fat. However, the comparison group in an ex post facto design is not an equivalent control group because these participants were not equivalent to those in the experimental group at the beginning of the study. This nonequivalence of groups limits the conclusions that can be drawn to those about differences between groups. No conclusions concerning causality can be made from the ex post facto design.

An example of an ex post facto design is a study conducted by Fuchs et al. (1995) on the effects of different levels of alcohol consumption on death from heart disease. These investigators began with a large group of healthy women, ages 34 to 59, and divided them into nondrinkers, light drinkers, moderate drinkers, and heavy drinkers. After 12 years, women in both the light drinking and the moderate drinking groups had lower death rates from cardiovascular disease than women who were nondrinkers, but heavy drinkers had a higher all-cause mortality rate than the nondrinkers.

In this study, the classification of women into nondrinkers, light drinkers, moderate drinkers, and heavy drinkers was ex post facto; that is, the participants were divided into groups according to criteria that the researchers selected rather than manipulated. The researchers then looked at death rates 12 years later and found a U-shaped relationship between level of alcohol consumption and cardiovascular death rate, meaning that nondrinkers and heavy drinkers had the highest death rates while light and moderate drinkers fared best.

Ex post facto designs allow comparisons between or among groups, but they do not permit researchers to determine that one variable causes changes in another variable. In the study on alcohol consumption, for example, the researchers could not conclude that light to moderate consumption caused the difference in death rates from cardiovascular disease, but the study does provide information about one risk factor for CVD.

RESEARCH METHODS IN EPIDEMIOLOGY

Many of the research methods used by psychologists are quite similar to those employed by epidemiologists. **Epidemiology** is a branch of medicine that investigates factors contributing to increased health or the occurrence of a disease in a particular population (Beaglehole, Bonita, & Kjellström, 1993). In both psychology and epidemiology, the researcher applies the scientific method to observe naturally occurring events or to conduct experimental studies. Both disciplines employ cross-sectional, longitudinal, and experimental designs; both test hypotheses, rely on statistical analyses, and draw inferences from their data. Although the procedures of psychology and epidemiology are similar, the terminology is not always the same.

THE FIELD OF EPIDEMIOLOGY

Epidemiology provides useful techniques for taking a first look at a health-related problem (Fraser, 1987). In ancient Greece and Babylon, observers first began to compare people who had a particular illness or characteristic to those who did not (Lilienfeld & Lilienfeld, 1980). However, epidemiology did not evolve as a science until the 19th century, when infectious diseases such as cholera, smallpox, and typhoid fever threatened the lives of millions of people. Many of these infectious diseases were controlled or conquered largely through the work of the epidemiologists who gradually and laboriously identified their causes.

A dramatic example is the work of John Snow, the brilliant English epidemiologist and anesthetist and one of the founding members of the London Epidemiological Society (Lilienfeld & Lilienfeld, 1980; Rosen, 1958). During the 1848 outbreak of cholera in London, Snow made careful observations of the distribution of cholera deaths in the southern section of the city. At that time, two different companies were supplying the residents of south London with drinking water. The water mains of the two companies were interwoven so that residences on the same side of the street were receiving their water from two separate sources. One water company was pumping its water from a polluted area of the Thames; the other had recently relocated its pumps to a less polluted area. Snow noted which houses received water from each company and calculated that the cholera death rate was more than five times higher in homes receiving their water from the Thames than in homes receiving water from the other south London company. He then compared both sets of death rates with those from the rest of London. Snow observed that the pattern of cholera deaths closely paralleled the distribution of polluted water. In 1855, without yet understanding the specific organism responsible for cholera, Snow published a report in which he suggested the existence of a cholera "poison" and expressed his views of how the disease started and how it spread. He also devised an ingenious plan of intervention: He simply turned off the source of polluted water. Not until 30 years later did Robert Koch isolate the cholera bacterium, thus establishing the essential validity of Snow's views.

Snow had identified a risk factor for a deadly disease; he had not discovered a specific cause. During the last half of the 20th century, epidemiological work has shifted from tracking infectious diseases to discovering factors associated with positive health or with chronic illnesses, but the procedures are quite like Snow's. Identifying these factors does not prove causation, but it is a necessary first step leading to the control or eradication of a particular disease.

Epidemiologists are interested in both the prevalence and the incidence of a disease. **Prevalence** refers to the proportion of the population that has a particular disease at a specific time; **incidence** measures the frequency of *new cases* of the disease during a specified period (Ahlbom & Norell, 1990). With both prevalence and incidence, the number of people in the *population at risk* is divided into either the number of people with the disease (prevalence) or the number of new cases in a particular time frame (incidence). For example, the prevalence of cardiovascular disease is greater than the incidence because people can live for years after a diagnosis.

In a given community, for example, the annual *incidence* of hypertension might be .025, meaning that for every 1,000 people in that community, 25 people per year will receive a diagnosis of high blood pressure. But because hypertension is a chronic illness, the *prevalence* in that community will be more than 25 per 1,000. On the other hand, for a disease such as influenza with a relatively short duration (due either to the patient's rapid recovery or quick mortality) the incidence per year will exceed the prevalence at any specific time during that year.

THE PURPOSES OF EPIDEMIOLOGICAL STUDIES

Lilienfeld and Lilienfeld (1980) identified three basic purposes of epidemiological studies. The first purpose is to determine the etiology or origins of a specific disease. For example, epidemiologists have looked at the prevalence of AIDS in certain populations and discovered possible causes of the disease. When researchers noted an increased prevalence of AIDS within the male homosexual communities and within a population of intravenous drug users, they hypothesized that the disease may somehow be transmitted through body fluids. Clinical tests have subsequently supported this hypothesis. In a similar fashion, John Snow discovered that the possible causes of cholera resided in polluted water, thus laying the groundwork for Koch's later discovery of a specific bacterium as the causal agent.

A second purpose is to determine whether hypotheses developed from other studies are consistent with epidemiological data. For example, physicians might notice that heart attack is more common in women who are overweight. Could obesity be related to heart disease in women? Only a large-scale epidemiological study could answer this question, and indeed, epidemiological studies have found such an association (Willett et al., 1995).

Also, epidemiological studies can be used to test more specific hypotheses regarding possible causes of a disease. For example, it has been noted that Seventh-Day Adventists have lower rates of CVD than the population in general. Could this lower rate be due to their vegetarian diet? Could it be their low rate of smoking? Do Seventh-Day Adventists have other behavioral differences from the general population that could lower their rate for CVD? Again, epidemiological studies can test these hypotheses by comparing Seventh-Day Adventists with others on

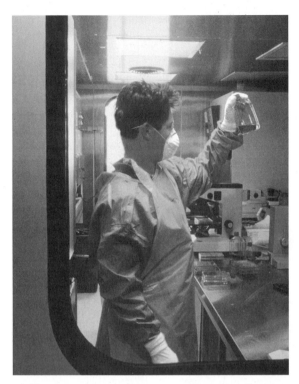

One purpose of epidemiology research is to determine the origins of a disease.

several possible factors that might logically relate to CVD.

A third purpose of epidemiological studies is to provide a basis for developing and evaluating various preventive procedures. Treatment programs developed to control CVD need to be tested to determine how well they work to prevent the development or progression of CVD. Testing that involves a large group of people would be necessary to demonstrate the overall rate of effectiveness.

AREAS OF EPIDEMIOLOGICAL STUDY

To achieve these purposes of epidemiological studies, researchers can use three broad methods: observational studies, "natural" experiments, and experimental epidemiology. Each method has its own requirements and yields specific information.

Observational Methods

Epidemiologists use observational methods to observe and analyze the occurrence of a specific disease in a given population. These methods do not show causes of the disease, but researchers can draw inferences about possible factors that relate to the disease. Observational methods are similar to correlational studies in psychology; both show an association between two or more conditions, but neither can be used to demonstrate causation.

Epidemiology studies have been used to identify psychosocial factors in cardiovascular disease. One such factor is the Type A behavior pattern, which has received extensive interest from both epidemiologists and psychologists. In one epidemiology study, Rosenman et al. (1975) found that men with the Type A behavior pattern were more than twice as likely as other men to experience coronary heart disease. Although this investigation did not use correlation coefficients, it suggested a correlation or association between Type A behavior and death from heart disease. In addition to being observational, this is an example of a prospective study.

Prospective studies begin with a population of disease-free participants and follow them over a period of time to determine whether a given condition, such as cigarette smoking or high blood pressure, is related to a later condition, such as cardiovascular disease or death. Prospective observational studies are identical to longitudinal studies in psychology: Both provide continuing information about a group of participants. **Retrospective studies** use the opposite approach; they begin with a group of people already suffering from a particular disease and then look backward for characteristics or conditions that marked them as being different from people who do not have that illness. For example, Mendes de Leon (1992) began with two groups of hospitalized patients; one consisted of men with heart disease, the other of men with diseases of the musculoskeletal system. Mendes de Leon found that one component of Type A behavior (the expression of anger) was related to coronary heart disease but not to musculoskeletal diseases. Retrospective studies such as this one are also referred to as **case-control studies** because cases (people affected by a disease) are compared to controls (people not affected). In general, prospective investigations provide more specific data than do retrospective studies, but prospective studies are expensive and time-consuming.

To compare retrospective studies to prospective designs, consider again the relationship between Type A behavior and heart disease. In the prospective study by Rosenman et al. (1975), the researchers measured Type A behavior of a large cohort (a group of participants starting an experience together) and then tracked the health of these participants to learn whether men with Type A behaviors would differ from other men in incidence of heart disease. The retrospective study by Mendes de Leon, in contrast, began with a group of heart disease patients and looked back at earlier records to determine whether their levels of anger expression differed from those of a matched group of controls. Both studies can show an association between a condition (such as Type A behaviors) and a subsequent illness (such as heart disease). The prospective study does so by looking forward whereas the retrospective study looks back in time.

Natural Experiments

A second area of epidemiological study is the natural experiment, in which the researcher can only select the independent variable, not manipulate it. Natural experiments are similar to the ex post facto designs used in psychology and involve the study of natural conditions that approximate a controlled experiment.

When John Snow compared death rates from cholera in two similar groups of houses, he was employing a natural experiment. Ethical considerations, of course, would have prevented him from purposely contaminating the water in one set of houses and supplying pure water for neighboring homes, as would be required for a true experiment.

When two similar groups of people naturally divide themselves into those exposed to a pathogen and those not exposed, natural experiments are possible. The study by Fuchs et al. (1995) described earlier as an ex post facto design also fits the description of a natural experiment. In this study, women who had preexisting rates of alcohol consumption were divided into four groups—nondrinkers, light drinkers, moderate drinkers, and heavy drinkers—and then compared for death rates from cardiovascular disease. Because these groups are alike in other important conditions, the researchers were able to conduct a natural experiment by merely selecting levels of alcohol consumption as the variable of interest and using CVD death rates as one dependent variable.

Experimental Investigations

The third type of epidemiological study, the experimental investigation, is essentially identical to experiments in psychology. With this method the researcher manipulates the independent variables rather than merely selecting them. Researchers match or randomly assign participants to an experimental or control group so that two (or more) groups are equated on all pertinent factors except the values of the independent variable. Although prospective studies are typically observational, some are experimental. The feature that makes a prospective study experimental is the selection of equal groups at the beginning of the investigation, the manipulation of an independent variable or variables, and long-term follow-up of the participants.

In studying the effects of a high-fat diet on cardiovascular disease, an experimental group would receive a diet high in fat content while a matched group would eat a lower fat diet. If the two groups are equal in other respects, differences between the two in rates of CVD might be attributed to the high-fat diet. Obviously, this study would present a major ethical problem with human participants. People are not always willing to be subjected, merely for scientific reasons, to such a potentially unhealthy behavior as eating a high-fat diet. True, many people already eat high-fat diets, but a valid experiment would need to begin with participants who were not currently doing so. People who volunteer for such an experiment must be willing to be placed in either the experimental group or the control group; that is, they must agree either to eat a high-fat diet or to continue with their usual low-fat diet.

On the other hand, if people were allowed to choose to be placed in either the experimental group or the control group, **self-selection** would be a problem. People who are willing to eat a high-fat diet are different from those who are not. This difference invalidates any experimental study that does not control for self-selection, and findings from such a study do not prove a cause-and-effect relationship.

Because of their scope and problematic ethical considerations, experimental prospective studies are quite rare. One such study, however, is the Multiple Risk Factor Intervention Trial (MRFIT), discussed as an example of a psychology experiment (Multiple Risk Factor Intervention Trial Research Group, 1977). The MRFIT study minimized the problem of self-selection because all the men had multiple risks for heart disease at the start of the study and all were free of any visible evidence of heart disease. Participants were randomly placed into two groups: those who received a special intervention and those who received usual health care. The intervention (experimental) group received three types of treatment: (1) hypertensive medication and advice on sodium restriction, (2) counseling on giving up cigarette smoking, and (3) dietary advice to reduce cholesterol levels. Both the treatment group and the control group were invited to return yearly for a medical history, physical examination, and laboratory work.

A 7-year follow-up showed a decline in heart disease risk factors for both groups (MRFIT Research Group, 1982). Mortality rates from coronary heart disease were 17.9 per 1,000 for men in the intervention group and 19.3 per 1,000 for men in the control (usual health care) group, a difference that was not statistically significant. During the next 3 years, the intervention group reported somewhat fewer deaths from coronary heart disease (MRFIT Research Group, 1990), a finding that suggested potential value in a program designed to change the behavior of men at risk for coronary heart disease.

Aside from prospective studies, there are two categories of experimental methods in epidemiology: clinical trials and community trials (Lilienfeld & Lilienfeld, 1980). *Clinical trials* test the effects of the independent variable on individuals whereas *community trials* (also called field studies) test the effects of the independent variable on a group of individuals. An example of a clinical trial would be an experiment designed to test the efficacy of a drug designed to lower cholesterol. In such an experiment, participants with high serum cholesterol are randomly assigned to either an experimental group that receives the active drug, such as lovastatin, or a control group that receives a placebo pill (Lovastatin Study Group III, 1988). Differences between the two groups in subsequent total cholesterol levels could be attributed to the differences in treatment — that is, the independent variable. Such an experiment would require a double-blind design in which neither the participants nor the people who administer the pills would know which pills contained the active ingredient and which were placebos. All drugs approved by the Food and Drug Administration (FDA) must first undergo extensive clinical trials of this nature.

In a field study, researchers compare one community to another. For example, people in one city might receive extensive information on the benefits of reducing cholesterol and high blood pressure whereas those in a city with similar characteristics would not be exposed to this information campaign. Winkleby, Flora, and Kraemer (1994) reported on such a study conducted as part of the Stanford Five-City Project. People in two experimental cities received increased educational messages from radio, newspapers, television, and other sources on the value of controlling coronary risk factors. People in the three control cities received no extra messages. After 6 years, people in the experimental cities had reduced their blood pressure and cholesterol somewhat more than people in the three control cities.

AN EXAMPLE OF EPIDEMIOLOGICAL RESEARCH

To give some idea of the way epidemiologists work, let's look at the Alameda County Study, an ongoing prospective community study designed to identify health practices that may protect against death and illness. We have seen that epidemiologists identify risk factors by studying large populations over some period of time and by sifting out behavioral, demographic, or inherent elements that show a relationship to subsequent disease or death. Dozens of large-scale community studies have been reported during the past 2 or 3 decades. Unlike community trials (which are experimental and compare one community with another), community studies are observational and look a single community. Examples of community studies include the Alameda County Study (Berkman & Breslow, 1983), the Framingham Heart Study (Dawber, 1980), the Honolulu Heart Program (Yano, Rhoads, Kagan, & Tillotson, 1978), the North Karelia Project in Finland (Pushka & Mustaniemi, 1975), the Seven Countries Study (Keys, 1980), and the Tecumseh

Community Health Study (Higgins, Kjelsberg, & Metzner, 1967). Some of these studies appear in later chapters. For now, a review of a single project, the Alameda County study, should reveal the flavor of community studies and the ways in which they have contributed to our knowledge of the influence of behavior and lifestyle in either promoting or endangering health.

The Alameda County study began as an attempt to identify the health practices and social variables that relate to mortality from all causes. In 1965, epidemiologist Lester Breslow and his colleagues from the Human Population Laboratory of the California State Department of Public Health began a survey of a sample of all the households in Alameda County (Oakland), California. After determining the number of adults living at these addresses, the researchers sent detailed questionnaires to each resident 20 years of age or older. Usable returns were eventually received from 6,928 people. Among other questions, these participants answered questions about seven basic health practices: (1) getting 7 or 8 hours of sleep daily, (2) eating breakfast almost every day, (3) rarely eating between meals, (4) drinking alcohol in moderation or not at all, (5) not smoking cigarettes, (6) exercising regularly, and (7) maintaining weight near the prescribed ideal.

At the time of the original survey in 1965, only cigarette smoking had been implicated as a health risk. Evidence that any of the other six practices predicted health or mortality was quite tenuous. Because several of these practices require some amount of good health, it was necessary to investigate the possibility that original health status might confound subsequent death rates. To control for these possible confounding effects, the Alameda County investigators asked residents about their disabilities, acute and chronic illnesses, physical symptoms, and current levels of energy.

A follow-up 5½ years later (Belloc, 1973) revealed that Alameda County residents who practiced six or seven of the basic health-related behaviors were far less likely to have died than those who practiced zero to three. This decreased mortality risk was independent of their 1965 health status, thus suggesting that healthy behaviors lead to lower rates of mortality (death). Surprisingly, these seven health

practices turned out to be better predictors of mortality than level of income.

In 1974, a major follow-up of living participants took place. At that time a new sample was also surveyed to determine whether the community in general had adopted a new lifestyle between 1965 and 1974. The 9-year follow-up determined the relationship between mortality and the seven health practices, considered individually as well as in combination (Berkman & Breslow, 1983; Wingard, Berkman, & Brand, 1982). Five of the health practices predicted mortality rates independently of participants' use of preventive health services and their physical health in 1965. Cigarette smoking, lack of physical activity, and alcohol consumption were strongly related to mortality, whereas obesity and too much or too little sleep were only weakly associated with increased death rates. As it turned out, skipping breakfast and snacking between meals were not significantly related to mortality.

Men who practiced zero to two health-related behaviors were nearly three times more likely to have died than were those who engaged in four to five of the behaviors. For women, the effect was even more dramatic: When compared to women who practiced four or five of these behaviors, those who engaged in zero to two were 3.2 times more likely to have died. In addition, a cumulative Health Practices Index predicted mortality independent of a wide range of factors, such as physical health at the time of the original survey, year of death, socioeconomic level, race, and use of preventive health services. The association between health practices and mortality appeared for participants in all age groups. Moreover, the number of close social relationships also predicted mortality: People with few social contacts were two and a half times more likely to have died than were those with many such contacts (Berkman & Syme, 1979).

An interesting finding was that a working woman's number of children seems to have little or no association with her mortality risk. Kotler and Wingard (1989) analyzed the effect of occupational, marital, and parental roles on mortality in Alameda County and found that for married working women, the number of children had virtually no effect on mortality. For single working women, having more children was slightly related to an increased risk of death, whereas housewives had a significantly elevated risk of mortality when they had four or more children. The number of children had no effect at all on mortality rates for men.

If some health practices are inversely related to mortality, then a second question would be how these same factors relate to morbidity or disease. A condition that predicts death need not also predict illness. Many disabilities, chronic illnesses, and illness symptoms do not inevitably lead to death. Therefore, it is important to know whether basic health practices and social contacts predict later physical health. Stated another way: Do health practices and social networks merely contribute to survival time, or do they also raise an individual's general level of well-being?

To answer this question, Camacho and Wiley (1983; Wiley & Camacho, 1980) studied a subset of the original sample of Alameda County participants. In their analysis of the data, Camacho and Wiley used social networks and only five of the health practices, eliminating eating breakfast and snacking between meals. They found that each of the five health behaviors predicted changes in health. Because change in health status was the dependent variable, former cigarette smokers actually fared better than nonsmokers; that is, the health of former cigarette smokers either improved more or did not deteriorate as much when compared to those who had never smoked. As expected, both former smokers and nonsmokers had better health than smokers.

With regard to alcohol consumption, moderate drinkers (17 to 45 drinks per month) did best, followed in order by heavy drinkers and finally abstainers. With regard to sleep, a curvilinear relationship appeared, with 7 or 8 hours per night being optimal; either more or less sleep was associated with negative changes in health status. As for exercise, both men and women who engaged in high levels of physical activity were healthier in 1974 than their more sedentary counterparts who had been their equals in health at the beginning of the survey. Weight, much like sleep, showed a curvilinear relationship to health status, with both overweight participants (30% or more above desirable weight) and underweight individuals (10% or more below desirable weight) reporting the greatest deterioration in health status.

Two indexes also predicted 9-year changes in health status. One was the Health Practices Index, which combined all the health behaviors, and the other was a Social Network Index, which combined marital status, contacts with friends and relatives and membership in church and other organizations. According to the findings, marriage did not have equal effects on the health of men and women. With both men and women, individuals who were formerly married—separated, divorced, or widowed—had greater negative changes in health, but women who had never been married were much healthier than were men who had never married. Never-married men had slightly negative health scores compared to married men, but never-married women had considerably higher health scores than either married or formerly married women. Marriage, it seems, agrees with men, but the single life is apparently healthier for women.

SUMMARY AND EVALUATION OF RESEARCH METHODS

Psychologists and epidemiologists employ similar designs to gather information on conditions that relate to health. Like other scientists, they use controlled observations, try to be objective and cautious in drawing conclusions, and conduct studies that they or others can replicate. They do not rely on opinions or testimonials in stating which factors might affect health. This approach contrasts with that of many people, such as Diane, and also with many advertisements in the popular media, which are directed at selling products. Figure 2.2 summarizes the broad areas of epidemiological study and shows their approximate counterparts in the field of psychology.

All psychological and epidemiological studies have weaknesses, and those pertaining to health psychology are not exceptions. A major limitation to most studies in this field is that they simply indicate an association between a behavior and a subsequent outcome. Much research shows a relationship between a single independent variable, such as the Type A behavior pattern, and later morbidity, such as heart disease. But by looking at a single illness outcome from a variety of perspectives and using multiple research methods, scientists learn much

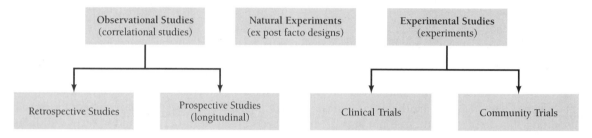

Figure 2.2 *Research methods in epidemiology with their psychology counterparts in parentheses.*

valuable information concerning that illness. We have seen that both psychology and epidemiology have examined cardiovascular disease from different angles and with a variety of methods. Such an approach has led to an increasingly better understanding of the behavioral factors in cardiovascular disease.

Nevertheless, little research exists showing how various psychological and behavioral factors interact with each other to influence the onset, progression, and severity of certain illnesses. In addition, researchers typically rely on limited assessment measures. Ideally, health psychologists and epidemiologists should use a variety of instruments, including self-reports and physiological indices, as well as measures that are both clinically and theoretically relevant. Such research is difficult, expensive, and time-consuming, but it is essential for a complete understanding of how behavioral and psychological factors influence illness and health.

DETERMINING CAUSATION

We have seen that both prospective and retrospective studies can identify risk factors in an illness, but they do not demonstrate causation. Obesity, hypertension, high total cholesterol, and cigarette smoking, for example, are all demonstrated risk factors for cardiovascular disease. People with one or more of these risks are more likely than people with none of these risks to develop CVD. However, some people with no known risks will develop cardiovascular disease and some people with multiple risks may never have CVD. This section looks at the risk factor approach as a means of suggesting causation and

then examines evidence that cigarette smoking *causes* illness.

THE RISK FACTOR APPROACH

The study that popularized the concept of risk factor was the Framingham Heart Study (Brown, 1988; Dawber, 1980), a large-scale epidemiology study that began in 1948 and included more than 5,000 men and women in the town of Framingham, Massachusetts. From its early years and continuing to the present, this study has allowed researchers to identify such risk factors for cardiovascular disease (CVD) as serum cholesterol, gender, high blood pressure, cigarette smoking, obesity, and the Type A behavior pattern. These risk factors do not necessarily cause cardiovascular disease, but they are related to it in some way. Obesity, for example, may not be a direct cause of heart disease, but it is generally associated with hypertension, which is strongly associated with cardiovascular disease. Because obesity is related to a known risk factor, it too is a risk factor for CVD.

Although risk factors do not derive from experimental studies, they can determine the *probability* that a person will develop a particular disease. Not all cigarette smokers will develop heart disease, but if you smoke, you are about twice as likely to die of cardiovascular disease than if you do not smoke (Centers for Disease Control and Prevention [CDC], 1993). Clearly, smoking cigarettes places one at risk for developing CVD. In a similar fashion, high cholesterol levels, high blood pressure, obesity, and stress are all risk factors for cardiovascular disease, but there is no *experimental* evidence that any of these conditions *cause* coronary heart disease or stroke.

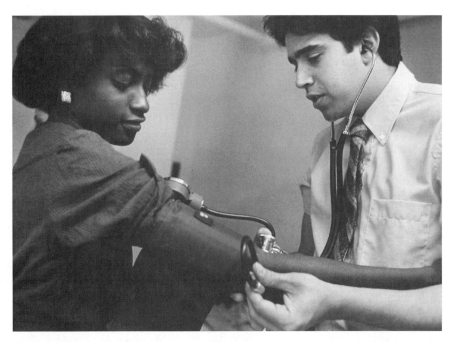

Blood pressure is a risk factor for cardiovascular disease, indicating that people with high blood pressure are at elevated risk but not that high blood pressure causes cardiovascular disease.

Although demonstration of causation is limited to experimental studies, epidemiologists have developed ways of inferring cause and effect relationships based on other types of evidence (Beaglehole et al., 1993: Susser, 1991). In modern epidemiology, a specific factor is neither necessary nor sufficient to suggest a causal relationship with a particular disease. If a condition were both necessary and sufficient, then causation would be absolutely established. For example, if all cigarette smokers died of lung cancer and no nonsmoker ever died of this disease, then cigarette smoking would be both a necessary and sufficient condition for lung cancer. This situation, of course, does not exist. Diseases ordinarily have many causes, and smoking is only one possible contributor to lung cancer.

How do epidemiologists infer causality through studies that are not experimental? Beaglehole et al. (1993) listed seven conditions that, if present, allow for inferences of causality. First, a dose-response relationship must exist between a possible cause and changes in the prevalence or incidence of a disease. A **dose-response relationship** is a direct, consistent relationship between an independent variable, such

as a behavior, and a dependent variable, such as an illness. For example, the mortality rate is greatest for heavy smokers, less so for moderate smokers, even less for light smokers, and still less for nonsmokers (U.S. Department of Health and Human Services [USDHHS], 1990b). This dose-response relationship suggests but does not, by itself, prove causality.

The second condition is that the prevalence or incidence of a disease should decline with the removal of the possible cause. For example, if people who quit smoking subsequently lower their chances of CVD, this second criterion would be met. Research (Ben-Shlomo, Smith, Shipley, & Marmot, 1994) has shown that quitting cigarette smoking lowered a person's risk of cardiovascular disease death.

A third and necessary criterion is that the possible cause must precede the disease. If an illness occurs before a condition, that condition cannot be the cause. For example, if a person takes up cigarette smoking only after developing heart disease, cigarette smoking could not have caused that person's heart disease.

Fourth, the cause-and-effect relationship between the condition and the disease must be plausible; that is, it must be consistent with other data and it must make sense from a biological viewpoint. Frequently, the physiology underlying the connection between a behavior and a disease is not known, but this is not necessary. Epidemiologists can infer causality without a known physiological connection, but such a connection must at least be a reasonable possibility.

Fifth, research data must be consistent; that is, a preponderance of the evidence must be on one side of the ledger. When data from well-controlled studies are in conflict, suspicion of causality arises. Beaglehole et al. (1993) pointed out that even consistently weak results might still suggest causation if a meta-analysis of those studies reveals significant results. **Meta-analysis** is a statistical technique for combining results of several studies when these studies have similar definitions of variables. Thus, when a dozen or so studies individually show only suggestive results, a meta-analysis of those studies may reveal significant results due to analyses of a larger number of participants. Other epidemiologists (Shapiro, 1994) have questioned the value of meta-analyses of nonexperimental studies and have further argued that if several studies produce only small effects, those results may be the result of a consistent bias and a meta-analysis would merely reinforce that spurious finding. Nevertheless, meta-analyses can be more useful for researchers than the results from a single study in inferring causation.

A sixth criterion is the strength of the association or the size of the relative risk. Epidemiologists use the term **relative risk** (RR) to refer to the ratio of the incidence or prevalence of a disease in an exposed group to the incidence or prevalence of that disease in the unexposed group. The relative risk of the unexposed group is always 1.00, so that a RR of 1.50 indicates that the exposed group is 50% more likely to develop the disease in question than the unexposed group. A relative risk of 0.70 means that the rate of disease in the exposed group is only 70% the rate in the unexposed group. For example, Klag et al. (1993) conducted a long-term follow-up of young men to determine the relationship between cholesterol levels and heart disease risks. They followed these men for an average of 30 years and found that the men with high cholesterol levels had a RR of 2.02 for dying of CVD compared with men

with low cholesterol levels; that is, those men with high cholesterol levels were more than twice as likely to die from cardiovascular disease as men with low cholesterol levels. On the other hand, Stampfer et al. (1993) found that a person could lower the relative risk of CVD by consuming vitamin E. That is, they found a RR of .66 for women with high versus low vitamin E intake.

The relative risk of 2.02 is quite high, but even RRs in the magnitude of 0.60 to 1.3 can suggest causality if they are consistent or if they are the result of a meta-analysis. Beaglehole et al. (1993) stated that a RR of 2.0 or greater is considered strong. Thus, cigarette smoking's relative risk of 9.0 for lung cancer (Lubin, Blot, et al., 1984) is extremely high, and because comparable relative risk figures have been reported in other studies, epidemiologists accept cigarette smoking as a causal agent for lung cancer.

The final criterion for inferring causality is the study's design. As previously stated, experimental designs reveal the clearest information on causality, but observational studies, if well designed, can also be suggestive. All studies, of course, should be confirmed by other researchers and in other locations. When these seven criteria are met, epidemiologists hold that a causal relationship has been established.

AN EXAMPLE OF DETERMINING CAUSATION

During the past 45 years, researchers have used nonexperimental studies to establish a link between cigarette smoking and several diseases, especially cardiovascular disease and lung cancer. Accumulated findings from these studies present an example of how nonexperimental studies can turn that link into a causal relationship.

In 1994, representatives from all the major tobacco companies came before the United States Congress House Subcommittee on Health to defend charges that cigarette smoking causes a variety of health problems, including heart disease and lung cancer. The crux of their argument was that no scientific study has ever proven that cigarette smoking causes heart disease or lung cancer in humans. Technically, their contention was correct because only experimental studies can absolutely demonstrate causation, and no such experimental study has ever been or ever will be conducted on humans.

However, experimental studies are not required before scientists can infer a causal link between the independent variable (smoking) and the dependent variables (heart disease and lung cancer). When a preponderance of ex post facto and correlational studies meet the seven criteria proposed by Beaglehole et al. (1993), causality is virtually certain. Does sufficient evidence exist to infer a cause-and-effect relationship between cigarette smoking and heart disease and lung cancer?

First, a multitude of studies (Doll & Hill, 1956; Kubik, 1984; Risch et al., 1993; USDHHS, 1990b) have consistently reported a *dose-response relationship* between both the number of cigarettes smoked per day and the number of years one has smoked and the subsequent incidence of heart disease and lung cancer.

Second, heart disease and lung cancer *incidences decline when people stop smoking*. Research (Ben-Shlomo et al., 1994; Kawachi et al., 1993; Rosenberg, Palmer, & Shapiro, 1990; USDHHS, 1990b) has consistently demonstrated that quitting cigarette smoking lowers one's risk of cardiovascular disease and greatly decreases one's risk of lung cancer. Moreover, quitting adds years to one's life (Fielding, 1985). People who continue to smoke continue to have increased risks of these diseases.

Third, cigarette *smoking almost always precedes incidence of disease*. (We have little evidence that people tend to begin cigarette smoking as a means of coping with heart disease or lung cancer.)

Fourth, although scientists may not completely understand the exact mechanisms responsible for the effect of cigarette smoking on the cardiovascular system and the lungs, such *a physiological connection is plausible*. It is not necessary that the underlying connection between a behavior and a disease be known, only that it be a possibility.

Fifth, research has produced remarkably *consistent evidence* of the relationship of cigarette smoking to cardiovascular disease and lung cancer. For nearly 50 years, evidence from ex post facto and correlational studies, as well as various epidemiological studies, has demonstrated a strong and consistent relationship between cigarette smoking and disease. As early as 1950, Doll and Hill noted a straight linear relationship between average number of cigarettes smoked per day and death rates from lung cancer. Although a positive correlation such as this is not sufficient to demonstrate causation, hundreds of additional correlational and ex post facto studies since that time have yielded overwhelming evidence to suggest that cigarette smoking causes disease.

Sixth, the *strength of the association* between cigarette smoking and cardiovascular disease is strong, with a relative risk of about 2.0 (CDC, 1993), and cigarette smoking's relative risk of about 9.0 for lung cancer is extremely high (Lubin, Blot, et al., 1984). Because other studies have found comparable relative risk figures, epidemiologists accept cigarette smoking as a causal agent for both CVD and lung cancer.

Finally, although no experimental designs with human participants have been reported on the relationship between cigarettes and disease, a sufficient number of *well-designed observational studies* have consistency revealed a close association between cigarette smoking and both cardiovascular disease and lung cancer. Because each of these seven criteria are clearly met by a preponderance of evidence, epidemiologists are able to discount the argument of tobacco company representatives that cigarette smoking has not been proven to cause disease. When evidence is as overwhelming as it is in this case, scientists infer a causal link between cigarette smoking and a variety of diseases, including heart disease and lung cancer.

RESEARCH TOOLS

Psychologists frequently rely on two important tools to conduct research: theoretical models and psychometric instruments. Many, but not all, psychology studies are driven by a theoretical model and are attempts to test hypotheses suggested by that model. In addition, many psychology studies rely on measuring devices to assess behaviors, physiological functions, attitudes, abilities, personality traits, and other independent and dependent variables. This section provides a brief discussion of these two tools.

THE ROLE OF THEORY IN RESEARCH

As the scientific study of human behavior, psychology shares with other disciplines the use of scientific methods to investigate natural phenomena. The work of science is not restricted to research methodology; it also involves constructing theoretical models to serve as vehicles for making sense of research findings. Health psychologists have developed a number of models and theories to explain health-related behaviors and conditions, such as stress, pain, smoking, alcohol abuse, and unhealthy eating habits. To the uninitiated, theories may seem impractical and superfluous, but scientists regard them as practical tools that give both direction and meaning to their research.

Scientific **theory** has been defined as "a set of related assumptions from which, by logical deductive reasoning, testable hypotheses can be drawn" (Feist, 1994, p. 9). Theories have an interactive relationship with scientifically derived observations. A theory gives meaning to observations, and observations in turn fit into and alter the theory erected to explain them. Theories, then, are dynamic and become more powerful as they expand to explain more and more relevant observations.

Near the beginning of this cycle, when the theoretical framework is still rudimentary and not yet sufficiently comprehensive to explain a large number of observations, the term **model** is more appropriate than theory. In practice, however, *theory* and *model* are sometimes used interchangeably.

The role of theory in health psychology is basically the same as it is in any other scientific discipline. First, a useful theory should generate research—both descriptive research and hypothesis testing. The goal of descriptive research is to expand the existing theory. This type of research deals with measurement, labeling, and categorization of observations. A useful theory of psychosocial factors in heart disease, for example, should generate a multitude of investigations that describe the psychological and social factors of people who have been diagnosed with heart disease. On the other hand, hypothesis testing is not specifically carried out to expand the theory but rather to contribute valid data to the body of scientific knowledge. Again, a useful theory of psychosocial factors in heart disease

should stimulate the formulation of a number of hypotheses that, when tested, produce a greater understanding of the psychological and social conditions that relate to heart disease. Results of such studies would either support or fail to support the existing theory; they ordinarily do not enlarge or alter it.

Second, a useful theory should organize and explain the observations derived from research and make them intelligible. Unless research data are organized into some meaningful framework, scientists have no clear direction to follow in their pursuit of further knowledge. A useful theory of the psychosocial factors in heart disease, for example, should integrate what is currently known about such factors and allow researchers to frame discerning questions that stimulate further research.

Third, a useful theory should serve as a guide to action, permitting the practitioner to predict behavior and to implement strategies to change behavior. A practitioner concerned with helping others change health-related behaviors is greatly aided by a theory of behavior change. For instance, a cognitive therapist will follow a cognitive theory of learning to make decisions about how to help clients and will thus focus on changing the thought processes that affect the clients' behaviors. Similarly, psychologists with other theoretical orientations rely on their theories to supply them with solutions to the many questions they confront in their practice.

Theories, then, are useful and necessary tools for the development of any scientific discipline. They generate research that leads to more knowledge, organize and explain observations, and help the practitioner (both the researcher and the clinician) handle a variety of daily problems, such as predicting behavior and helping people change unhealthy practices. Later chapters discuss several theoretical models that are frequently used in health psychology.

THE ROLE OF PSYCHOMETRICS IN RESEARCH

From the work of Sir Francis Galton (1879, 1883) during the 19th century until the present time, psychology has had a close relationship with the measurement of human abilities and behaviors. Indeed, one of psychology's most important contributions to behavioral medicine and behavioral health is its sophistication in assessment techniques. Nearly every important issue in health psychology demands the measurement of the phenomenon being investigated. Psychologists have reacted to this demand by constructing a number of instruments to assess such behaviors and conditions as stress, pain, the Type A behavior pattern, eating habits, and personal hardiness.

For these or any other measuring instruments to be useful, they must be both **reliable** (consistent) and **valid** (accurate). The problems of establishing reliability and validity are critical to the development of any measurement scale.

Establishing Reliability

The reliability of a measuring instrument is the extent to which it yields consistent results. Reliability can be determined by (1) comparing scores on two or more administrations of the same instrument (test-retest reliability); (2) comparing scores yielded by parallel forms of the same instrument (alternate form reliability); (3) comparing half the test items with the other half (split-half reliability); (4) examining the consistency of individual items through the use of an interitem consistency technique such as the Kuder-Richardson Formula 20 (Kuder & Richardson, 1937); or (5) comparing ratings obtained from two or more judges observing the same phenomenon (interrater reliability).

Reliability is most frequently expressed in terms of either correlation coefficients or percentages. The correlation coefficient, which expresses the degree of correspondence between two sets of scores, is the same statistic used in correlational studies. High reliability coefficients (such as .80 to .90) indicate that participants have obtained nearly the same scores on two administrations of a test. Percentages can be used to express the degree of agreement between the independent ratings of observers. When two or more interviewers rate the same participants, or when a single interviewer rates the same participants two or more times, the percentage of agreement between ratings can be determined. High percentages (such as 85% to 95%) indicate that the instrument is capable of eliciting nearly the same ratings from two or more interviewers or that the same observer rated a participant in a similar fashion at two or more separate points in time.

Establishing reliability for the numerous assessment instruments used in health psychology is obviously a formidable task, but it is an essential first step in developing useful measuring devices.

Establishing Validity

A second step in constructing assessment scales is to establish their validity. Measuring scales may be reliable and yet lack validity, or accuracy. Validity is the extent to which an instrument measures what it is designed to measure.

Psychologists determine the validity of a measuring instrument by comparing scores from that instrument with some independent or outside criterion—that is, a standard that has been assessed independently of the instrument being validated. Selection of an appropriate criterion is not only critical but often troublesome. Many validity investigations in health psychology are hampered by the problem of criterion selection. For instance, what might constitute a satisfactory criterion for assessing adherence to prescribed medical regimens? What criterion would be appropriate for determining whether patients are taking medication in the recommended manner? One possible approach would be to count the number of pills remaining after a certain time. Such a procedure has the advantage of being simple, direct, and easily quantifiable. However, counting pills as an index of patient behavior is not without problems. First, pills may have been consumed by someone other than the patient. Second, the patient may have destroyed some pills to give the appearance of compliance. Third, the patient may have taken all the medication but not in the prescribed manner. If pill count is an unsuitable criterion for compliance, then what about changes in health status? Health status has the advantage of being a direct measure of a biological condition, but it is inappropriate as the sole criterion for assessing levels of compliance because many factors other than adherence to prescribed medical recommendations may affect it.

Health psychologists are often interested in three types of validity: construct, current, and predictive. **Construct validity** is the extent to which an instrument measures some hypothetical construct—for example, the Type A behavior pattern, the cancer-prone personality, stress, or personal control. These concepts are constructs because they do not literally exist in a physical sense and can be observed only indirectly through measures of behavior (Murphy & Davidshofer, 1994). **Concurrent validity** is the degree to which an inventory meets some existing standard, such as another inventory or the rating of experts. For example, the concurrent validity of a stress inventory could be determined by checking its scores against an older, established test or by comparing its results with judgments of psychologists or other health care professionals. **Predictive validity** is an estimate of the instrument's ability to predict which participants will develop a particular condition and which ones will remain disease free. For example, life events scales (see Chapter 3) have been used to measure stress and to predict future mortality or morbidity. For such a scale to demonstrate predictive validity it must be administered to participants who are currently free of illness. If people who score high on the scale eventually have higher rates of death or illness than participants with low scores, then the scale can be said to have predictive validity; that is, it differentiates between participants who will remain disease free and those who will die or become ill.

CHAPTER SUMMARY

In recent years, a wealth of material has emerged dealing with the effects of behavior and lifestyle on health and illness. Although some of this material has been biased and self-serving, much of it has a basis in solid scientific research.

A continuing problem with experimental designs is the participants' awareness that they are taking part in a study. To minimize this problem, researchers attempt to balance the effects on the control group by administering a *placebo,* an inactive substance or condition that has the appearance of a treatment. A placebo itself may cause participants to improve or change their behavior because of their belief in the placebo's efficacy. Although the placebo effect is a problem in research, it can be an advantage in treatment, just as the nocebo can be a disadvantage.

Two disciplines—psychology and epidemiology—have been responsible for much of the information now available about the effects of lifestyle and behavior on physical and psychological health. Psychology and epidemiology use research methods that are quite similar.

At least five psychology research methods have contributed to health psychology: (1) case studies, (2) correlational studies, (3) cross-sectional studies and longitudinal studies, (4) experimental designs, and (5) ex post facto studies. Each of these makes its own unique contribution to the understanding of behavior and health. The *case study* is an intensive investigation of one person. *Correlational studies* indicate the degree of association or correlation between two variables, but by themselves, they cannot be used to determine a cause-and-effect relationship. *Cross-sectional studies* investigate a group of people at one point in time whereas *longitudinal studies* follow the participants over an extended period. In general, longitudinal studies are more likely to yield useful and specific results, but they are more time-consuming and expensive than cross-sectional studies. With *experimental designs,* researchers manipulate the independent variable so that any resulting differences between experimental and control groups can be attributed to their differential exposure to the independent variable. *Ex post facto studies* are similar to experimental designs in that researchers compare two or more groups and then record group differences in the dependent variable. However, in the ex post facto study, the experimenter merely selects a subject variable on which two groups have naturally divided themselves rather than creating differences through manipulation.

Many of the research methods used in psychology are quite similar to those used in epidemiology, a branch of medicine that investigates factors contributing to the occurrence of a disease in a particular population. Epidemiologists use at least three basic kinds of research methodology: (1) observational studies, (2) natural experiments, and (3) experimental studies. *Observational studies,* which parallel the correlation studies used in psychology, are of two types: retrospective and prospective. *Retrospective studies* begin with a group of people already suffering from a disease and then look for characteristics of these people that are different from those of people who do not have that disease; *prospective studies* are longitudinal designs that follow the forward development of a population or sample. *Natural experiments,* which are similar to ex post facto studies, involve selection rather than manipulation of the independent variable. Epidemiologists also use *experimental designs,* the two most common of which are *clinical trials* and *community trials.* Occasionally, experimental epidemiological studies are also longitudinal, and these demonstrate cause-and-effect relationships.

Most epidemiological investigations, such as the Alameda County Study, do not demonstrate causation. Instead, they point to specific risk factors that are associated with a particular disease or disorder. A *risk factor* is any characteristic or condition that occurs with greater frequency in people with a disease than it does in people free from that disease.

However, epidemiologists are able to infer causality by looking at evidence from several well-designed observational studies that produce consistent results. Perhaps the clearest example of a nonexperimental cause and effect relationship in health psychology is the determination that cigarette smoking causes a number of diseases, including cardiovascular disease and lung cancer.

Two important tools—theories and psychometric instruments—help psychologists conduct research in many fields, including health. Theories generate research, give meaning to research data, and help the practitioner solve a variety of problems. Psychometric instruments, to be useful, must be both reliable and valid. *Reliability* is the extent to which an assessment device measures consistently, and *validity* is the extent to which an assessment instrument measures what it is supposed to measure.

SUGGESTED READINGS

Beaglehole, R., Bonita, R., & Kjellström, T. (1993). *Basic epidemiology.* Geneva, Switzerland: World Health Organization. An introduction to basic epidemiological methods, including types of studies, definitions, and an insightful discussion of the necessary and sufficient conditions for establishing causes of a disease.

Evans, F. J. (1985). Expectancy, therapeutic instructions, and the placebo response. In L. White, B. Tursky, & G. E. Schwartz (Eds.), *Placebo: Theory, research, and mechanisms* (pp. 215–228). New York: Guilford Press.

Evans provides an interesting discussion of placebos, especially their influence on the experience of pain.

Susser, M. (1991). What is a cause and how do we know one? A grammar for pragmatic epidemiology. *American Journal of Epidemiology, 133,* 635–648. Since the 1950s, epidemiologists have developed ways of showing causality in nonexperimental designs, and in this practical article, Susser presents criteria for making these causal inferences.

2 Behavior and Illness

3

Defining and Measuring Stress

Three years ago, Rick's life was so filled with stress that he did not see how he was going to manage. When he was 28 years old, he separated and then divorced his wife and was involved in a bitter custody battle over his daughter. Both his father and a close friend died within weeks of each other. He lost his job and had to work at two and sometimes three jobs to meet his financial commitments.

His work was also a source of stress. Rick was in law enforcement, and his patrol duties and dealings with prisoners were sometimes dangerous and often difficult experiences. He also worked in a large discount store part time, and the constant activity and many demands of that work situation were quite difficult. Rick did not feel that he could cut back on the jobs because he needed the money.

His divorce and the death of his father and friend changed Rick's social life. According to Rick, his so-

cial network "fell apart," leaving him more isolated than he had ever been. In addition, he felt a great deal of animosity toward his ex-wife and her family. In the custody battle, his ex-wife and her family tried to alienate Rick from his daughter and keep him from seeing her. Rick was angry, but he felt that it was important not to lose control, so he suppressed his emotions.

No facet of Rick's life was untouched, and his health-related behaviors changed. Although he had never smoked and drank only occasionally, his diet became less healthy and he did not have time to exercise in any regular program. He experienced problems in sleeping, but a more serious development was that the headaches he had experienced for about 3 years became more severe and more frequent. Rick's headaches related to two neck injuries, but he also believes that stress played a major role in their developing into a chronic pain problem. There were times when his pain interfered with working, and Rick was tense at the prospect of getting a severe headache, a condition that he knew made the headaches more likely.

For more than a year Rick experienced incessant, overabundant stress. To cope with the pressure and social isolation, he started college and became active in his church, activities that helped Rick build a new social life and career. He still experiences the "normal" stresses of taking tests and juggling work and school, but he contrasts his life now with 3 years ago and admits that the difference is enormous.

This chapter looks at what stress is and how it can be measured. Chapter 4 examines the question of whether stress, like Rick's, can cause illness or premature death. But first, this chapter discusses the physiology of the peripheral nervous system and the neuroendocrine system to help you understand the biological bases of stress.

THE NERVOUS SYSTEM AND THE PHYSIOLOGY OF STRESS

The basic function of the nervous system is to integrate all the body's systems. Small, simple organisms do not need (nor do they have) nervous systems. In larger and more complex organisms, nervous systems provide internal communication and relay information to and from the environment.

The human nervous system contains billions of individual cells called **neurons.** The action of neurons is electrochemical. Within each neuron, electrically charged ions hold the potential for an electrical discharge. This discharge, a minute electrical current, travels the length of the neuron. The electrical charge leads to the release of chemicals called **neurotransmitters** that are manufactured within each neuron and stored at the ends of the neurons. The released neurotransmitters diffuse across the **synaptic cleft,** the space between neurons.

A number of different neurotransmitters have been identified; many more remain unidentified. Of those that are understood, the chemical action is quite complex. Some neurotransmitters produce an excitatory action, which promotes the development of the neurons' electrical potential. Other neurotransmitters inhibit transmission, making neurons more difficult to activate. When a neuron is stimulated and releases its transmitter chemical, the excitatory and inhibitory messages have a cumulative effect. The next neuron's threshold must be exceeded for it to be activated. If the threshold is reached, then the next neuron "fires." If the threshold is not reached, then the next neuron will not be activated.

Neurons do not form an end-to-end chain; rather, they are more like a net, with each neuron having as many as several hundred synaptic connections. One neuron may form multiple connections with another neuron and, in addition, it may synapse with several other neurons. With the many avenues for communication among neurons, excitatory and inhibitory effects, and billions of neurons in each person's nervous system, great complexity in neural transmission is assured.

The billions of neurons fall into three types. **Afferent neurons** (sensory neurons) relay information from the sense organs toward the brain. The action of **efferent neurons** (motor neurons) results in movement of muscles or stimulation of organs or glands. **Interneurons** connect sensory neurons to motor neurons.

The nervous system is organized hierarchically, with major divisions and subdivisions. The two major divisions of the nervous system are the **central nervous system (CNS)** and the **peripheral nervous system (PNS).** The CNS is composed of the brain and the spinal cord, and the PNS consists of all other neurons. The divisions and subdivisions of the nervous system are illustrated in Figure 3.1.

The next section describes the nervous system from the bottom of its organizational hierarchy to the top—that is, beginning with the PNS and ending with the brain. This approach traces the path of information from the periphery of the nervous system to the brain.

THE PERIPHERAL NERVOUS SYSTEM

The peripheral nervous system, that part of the nervous system lying outside the brain and spinal cord, is divided into two parts: the **somatic nervous system** and the **autonomic nervous system (ANS).** The somatic nervous system has both sensory and motor components, primarily serving the skin and the voluntary muscles. The autonomic nervous system primarily serves internal organs.

The Somatic Nervous System

The somatic division of the peripheral nervous system serves muscles and skin. Sensory impulses begin with stimulation of the skin and muscles, and these neural impulses travel toward the spinal cord by way of sensory nerves in the somatic nervous system. Motor messages that originate in the brain travel down the spinal cord, are relayed to muscles, and initiate muscle movement. The motor nerves that activate those muscles are part of the somatic nervous system.

Sensory and motor impulses in the head and neck region do not travel through the spinal cord. Instead, 12 pairs of cranial nerves enter and exit directly from the lower part of the brain. The cranial nerves are also part of the somatic nervous system. They function like the sensory and motor neurons that run through the spinal cord.

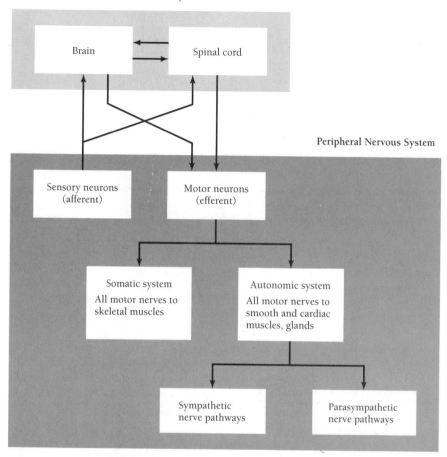

Figure 3.1 *Divisions of the human nervous system.* SOURCE: Based on *Biological Psychology* (2nd ed.) by J. W. Kalat, 1984, Belmont, CA: Wadsworth. Copyright 1984 by Wadsworth Publishing Company. Reprinted by permission of Brooks/Cole Publishing Company.

The Autonomic Nervous System

The term *autonomic* means "self-governing." It has been applied to this division of the peripheral nervous system because, traditionally, the autonomic nervous system has been considered outside the realm of conscious or voluntary control. Although the functions of the ANS do not require conscious thought, we now know it is possible for people to learn to exert conscious control over many ANS functions. Neal Miller's (1969) famous experiments with biofeedback demonstrated that rats could learn to accelerate or decelerate their heart rate, a function under autonomic control. Many types of biofeedback have been developed, and several have clinical appli-

cations in health psychology (as Chapter 6 explains). Learning to control autonomic functions requires both effort and training, but some control of the ANS is within the realm of human capability.

The ANS allows for a variety of responses through its two divisions: the **sympathetic nervous system** and the **parasympathetic nervous system**. These two subdivisions differ anatomically as well as functionally. They, along with their target organs, are shown in Figure 3.2.

The sympathetic division of the ANS mobilizes the body's resources in emergency, stressful, and emotional situations. Walter Cannon (1932) termed this configuration of responses the "fight or flight"

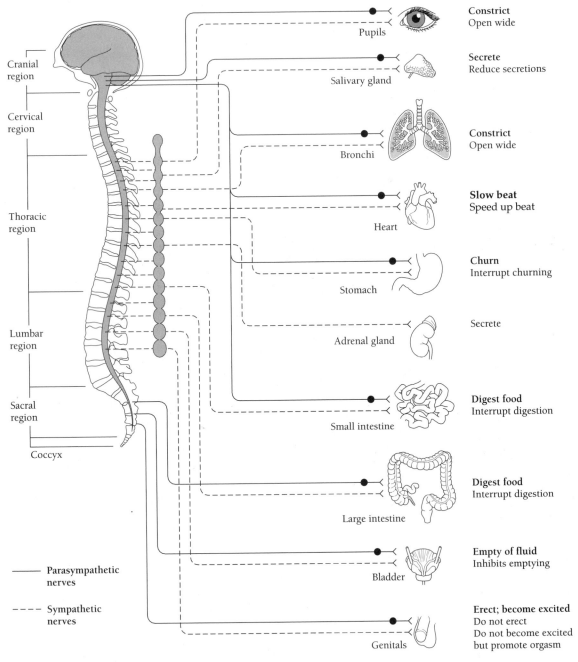

Figure 3.2 Autonomic nervous system and target organs. SOURCE: From *Biological Psychology* (2nd ed., p. 18) by J. W. Kalat, 1984, Belmont, CA: Wadsworth Publishing Company. Reprinted by permission of Brooks/Cole Publishing Company.

reaction. Sympathetic activation prepares the body for intense motor activity, the sort necessary for attack, defense, or escape. The reactions include an increase in the rate and strength of cardiac contraction, constriction of blood vessels in the skin, a decrease of gastrointestinal activity, an increase in respiration, stimulation of the sweat glands, and dilation of the pupils in the eyes.

The parasympathetic division of the ANS, on the other hand, promotes relaxation and functions under normal, nonstressful conditions. The parasympathetic and sympathetic nervous systems serve the same target organs, but they tend to function reciprocally, with the activation of one increasing as the other decreases. For example, the activation of the sympathetic division reduces the secretion of saliva, producing the sensation of a dry mouth, whereas activation of the parasympathetic division promotes secretion of saliva.

As in other parts of the nervous system, neurons in the ANS are activated by neurotransmitters. Neurotransmission in the ANS is conducted mainly by two chemicals, **acetylcholine** and **norepinephrine**, which have complex effects. Each of these neurotransmitters has different effects in different organ systems because the organs contain different neurochemical receptors. In addition, the balance of these two main neurotransmitters, as well as their absolute quantity, is important. Therefore, even though there are only two major ANS neurotransmitters, they produce a wide variety of responses.

At its optimum, the autonomic nervous system adapts smoothly, rapidly mobilizing resources by sympathetic activation and adjusting to normal demands by parasympathetic activation.

THE NEUROENDOCRINE SYSTEM

The **endocrine system** consists of ductless glands distributed throughout the body (see Figure 3.3). The **neuroendocrine system** consists of those endocrine glands that are controlled by the nervous system. Glands of the endocrine and neuroendocrine systems secrete chemicals known as **hormones**, which move into the bloodstream to be carried to different parts of the body. Specialized receptors on target tissues or organs allow hormones to have specific effects, even though the hormones circulate throughout the body. At the target, hormones may have a direct effect, or they may cause the secretion of another hormone.

The endocrine and nervous systems can work closely together because they have several similarities, but they also differ in important ways. Both systems share, synthesize, and release chemicals. In the nervous system these chemicals are called *neurotransmitters*. In the endocrine system they are called *hormones*. The activation of neurons is usually rapid and the effect is short term; the endocrine system responds more slowly, and its action persists longer. In the nervous system, neurotransmitters are released by stimulation of neural impulses, flow across the synaptic cleft, and are immediately either reabsorbed or inactivated. In the endocrine system, hormones are synthesized by the endocrine cells, are released into the blood, reach their targets in minutes or even hours, and have prolonged effects. The endocrine and nervous systems both have communication and control functions, and both work toward integrated, adaptive behaviors. The two systems are related in function and interact in neuroendocrine responses.

The Pituitary Gland

Located within the brain, the **pituitary gland** is an excellent example of the intricate relationship between the nervous and endocrine systems. The pituitary is connected to the hypothalamus, a structure in the forebrain. These two structures work together to regulate and produce hormones. The pituitary has been referred to as the "master gland" because it produces a number of hormones that affect other glands and prompts the production of other hormones.

Of the seven hormones produced by the anterior portion of the pituitary gland, **adrenocorticotropic hormone (ACTH)** plays an essential role in the stress response. When stimulated by the hypothalamus, the pituitary releases ACTH, which in turn acts on the **adrenal glands**.

The Adrenal Glands

The adrenal glands are endocrine glands located on top of each kidney. Each gland is composed of an outer covering, the **adrenal cortex**, and an inner part, the **adrenal medulla**. Both secrete hormones that are important in the response to stress. ACTH from the pituitary stimulates the adrenal cortex to release **glucocorticoids**, one type of hormone. **Cortisol** is the most important of these hormones and is so closely associated with stress that the level of cortisol circulating in the blood is used as an index of stress.

The adrenal medulla is activated by the sympathetic nervous system and secretes **catecholamines**, a class of chemicals containing **epinephrine** and norepinephrine. Epinephrine (sometimes referred to as adrenaline) is produced exclusively by the adrenal medulla and accounts for about 80% of the hormone

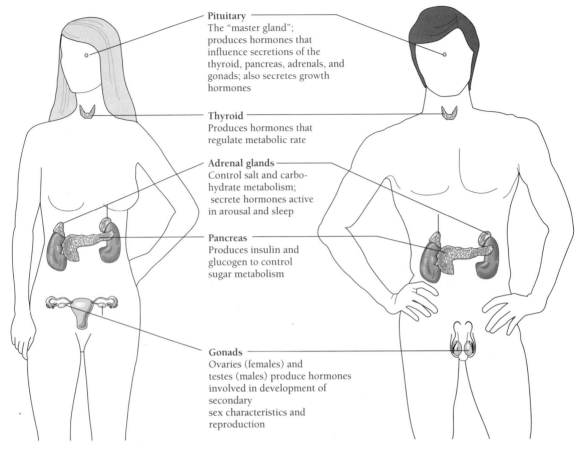

Figure 3.3 *Some important endocrine glands.*

production of the adrenal glands. Norepinephrine is also a neurotransmitter and is produced in many places in the body besides the adrenal medulla. Both of these hormones act slower than other neurotransmitters and their action is more prolonged.

PHYSIOLOGY OF THE STRESS RESPONSE

The sympathetic division of the autonomic nervous system controls mobilization of the body's resources in emotional, stressful, and emergency situations. Through the effects of various hormones, stress initiates a complex series of events within the neuroendocrine system. The anterior pituitary (the part of the pituitary gland at the base of the brain) secretes adrenocorticotropic hormone (ACTH), which stimulates the adrenal glands to secrete glucocorticoids, including cortisol. Its secretion mobilizes the body's

energy resources, raising the level of blood sugar to provide energy for the cells. Cortisol also has an anti-inflammatory effect, giving the body a natural defense against swelling from injuries that might be sustained during a fight or a flight.

Activation of the adrenal medulla results in the secretion of catecholamines, the class of chemicals that includes norepinephrine and epinephrine. Norepinephrine, however, is also one of the neurotransmitters of the autonomic nervous system. Neurotransmitters work at the synapse whereas hormones circulate through the blood. Norepinephrine has both actions and is produced at many places in the body, not exclusively in the adrenal medulla.

Epinephrine, on the other hand, is produced exclusively in the adrenal medulla. It is so closely and uniquely associated with stress that it is sometimes used as an index of stress. The amount of epinephrine

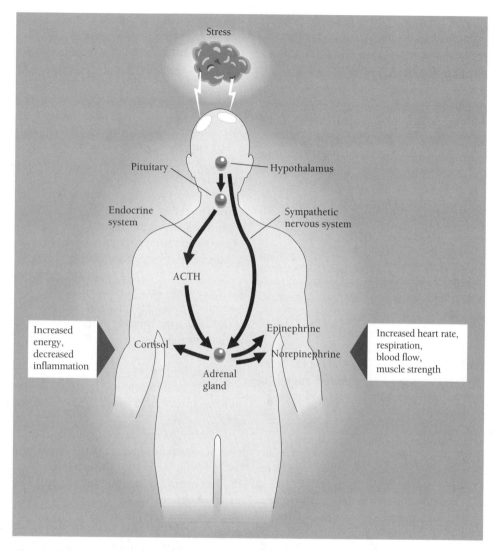

Figure 3.4 *Physiological effects of stress.*

secreted can be determined by assaying a person's urine, thus measuring stress by tapping into the physiology of the stress response. Such an index can be helpful because it does not rely on personal perceptions of stress and its use as a measure of stress can give an alternative perspective.

SUMMARY OF THE PHYSIOLOGY OF STRESS

The physiology of the stress response is extremely complex, and Figure 3.4 illustrates these nervous and endocrine responses. When a person perceives

stress, the sympathetic division of the autonomic nervous system rouses the person from a resting state by way of stimulating the adrenal medulla, which produces catecholamines. The pituitary releases ACTH, which in turn affects the adrenal cortex. Glucocorticoid release prepares the body to resist the stress and even to cope with injury by the release of cortisol. The ANS activation is rapid, as is all neural transmission, whereas the action of the neuroendocrine system is slower. Together the two systems form the physiological basis for the stress response as well as the potential for illness.

An understanding of the physiology of stress does not completely clarify the meaning of stress. Thus several models have been constructed in an attempt to better define and explain stress.

THEORIES OF STRESS

Despite a great deal of scientific research on the subject and the widespread use of the term in everyday conversation, *stress* has not been precisely defined. When some people talk about *stress,* they are referring to an environmental *stimulus,* as in "I have a high-stress job." Others consider stress a *response* to environmental stimuli, as in "I feel a lot of stress whenever I have to make important decisions at work." Still others consider the *interaction* between the environmental stimuli and the response to be the defining characteristic of stress.

The view of stress as an external event was the first approach taken by stress researchers, the most prominent of whom was Hans Selye. The most influential view has been the interactionist approach, proposed by Richard Lazarus.

SELYE'S VIEW

Beginning in the 1930s and continuing until his death in 1982, Hans Selye (1956, 1976, 1982) researched and popularized the concept of stress, making a strong case for its relationship to physical illness and bringing the importance of stress to the attention of the public. Although he did not originate the concept of stress, he researched the effects of stress on physiological responses and tried to connect these reactions to the development of illness.

Over the course of his career, Selye first considered stress to be a stimulus and later saw it as a response. His original position was that stress was a stimulus, but in the 1950s, he started to use the term *stress* to refer to a response that the organism makes. To distinguish the two, Selye started using the terms *stressor* to refer to the stimulus and *stress* to mean the response.

Selye's contributions to stress research included a concept of stress and a model for how the body defends itself in stressful situations. Selye conceptualized stress as a nonspecific response, repeatedly insisting that stress is a general physical response caused by any of a number of environmental stressors. He believed that a wide variety of different situations could prompt the stress response, but that response would always be the same.

The General Adaptation Syndrome

The body's generalized attempt to defend itself against noxious agents became known as the **general adaptation syndrome (GAS)**. This syndrome is divided into three stages, the first of which is the **alarm reaction**. During alarm, the body's defenses against a stressor are mobilized through activation of the sympathetic nervous system. This division activates body systems to maximize strength and prepares them for the "fight or flight" response. Adrenaline (epinephrine) is released, heart rate and blood pressure increase, respiration becomes faster, blood is diverted away from the internal organs toward the skeletal muscles, sweat glands are activated, and the gastrointestinal system decreases its activity. As a short-term response to an emergency situation, these physical reactions are adaptive, but many modern stress situations involve prolonged exposure to stress.

Selye called the second phase of the GAS the **resistance stage**. In this stage the organism adapts to the stressor. How long this stage lasts depends on the severity of the stressor and the adaptive capacity of the organism. If the organism can adapt, the resistance stage will continue for a long time. During this stage, the person gives the outward appearance of normality, as Rick did following his father's death and during his divorce, but physiologically the body's internal functioning is not normal. Continuing stress will cause continued neurological and hormonal changes. Selye believed that these demands take a toll, setting the stage for what he described as *diseases of adaptation,* those diseases related to continued, persistent stress.

Among the diseases Selye considered to be the result of prolonged resistance to stress are peptic ulcers and ulcerative colitis, hypertension and cardiovascular disease, hyperthyroidism, and bronchial asthma. In addition, Selye hypothesized that resistance to stress would cause changes in the immune system, making infection more likely.

The capacity to resist stress is finite, and the final stage of the GAS is the **exhaustion stage**. At the end, the organism's ability to resist is depleted, and a breakdown results. This stage is characterized by activation of the parasympathetic division of the autonomic nervous system. Under normal circumstances, parasympathetic activation keeps the body functioning in a balanced state. In the exhaustion stage, however, functioning is at an abnormally low level to compensate for the abnormally high level of sympathetic activation that has preceded it. According to Selye, exhaustion frequently results in depression and sometimes even death.

Evaluation of Selye's View

Selye concentrated on the physical aspects of stress and largely ignored psychological factors, including the emotional component and the individual interpretation of stressful events. John Mason (1971, 1975) criticized Selye for ignoring the element of emotion in stress and hypothesized that the consistency in the stress response is due to this underlying element of emotion.

Selye's emphasis on the physiology of stress resulted in his experimentation using nonhuman animals, and he downplayed the differences between humans and other animals. Thus, he neglected the factors unique to humans, such as perception and interpretation of stressful experiences. Although Selye's view has had a great influence on the popular conception of stress, an alternative model formulated by psychologist Richard Lazarus has had a greater impact among psychologists.

LAZARUS'S VIEW

In Lazarus's view, the interpretation of stressful events is more important than the events themselves. It is neither the environmental event nor the person's response that defines stress, but rather the individual's *perception* of the psychological situation. This perception includes potential harms, threats, and challenges as well as the individual's perceived ability to cope with them.

Psychological Factors

Lazarus's emphasis on interpretation and perception differs from that of Selye. Also, Lazarus has worked largely with humans rather than nonhuman ani-

mals. The ability of people to think about and evaluate future events makes them vulnerable in ways that other animals are not. Humans encounter stresses because they have higher-level cognitive abilities that other animals lack.

According to Lazarus (1984a, 1993), the effect that stress has on a person is based more on that person's feelings of threat, vulnerability, and ability to cope than on the stressful event itself. For example, losing a job may be extremely stressful for someone who has no money saved or no confidence in finding another job. But to a person who has either another source of income or confidence in finding a new job, loss of a job may be only mildly stressful. In Lazarus's view, a life event is not what produces stress; rather, it is one's view of the situation that causes an event to become stressful. Rick's loss of his job was especially stressful because he was involved in a divorce and needed extra money. He appraised this life event (job loss) as threatening to his career and financial position.

Lazarus and Susan Folkman defined psychological stress as *"a particular relationship between the person and the environment that is appraised by the person as taxing or exceeding his or her resources and endangering his or her well-being"* (1984, p. 19). You should note several important points in this definition. First, Lazarus and Folkman take a *transactional* position, holding that stress refers to a relationship between person and environment. Second, they believe that the key to that transaction is the person's appraisal of the psychological situation. Third, they believe the situation must be seen as threatening, challenging, or harmful.

Appraisal

Lazarus and Folkman (1984) recognized that people use three kinds of appraisal to assess situations: primary appraisal, secondary appraisal, and reappraisal. **Primary appraisal** is not necessarily first in importance, but it is first in time. A person who first encounters an event, such as an offer of a job promotion, appraises it in terms of its effect on his or her well-being. An event may be viewed as irrelevant, benign-positive, or stressful. It is unlikely that an offer of a job promotion would be seen as irrelevant, but many environmental events, such as a snowstorm in another state, have no implications for a person's well-being. A benign-positive appraisal means that the event is seen as having good implications. A stressful appraisal can mean that the event is seen as harmful, threatening, or challenging. Each of these three—harm, threat, and challenge—is likely to generate an emotion. Lazarus (1993) defined *harm* as the psychological damage that has already been done, such as an illness or injury; *threat* as the anticipation of harm; and *challenge* as a person's confidence in overcoming difficult demands. An appraisal of harm may produce anger, disgust, disappointment, or sadness; an appraisal of threat is likely to generate worry, anxiety, or fear; an appraisal of challenge may be followed by excitement or anticipation. It is important to remember that these emotions do not produce stress; instead, they are generated by the individual's appraisal of an event.

After a person's initial appraisal of an event, that person forms an impression of his or her ability to control or cope with harm, threat, or challenge, an impression called **secondary appraisal.** A person asks three questions in making secondary appraisals. The first is "What options are available to me?" The second is "What is the likelihood that I can successfully apply the necessary strategies to reduce this stress?" As an example, let's look at Jill, who has just lost her job. Her secondary appraisal would begin with an assessment of her ability to make a favorable impression that would lead to a job offer.

The third question a person asks is "Will this procedure work? That is, will it alleviate my stress?" Even if Jill believes that she makes a sufficiently good impression to get a job offer, she may not believe that a favorable impression will lead to another job. When people believe they can do something that will make a difference—when they believe they can successfully cope with a situation—stress is reduced.

The third type of appraisal is **reappraisal.** Appraisals change constantly as new information becomes available. Jill may recall some advice on writing an attractive letter of application or relaxing during a job interview and gain more confidence in her ability to cope, thereby reducing her stress. Or reappraisal may follow from an environmental source, as when Jill reads a newspaper article about the strong demand for employees with her training

and experience. This new information may allow Jill to reappraise her employment situation and turn her previously stressful appraisal into a benign-positive one.

Reappraisal does not always result in less stress; sometimes it increases stress. A situation previously assessed as benign or irrelevant can take on a threatening, harmful, or challenging aspect if the environment changes or the person begins to see the situation differently. For example, a husband who has been satisfied with his marriage for years may begin seeing his relationship with his wife as stressful when his wife begins college course work.

Vulnerability

Stress is most likely to be aroused when a person is vulnerable, when he or she lacks resources in a situation of some personal importance. These resources may be either physical or social, but their importance is determined by psychological factors, such as perception and evaluation of the situation. An arthritic knee, for example, would produce physical vulnerability in a professional athlete but would be a minor inconvenience to the professional life of someone who works behind a desk.

Lazarus and Folkman (1984) insisted that physical or social deficits alone are not sufficient to produce vulnerability. What matters is whether one considers the situation personally important. Vulnerability differs from threat in that it represents only the *potential* for threat. Threat exists when one perceives that his or her self-esteem is in jeopardy; vulnerability exists when the lack of resources creates a potentially threatening or harmful situation.

Coping

An important ingredient in Lazarus's theory of stress is the ability or inability to cope with a stressful situation. Lazarus and Folkman defined coping as "*constantly changing cognitive and behavioral efforts to manage specific external and/or internal demands that are appraised as taxing or exceeding the resources of the person*" (1984, p. 141). This definition spells out several important features of coping. First, coping is a process, constantly changing as one's efforts are evaluated as more or less successful. Second, coping is not automatic; it is a learned pattern of responding to stressful situations. A response that is automatic (such as closing one's eyes to block out intense light) or that becomes automatic through experience (such as shifting one's weight while riding a bicycle) would not be considered coping. Third, coping requires effort. A person need not be completely aware of his or her coping response, and the outcome may or may not be successful, but effort must have been expended. Fourth, coping is an effort to *manage* the situation; control and mastery are not necessary. For example, most of us make an effort to manage our physical environment by striving for a comfortable air temperature. Thus we cope with our environment even though complete mastery of the climate is impossible.

How well people are able to cope depends on several factors. Lazarus and Folkman (1984) listed *health and energy* as one important coping resource. Healthy, robust individuals are better able to manage external and internal demands than are frail, sick, tired people. A second resource is a *positive belief*— the ability to cope with stress is enhanced when people believe they can successfully bring about desired consequences. This ability is related to the third resource: *problem-solving skills*. Knowledge of anatomy and physiology, for example, can be an important source of coping when a person is receiving information about her or his own health from a physician who is speaking in technical terms. A fourth coping resource is *social skills*. Confidence in one's ability to get other people to cooperate can be an important source of stress management. Closely allied to this resource is *social support*, or the feeling of being accepted, loved, or prized by others. (Chapter 4 shows the importance of social support in reducing the chances of developing a physical or psychological disorder following periods of intense stress, and Chapter 6 presents information on the importance of social support in coping.) Finally, Lazarus and Folkman list *material resources* as an important means of coping. Having the money to get one's car repaired decreases the stress of having a transmission problem.

In Lazarus's transactional view, of course, material and social resources by themselves are not so important as one's personal belief about these resources. Perceiving that you can manage or alter a stressful environmental situation and feeling confident that you can regulate your own emotional distress are the two main ways to cope with stress. The ways people cope with stressful life events, including daily annoyances, play a leading role in stress-related illnesses.

In summary, Lazarus holds a cognitively oriented, transactional view of stress and coping. Stressful encounters are dynamic and complex, constantly changing and unfolding, so that the outcomes of one stressful event alter the subsequent appraisal of new events. Individual differences in coping strategies and in the appraisal of stressful events are crucial to a person's experience of stress; therefore, the likelihood of developing any stress-related disorder also varies with individuals. The relationship between stressful events and subsequent health is complex, according to Lazarus, and any attempt to measure stress and a person's attempts to cope with it must also be complex.

SOURCES OF STRESS

Different theoretical views propose different sources and severity of stress. In each theory, however, both environmental and personal sources contribute to stress. And both sources of stress have been linked to health.

ENVIRONMENT

Many people associate environmental sources of stress with urban life. They think of noise, pollution, crowding, fear of crime, and personal alienation as being associated with city living. However, adverse environmental factors are not limited to large metropolitan communities, although they are frequently more concentrated there. Rural life can also be noisy, polluted, hot, cold, humid, or even crowded, with many people living in a one- or two-room dwelling. The noise from farm machinery is often louder than any experienced by urban dwellers. And although air and water pollution usually originate in urban or industrial settings, they may then disperse to other parts of the world.

Therefore, environmental sources of stress are not limited to urban settings, but the crowding, noise, pollution, fear of crime, and personal alienation combine to produce an urban environment that is stressful to many city dwellers. Not only can each source of stress be considered separately, but the combination of these stressors occurs in a natural context.

Crowding

Experiments with animals have revealed a variety of adverse effects from high-density living conditions, but research on human health is not as clear. Calhoun (1956, 1962, 1971) reported on a series of studies involving the effects of high population density in rats. Calhoun conducted a number of experiments to determine the effects of crowding on behavior. In one study, Calhoun provided ideal living conditions to a group of rats to see how quickly they would become overcrowded. He found that, despite rats' ability to multiply quickly, their total population did not reach "standing room only" levels. He did find, however, that their behavior changed with the population density. When the number of rats was few, their behavior was normal, with the rats forming social groups and mating.

When the population reached a certain level, however, things began to change. Fighting increased, and social strata emerged, with the two dominate male rats staking out their own "private" pens and maintaining a low population density within these pens. The remainder of the population was concentrated in the two pens not claimed by the dominant male rats. But even in these somewhat crowded pens, the population did not skyrocket because infant mortality increased sharply, female rats became less sexually receptive, some male rats became cannibalistic, and some male rats became sexually "deviant," attempting to mate with other male rats or with female rats not in estrus. As a result, the total adult population tended to remain about the same after an initial period of rapid increase.

These studies demonstrate that physical, emotional, and social health is disrupted by high-density living conditions and that crowding in rats is stressful in a variety of ways. But what about crowding among humans? Do high-density populations produce equally deleterious effects in humans?

Answering these questions requires a distinction between the concepts of *population density* and *crowding*. In 1972, Daniel Stokols defined **population density** as a *physical* condition in which a large population occupies a limited space. **Crowding,** however, is a *psychological* condition that arises from a person's perception of the high-density environment in which that person is confined. Thus, density is necessary for crowding but does not automatically produce the feeling of being crowded. The crush of people in the lobby of a theater during intermission of a popular play may not be experienced as crowding, despite the extremely high population density. Conversely, however, a reclusive early American pioneer who migrated westward when a new resident came into his county would also not be crowded. He may have felt uncomfortable living within 10 miles of another person, but because the population was not dense, his experience would not meet Stokol's definition of being crowded. The distinction between density and crowding means that personal perceptions must be considered whenever investigators study the effects of crowding.

Unquestionably, density and crowding affect human behavior, but the effect on health is less clear. A review of laboratory and field studies on crowding (Sundstrom, 1978) showed that density and crowding were associated with increased aggression, lowered performance on complex tasks, greater withdrawal from interpersonal relations, increased crime rates, and a number of other negative factors.

If crowding is defined as one's view of high-density living conditions, people's perception of being crowded is related to their feelings of stress. Evans, Palsane, Lepore, and Martin (1989) studied residential density and its effects on the psychological health of male heads of household living in crowded conditions in India. They found that density led to excessive, unwanted social interactions and insufficient privacy—conditions that in turn led to social withdrawal as a means of coping. The researchers hypothesized that social withdrawal could lead to a breakdown in socially supportive relationships and that this breakdown could account for some of the negative consequences of chronic high-density living conditions. The combination of insufficient privacy, unwanted social contacts, and crowded living conditions seemed to produce more stress and social withdrawal than could be accounted for by crowding alone.

One study that weighs directly on the issue of health and crowding was conducted within a prison environment. Paulus, McCain, and Cox (1978) believed that prison inmates might find crowding particularly unpleasant because they have no control over the type and duration of their housing. In one phase of this study, the researchers examined the mortality rates in a prison psychiatric unit over a 16-year period during times of high- and low-density living conditions. Figure 3.5 shows nearly identical curves for the average yearly population and the death rate of inmates. As population rose, so did rate of mortality, and as conditions became less crowded, the death rate dropped correspondingly.

In summary, the relationship between high-density human population and stress seems to be positive. When the psychological factor of crowding is considered, the influence is even stronger. In addition, the factor of lack of personal control (Altman, 1978; Epstein, 1982; Rodin & Baum, 1978) may interact with high population density to produce a number of negative consequences, including illness and death.

Pollution

Pollution is a second environmental condition that may produce stress, but pollution exerts health effects directly as well as through increased stress. Although pollution of the environment has become an important concern, it is not a recent phenomenon. Both air and water pollution predate history (Eckholm, 1977). Modern technology has given us more pollutants and speeded their dispersion, but it did not originate the practice of adding harmful substances to the air, water, and soil.

Modern technology has increased not only the amount of pollution but also the potential for accidents in the storing or handling of dangerous nuclear or chemical pollutants. An accident with toxic chemicals could create extreme feelings of helplessness because such accidents are beyond the control of many of the affected people. Indeed, these accidents may occur quite randomly, as in a train derailment or a tank-car accident, and thus quite unpredictably. Furthermore, the fear of accidents may pervade the entire neighborhood surrounding industries where dangerous chemicals are used or manufactured, providing long-lasting stress for the residents (Baum, Gatchel, & Schaeffer, 1983).

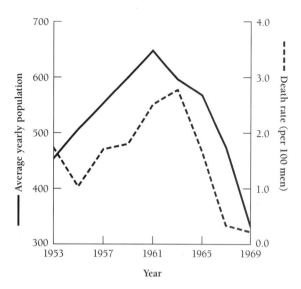

Figure 3.5 *Total population and death rates per 100 men for a psychiatric prison.*
SOURCE: Adapted from "Death Rates, Psychiatric Commitments, Blood Pressure and Perceived Crowding as a Function of Institutional Crowding," by P. B. Paulus, G. McCain, & V. C. Cox, 1978, *Environmental Psychology and Nonverbal Behavior, 3,* p. 110. © 1978 by Human Science Press.

Studies on the psychological effects of pollution have implications for stress and health, and several of these studies deal with feelings of personal control and perceived severity of the pollution. According to an early study (Rankin, 1969), people who are concerned about air pollution in their community frequently do not complain because they believe their protests will do no good; that is, they feel helpless. Another study (Rotton, Yoshikawa, & Kaplan, 1979) investigated the effect of control over air quality on tolerance for frustration and found that the perception of control is more crucial than the level of pollution in making the experience stressful.

Long-term Los Angeles residents tested on their attitudes, behaviors, and biochemical response in connection with air pollution were less sensitive to pollution than people who had recently moved to Los Angeles, both in their perception of it and in their biochemical response to it. In addition, long-time residents tended to take less active measures to cope with unpleasant air pollution, demonstrating that those who live in polluted cities may become both psychologically and physiologically adapted to their polluted environment. Therefore, pollution is a source of stress, but its health effects are mostly direct results of their toxic effects rather than indirect effects through increasing stress levels.

Noise

In addition to crowding and pollution, exposure to noise may produce stress. Noise is considered a type of pollution because it is a noxious, unwanted stimulus that intrudes into a person's environment. Evidence also shows a relationship between noise and health problems, but again, the health effects of noise might be direct influences of noise rather than indirect effects produced by increased stress. In addition, noise is quite difficult to define in any objective way. Definitions are invariably subjective because noise is a sound that a person does not want to hear. Noise can be loud, soft, or somewhere between. One person's music is another person's noise.

The importance of subjective attitude toward noise was illustrated by Nivision and Endresen (1993), who asked residents living beside a busy street about their health, sleep, anxiety level, and attitude toward noise. These researchers found no relationship between objective noise levels and either health or sleep. However, they found a strong association between residents' subjective view of noise and the number of their health complaints.

Defined by the objective criterion of volume, noise can produce detrimental health effects. For example, Cohen, Glass, and Phillips (1977) found that workers exposed to high levels of noise tended to report more nausea, headaches, impotence, argumentativeness, and moodiness. In a naturalistic study of residents in the Los Angeles airport area, researchers found that children living in a high-noise area had significantly higher blood pressure than those living in a lower-noise area (Cohen, Krantz, Evans, & Stokols, 1982). In addition, children living in the high-noise area performed less well academically in school, were more easily distracted, had a lower frustration tolerance, and tended to give up in their attempts to solve difficult puzzles.

Potential for control also seems to be a factor in perception of stress from noise. A laboratory study by Glass and Singer (1972) allowed one group of participants the possibility of controlling a loud, distracting noise but offered no such possibility to another group. The results indicated that personal control was an important factor in appraising the stressful effects of noise. The performance of the group exposed to uncontrollable noise was worse than those not given the option of control, even though these participants never exercised their control. Therefore, the possibility of control seemed to act as a buffer against the problems created by noise.

Urban Press

Crowding, pollution, and noise can occur in any social context, but these factors are a commonplace combination in the urban environment. Eric Graig (1993) used the term *urban press* to refer to the many sources of environmental stressors that affect city living. Commuting hassles and fear of crime add to the urban dwellers' experience with crowding, pollution, and noise. Graig pointed out that the laboratory studies on crowding, noise, and pollution fall far short of capturing the experience of actually living with these stressors.

Graig also noted that not only are all these sources of stress combined in city life but that they tend to be beyond personal control. For example, traffic noise is not something that commuters or residents can control. Laboratory studies on noise and pollution indicate that lack of control tends to make people feel stressed, and this principle may apply to these factors in the urban environment.

Crime is not unique to urban life, but fear of crime has become part of the urban environment (Riger, 1985), and these fears can affect behavior, such as installing locks on the doors and bars on the windows and avoiding locations perceived as high-crime areas. Crime victimization is unlikely for any individual (see box Would You Believe . . . ?), but the fear of crime is much more common.

One factor in that perception is the newspaper coverage given to crime. Williams and Dickinson (1993) studied the relationship between the fear of crime and the amount of space and prominence given to newspaper reports of crime. The researchers found that independent of demographic factors such as income and age, there was a significant positive correlation between people's fear of crime and the media's reporting of crime information. Other re-

WOULD YOU BELIEVE . . . ?

Declining Murder Rate

Would you believe that the murder rate in the United States is now lower than it was 60 years ago? During the mid-1990s, former U. S. Surgeon General Joycelyn Elders named gun violence as the leading public health issue of our time. Her words have been echoed by almost daily reports from newspapers and television that feature stories on the escalating rise of murder and other crimes in the United States. Results from various opinion polls seem to show that crime is the most serious problem facing this country. How accurate are these perceptions? Just how rapidly are crime rates rising?

With regard to crime rates, popular perception diverges from reality. During the 13-year period from 1980 to 1992, the United States experienced slight increases in robbery, forcible rape, and theft. The largest increase was in forcible rape with an annual rise of about 2%, and this increase may be due mostly to a greater trend in reporting rape rather than to an actual increase in the crime. During this same period, robbery

increased 2% a year and the rate of theft rose less than 1% per year. On the other hand, reported burglaries *decreased* during this time and homicide rates remained about the same. As for Elders's concerns about gun violence, murder victims were slightly more likely to have been shot in 1992 than were murder victims in 1980, but the homicide rate was slightly higher in 1980 than in 1992 (USBC, 1995).

For some groups of people, particularly young African American men, becoming a victim of homicide is rightly considered to be a serious problem. Although only about one in eight people in the United States is African American, slightly more African Americans than Whites are murdered each year. Before the age of 10 and especially after the age of 40, murder victims are more likely to be White. However, for homicide victims from age 15 to 24, more than 60% are African Americans, even though they make up only about 12% of the population (USBC, 1995).

In spite of these data, many other people live in nearly constant fear of physical assault or murder. Are these fears justified? According to government statistics, less than one person per 10,000 will become a murder victim in any one year (USBC, 1995). Actually, homicide rates have decreased during the past 65 years. In 1930, the murder rate was 12.4 per 100,000 persons; that number had dropped to 9.3 in 1992 (USBC, 1973, 1995). In more recent years, the homicide rate has remained quite steady, especially for Whites. In addition, fewer people were touched by crime in 1992 than in 1990 (USBC, 1995).

Although crime, like any health problem, is a serious concern for those people directly affected, recent government figures suggest that the United States is not experiencing a rapid rise in murder, rape, robbery, burglary, or theft. Would you believe that the constant clamoring of politicians and the media over the escalating trends in crime does not reflect reality?

searchers (Liska & Baccaglini, 1990) found more complex relationships between newspaper reports and people's fear of crime, but these researchers found that the information in official crime statistics was mediated through newspaper coverage. Such studies demonstrate the power of the press to increase or decrease the fear of crime.

When people fear victimization, their behavior changes. One change is a restriction of activities that might take them into areas considered dangerous. Forde (1993) found that people who are concerned with increasing crime avoided walking alone at night, and Bazargan (1994) found that elderly African Americans limited their mobility out of fear of crime. Although giving up walking alone at night may not seem much of a sacrifice, it reflects the feel-

ing of restriction that occurs in people's lives when they feel that they must think about their safety. When elderly people feel that they must limit how much they go out of their homes, this attitude reflects a serious national problem. Krause (1991) explored this possibility and concluded that chronic stress tends to promote distrust of others in the elderly, and distrust can contribute to isolation.

Ross (1993) researched the connection between fear of victimization and health. She surveyed over 2,000 people varying in age from 18 to 90 years and concluded that fear of crime affects both psychological and physical health. People who were afraid of being assaulted, robbed, or physically injured reported worse health than people who had no such fears. Ross suggested that restriction from outdoor activities and exercise may explain the relationship between poor health and fear of crime. Therefore, crime is not only a factor in the urban environment, but fear of crime is also a stressor that can have indirect effects on health.

OCCUPATION

Do business executives who must make many decisions every day suffer more from a high level of stress than do their employees who merely carry out those decisions? Most executives have jobs in which the demands are high but so is their level of control, and research indicates that lack of control is more stressful than the burden of decision making. Smith, Colligan, Horning, and Hurrel (1978) reported that lower-level occupations are actually more stressful than executive jobs. Using stress-related illnesses as a criterion, they found that the jobs of construction worker, secretary, laboratory technician, waiter or waitress, machine operator, farm worker, and painter are among the most stressful. These jobs all share a high level of demand combined with a low level of control. Another highly stressful job is middle-level manager, such as foreman or supervisor. Middle managers must meet demands from two directions: their bosses and their workers. Thus, they have more than their share of stress and stress-related illnesses.

Several studies have confirmed that the combination of high demands and low control produces job stress and is also related to heart disease. Vitaliano et al. (1988) found that physicians, whose jobs include a very high level of demands but also a high degree of control, suffer less from stress than medical students, who are burdened with the undesirable combination of high demands and low control. Alterman, Shekelle, Vernon, and Burau (1994) found that the more latitude men had in making decisions on the job, the lower was their death rate from coronary heart disease. In addition, workers in high demand/low decision jobs had an elevated risk of heart disease mortality and this risk was greater for white-collar workers than for blue-collar workers.

Not only is the high demand-low control combination related to coronary heart disease (Karasek et al., 1988; Krantz, Contrada, Hill, & Friedler, 1988) but social support is also a factor that can increase

or decrease risk. One study (Johnson & Hall, 1988) showed that people in jobs with high demands, low control, and low social support were at double risk for cardiovascular disease when compared to those in jobs with low demands, high control, and high support from co-workers. In a case-control study of male workers, Schnall et al. (1990) found that the combination of high demands and low opportunity to make decisions was significantly related to hypertension.

In reviewing the research on the link between job demands and control and coronary heart disease, Repetti (1993a) found strong evidence that jobs with the combination of high demand and low control constitute a risk factor for hypertension and heart disease. These conditions applied to Rick's job in law enforcement, which was filled with occasional danger but almost constant demands from superiors and those who were arrested or victimized.

The social environment at work is a second factor that contributes to stress on the job, playing a role in both physical and mental health (Repetti, 1993a). Repetti also mentioned the existence of a relationship between poor supervisor relationships and workplace stress. Further research by Repetti (1993b) showed that workers experienced more negative moods on days when they had distressing interactions with supervisors or co-workers. Therefore, negative interactions and poor relationships at work are further sources of occupational stress.

High demands and low control also combine with other workplace conditions to increase on-the-job stress. Neither noise nor danger of chemical exposure is sufficient to produce stressful work conditions (Cottington & House, 1987), but the combination of a noisy workplace and rotating shiftwork can produce a higher level of epinephrine excretion, a physiological index of stress. In addition, shiftwork can lead to a variety of physical complaints, including sleep and gastrointestinal problems, and rotating shifts can interfere with family life (Holt, 1993).

The conflict between work demands and family obligations affects both men and women, but the increase in employment for women has sparked more research on their potential sources of job stress. Contrary to what many people had assumed, women who pursue careers are not at increased risk

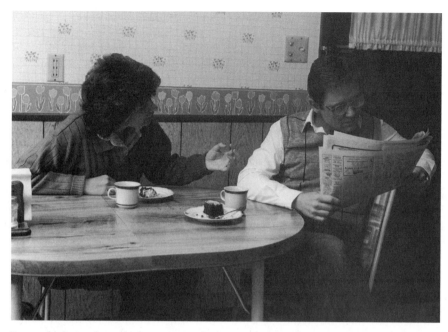

Personal relationships can be a source of stress, and physical stress reactions are related to marital instability.

for coronary heart disease (Haynes, Feinleib, & Kannel, 1980). However, factors in their careers and home life may increase their risks by increasing their stress, and women who have employment and child care obligations experience more stress than women who are not employed (Cottington & House, 1987; Haynes, 1989; Verbrugge, 1983). However, they also experience more satisfaction.

Verbrugge's (1983) study indicated that women who had young children and a job, but who were not married, had an elevated risk for poor health. In contrast, both employment and marriage were generally positive factors in health. These findings indicate that filling multiple obligations is not necessarily stressful for women, but that some combinations of roles can produce stress and poorer health.

LaCroix and Haynes (1987) reviewed the research on workplace roles and concluded that employed women are generally healthier than nonemployed women. They pointed out that women are more likely than men to occupy jobs with a combination of high demands and low control, so women may encounter more stress at work than men do. But the stress is due to the types of jobs they hold rather than the fact that they are employed.

Do women who hold executive positions benefit from the high degree of control their jobs offer? The results of one study (LaRosa, 1990) indicated that they do. The female executives in this study had excellent physical health and reported greater life satisfaction than other employed women. The health and positive attitude of these executives support the view that women's workplace stress is related more to type of job than to gender.

PERSONAL RELATIONSHIPS

Personal relationships are another potential source of stress, but they can also buffer against stress; that is, people who have fewer personal relationships are at increased health risk compared to those with more relationships (Berkman & Syme, 1979; Hobfoll & Vaux, 1993). Relationships do not automatically provide benefits. As the research on social support at work suggests, problems in personal relationships can create stress, but supportive relationships can protect against stress. These effects are not unique to the workplace but apply to other relationships as well. In Rick's case, his relationship with his wife was a major source of stress, and the loss of a supportive wife and family added to his stress.

In a survey of college students, a third of the stress events involved relationships (Ptacek, Smith, & Zanas, 1992). The frequency of this source of stress should not be surprising considering the number of potential relationships — co-workers, supervisors, friends, and romantic partners as well as family relationships that include parents, children, spouses, aunts, uncles, and cousins. For the college students in the Ptacek et al. survey, nonfamily relationships were a more frequent source of stress than family relationships, but perhaps the social circumstances of college students tend to create more nonfamily interactions and stresses.

For married or cohabiting couples, relationships within the family provide sources of stress that interact with other life circumstances. For example, the demands of employment and family life can create stress when these are in conflict (Aneshensel & Pearlin, 1987). Such stresses tend to differ for men and women, who occupy different roles and who are faced with different expectations within the family. Women often encounter stress because of the increased burden of doing the work associated with their multiple roles as employee, wife, and mother (Hochschild, 1989).

Occupying multiple roles is not necessarily stressful, but conflict and difficulties connected with fulfilling each role can result in stress. For example, husbands who do not support their wives' employment can create stress in the lives of both by failing to perform a fair share of household work and child care, leading to the perception of inequity that can escalate into conflict (Blumstein & Schwartz, 1983; Thompson & Walker, 1989). Indeed, disagreement over the inequitable distribution of household work is a point of conflict and stress for many couples, and research (Gottman, 1991) has indicated that men who do housework are healthier than those who do not.

Many men are not completely supportive of their wives' employment because employed wives gain power in the relationship. In addition, husbands may feel that they are not receiving the care they believe wives should supply (Rosenfield, 1992). This attitude can contribute to husbands' stress, which can lead to their failure to support their wives' efforts. Both wives and husbands who spend many hours devoted to their jobs and who feel a lack of support from their spouses tend to experience stress (Greenberger & O'Neil, 1993). Therefore, multiple commitments to employment and family can produce stress for both men and women, and this stress is increased by feelings of lack of support from spouses.

Gottman (1991) has found that couples whose interactions provoked the physiological responses associated with stress tended to have marriages that dissolved. Thus, stress responses were a good predictor of marital stability. "Couples whose hearts beat faster, whose blood flowed faster, who sweated more and moved more during marital interaction or even when they were just silent but anticipating marital conflict, had marriages that deteriorated in satisfaction" (Gottman, 1991, p. 4). These physiological measures were 95% accurate in predicting which couples would stay together and which would separate. Later research (Malarkey, Kiecolt-Glaser, Pearl, & Glaser, 1994) demonstrated that hostile marital interaction was associated with neuroendocrine measures of stress. These studies show that marital relationships can arouse stress responses and that stress-related physiological arousal is strongly related to relationship stability.

Blumstein and Schwartz's (1983) survey of couples shows that work, money, and sex were all potential sources of stress for married as well as cohabiting, and gay as well as heterosexual couples. Differing attitudes in any of these (or other) areas can lead to conflict, which can result in couples' failing to support each other. Lack of support increases feelings of stress and negates some of the benefits of personal relationships.

SLEEP PROBLEMS

Sleep problems can take several forms and affect a large number and wide variety of people. Some people experience **insomnia**, the inability either to fall asleep or to stay asleep, whereas others voluntarily deprive themselves of sleep to have more time to do other things. Whether voluntary or involuntary, sleep deprivation is associated with a variety of behavioral and health problems.

People who do not get sufficient sleep often feel tired, anxious, drowsy, weary, and fatigued, and the

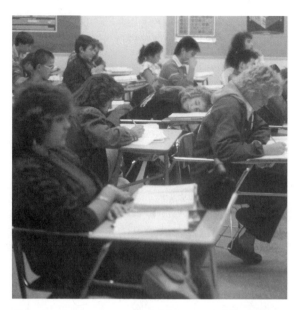

Sleep deprivation may cause adolescents to fall asleep in class and adults to work less efficiently.

quirements rather than try to make it serve our paltry demands" (cited in Goleman, 1982, p. 28). According to this view, the type of sleep deprivation that most people experience is self-imposed and self-limiting. Sleep deprivation researcher David Dinges voiced another view: "Sleep loss is pervasive and insidious. We keep shrinking the amount of time we sleep and shifting the time we sleep. And we continue to behave as if there is no cost" (cited in Hellmich, 1995, p. D2). This view holds that many people continue to function at diminished capacity due to chronic sleep deprivation.

Although many people voluntarily decrease the amount of sleep they get, others have difficulty in getting to sleep or staying asleep for a sufficient time to feel rested. Both problems are typical of people classified as having *primary insomnia* (American Psychiatric Association, 1994). Stress and anxiety can be both a cause and an effect of such sleep problems (Fichten et al., 1995). Some of the other sources of stress—work, noise, and personal relationships—may interfere with sleep, as they did for Rick. Intrusive thoughts concerning work or interpersonal relationships and environmental factors such as noise, odors, or lights are common sources of sleep onset or sleep maintenance problems (Bennett, Goldfinger, & Johnson, 1987). Depression and other psychological disorders can also contribute to sleep problems (Benca, Obermeyer, Thisted, & Gillin, 1992). Changing these conditions or adopting other methods of coping with stress can improve sleep.

Another cause of sleep problems involves changes in a person's normal sleep cycle. Such alterations can occur with rotating work schedules, travel across time zones, and weekend activities. The resulting sleep difficulty is labeled *circadian rhythm sleep disorder* (American Psychiatric Association, 1994). People who suffer from "Sunday night insomnia" can solve the problem by adhering to a regular sleep schedule, even on weekends. Travelers and shift workers, however, have greater difficulties in adjusting, and they not only exhibit sleep difficulties but also lose some ability to function effectively. For shift workers, inattention and difficulty in concentrating has been associated with accidents (Åkerstedt, 1988). Research by Czeisler and his colleagues (1990) has offered some promise of treatment for this type of sleep problem. They found that exposing shift workers to bright light during the night and

number of people affected has been estimated at between 30% and 50% of the population (Hellmich, 1995). Adolescents make time to work, study, and socialize by skipping sleep; and adults decrease their sleep time to do more work and to spend time with family. Additionally, many jobs require shift work and changes in workers' sleep schedules. Deprived of sleep, adolescents may fall asleep in class and adults may be too fatigued to work efficiently. Both groups have an increased risk for accidents resulting from fatigue, impaired coordination, and altered judgment.

Much of the knowledge about sleep deprivation comes from case studies and experimental studies in which people voluntarily go without sleep or reduce the amount of time they sleep. Horne (1988) reviewed these case studies as well as experiments that subjected groups of participants to sleep deprivation. Most of the group experiments prevented participants from sleeping for 60 to 120 hours and then measured their psychological and physiological responses, revealing that extreme sleep deprivation diminishes people's ability to perform physical tasks, impairs attention and concentration, and may produce hallucinations.

Wilse Webb, one of the leading authorities on sleep, said that "sleep is a fixed, biological gift we are given, and we had better learn to adjust to its re-complete darkness during the day increased both their alertness and their cognitive performance.

An increasing body of research indicates that sleep problems are associated with changes in the immune system and possibly with illness and death. Early research (Palmblad, Petrini, Wasserman, & Åkerstedt, 1979) indicated that certain immune system responses decreased during sleep deprivation, but later research (Dinges et al., 1994; Moldofsky, Lue, Eisen, Keystone, & Gorczynski, 1986) has demonstrated that some immune system responses decrease while others increase during sleep deprivation. Even partial sleep deprivation can negatively affect immune system function (Irwin et al., 1994). These increases and decreases in immune function suggest a complex relationship between sleep deprivation and the immune system, allowing for the possibility that sleep loss may mobilize the immune system in a way similar to the effect of pathogens and yet depress other immune system responses. These changes present the possibility that sleep loss can lead to increased chances for illness, just as people commonly assume.

In summary, sleep deprivation can be both a cause of stress and a result of stress, with effects on both psychological and physiological functioning. Some people voluntarily restrict their sleep whereas others have trouble getting to sleep or staying asleep. Both may experience the negative effects of sleep deprivation. Health effects of sleep deprivation come from the increased risk of accidents and changes in immune system function.

MEASUREMENT OF STRESS

Several procedures have been developed for measuring stress. This section discusses some of the more widely used methods and addresses the problems in determining their reliability and validity.

METHODS OF MEASUREMENT

Researchers have used a variety of approaches to measure stress, but most fall into three broad categories: performance tests, physiological measures, and self-reports, including those that measure life events or daily hassles. Health psychologists rely most heavily on self-report procedures, but all three

approaches hold some potential for investigating the effects of stress on individuals' illness and health.

Performance Tests

People under stress perform differently from those not experiencing stress. On rare occasions, stress actually enhances some kinds of performance, but in most cases it impairs performance. Because stress changes performance, one method of assessing stress is to measure performance.

Performance tests typically measure the after-effects of exposure to a stressor. If people show lowered ability to perform certain tasks after having been exposed to such stressors as loud noises, crowding, or electric shock, we may assume that the impaired performance was a result of the stress. Cohen (1980) reviewed the literature dealing with impaired performance after a period of stress. He found that the literature could be interpreted as generally supporting Selye's notion that prolonged exposure to a stressor drains a person's adaptive reserves and leads to exhaustion. In addition, impaired performance persists even after the removal of the stressful stimuli. For example, an early study (Glass & Singer, 1972) reported that prolonged exposure to unpredictable and uncontrollable stressors, such as loud noise, lowered performance on such simple cognitive tasks as proofreading and recognizing color. However, environmental and personal factors, such as fatigue, illness, and personal incentive, can also raise or lower performance. Therefore, performance tests should not be used alone as an indicator of stress but should be supplemented by other measurements, such as self-report inventories and physiological measures.

Physiological Measures

A second method of measuring stress uses various physiological and biochemical measures. Physiological indexes include blood pressure, heart rate, galvanic skin response, and respiration rate whereas biochemical measures include secretion of glucocorticoids and catecholamines. These measures of stress have the advantage of being direct, highly reliable, and easily quantified. A disadvantage is that the mechanical and electrical hardware and clinical settings that are frequently used may themselves produce stress. Physicians and nurses have long been aware that a person's blood pressure, for example, may rise as a result of the clinical setting in which blood pressure measures have traditionally been taken. Some measuring instruments have been miniaturized and used in settings away from the laboratory or clinic (Carruthers, 1983). Such portable devices have an advantage over laboratory-based equipment because they are less intrusive and therefore less likely to induce stress while trying to measure it.

Life Events Scales

Since the late 1950s and early 1960s, researchers have developed a number of self-report instruments to measure stress. The most widely used of these self-report procedures is the Social Readjustment Rating Scale (SRRS), developed by Thomas H. Holmes and Richard Rahe in 1967. This scale is simply a list of 43 life events arranged in rank order from most to least stressful (see Table 3.1). Each event carries an assigned value, ranging from 100 points for death of a spouse to 11 points for minor violations of the law. Respondents check the items they have experienced during a recent period, usually the previous 6 to 24 months. Adding each item's point value and totaling scores yields a stress score for each person. These scores can then be correlated with future events, such as incidence of illness, to determine the relationship between this measure of stress and the occurrence of physical illness.

Because the SRRS has a deceptively simple format, it has often been misused by people looking for an easily administered scale to predict future health or illness. Life events scales like the SRRS have

Table 3.1 **Social Readjustment Rating Scale (SRRS)**

Rank	Life event	Mean value	Rank	Life event	Mean value
1.	Death of spouse	100	23.	Son or daughter leaving home	29
2.	Divorce	73	24.	Trouble with in-laws	29
3.	Marital separation	65	25.	Outstanding personal achievement	28
4.	Jail term	63	26.	Wife begins or stops work	26
5.	Death of close family member	63	27.	Begin or end school	26
6.	Personal injury or illness	53	28.	Change in living conditions	25
7.	Marriage	50	29.	Revision of personal habits	24
8.	Fired at work	47	30.	Trouble with boss	23
9.	Marital reconciliation	45	31.	Change in work hours or conditions	20
10.	Retirement	45	32.	Change in residence	20
11.	Change in health of family member	44	33.	Change in schools	20
12.	Pregnancy	40	34.	Change in recreation	19
13.	Sex difficulties	39	35.	Change in church activities	19
14.	Gain of new family member	39	36.	Change in social activities	18
15.	Business readjustment	39	37.	Mortgage or loan less than $10,000	17
16.	Change in financial state	38	38.	Change in sleeping habits	16
17.	Death of close friend	37	39.	Change in number of family get-togethers	15
18.	Change to different line of work	36	40.	Change in eating habits	15
19.	Change in number of arguments with spouse	35	41.	Vacation	13
20.	Mortgage over $10,000	31	42.	Christmas	12
21.	Foreclosure of mortgage or loan	30	43.	Minor violations of the law	11
22.	Change in responsibilities at work	29			

SOURCE: From The Social Readjustment Rating Scale by T. H. Holmes and R. H. Rahe, 1967. *Journal of Psychosomatic Research, II*, p. 216. Reprinted by permission of Pergamon Press and Thomas H. Holmes.

sometimes appeared in the popular press with the implication that people should count their stress points and use care to avoid additional stress that might put them beyond some critical total, usually 300 points on the SRRS. This advice ignores the fact that many people accumulate far more than 300 points in a year and never become ill. Rick, in our case study, scored over 700 on the SRRS and his chronic headaches got substantially worse. He did not develop any major illnesses during the year following his assessment, but his physician believed that Rick was in danger and told him that he had to cut down on the number of hours he was working to decrease his stress.

Holmes and Rahe developed their scale by assuming that *change* in life adjustment is a key ingredient in stress. As Table 3.1 shows, not all stressful life events result in undesirable changes. For example, marriage, outstanding personal achievement, and marital reconciliation are usually regarded as desirable or positive changes yet they appear on the SRRS. A number of other items, such as business readjustment and change in the number of arguments with one's spouse, could be either positive or negative. On the SRRS, however, either increasing or decreasing the number of arguments with one's spouse is worth the same number of points, and the experience of *change* is the critical factor in this view of stress.

Since the development of the Holmes and Rahe scale, considerable debate has arisen over the number and nature of items that should included in life events scales. Holmes and Rahe began by observing which life events preceded the onset of disease in about 5,000 patients and came up with only 43 items. These life events were then weighted by a different group of people, who were asked to rate them according to the degree of readjustment each required (Holmes & Masuda, 1974). This "average person" scaling system gives each item a constant weight, with no consideration for an item's subjective meaning to a particular individual. For example, death of a spouse is weighted at 100 points for everyone, regardless of length of marriage, number of previous spouses, or degree of dependency. Some investigators (Lazarus & Folkman, 1984; Sarason, Sarason, & Johnson, 1985) have criticized any approach that does not permit the individual's subjective appraisal of the stressful situation.

Holmes and Rahe regarded any change—desirable or undesirable—to be stressful, because change in one's life requires some type of social readjustment. This emphasis on change is consistent with Selye's view of stress, but it has been criticized by investigators who have found that undesirable changes are more highly related to illness than are desirable changes (Crandall & Lehman, 1977; Paykel, Prusoff, & Uhlenhuth, 1971). In addition, some other researchers have argued that a longer list of life events would be more representative of all the experiences that help define stress. Consequently, a number of other life events scales have been developed since the first Holmes and Rahe inventory.

A more sophisticated life events inventory is the Psychiatric Epidemiology Research Interview (PERI) Life Events Scale, developed by Barbara Dohrenwend and her colleagues (Dohrenwend, Krasnoff, Askenasy, & Dohrenwend, 1978, 1982). This 102-item inventory avoids many of the problems of inadequate sampling common to nearly all previous scales. Earlier scales, with very few exceptions, also failed to consider that social class and other cultural factors would make a difference in the way life experiences are perceived. Some evidence is available that people from different cultural backgrounds perceive life events differently (Miller, Bentz, Aponte, & Brogan, 1974). Although the norm group for the PERI is limited geographically to the New York City area, it is based on a sample stratified for gender, age, marital status, educational level, ethnic group, and socioeconomic level. It is also distinguished from most of the newer scales by its generous use of desirable life event changes. In fact, nearly half the items have either positive or indeterminate value. This emphasis on change, of course, agrees with Holmes and Rahe and also with Selye's formulation of stress as a homeostatic readjustment to life changes.

In addition to the Social Readjustment Rating Scale and the Psychiatric Epidemiology Research Interview, another instrument is the newer Undergraduate Stress Questionnaire (USQ) developed by Christian Crandall, Jeanne Preisler, and Julie Aussprung (1992). As the name implies, the USQ is designed to measure stress among undergraduate students. It includes some major events, such as death of family members, but it also contains everyday hassles in the lives of students, such as sitting through a boring class, cramming for a test, or dealing with incompetence at the registrar's office. Each of the 83 items on the questionnaire is rated for (1) *severity*, or how stressful the event would be to undergraduates (4-point scale); (2) *commonness*, or how frequently the event occurs over a long period of time in the lives of undergraduates in general (5-point scale); and (3) *frequency*, or the number of times people have experienced that event during the past week. This scale has not yet generated much research, but Crandall et al. reported that the Undergraduate Stress Questionnaire is valid, reliable, and easy to administer.

The Daily Hassles Scale

Richard Lazarus and his associates have pioneered an approach to stress measurement that looks at daily hassles rather than major life events. Daily hassles are "experiences and conditions of daily living that have appraised as salient and harmful or threatening to the endorser's well-being" (Lazarus, 1984a, p. 376).

Recall from the discussion of theories of stress that Lazarus views stress as a transactional, dynamic complex shaped by people's *appraisal* of the environmental situation and their *perceived capabilities to cope* with this situation. Consistent with this view, Lazarus and his associates insisted that measurement instruments must not conceptualize stress as an objective environmental stimulus but instead must allow for subjective elements such as personal appraisal, beliefs, goals, and commitments (Lazarus, DeLongis, Folkman, & Gruen, 1985).

As a consequence, Lazarus and his associates (Kanner, Coyne, Schaefer, & Lazarus, 1981) developed the Hassles Scale, which consists of 117 items of annoying, irritating, or frustrating ways in which people may feel hassled. This scale first requires respondents to check any hassle that happened to them during the past month. Next, respondents indicate on a 3-point scale how severe each of the checked hassles was during that time. This second step is consistent with Lazarus's belief that an individual's *perception* of stress is more crucial than the objective event itself. Table 3.2 shows the 10 most frequently checked hassles reported by a sample of 100 middle-aged people.

Does the Hassles Scale measure the same kind of stress revealed by life events scales? Kanner et al. (1981) found that hassles and life events were only modestly correlated. This slight overlap between life

Table 3.2 Ten most frequently checked hassles (n = 100)

Item	Percentage of Times Checked
1. Concerns about weight	52.4%
2. Health of a family member	48.1
3. Rising prices of common goods	43.7
4. Home maintenance	42.8
5. Too many things to do	38.6
6. Misplacing or losing things	38.1
7. Yard work or outside home maintenance	38.1
8. Property, investment, or taxes	37.6
9. Crime	37.1
10. Physical appearance	35.9

SOURCE: From "Comparison of Two Modes of Stress Measurement: Daily Hassles and Uplifts Versus Major Life Events" by A. D. Kanner, J. C. Coyne, C. Schaefer, and R. S. Lazarus, 1981, *Journal of Behavioral Medicine, 4,* p. 14. Copyright 1981 by Plenum. Adapted by permission.

events and daily hassles was explained by Lazarus (1984a) as evidence that major life events have some effect on day-to-day routines but that many daily hassles are independent of life events. As a predictor of psychological health, the Hassles Scale was more accurate than the life events scale, a finding that Kanner et al. (1981) interpreted to mean that the Hassles Scale supplements life events scales as a measure of stress and that the life events scale added little to the predictive value of the Hassles Scale.

Nevertheless, the Hassles Scale has been criticized for including contaminated items—that is, items such as concerns about weight that might reflect illness rather than predict it (Dohrenwend, Dohrenwend, Dodson, & Shrout, 1984; Green, 1986; Kohn, Lafreniere, & Gurevich, 1991). To avoid this problem, Paul Kohn and his associates at York University in Ontario, Canada, have developed two decontaminated scales that purport to measure stress indirectly: the Inventory of College Students' Recent Life Experiences (Kohn, Lafreniere, & Gurevich, 1990) and the Survey of Recent Life Experiences (Kohn & Macdonald, 1992).

The Inventory of College Students' Recent Life Experiences (ICSRLE) consists of 49 items, each of which was written to reflect students' life experiences rather than their physical and psychological distresses. Some items refer specifically to college students' problems, such as "Finding courses too demanding"; others are more general, such as "Too many things to do at once." Respondents rate the extent of their experiences with each item over the past month on a 4-point scale from *not at all part of my life* to *very much part of my life*. Factor analysis of ICSRLE scores produced seven relatively independent factors, which Kohn et al. (1990) cited as evidence that their scale is relatively uncontaminated by students' feelings of a generally stressful life. Kohn et al. (1990) also claimed that the ICSRLE has adequate reliability and validity. In addition, Kohn and his associates (Kohn, 1991; Kohn & Gurevich, 1993; Kohn et al., 1991) have found that ICSRLE scores predict both perceived stress and physical and psychological ailments.

The Survey of Recent Life Experiences (SRLE) was developed by Kohn and Macdonald (1992) as a decontaminated hassles scale for adults. The SRLE parallels the college students' scale and contains some of the same items. Respondents indicate the extent of their experience over the past month with each of the 51 items of the SRLE, using the same 4-point scale as the college students' inventory. Although Kohn and Macdonald reported some reliability and validity for the Survey of Recent Life Experiences, little evidence exists from independent investigators that either the ICSRLE or the SRLE is reliable and valid.

Sheldon Cohen, Tom Kamarck, and Robin Mermelstein (1983) developed the Perceived Stress Scale (PSS), another alternative to the Hassles Scale of Kanner et al. The PSS is a 14-item scale that attempts to measure the degree to which situations in people's lives are appraised as "unpredictable, uncontrollable, and overloading" (Cohen et al., 1983, p. 387). The scale assesses three components of stress: (1) daily hassles, (2) major events, and (3) changes in coping resources. Respondents answer "never," "almost never," "sometimes," "fairly often," or "very often" to items that ask about their stressful situations during the past month. Cohen et al. reported acceptable reliability of the Perceived Stress Scale but a correlation of only .14 between scores of a group of college students and their subsequent

physiological ailments. Later researchers (Hewitt, Flett, & Mosher, 1992; Pbert, Doerfler, & DeCosimo, 1992) have found some ability of the Perceived Stress Scale to predict psychiatric and physical symptoms.

Clearly, more research on the reliability and validity of the Inventory of College Students' Recent Life Experiences, the Survey of Recent Life Experiences, and the Perceived Stress Scale is necessary before the usefulness of these scales can be assessed. The following section discusses the problems in establishing reliablity and validity of stress measures.

RELIABILITY AND VALIDITY OF STRESS MEASURES

The usefulness of stress measures rests on their ability to predict some established criterion consistently. For our purposes, that criterion is illness. Chapter 4 examines the evidence on the relationship between stress and specific illnesses.

In general, the purpose of self-report inventories is not only to assess current levels of stress but also to predict some future behavior or condition. To predict the future, these instruments must be both reliable and valid. Reliability is the consistency with which an instrument measures whatever it measures, and validity is the extent to which it measures what it is supposed to measure.

The reliability of self-report inventories is most frequently determined by either the paired-associate method or the test-retest technique. In the paired-associate method, close associates (usually a spouse) fill out the inventory, answering as if the item applied to their associate. Responses are then matched with those of that associate. The degree of agreement between the two associates is usually quite high for moderately or severely stressful events. Slater and Depue (1981), for example, found 93% agreement in paired-associate responses for moderately and severely stressful items, such as death of a close friend or marital separation. Understandably, the overlap decreases with less stressful experiences (Zimmerman, 1983). Respondents and associates tend to agree only moderately well when asked to check life events that are merely mildly stressful, such as change in social activities.

The second approach to determining the reliability of self-report inventories is the test-retest technique, in which the same person completes the stress inventory at two different times. Inaccuracies in memory are the main reason for less than perfect agreement. A review of test-retest reliability studies revealed that the relationship is far from perfect, even when participants were asked to recall the same time period (Neugebauer, 1984). In most of the reviewed studies, people were asked to report stressful life events on only two occasions covering the same period of time.

Other studies have used a somewhat different approach to measure the reliability of life events scales. Rather than asking people to fill out a scale only twice, Klein and Rubovits (1987) required college students to complete a life events questionnaire once every 5 weeks for 20 weeks. Immediately after the last administration, the students filled out the scale once again but this time for the entire 20-week period. The correlation between the number of events reported during the four 5-week periods and the number reported in the 20-week assessment was .63, indicating only moderate reliability. Looking at the data from a different angle, these authors found that 26% fewer events were reported over the single long period than in the four shorter periods.

Using a similar design, Raphael, Cloitre, and Dohrenwend (1991) assessed the reliability of the checklist method of measuring stressful life events. Two groups of women (pain patients and healthy subjects) reported their life events once every month for 10 months. Then, at the end of the study, participants reported their life events over the same 10-month period. Only 25% of the event categories appeared in both reports. Far more events were reported on a monthly basis than on the 10-month retrospective report. These results prompted the authors to caution against relying on life events checklists to measure the relationship between stress and illness. If self-reports of stress are not reliable, then they cannot validly predict illness—even if stress causes illness.

These findings confirm those of earlier reviews (Neugebauer, 1984; Thoits, 1983)—that life events scales had limited usefulness as an independent measure of stress. When a scale's reliability is limited, its validity is also questionable.

To consider the *validity* of self-report inventories, we must begin with the question "What are these instruments supposed to measure?" At least three approaches to answering this question are possible. First, the scales should measure life events; that is, the items in the inventories should accurately represent all the life events experienced by the respondents. Second, these scales are supposed to measure stress. Thus, scores on self-report inventories should correlate with some other measure of stress, such as judgments of a spouse or close associate or physical measurements of stress. Third, as they are most frequently used, self-report inventories are supposed to measure or predict the incidence of future illness.

Let's consider the three possible approaches in more detail. First, do self-report inventories accurately represent all experiences of stressful life events? Monroe (1982) suggested that some people tend to underreport on life events scales; that is, they omit some events. Other critics (Rabkin & Struening, 1976) contended that sick people overreport life events, providing a kind of justification for their illness. If people either overreport or underreport items on life events scales, then obviously the scales are not totally valid measures of life events.

The second approach asks how one can determine the degree to which a person is accurately reporting stressful events. One method is to compare reports from a spouse or close associate. But the result generally yields significant levels of disagreement between partners, especially when mildly distressful events are included. One study, for example, found that the partners of psychiatric patients and nonpatients failed to confirm about two-thirds of all reported life events (Yager, Grant, Sweetwood, & Gerst, 1981).

The third and most useful type of validity for stress inventories is the extent to which they predict future illnesses or disorders. If self-report scales can demonstrate predictive validity, they will play a valuable role in determining who may be at risk for stress-related illnesses. One problem in measuring the relationship between stress inventories and illness is the confounding of items on the major life events scales with the presence of physical disorders. Being ill can be stressful, of course, but it can also lead to answers that have been included in the Social Readjustment Rating Scale, such as sex difficulties, revision of personal habits, change in sleeping habits, and change in eating habits. Therefore, a high score on the SRRS or other similarly constructed life events scale may be a consequence rather than a cause of illness. Hudgens (1974) reported that 29 of the 43 events on the SRRS are frequently symptoms or consequences of physical disorders. The next chapter reviews several studies dealing with the relationship between stress and illness, but conclusions from this research must be tempered by a consideration of reliability, validity, and confounding problems of the various measures of stress.

CHAPTER SUMMARY

The nervous system plays a central role in the physiology of stress. When a person perceives stress, the sympathetic division of the autonomic nervous system stimulates the adrenal medulla, producing catecholamines and arousing the person from a resting state. The pituitary gland releases the adrenocorticotropic hormone (ACTH), which in turn affects the adrenal cortex. This release prepares the body to resist stress. The autonomic nervous system and the neuroendocrine system form the physiological foundation for both stress and illness.

Hans Selye and Richard Lazarus have both proposed theories of stress. Selye defined stress as a nonspecific or generalized response to a variety of environmental stressors. Whenever the body encounters a disruptive stimulus, it mobilizes itself in a generalized attempt to adapt to that stimulus. This mobilization is called the general adaptation syndrome. The GAS has three stages—alarm, resistance, and exhaustion—and the potential for trauma or illness exists at all three stages. Lazarus has insisted that a person's perception of a situation is the most significant component of stress. To Lazarus, stress depends on one's appraisal of an event rather than the event itself. Whether stress produces illness is closely tied to one's vulnerability as well as to one's perceived ability to cope with the situation.

Several possible sources of stress have been suggested, but the level of stress people experience depends in large part of their perception of these sources and on their perceived ability to cope. Stressors can be either environmental or personal. One possible source of environmental stress is crowding, and the *feeling* of being crowded, which can be more stressful than population density itself. Lacking the means to avoid a crowded environment adds to the stress. The potential for accidents with toxic chemicals is another environmental stressor, and again, its effects are most severe when people feel that they have little or no control of the situation, which is often the case with a polluted environment. Noise can also be stressful, but the greatest health risk of loud noise is a direct effect—loss of hearing—rather than the indirect effect of stress. The combination of stress from crowding, pollution, and noise may combine in urban settings with commuting hassles and fear of crime to create a situation described as urban press.

Some jobs are more stressful than others, but the number of decisions made on the job is not a valid indicator of stress. People who have some control over their work, such as executives of large corporations, have less stressful jobs than food service workers and middle-level managers. Personal relationships on the job offer the potential for stress or can provide a buffer against stress, and this potential also applies to personal relationships with friends and family. Surveys of stressful experiences list personal interactions as an important source of stress. Family relationships and the multiple roles that both women and men fulfill can be sources of stress, especially when people feel that their partners are not supportive.

Sleep problems may cause stress, and stress may cause problems in sleep. Some people voluntarily limit their sleep, whereas others have difficulty going to sleep or staying asleep. Either cause of sleep deprivation can limit a person's ability to function, increasing the risk of accidents. In addition, a growing body of research indicates that sleep deprivation affects the immune system in complex ways, suggesting that sleep problems adversely affect health.

Stress has been assessed by several methods, including physiological and biochemical measures, performance tests, and self-reports of stressful life events. Most life events scales are patterned after Holmes and Rahe's Social Readjustment Rating Scale. Some of these instruments include only undesirable events; others are based on the premise that any major change is stressful. Lazarus has pioneered a scale that measures daily hassles and emphasizes the *severity* of the event as perceived by the person.

The reliability of self-report inventories of stress is most often determined by having people fill out the questionnaire a second time on a later occasion or by having a close associate, such as a spouse, fill out the inventory as if answering for the subject. Although most self-report inventories have acceptable reliability, their ability to predict illness remains to be established. For these stress inventories to predict illness, two conditions must be met: First, they must be valid measures of stress; second, stress must be related to illness. Chapter 4 takes up the question of whether stress causes illness.

SUGGESTED READINGS

Cottington, E. M., & House, J. S. (1987). Occupational stress and health: A multivariate relationship. In A. Baum & J. E. Singer (Eds.), *Handbook of psychology and health: Vol. 5. Stress* (pp. 41–62). Hillsdale, NJ: Erlbaum. This article reviews the extensive research on the relationship between occupational stress and health and attempts to organize the results. The authors consider individual differences and both the work and nonwork environments. They also critically review existing research results and suggest directions for future research.

Graig, E. (1993). Stress as a consequence of the urban physical environment. In L. Goldberger & S. Breznitz (Eds.), *Handbook of stress: Theoretical and clinical aspects* (2nd ed., pp. 316–332). New York: Free Press. Graig discusses the many stressful conditions associated with living in large urban areas. These conditions include noise, pollution, commuting problems, and fear of crime.

Lazarus, R. S., & Folkman, S. (1984). *Stress, appraisal, and coping.* New York: Springer. A comprehensive treatment of Lazarus's views of stress, cognitive appraisal, and coping, this book discusses Lazarus's psychological model of stress and the relevant literature.

Selye, H. (1982). History and present status of the stress concept. In L. Goldberger & S. Breznitz (Eds.), *Handbook of stress: Theoretical and clinical aspects* (pp. 7–17). New York: Free Press. This brief article, written shortly before Selye's death, gives a review of stress as conceptualized by the most influential person in the field.

Understanding Stress and Illness

Chapter 3 introduced Rick, who had undergone a period of extreme stress because of the deaths of his father and a close friend; he also had experienced a bitter divorce and custody dispute. As a consequence of these problems, Rick was left without family and social support, felt alienated from people at work, believed that he needed to hold at least two jobs to pay his bills, and began to have trouble sleeping. Did all these changes in lifestyle, most of which are negative, place Rick at risk for stress-related illnesses?

This chapter reviews the evidence relating to stress as a possible cause of disease and follows Rick to see whether his high levels of stress place him at an elevated risk for illness or death. First, let's look at how stress, a psychological factor, might influence physical disease. We begin with a discussion of the immune system, which protects the body against stress-related illnesses.

PHYSIOLOGY OF THE IMMUNE SYSTEM

The immune system consists of tissues, organs, and processes that protect the body from invasion by foreign material, such as bacteria, viruses, and fungi. In addition, the immune system performs housekeeping functions by removing worn-out or damaged cells and patroling for mutant cells. Once the invaders and renegades are located, the immune system activates processes to eliminate them.

ORGANS OF THE IMMUNE SYSTEM

Rather than being a centralized system like the heart or the brain, the immune system is spread throughout the body in the form of the **lymphatic system**. The tissue of the lymphatic system is **lymph**; it consists of the tissue components of blood except red cells and platelets. In the process of vascular circulation, fluid and *leukocytes* (white blood cells) leak from the capillaries. These blood components routinely escape from the circulatory system in the process of capillary diffusion. In addition, fluid is also secreted from body cells. This tissue fluid is referred to as *lymph* when it enters the lymph vessels, which circulate lymph and eventually return it to the bloodstream.

The structure of the lymphatic system (see Figure 4.1) roughly parallels the circulatory system for blood. Lymph also circulates, but it does so by entering the lymphatic system and then reentering the bloodstream rather than staying exclusively in the lymphatic system. In its circulation, all lymph trav-

which are T-lymphocytes, or **T-cells**; B-lymphocytes, or **B-cells**; and **natural killer (NK) cells**. Lymphocytes arise in the bone marrow, but they mature and differentiate in other structures of the immune system. In addition to lymphocytes, two other types of leukocytes exist: granulocytes and monocytes/macrophages. These leukocytes are involved in the nonspecific response of the immune system whereas lymphocytes are involved in specific immune system responses (discussed more fully below).

The **thymus**, which has endocrine functions, secretes a hormone called **thymosin**. This hormone seems to be involved in the maturation and differentiation of the T-cells. Interestingly, the thymus is largest during infancy and childhood and then atrophies during adulthood. Its function is not entirely understood, but the thymus is clearly important in the immune system because its removal impairs immune function. Its atrophy also suggests that the immune system's production of T-cells is more efficient during childhood and that aging is related to lowered immune efficiency. The **tonsils** are masses of lymphatic tissue located in the throat. Their function seems to be similar to that of the lymph nodes: trapping and killing invading cells and particles. The **spleen**, an organ near the stomach in the abdominal cavity, is one site of lymphocyte maturation. In addition, it serves as a holding station for lymphocytes as well as a disposal site for worn-out blood cells.

The surveillance and protection that the immune system offers is not limited to the lymph nodes but takes place in other tissues of the body that contain lymphocytes. Therefore, the organs of the immune system may be considered all those structures that manufacture, differentiate, store, and circulate lymph; but immune function relies on more than these structures and is not confined to the lymphatic system. To protect the entire body, immune function must occur in all parts of the body.

FUNCTION OF THE IMMUNE SYSTEM

The immune system's function is generally to protect against injury and specifically to maintain vigilance against foreign substances that the body has encountered. As R. J. Glasser (1976) pointed out, the immune system must be extraordinarily effective to

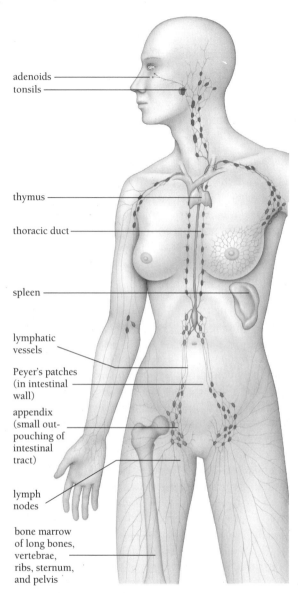

adenoids
tonsils
thymus
thoracic duct
spleen
lymphatic vessels
Peyer's patches (in intestinal wall)
appendix (small outpouching of intestinal tract)
lymph nodes
bone marrow of long bones, vertebrae, ribs, sternum, and pelvis

Figure 4.1 Lymphatic system. SOURCE: From Ingraham & Ingraham, 1995, p. 407.

els through at least one **lymph node**. The lymph nodes are round or oval capsules spaced throughout the lymphatic system that help clean lymph of cellular debris, bacteria, and even dust that has entered the body.

Lymph gets its name from the **lymphocytes**, a type of white blood cell found in lymph. There are several types of lymphocytes, the most fully understood of

prevent 100% of the invading bacteria, viruses, and fungi from damaging our bodies. Few other body functions must operate at 100% efficiency. Glasser emphasized that the immune system must perform at that level for people (and other animals) to remain healthy.

Invading organisms have many ways to enter the body, and the immune system has a means to combat each type of entry. In general, immune system responses to invading foreign substances are of two types: general (nonspecific) and specific responses.

Nonspecific Immune System Responses

Intact skin and mucous membranes are the first line of defense against foreign substances, but some invaders regularly bypass them and enter the body. Those that do face two general (nonspecific) mechanisms. One is **phagocytosis**, the attack of foreign particles by cells of the immune system. Two types of leukocytes perform this function. **Granulocytes** contain granules filled with chemicals. When these cells come into contact with invaders, they release their chemicals, which attack the invaders. **Macrophages** perform a variety of immune functions, including scavenging for worn-out cells and debris, assisting in the initiation of specific immune response, and secreting a variety of chemicals involved in the immune response. Several chemical substances, called *complement,* are involved in breaking down the cell membranes of the invaders. Therefore, phagocytosis, which is part of the nonspecific immune system response, involves several mechanisms that can quickly result in the destruction of invading bacteria, viruses, and fungi. However, some invaders escape this nonspecific action.

Inflammation is a second type of nonspecific immune system response. Inflammation works to restore tissues that have been damaged by invaders. When an injury occurs, blood vessels in the area of injury contract temporarily. Later they dilate, increasing blood flow to the tissues and causing the warmth and redness that accompany inflammation. The damaged cells release enzymes that help destroy invading microorganisms; these enzymes can also aid in their own digestion, should the cells die. Both granulocytes and macrophages migrate to the site of injury to battle the invaders. Finally, tissue repair begins. Figure 4.2 illustrates the process of inflammation.

Specific Immune Systems Responses

Two types of lymphocytes, T-cells and B-cells, carry out specific immune responses—that is, an immune response that is specific to one invader. When a lymphocyte encounters a foreign substance for the first time, both the general response and a specific response are initiated. Invading microorganisms are killed and eaten by macrophages, which present fragments of these invaders to T-cells that have moved to the area of inflammation. This contact sensitizes the T-cells; they acquire specific receptors on their surfaces so they can recognize the invader. An army of *cytotoxic T-cells* forms through this process, and it soon mobilizes a direct attack on the invaders. This process is referred to as *cell-mediated immunity* because it occurs at the level of the body cells rather than in the bloodstream. Cell-mediated immunity is especially effective against fungi, viruses that have already entered the cells, parasites, and mutations of body cells.

The other variety of lymphocyte, the B-cells, mobilize an indirect attack on invading microorganisms. With the help of one variety of T-cell (the *helper T-cell*), B-cells differentiate into **plasma cells** and secrete **antibodies.** Each antibody is specifically manufactured in response to a specific invader. Foreign substances that provoke antibody manufacture are called **antigens** (for *anti*body *gen*erator). Antibodies circulate, find their antigens, bind to them, and mark them for later destruction. Figure 4.3 shows the differentiation of T- and B-cells.

The specific reactions of the immune system constitute the *primary immune response.* Figure 4.4 shows the development of the primary immune response and depicts how subsequent exposure activates the *secondary immune response.* During initial exposure to an invader, some of the sensitized T-cells and B-cells replicate, and rather than going into action, they are held in reserve. These *memory lymphocytes* form the basis for a rapid immune response on second exposure to the same invader. Memory lymphocytes can persist for years. They will not be activated unless the antigen invader reappears. If it does, then the memory lymphocytes initiate the same sort of direct and indirect attacks that occurred at the first exposure, but much more rapidly. This specifically tailored

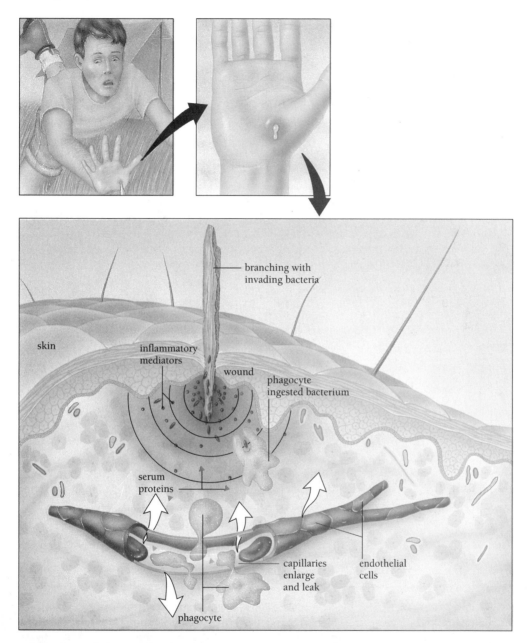

Figure 4.2 Acute inflammation is initiated by a stimulus such as injury or infection. Inflammatory mediators are produced at the site of the stimulus. They cause blood vessels to dilate and increase their permeability; they also attract phagocytes to the site of inflammation and activate them.
SOURCE: From Ingraham & Ingraham, 1995, p. 407.

rapid response to foreign microorganisms that occurs with repeated exposure is what most people consider **immunity**.

This system of immune response through B-cell recognition of antigens and their manufacture of an- tibodies is called **humoral immunity**, because it happens in the bloodstream. The process is especially effective in fighting against bacterial invaders and viruses before they enter the cells — that is, while they are still circulating in the blood.

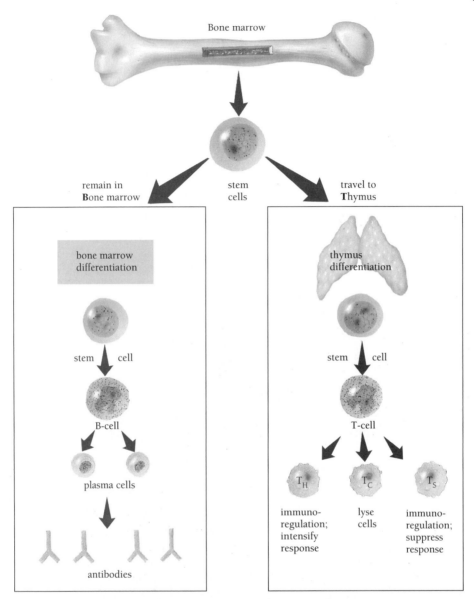

Figure 4.3 Origins of B-cells and T-cells. Lymphocytes, like all blood cells, arise from stem cells in the bone marrow. B-cells differentiate there. Later, as mature B-cells, some differentiate further into plasma cells if the body is under microbial attack. T-cells, on the other hand, travel to the thymus where they differentiate. SOURCE: From Ingraham & Ingraham, 1995, p. 407.

Creating Immunity

One widely used method to induce immunity is **vaccination**. In vaccination, a weakened form of a virus or bacteria is introduced into the body, stimulating the production of antibodies. These antibodies then confer immunity for an extended period. Smallpox, which once killed thousands of people each year, has been eradicated through the use of vaccination. Now smallpox is a scientific curiosity confined to laboratory cultures. Other vaccines exist for a variety of diseases. They are especially useful in the prevention of viral infections. However, immunity must be created for each specific virus, and thousands of viruses exist. Even viral illnesses that produce simi-

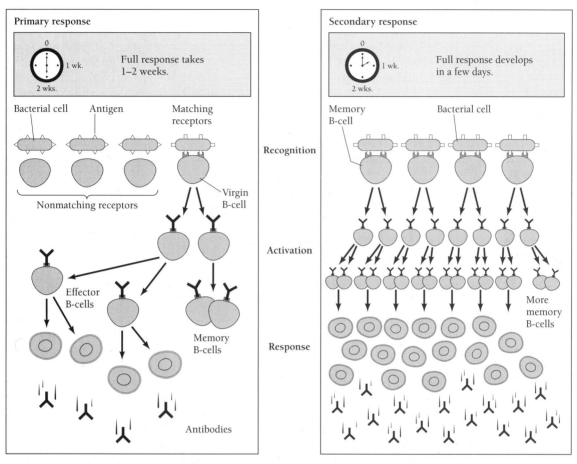

Figure 4.4 *Primary versus secondary immune response. The first time a person encounters an antigen, virgin B-cells mount a primary immune response by producing antibodies and some memory B-cells. If a person encounters the same antigen again, the memory B-cells initiate a secondary immune response, which is more rapid and effective than a primary response.*

lar symptoms, like the common cold, may be caused by many different viruses. Therefore, immunity for colds would require many vaccinations, and the development of these has not proven practical.

Cells that are infected with a virus produce **interferon**, a type of protein chemical messenger. Interferon travels to other cells and prevents them from becoming infected by a virus. The protection is not specific to the infecting virus because infection from one virus confers immunity against others. The finding that interferon stimulates immunity against viral infection seems promising because viral infections are difficult to treat, and vaccination produces only specific immunity.

Nonspecific immunity against viral infection offers the promise of treatment for diseases as diverse as the common cold and cancer. In the past, however, optimism was tempered by the practical problems in research with interferon. First, interferon apparently differs from species to species, so it is not possible to use interferon from other species to treat humans. Second, it could be obtained only in small quantities. Third, it is difficult to purify. The scarcity of interferon, therefore, was a significant problem in assessing its effectiveness in clinical treatment.

In later years, however, a technique using *recombinant DNA* allowed the synthesis of human interferon, thus making more interferon available for research (Schindler, 1992). Currently researchers are avidly studying the effectiveness of interferon in preventing viral diseases. Interferon's ability to enhance natural immune responses offers the advantages of vaccination without the potential side effects.

IMMUNE SYSTEM DISORDERS

Immune deficiency, an inadequate immune response, may occur for several reasons. For example, it is a side effect of most drugs used for cancer chemotherapy. Immune deficiency also occurs naturally. Although the immune system is not fully functional at birth, infants are protected by antibodies they have received from their mothers through the placenta, and infants who breast-feed receive antibodies from their mother's milk. These antibodies offer protection until the infant's own immune system develops during the first months of life.

In rare cases, the immune system fails to develop, leaving the child without immune protection. Physicians can try to boost immune function, but the well-publicized "children in plastic bubbles" still show the results of immune deficiency. Exposure to any virus or bacterium can be fatal to these children. They are sealed into sterile quarters to isolate them from the microorganisms that are part of the normal world.

An even more publicized type of immune deficiency is **acquired immune deficiency syndrome (AIDS)**. This disease is caused by a virus, the human immunodeficiency virus (HIV), which acts to destroy the T-cells and macrophages in the immune system (O'Leary, 1990). Those who are infected with HIV are thus vulnerable to a wide range of bacterial, viral, and malignant diseases. The disease is known to be contagious but not easily transmitted from person to person. The highest concentrations of the virus are found in blood and in semen. Blood transfusions from an infected person, intravenous injection with a contaminated needle, and sexual intercourse seem to be the most common routes of infection. Treatment consists of the management of the diseases that develop because of immune deficiency. As of 1995, the only direct treatment for the AIDS virus consisted of administering drugs that affect viral infections, a treatment that slows the progress of the disease but does not cure it.

Allergies constitute another immune system disorder. An allergic response is an abnormal reaction to a foreign substance that normally elicits little or no immune reaction. People with allergies are hypersensitive to certain substances. A wide range of substances cause allergic reactions, and the severity of the reactions also varies widely. Some allergic reactions may be life threatening whereas others merely cause runny noses. Some cases of allergy are treated by introducing regular, small doses of the allergen. This process desensitizes the person to the allergen, alleviating the allergic response. Other cases of allergy are treated by teaching allergic individuals to recognize and avoid their allergens.

Autoimmune diseases occur when the immune system attacks the body, for reasons not well understood. Part of the function of the immune system is to recognize foreign invaders and mark them for destruction. In some people, the person's own body cells are marked for destruction. In these cases the immune system appears to have lost the ability to distinguish the body from an invader, and it mounts the same vicious attack against itself that it would against an intruder. Lupus erythematosus and rheumatoid arthritis are autoimmune diseases, and multiple sclerosis may also be.

Transplant rejection is not really an immune disorder, but it is a problem caused by the immune system's activity. When working efficiently, the immune system has the ability to detect foreign substances. With the exception of identical twins, no two humans have the same biochemistry. Therefore, the immune system normally recognizes any foreign tissue as an invader. A transplanted heart, liver, or kidney will be recognized as foreign tissue because the biochemical markers from its donor differ from those of its host. Thus, the host's immune system will try to destroy the transplant. In an effort to prevent this reaction, drugs are administered that suppress immune system function. This strategy often works, but unfortunately the suppression is not specific to the transplanted organ. The entire immune response is affected, leaving the person vulnerable to infection. Currently, people who have received successful organ transplants must adapt their lifestyles to minimize the risk of infection due to their weakened immune system. Modification of lifestyle and compliance with medical regimens are topics of interest to health psychologists and other health professionals who use them in the treatment of organ transplant patients.

According to the **immune surveillance theory**, cancer is also the result of an immune system dysfunction. This view holds that the cellular mutations that initiate cancer occur quite frequently, but that these mutations are normally identified and killed by the T-cells in the immune system. Cancer develops when the immune system fails to identify and destroy mutant cells. Researchers who are investigating this theory are interested in discovering methods of stimulating immune system function as a treatment for cancer. If this theory is supported by future research, a vaccine against cancer may be possible. As in the case of smallpox, cancer could someday become an object of laboratory study rather than the killer of thousands.

PSYCHONEUROIMMUNOLOGY

The previous section examined the function of the immune system as well as its tissues, structure, and disorders. Physiologists have traditionally taken a similar approach, studying the immune system as separate and independent of other body systems. Recently, however, evidence has accumulated suggesting that the immune system interacts with the central nervous system (CNS) and the endocrine system and that the CNS, endocrine system, and immune system can be affected by psychological and social factors. In addition, immune function can affect neural function, providing the potential for the immune system to alter behavior and thought (Maier, Watkins, & Fleshner, 1994). This recognition has led to the founding and rapid growth of the field of **psychoneuroimmunology**, a multidisciplinary field that focuses on the interactions among behavior, the nervous system, the endocrine system, and the immune system.

HISTORY OF PSYCHONEUROIMMUNOLOGY

George Solomon and Rudolph Moos first used the term *psychoneuroimmunology* in a publication in 1964. In that article and in his research in the 1960s, Solomon laid the groundwork for the field of psychoneuroimmunology (Kiecolt-Glaser & Glaser, 1989).

One event that dramatically shaped the field of psychoneuroimmunology was the 1975 publication of an article by Robert Ader and Nicholas Cohen on classical conditioning of the immune system. This research demonstrated how the nervous system, the immune system, and behavior could interact. Ader and Cohen conditioned rats to associate a novel, conditioning stimulus (CS)—a saccharine and water solution—with an unconditioned stimulus (UCS) that naturally produces an unconditioned response (UCR). In Ader and Cohen's procedure, a drug that suppresses the immune system was the UCS. The rats were allowed to drink the saccharin solution and then were injected with the drug. The response was the expected suppression of the immune system. However, the rats later showed immune suppression when they were given the saccharin solution alone. That is, their immune systems had been conditioned to respond to the saccharin solution in much the same manner that it reacted to the drug. This type of conditioning is not so surprising when one recalls Pavlov's classical experiment in which dogs learned to associate ringing bells with meat powder. But Ader and Cohen demonstrated that the immune system was subject to the same type of associative learning as other body systems.

Until Ader and Cohen's 1975 report, most physiologists believed that the immune system and the nervous system did not interact. Ader and Cohen's results were not immediately accepted (Kiecolt-Glaser & Glaser, 1989, 1993), but after many replications of their findings, physiologists now believe that the immune system and other body systems are interdependent. This belief has spurred researchers to explore the physical mechanisms by which behavior might affect the immune system.

Despite difficulties, psychoneuroimmunology research grew rapidly during the 1980s. As Kiecolt-Glaser and Glaser (1989) pointed out, many psychologists became interested in research in the area, but few had the required knowledge of immunology and the resources to conduct the immunological assays that are necessary to measure immune system function. On the other hand, advances in the field of immunology excited many researchers, and the AIDS epidemic focused public attention (and federal funding) on how behavior influences the immune system and therefore health. The vitality of the new field of psychoneuroimmunology was demonstrated by the appearance in 1987 of a journal, *Brain, Behavior, and Immunity,* devoted to reporting its research.

RESEARCH IN PSYCHONEUROIMMUNOLOGY

According to Ratliff-Crain, Temoshok, Kiecolt-Glaser, and Tamarkin, "the long-range goal of this research is to provide a comprehensive understanding of the role that behavior might play in promoting health and provoking illness" (1989, p. 747). To reach this goal, researchers must establish a connection between psychological factors and changes in immune function and also establish a relationship between impaired immune function and changes in health status. Ideally, research should include all three components—psychological distress, immune system malfunction, and development of illness—in order to establish the connection between stress and illness (Kiecolt-Glaser & Glaser, 1988). This task is difficult for several reasons.

First, not all people whose immune system malfunctions will become ill (Kiecolt-Glaser & Glaser, 1988). Illness is a function of both the immune system's competence and the person's exposure to pathogens, the agents that produce illness. Second, the development of illness can be investigated only through longitudinal studies that follow people for a period of time after they have experienced a decline in immunocompetence resulting from stress. Only a few studies have included all three components, and most have been restricted to nonhuman animals.

The majority of research in psychoneuroimmunology has focused on the relationship between various stressors and altered immune system function. Also, most studies measure the immune system's function by testing blood samples rather than by testing immune function in people's bodies (Stein & Miller, 1993). Some research has concentrated on the relationship between altered immune system function and the development of illness or spread of cancer, but such studies are in the minority. Furthermore, the types of stressors, the species of animals, and the facet of immune system func-

tion have varied, producing an abundance of varied studies as well as varied results (Ader & Cohen, 1993).

An early study by Laudenslager, Ryan, Drugan, Hyson, and Maier (1983) demonstrated that the nature of the stressor makes a difference in immune system response. Using rats, they showed that inescapable stress—in the form of electric shock—resulted in decreased immune responses, a reaction not found in rats that could escape the shocks. Even with similar physical stress, different immune system responses occurred, depending on the psychological factor of the organism's ability to cope actively with the stressor. Another study with rats (Fleshner, Laudenslager, Simons, & Maier, 1989) confirmed the role of control in immune response by measuring immune function in rats that had been attacked by other rats in dominance challenges. Rats that had been bitten did not necessarily experience immune alterations, but those that had been defeated did. Thus, defeat and not physical attack was associated with the inhibition of antibodies.

Some researchers have manipulated short-term stressors in a laboratory situation, such as electric shock, loud noises, or complex cognitive tasks; others have used naturally occurring stress in people's lives to test the effect of stress on immune system function. Jemmott et al. (1983) used the naturally occurring stress of school exams to study immune function in dental students. By measuring levels of immunoglobulin A (IgA), an antibody that protects the upper respiratory tract from infection and also plays a role in fighting dental cavities, the researchers found that dental students had lower antibody levels during periods of school stress than they did during vacations from school. Lowered levels of IgA should produce an increase in illness, but this study did not measure illness consequences. In a subsequent study, Jemmott and Magloire (1988) measured levels of IgA before, during, and after final exams and found that levels of IgA were lower during the final exam period.

In addition to immune function, these researchers measured psychological factors that moderated the influence of academic stress, finding that students who were motivated more by power needs than by friendship needs secreted less IgA during exams (Jemmott et al., 1983) and that social support was a factor in immune suppression (Jemmott & Magloire, 1988). Jemmott and his colleagues (1990) also found that those with a strong need for power and influence over others had less natural killer cell activity than people with a strong need for affiliation. This research indicated that not only stressful events but also the interaction of personal factors and stressful events is related to immune function.

Another psychological variable, loneliness, can also influence immune function in medical students. Kiecolt-Glaser, Speicher, Holliday, and Glaser (1984) found that examination stress affected the function of B-lymphocytes and that lonely students had poorer immunocompetence than those who were less lonely. Kiecolt-Glaser and Glaser (1988) summarized their research with medical students by reporting differences in immunocompetence measured by number of natural killer cells, percentages of T-cells, and percentages of total lymphocytes. A longitudinal assessment of these medical students revealed a trend toward more symptoms of infectious disease before and after exams.

Exam stress is typically a short-term stress, but chronic stress has also been related to decreases in immune competence. Kiecolt-Glaser et al. (1987) found that recently separated women had lower immune system function than married women. This finding is consistent with that of Parkes (1964), who found a higher mortality rate among women whose husbands had recently died, and with that of Schleifer, Keller, Camerino, Thorton, and Stein (1983), who found significant suppression of the immune system in men whose wives had died recently.

Immune function and chronic stress were also the focus of a study by McKinnon, Weisse, Reynolds, Bowles, and Baum (1989), who measured immune system activity in residents who lived near the Three Mile Island nuclear plant at the time of the accident at that facility. These residents were matched to a group of controls on measures of various types of immune system cells and on assessment of antibody responsiveness. The study found that people who lived near the Three Mile Island plant had fewer B-cells, T-cells, and natural killer cells.

Chronic stress can also come from caring for someone with Alzheimer's disease (see Chapter 11 for more about the disease and the stress of care-

giving). Kiecolt-Glaser and her colleagues (Esterling, Kiecolt-Glaser, Bodnar, & Glaser, 1994; Kiecolt-Glaser, Dura, Speicher, Trask, & Glaser, 1991; Kiecolt-Glaser, Marucha, Malarkey, Mercado, & Glaser, 1995) studied a group of Alzheimer's caretakers over a period of years. These researchers found that, compared to a control group with similar demographic characteristics who were not caretakers for someone with a chronic illness, Alzheimer's caretakers had poorer psychological and physical health, longer healing times for wounds, and lowered immune function. Furthermore, the death of the Alzheimer's patient did not improve the psychological health or immune system functioning of the former caretaker. Both caretakers and former caretakers were more depressed and showed lowered immune system functioning, suggesting that this stress continues after the caregiving is over. Thus, chronic stress can affect not only immune system function but also physical and psychological health.

Chronic stress can also influence immune system reaction to acute stressors. Jennifer Pike and her colleagues (Pike, Smith, Hauger, Nicassio, & Irwin, 1994) presented a laboratory stressor to young men who either were or were not chronically stressed and measured their distress as well as several measures of endocrine and immune function. The results indicated that the participants who were under chronic stress at the time of the laboratory stress reacted much more strongly to the laboratory stressor. These results suggest that chronic stress sensitizes people so that their responses to other stressors are exaggerated.

Levy and her colleagues (1989) studied a group of healthy young adults for 6 months to determine the relationship among immune system activity, mood, and physical health. They found that about a third of the group had natural killer cell *activity* below normal, although the *number* of these cells was within the normal range. Those people with lower natural killer cell activity reported more infection-related illness during the study. Younger individuals who reported stronger responses to stress seemed to be particularly vulnerable to illnesses.

After conducting a meta-analysis of studies on stress and immunity, Herbert and Cohen (1993b) concluded that substantial evidence exists for a relationship between stress and decreased immune

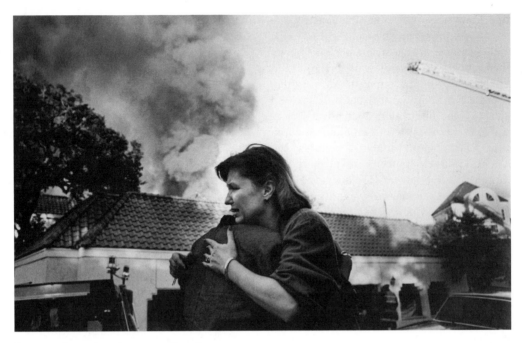

Stress can lower immune system function.

function. This meta-analysis showed that many types of immune system function are related to stress and that immune suppression varies with duration and intensity of the stressor.

Some of the psychoneuroimmunology research that has most clearly demonstrated the three-way link among stress, immune function, and disease has used rats as subjects. In one such study (Ben-Eliyahu, Yirmiya, Liebeskind, Taylor & Gale, 1991), researchers injected rats with tumor material and observed the resulting change in natural killer cell activity and tumor metastases. The results showed that stress increased the metastases when the rats received the tumor material and experienced the stress within 1 hour of each other but not when a 24-hour gap occurred between the stress and the exposure to the malignancy. Thus, this study demonstrated that stress affected both immune function and a disease-related condition.

Bonneau, Sheridan, Feng, and Glaser (1991) used a different disease and a different laboratory stressor but obtained similar results. These researchers exposed rats to the herpes simplex virus, stressed the rats, and observed the changes in immune function. They found that the rats' immune systems were inhibited by the stress, making them less resistant to subsequent infection.

In summary, researchers in the field of psychoneuroimmunology have demonstrated that various functions of the immune system respond to both short-term and long-term psychological stress. In addition, research has revealed that the psychological variables of power motivation, social support, and loneliness affect the immune system. The field of psychoneuroimmunology has therefore made progress toward linking psychological factors, immune system function, and illness, but few studies have included all three elements. The studies that have done so provide evidence for a three-way link among stress, immune function, and disease.

PHYSICAL MECHANISMS OF INFLUENCE

"Psychosocial factors do not influence disease in some mystic fashion. Rather, the physiological status of the host is altered in some way" (Plaut & Friedman, 1981, p. 5). The previous section presented studies showing that such influence occurs but did not explore the physiology underlying that influence.

Immunosuppression may be either part of the body's response to stress or a result of the effects of the stress response (Baum, Davidson, Singer, & Street, 1987). In other words, it may be either a direct or an indirect effect of stress. The effects of stress can occur through the relationship of the nervous system to the immune system through two routes— through the peripheral nervous system and through the secretion of hormones.

According to Maier et al. (1994), evidence exists for connection through both routes. The connection between the nervous system and the immune system occurs through the peripheral nervous system, which has connections to immune system organs such as the thymus, spleen, and lymph nodes. The brain can also communicate with the immune system by producing releasing factors, hormones that stimulate endocrine glands to secrete hormones. These hormones travel through the bloodstream and affect target organs, such as the adrenal glands. (Chapter 3 included a description of these systems and the endocrine component of the stress response.) T- and B-cells have receptors for the glucocorticoid hormones, and lymphocytes have catecholamine receptors.

When the sympathetic nervous system is activated, the adrenal glands release several hormones. The adrenal medulla releases epinephrine and norepinephrine, and the adrenal cortex releases cortisol. The modulation of immunity by epinephrine and norepinephrine seems to come about through the autonomic nervous system rather than through a direct link with the immune system (Hall & Goldstein, 1981).

The release of cortisol from the adrenal cortex results from the release of adrenocorticotropic hormone (ACTH) by the pituitary in the brain. Another brain structure, the hypothalamus, stimulates the pituitary to release ACTH. Elevated cortisol is associated with a number of physical and emotional distress conditions (Baum et al., 1987), and it exerts an anti-inflammatory effect. Cortisol and the glucocorticoids tend to depress immune responses, phagocytosis, and macrophage activation (Cunningham, 1981).

Stein, Schleifer, and Keller (1981) argued that the hypothalamus plays a central role in the modification of immune responses by psychological factors.

They hypothesized that the hypothalamus plays a unique role because of its involvement in regulation of the endocrine system and its role in neurotransmitter processes. The evidence concerning the role of the hypothalamus in both humoral- and cell-mediated immunity suggests a feedback loop between the hypothalamus and the immune response.

The brain might also modulate the immune response through its secretion of neurochemicals (MacLean & Reichlin, 1981). As Jemmott and Locke (1984) pointed out, lymphocytes have receptors for beta-endorphin, one of the brain's opoid peptides that has been shown to relate to immunosuppression. Moreover, the release of the opoid peptides occurs through the same stimuli—stress and distress—that trigger the release of hormones in the interaction between the pituitary and adrenal glands (Baum et al., 1987). The similarity of the situations that prompt release and the physical mechanisms for reception suggests that neurochemicals are a possible mechanism by which the brain influences the immune response.

Maier et al. (1994, p. 1007) summarized the relationship between nervous and immune systems:

> Destruction or stimulation of neural pathways that are connected to the immune system do, in fact, alter the function of the immune system, and so the connection between the CNS is of real significance, not merely an anatomic curiosity. Similarly, blocking the hormone receptors on lymphocytes alters the course of immunity.

Although psychoneuroimmunology research has concentrated on the potential for influence of the nervous system on the immune system, Maier et al. argued that the physical mechanisms of influence also act in the other direction: The immune system has the power to alter behavior through affecting the nervous system. The response to immune system activation is equivalent to the peripheral nervous system's stress response. Thus, the interrelationship between nervous system and immune system is complex, with possibilities for influence of each on the other.

THERAPEUTIC EFFECTS

Most studies in psychoneuroimmunology have demonstrated that immune system activity decreases following psychological changes. A basic assumption of many psychoneuroimmunologists is that increases in psychological distress lead to immunological changes and that these changes lead to illness (Kiecolt-Glaser & Glaser, 1988). If this reasoning is correct, then the field of psychoneuroimmunology can spell out conditions that produce illness. But is it possible to boost immunocompetence through changes in behavior? Would this boost enhance health? A few studies have suggested that therapeutic uses of psychoneuroimmunology may be possible but that boosting immune function above normal good functioning is probably not possible (Kiecolt-Glaser & Glaser, 1993). However, many people have compromised immune system function, and improvements could make a difference for them.

Kiecolt-Glaser et al. (1985) improved immune system function in a group of elderly people, who are especially at risk because the immune system loses some of its effectiveness with age. The elderly people in this study received relaxation training, which appeared to help boost their immune system function.

Pennebaker, Kiecolt-Glaser, and Glaser (1988) investigated the relationship between immune function and methods of dealing with troubling experiences by comparing two groups of healthy college students. One group wrote about troubling experiences, and the other group wrote about superficial topics. The rationale for the comparison was that writing about troubling experiences would constitute a confrontation with them. The results suggested that college students benefited from confronting traumatic experiences simply by writing about them. They demonstrated increased cellular immune system function and reported fewer visits to the health center.

Michael Antoni and his colleagues (Antoni, 1993; Antoni et al., 1990; Antoni et al., 1991) have explored another possibility for beneficial psychological interventions. Their research concentrated on individuals infected with the HIV virus and those who were at high risk for infection who had not yet developed AIDS or learned of their HIV status. The researchers' purpose was to determine whether such interventions as aerobic training and stress management could boost immune function in these at-risk individuals and thereby delay the onset of AIDS

symptoms in infected men. Although complex, results from their program of research suggest that the intervention positively affected immune system function, holding some potential that such interventions could slow the progress of AIDS.

Another study (Levy, 1989) showed that a cognitive-behavioral intervention with cancer patients after surgery was capable of affecting the immune system. In this study, both the percentage and the killing ability of natural killer cells was significantly higher in the intervention (cognitive-behavioral) group than in the control group.

Another potential application involves depression of immune system function. In 1975, Ader and Cohen demonstrated that immune function could be classically conditioned, and in a subsequent study, Ader and Cohen (1982) showed that conditioned immunosuppression could be used therapeutically. Their subjects consisted of mice that were genetically prone to lupus erythematosus, an autoimmune disease. This disease can be controlled with a drug that suppresses the immune system, slowing the body's attack on itself. Using the same procedure as in their 1975 study, Ader and Cohen conditioned the mice to respond a saccharin solution with immunosuppression; the saccharin solution was the conditioning stimulus, the immunosuppressant drug was the unconditioned stimulus—and immune suppression was the unconditioned response. The magnitude of the immune system suppression from the conditioning alone was not sufficient to produce therapeutic effects. However, administering the saccharin solution *and* a low dose of the drug (which would not have produced therapeutic effects by itself) brought about sufficient immunosuppression to produce therapeutic effects. Ader and Cohen were able to demonstrate that conditioned immune suppression allowed a lower dose of a drug to have therapeutic effects. This provocative result suggests potential treatment for autoimmune diseases.

SUMMARY OF PSYCHONEUROIMMUNOLOGY RESEARCH

Research in the field of psychoneuroimmunology attempts to link psychological factors, immune system changes, and changes in health status. Although the history of this field is short, the research has succeeded in demonstrating that distress and other psychological factors can depress immune system function, both in the number of immune system cells and in the activity of particular types of antibodies. Some research has been successful in linking immune system changes to changes in health status, and this link is necessary to complete the chain between psychological factors and physical illness.

In addition to establishing links between psychological factors and immune system changes, theorists and researchers in the field of psychoneuroimmunology have attempted to specify the physical mechanisms through which these changes occur. The possibilities for the mechanisms include direct connections between nervous and immune systems and an indirect connection through the neuroendocrine system, and evidence exists for both. A complete understanding of these mechanisms will reveal how psychological factors affect the nervous system and how the nervous system influences specific immune system structures and functions.

The promise of psychoneuroimmunology comes not only from an understanding of the relationships among behavior, the nervous system, and the immune system but also from therapeutic applications in the form of behavioral interventions for people whose immune systems are not functioning effectively.

PERSONAL FACTORS AFFECTING STRESS AND ILLNESS

Why does stress affect some people, apparently causing them to get sick, while leaving others unaffected? The relation between stress and illness is far from perfect, and some high-stress individuals become sick while others remain healthy. Then, too, some low-stress people develop an illness while others do not. Why do some people fall ill from stress while other people stay well? This section looks at three possible explanations for this question. First, the *diathesis-stress model* suggests that some people are more inherently vulnerable to the effects of stress; second, the *hardy personality model* holds that psychologically healthy individuals are buffered against the harmful effects of stress; and third, the

identity disruption model proposes that psychologically unhealthy people are placed in danger of illness whenever they experience positive life events that are incongruent with their negative view of themselves.

THE DIATHESIS-STRESS MODEL

The **diathesis-stress model** suggests that some individuals are vulnerable to stress-related illnesses because either genetic weakness or biochemical imbalance inherently predisposes them to those illnesses (Gatchel, 1993). The diathesis-stress model has a long history in psychology, particularly in explaining the development of psychological disorders. During the 1960s and 1970s, the concept was used as an explanation for the development of psychophysiological disorders (Levi, 1974; Sternbach, 1966) as well as schizophrenic episodes, manic-depressive disorders, anxiety disorders, and other forms of neurotic and psychotic conditions (Rosenthal, 1970; Zubin & Spring, 1977).

Applied to either psychological or physiological disorders, the diathesis-stress model holds that some people are predisposed to react abnormally to environmental stressors. This predisposition (diathesis) is usually thought to be inherited through biochemical or organ system weakness, but some theorists (Sternbach, 1966; Zubin & Spring, 1977) also have included acquired propensities as components of vulnerability. Whether inherited or acquired, the vulnerability is relatively permanent. What varies over time are environmental stressors, which may account for the waxing and waning of illnesses.

Thus, the diathesis-stress model assumes that two factors are necessary to produce illness. First, the person must have a relatively permanent predisposition to the illness, and second, that person must experience some sort of stress. Diathetic individuals respond pathologically to the same stressful conditions with which most people can easily cope. For those people with a strong predisposition to an illness, even a mild environmental stressor may be sufficient to produce an illness episode. The illness does not flow from an interaction between personality and stress but from the interaction of *personal physiology* and stress (Cotton, 1990).

Sternbach (1966) explained the development of illness in terms of a stereotypical pattern of physical responses to life situations. These stereotypical patterns vary from person to person but are consistent within each person, placing people who exhibit these patterns in danger of developing a stress-related illness. For example, people who have developed a pattern of responding to stress by increased gastric activity become vulnerable to gastrointestinal problems if they experience many stress situations. The repeated activation of that organ system creates wear and tear, which can permanently damage the system. Different people have different vulnerabilities, resulting in a variety of possibilities for damage due to diathesis combined with stress.

THE HARDY PERSONALITY MODEL

The converse of the diathesis-stress model would hold that psychologically healthy people are buffered against levels of stress that might lead to an illness in less healthy individuals. In 1977, Suzanne Kobasa and her mentor Salvatore Maddi proposed the notion of the hardy personality as an explanation for why stress relates to illness in some people but not others. The **hardy personality model** grew out of existential personality theory, which emphasizes the idea of an authentic person in control of his or her life. Kobasa and Maddi (1977) hypothesized that hardiness buffers the harmful effects of stress and thus protects the hardy personality from stress-related illness. In her original study, Kobasa (1979) looked at middle-aged, mostly White, Protestant executives who had filled out Holmes and Rahe's Social Readjustment Rating Scale. She followed these middle- and upper-level managers for 3 years, monitoring both their level of stress and their incidence of illness. As a result, she was able to identify two groups: high-stress/low-illness executives and high-stress/high-illness executives.

Kobasa used the term *hardiness* to describe those people who were able to withstand stress and not succumb to illness. Hardy executives differed from those who became sick in three important ways. First, they expressed a stronger sense of *commitment* to self; second, they demonstrated an internal locus of *control* over their lives; and third, they were more likely to view necessary readjustments as a *challenge*

rather than a stress. These three factors—commitment, control, and challenge—separated the hardy executives from those who became ill even though both groups experienced equal amounts of stress. Those who became ill were characterized by external locus of control or the belief that important factors in their lives are beyond their personal control, a sense of nihilism or meaninglessness of life, a feeling of powerlessness, alienation from self, and a lack of vigor or active involvement with their surroundings. These findings suggest that hardiness may act as a buffer against the harmful effects of stress.

Later, Kobasa and her colleagues (Kobasa, Maddi, & Courington, 1981; Kobasa, Maddi, & Kahn, 1982) investigated the hypothesis that hardy male executives are able to fend off the effects of stress and thus avoid subsequent illness. At 1-year intervals over a 2-year period, male executives who had previously been classified as to their hardiness filled out a modified Holmes and Rahe Social Readjustment Rating Scale and a questionnaire asking about illness symptoms. The investigators found that hardiness—defined as commitment, control, and challenge—was related to a decrease in illness, thus suggesting that hardiness protected high-stressed executives against illness.

However, Kobasa's hardiness hypothesis has received only mixed support from other investigators. In a study with undergraduate women, Ganellen and Blaney (1984) found that hardiness by itself did not offer much protection against stress, but when combined with social support (see Chapter 6), hardiness buffered these women against the harmful consequences of stress. In addition, a study by Schmied and Lawler (1986) of female secretaries showed no support for the notion that a hardy personality provides a buffer between stress and illness. These authors offered several possible reasons for the discrepancy between their findings and those of Kobasa. First, hardiness may not generalize to women, at least for physical symptoms. Second, the jobs of clerical workers may not lend themselves to the buffering effect. Third, hardiness may simply be defined differently for women than it is for men. Fourth, because they found that the hardier secretaries were older and better educated, the authors suggested that age and education may have confounded their results.

Also, Funk and Houston (1987), Allred and Smith (1989), and Funk (1992) contended that *neuroticism,* or general maladjustment, may account for any relationship between hardiness and self-reports of illness. These authors contended that neuroticism overlaps substantially with measures of hardiness and probably accounts for most of the correlation between hardiness scores and subsequent illness, especially psychological problems. Williams, Wiebe, and Smith (1992) supported this contention in a study that showed hardiness, coping, and self-reported illness to be correlated with neuroticism. In other words, hardiness may simply measure the broad dimension of neuroticism, an underlying personality factor highly related to subjective reports of illness but not necessarily to objective accounts. Williams et al. further suggested that hardiness is not a unitary construct and that commitment and control are more significant than challenge in predicting which people are most likely to use adaptive coping behaviors in response to stress.

Nevertheless, some studies have provided at least partial support for Kobasa's hardiness concept. Holahan and Moos (1985) investigated a random sample of families in the San Francisco area and found that people who remained healthy despite high stress were more relaxed, felt positive about change, were motivated to achieve and endure, and felt influential rather than helpless. In a later study, Contrada (1989) looked at the *interaction* of hardiness with the Type A behavior pattern (see Chapter 9) to assess its effects on cardiovascular response. Contrada assessed male college students for hardiness and the Type A behavior pattern and then gave them a frustrating psychomotor task. In general, Type A students showed increases in both systolic and diastolic blood pressure after being frustrated, but Type A students with high hardiness scores did not show as large an increase in diastolic blood pressure. This finding suggests that hardiness may be a buffer for diastolic blood pressure but not systolic blood pressure. However, Allred and Smith (1989) found almost the opposite results—that hardiness was associated with *increased* cardiovascular responsiveness. In this study, hardy people had higher than expected levels of systolic blood pressure after being exposed to a challenging task. Allred and Smith suggested that the increased cardiovascular responsiveness

may have resulted from increased coping efforts by hardy individuals.

The notion that some people possess personal traits that help protect them against the harmful effects of stress is an appealing one. Nonetheless, Kobasa's hardiness concept has been seriously questioned. In critiquing the concept, Hull, Van Treuren, and Virnelli (1987) and Funk (1992) concluded that hardiness probably does not provide a buffer against stress. Hull et al. contended that the challenge component has little, if any, relationship to health. The other two variables, control and commitment, have a direct rather than a buffering effect on health because lack of control and lack of commitment are themselves psychologically stressful. Funk also suggested that the use of self-reports to assess physical illness was a potentially serious methodological weakness in Kobasa's studies, as people who score low on the hardiness scales have a tendency to see themselves as having numerous physical symptoms, even when they are not sick. Objective measures of health, such as physician diagnoses, would eliminate this problem.

Orr and Westman (1990) reviewed much of the hardiness literature and concluded that, at best, hardiness offers little substantiated protection against physical illness, although it may buffer against some psychological disorders. In addition, they found that Kobasa's three components—commitment, control, and challenge—were not independent, with commitment and control being highly interrelated. They also noted that the challenge component offered no additional power to the hardiness concept. In addition, Wiebe and Williams (1992) reviewed the literature on hardiness and reported that the research is largely inconsistent regarding the ability of hardiness to buffer the effects of stress on physical health.

However, Kobasa (who has also published under the names S. C. Ouellette and S. C. Ouellette Kobasa) has pointed out that many of the inconsistent findings on hardiness are the result of different measures of the hardy personality (Ouellette, 1993). She contended that many investigators have attempted to extend the concept to inappropriate populations— for example, college undergraduates. Hardiness, with its origins embedded in existential philosophy and psychology, is probably most applicable to people who are searching for a sense of meaning or purpose in life, who are motivated by responsibility and freedom, who view subjective experience as reality, and who believe that they are capable of significantly shaping society (Ouellette, 1993).

Because an important function of any theory is to generate research, the hardy personality theory has been at least partially successful. To date, more than 100 research papers have been published on this concept. Moreover, the notion that some people, for whatever reason, are buffered against the deleterious effects of stress has led others to hypothesize alternative models. For example, Aaron Antonovsky (1987) suggested that a sense of coherence helps people manage stress and stay well; Michael Rosenbaum (1988, 1990) proposed the notion of learned resourcefulness as the force that distinguishes people who will get sick from those who will not; and Greg Feist (Feist, Bodner, Jacobs, Miles, & Tan, 1995) found that subjective well-being (along with one's worldview and one's ability to cope constructively with life's experiences) acts as both a cause and an effect of one's physical health status. Each of these models rests on assumptions that the relationship between stress and subsequent illness is complex and that personal qualities influence people's view of stress, their personal ability to cope, and their perception of when they are sick.

THE IDENTITY DISRUPTION MODEL

A third attempt to relate personal factors to stress was proposed by Jonathon Brown and Kevin McGill (1989), who were interested in discovering why positive life events might produce negative health consequences. Remember, some items of the Social Readjustment Rating Scale are basically positive — for instance, marriage, marital reconciliation, and outstanding personal achievement — and yet show some relationship to health problems. Brown and McGill's **identity disruption model** suggests that people with low self-esteem have difficulty accepting the good things that happen to them because positive events lie outside their sense of identity. In contrast, when good things happen to people with high self-esteem, their identity is not disrupted. The more that life events force people to change what

they think about themselves, the greater is their risk of developing an illness.

The identity disruption model follows a two-step process. First, life events can change one's sense of identity by forcing an abandonment of one's existing view of self. For example, when students graduate from college and enter a profession, they no longer see themselves as students but as teachers, nurses, businesspeople, and so forth. Similarly, marriage changes one's identity from a single person to a married person with a spouse. Second, identity disruption has a negative impact on health. Earlier personality theorists, such as Prescott Lecky (1945) and George Kelly (1955), emphasized the self-consistency of personality. Any event that is inconsistent with the self-concept is seen as a threat to the person's identity. Therefore, any change, whether positive or negative, will force a person to devote extra attention to this threat, thereby lowering his or her ability to withstand stress.

If the identity disruption model is valid, then positive events will be easily accepted by people with high self-esteem but will force an identity reorganization in people with low self-esteem. More specifically, positive life events will combine with low self-esteem to produce illness. To test this hypothesis, Brown and McGill (1989) conducted two separate investigations. In their first study, they measured life events, self-esteem, and physical health of high school girls at the beginning of the school year and assessed their health again 4 months later. In support of the identity disruption hypothesis, they found that positive life events were linked to increases in illness only for students who were low in self-esteem. For girls with high self-esteem, illness declined as positive life events rose.

A weakness of this study was the authors' use of self-reports of illness. As discussed in connection with the hardiness studies, self-reports can contaminate results because people with low hardiness may be more sensitive to physical symptoms and thus tend to overreport illnesses. Similarly, people with low self-esteem may tend to overreport physical symptoms. To avoid this limitation, Brown and McGill conducted a second study that used a more objective measure of illness; namely, visits to a health facility. Participants in this second investigation were female and male college students who were assessed during the fall semester on life events, self-esteem, and illness symptoms and then measured again during the spring for physical illness. Results of this study paralleled those of the study on high school girls. College students with high self-esteem enjoyed good health following positive life events, but those with low self-esteem had more illness symptoms after reporting positive life events.

The identity disruption model is based on the logical assumption that personal identity is threatened by positive life experiences for people who see themselves as somehow undeserving of such experiences. Unlike the hardiness concept, however, the identity disruption model has failed to generate much research. Indeed, the little research that has appeared is not very supportive of Brown and McGill's hypothesis. For example, Kaniasty and Norris (1993) studied older adults and found no support for the identity disruption model among people 55 and older. Perhaps the model does not extend to older adults, or perhaps the identity disruption hypothesis is not the answer to why positive events bring about negative health consequences.

The diathesis-stress model, the hardiness concept, and the identity disruption model offer three possible explanations for why some people are adversely affected by stress while others remain free from illness. All three adopt a biopsychosocial approach, which assumes that psychological, social, and biological factors interact to contribute to illness. At present, however, none of the three models offers a satisfactory explanation for why some people develop stress-related illnesses while others stay well.

DOES STRESS CAUSE ILLNESS?

Illness is caused by many factors, and stress may be one of those factors. Due to the variety and combinations of influences, the relationship between measures of stress and illness should be no more than modest. Indeed, most research substantiates this expectation. A typical study found a correlation of about .20 between life events and depression, with a slightly stronger relationship when only undesirable events were included (Tausig, 1982).

In any consideration of the association between illness and major life events or daily hassles, it is well to remember that most people at risk from stressful experiences do *not* develop an illness. Furthermore, in contrast to other risk factors—such as having high cholesterol levels, smoking cigarettes, or drinking alcohol—the risks conferred by life events are usually temporary. As Rahe (1984, p. 49) expressed it, "Most individuals with high recent life-change totals do not remain at such levels for more than a year or two before returning to baseline levels which connote far less risk."

In this section, we review the evidence concerning the link between stress and several physical illnesses, including headache, infectious illness, cardiovascular disease, diabetes mellitus, premature delivery, asthma, and rheumatoid arthritis. In addition, stress shows some relationship to negative moods and mood disorders such as depression and anxiety disorders.

STRESS AND PHYSICAL ILLNESS

What is the evidence linking stress to illness? Which illnesses have been implicated? What physiological mechanism might mediate the connection between stress and illness?

Herbert and Cohen (1994) discussed several possibilities for pathways through which stress could produce illness. Direct influence could occur through the effects of stress on the nervous and endocrine systems as well as on the immune system. Because any or all of these systems can create physical illness, sufficient physiological foundations exist to provide a link between stress and illness. In addition, indirect effects could occur through changes in health practices that increase risks. Therefore, possibilities exist for both direct and indirect effects of stress on illness. Does the evidence support these hypothetical relationships?

Selye's concept of stress (see Chapter 3) includes suppression of the immune response, but until recently no evidence existed to support this hypothesis. Now a growing body of evidence suggests interactions among the nervous, endocrine, and immune systems. This interaction is similar to the responses hypothesized by Selye and provides strong evidence

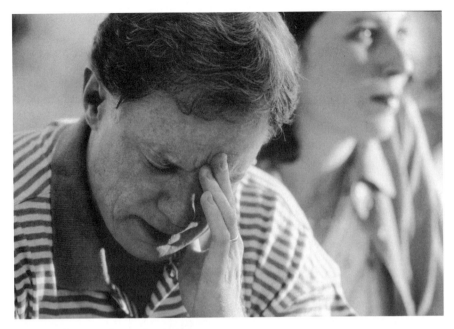

Stress is a factor in chronic headaches.

that stress could cause headaches, viral illnesses, cardiovascular disease, and a variety of other physical ailments.

Headaches

For most people, headaches are a minor problem that require little more than over-the-counter medication, but headache is also one of the most frequent causes of visits to physicians (Hatch, 1993). Headache can signal serious medical conditions, but most often the pain associated with the headache is the problem. The majority of those who seek medical assistance for headaches are plagued by the same sorts of headaches as those who do not; the difference stems from the frequency and severity of the headaches or from personal factors involved in seeking assistance.

Although over 100 types of headaches exist, distinguishing among them has become controversial, and the underlying causes for the most common types remain unclear (Hatch, 1993). Nevertheless, diagnostic criteria have been devised for several types of headaches. The most frequent type of headache is *tension headache,* usually associated with increased muscle tension in the head and neck region. Tension is also a factor in vascular headache.

Holroyd, Appel, and Andrasik (1983) discussed the difficulty in separating the two, contending that many tension headaches have vascular components and vice versa. The most notorious of the vascular headaches are *migraine headaches,* hypothesized to be caused by changes in constriction of the vascular arteries and associated with throbbing pain localized in one side of the head.

Stress is recognized as a factor in both tension and vascular headaches (Rasmussen, 1993). However, de Benedittis and Lorenzetti (1992) found that the type of stress associated with headaches was not traumatic life events but rather the sorts of occurrences that Lazarus and his colleagues labeled daily hassles. By administering stress scales to a group of chronic headache patients and contrasting them with a group who did not have headaches, de Benedettis and Lorenzetti found that people with tension and mixed headaches were more likely than those with migraines to report more and more intense daily hassles.

Like most people, Rick had always experienced occasional headaches, but several years before his divorce, his headaches became more frequent and more severe. He traces this change to a neck injury, but he also believes that tension is the basis for his headaches and that they are exacerbated by stress. Indeed, headaches were a major problem during the 18 months in his life when he was under exceedingly high levels of stress.

Infectious Illness

Are people under stress more likely than non-stressed individuals to develop infectious illnesses such as the common cold? Research suggests that the answer may be yes. Stone, Reed, and Neale (1987) studied married couples who kept diaries on their own and their spouse's desirable and undesirable daily life experiences. Participants developed somewhat more infectious illnesses (colds or flu) 3 and 4 days after a decline in desirable events and 4 and 5 days after an increase in undesirable events. Although these associations were not strong, this study was the first prospective design to show a relationship between daily life experiences and subsequent illness, when both the life events and the illness were measured on a daily basis. In a later study, Stone et al. (1992) intentionally inoculated 17 University of Virginia undergraduate students (who were each paid $350 for their participation) with a cold virus. Although all students were infected, only 12 developed clinical colds. Stone et al. found no difference between those who developed colds and those who did not on current mood and perceived stress. However, students who developed colds reported significantly more positive and negative major life events during the previous year. Results of this experimental study suggest that a high level of life events (either positive or negative) may lead to the development of colds.

Using a similar design, Sheldon Cohen and his colleagues (Cohen, Tyrrell, & Smith, 1991, 1993) intentionally exposed healthy participants in Salisbury, England, to various common cold viruses to see who would develop a cold and who would not. Cohen et al. (1991) used three measures of psychological stress: (1) number of major stressful life events during the past year; (2) perception that demands exceed a person's ability to cope; and (3) current level of negative affect—that is, a person's self-ratings on 15 emotional states, such as hostile, scared, and angry at self. The experimenters combined the three stress measures into a single stress index and then assessed the level of psychological stress in nearly 400 healthy male and female participants. Next, they gave nasal drops containing one of five respiratory viruses to people in an experimental group and placebo saline nasal drops to people in a control group. They found that the degree of psychological stress was related in a dose-response manner to the number of both respiratory infections and clinical colds the participants developed. In other words, the higher the person's stress, the more likely it was that he or she would become ill. The associations were similar for all five viruses and could not be explained by other health-related habits and conditions, including smoking, alcohol, exercise, diet, quality of sleep, and white blood cell count. Also, the personal qualities of self-esteem, personal control, and introversion/extraversion were unrelated to the number of infections and colds that the participants developed. Moreover, the relationship between stress and colds was not affected by whether the participants shared housing with an infected person. Later, Cohen, Tyrell, and Smith (1993) analyzed the relationship between the common cold and the three individual measures of stress. Each of the three measures independently predicted a person's risk of developing a cold.

The findings of Stone et al. and Cohen et al. suggest that stress may be a more important contributor to the common cold than diet, lack of sleep, or even white cell count. To develop a cold, one must be exposed to a cold virus, but exposure alone cannot predict who will develop a cold and who will not. Psychological stress now seems to be the best predictor.

Cardiovascular Disease

Cardiovascular disease (CVD) has a number of behavioral risk factors, some of which are related to stress. Chapter 9 examines these behavioral risk factors in more detail; in this section we look only at stress as a contributor to CVD. Although some people assume that stress is a major cause of heart disease, the available evidence is less clear.

Studies from the 1970s seemed to support the notion that stress leads to heart disease; their findings indicated that people who died of a sudden heart attack had experienced more stressful life events in the 6 months preceding the attack than did those who survived (Rahe, Romo, Bennett, & Siltanen, 1974). In addition, specific stresses such as bereavement, loss of prestige, and loss of employment have been found to be risks for heart attack (Kavanagh & Shepard, 1973).

However, later studies have yielded less consistent results. A follow-up of the Multiple Risk Factor Intervention Trial (MRFIT) demonstrated that stressful life events during each of the 6 previous years were positively related only to angina but not to risk of coronary heart disease or to nonfatal heart attack (Hollis, Connett, Stevens, & Greenlick, 1990). Unexpectedly, this study showed that stressful life events were *inversely* related to all-cause mortality; that is, the men with lower levels of stress were more likely to die than those with higher levels.

Rosengren, Tibblin, and Wilhelmsen (1991) found only a modest relationship between stress and coronary artery disease (CAD) in middle-aged men. These investigators divided men with no prior history of heart disease into six levels of psychological stress, followed them for 12 years, and noted different rates of coronary artery disease. They defined psychological stress as feelings of tension, irritability, or anxiety, or sleep difficulties as the result of work. Compared with men in the four lowest levels of stress, those in the two highest levels had about a 50% greater likelihood of CAD. However, there was no increased risk from level 1 to level 4, suggesting that only *substantial* psychological stress contributes to coronary artery disease. In a second part of this study, the researchers found no significant relationship between stressful life events and CAD in a sample of 50-year-old men.

In Chapter 3 we cited a study by Karasek et al. (1988) that reported that job strain, defined as jobs low in decision latitude and high in psychological work load, was related to an increased risk of heart attack. However, these risks were modest—about 25% excess deaths in one sample and about 33% in another. Using the definition of job strain developed by Karasek et al., researchers in Sweden found a 70% increase in all-cause mortality for men with jobs low in control and high in psychological demand (Falk, Hanson, Issacsson, & Ostergren, 1992). The study indicated that high job strain combined with a weak social network and low social support resulted in an increase of relative risk that was more than four times the rate of men who had low job strain and adequate social supports. Thus, it appears that job strain may have a synergistic effect with a weak social network and low social support to contribute to death rates. (A **synergistic effect** means that the total impact exceeds the sum of two or more individual effects; that is, the combination of job strain, a weak social network, and low social support would have a much higher risk than their separate risks added together.)

This increased risk, however, does not hold for all groups. In the Honolulu Heart Program (Reed, LaCroix, Karasek, Miller, & MacLean, 1989), no significant relationship appeared between job strain (high psychological demands and low job control) and coronary heart disease in men of Japanese ancestry in Hawaii. For the men who had adopted a more Westernized lifestyle, there was a slight inverse trend; that is, men high in job strain had slightly lower CHD.

These somewhat inconsistent results suggest that individual factors such as social support and a traditional lifestyle may interact with job strain either to buffer the risk for heart disease and all causes of mortality or to contribute to them. Also, physical fitness may moderate the effects of stress on disease. Brown (1991), for example, studied male and female undergraduate students and found that those who were physically fit were less vulnerable to the adverse effects of stress. Although heart disease was not used as the dependent variable in this study, a major conclusion was that "life stress had little ill effects among subjects whose fitness level was relatively high" (Brown, 1991, p. 560).

Hypertension. Hypertension is a cardiovascular disorder that is sometimes assumed to be related to stress, but the evidence for this relationship is mostly circumstantial (Holroyd et al., 1983). Situational factors such as noise can elevate blood pressure, but most studies have shown that blood pressure returns to normal when the situational stimulus is removed.

In contrast, one study concerned the effect of *chronic* exposure to noise on hypertension (Talbott et al., 1985). This study measured the blood pressure of men working in two plants—one with a high noise level and the other with a low noise level. The average blood pressure of the two groups did not differ, except for men over 55 years old who had noise-induced hearing loss. A significant relationship was found between blood pressure and exposure to noise sufficient to cause hearing loss. This study suggests that when repeated exposure to noise is sufficient to induce hearing loss, chronic hypertension may result, at least in certain age groups.

Further clarification of the role of stress in hypertension has come from Light and her associates (Light, Kopke, Obrist, & Willis, 1983). After finding that stress situations were capable of inducing kidney retention of salt and that the amount of such retention was greater in rats that developed high blood pressure, the researchers performed an analogous experiment on humans. They chose people who had normal blood pressure but who were at high risk for developing hypertension and compared them with people whose blood pressure was in the normal range and who were not at high risk. After some testing, the researchers were able to divide each group of participants into those whose sympathetic nervous systems responded strongly to the stress situations and those who showed no such response. The high-risk participants with a strong sympathetic response retained sodium during the testing, but the low-risk participants did not. This finding suggests that stress can cause sodium retention in a particular type of person.

A review of research on stress and sodium intake (Haythornthwaite, 1992–93) showed that both factors can affect blood pressure and that the two in combination may have a synergistic effect. In studies using both human and nonhuman animals, the combination of stress and sodium in the diet has resulted in elevations in blood pressure.

Therefore, the relationship between stress and temporary increases in blood pressure is stronger than the evidence for stress as a factor in chronic hypertension. Some evidence exists showing that chronic stress may be related to hypertension, but other factors, such as sodium intake, may interact with stress to raise the risk for hypertension.

Reactivity. The idea that some people react more strongly to stress than other people has received considerable attention in recent years. This response, called *reactivity,* may be an important stress-related factor in the development of cardiovascular disease. Matthews (1986a, p. xi) defined reactivity "as the magnitude of an array of physiological responses to discrete, environmental stressors—for example, performing a challenging mental task or exercising strenuously." For such responses to play a role in the development of cardiovascular disease, they must be relatively stable within an individual and be prompted by events that occur frequently in the individual's life. Matthews (1986b) hypothesized that people are probably reactive to a specific class of stressors—for example, interpersonal situations, competition, public speaking, alcohol, caffeine, or nicotine. Researchers have investigated the stability of reactivity and have also tried to discover those events that prompt it. Exercise, competition, cigarette smoking, cold temperatures, video games, and arguments are some of the situations that have been considered as possible stressors. In addition, researchers have measured an array of cardiac responses, including diastolic blood pressure, systolic blood pressure, heart rate, and catecholamine excretion as indexes of reactivity.

With such a variety of independent and dependent variables, unambiguous results would be surprising. Kamarck and his colleagues (Kamarck, Jennings, Pogue-Geile, & Manuck, 1994) made sense of the variety of measurements by conducting a factor analysis of stress-related measures of reactivity, revealing two factors: vascular reactivity and cardiac reactivity. Their research showed that the patterns of responses for these factors were stable over time for the same people and for similar tasks on different people. This research demonstrated one of the necessary conditions for demonstrating a relationship between reactivity and cardiovascular disease: a stable pattern of responding to similar stresses over time for the same individual.

Smith and Allred (1989) investigated the role of hostility in blood pressure reactivity. They measured men's hostility level and then exposed them to confrontation and argument. They found that the high-hostility group showed greater systolic and diastolic blood pressure responses and concluded that hostility is associated with greater responses to an interpersonal stressor.

In addition to hostility, reactivity is also related to aggression, anxiety, and locus of control (Houston, 1986), but coping style and outlook can also influence cardiac reactivity. Dolan, Sherwood, and Light (1992) found that young men who were high in the tendency to cope with stress by keeping to themselves and blaming themselves showed higher blood pressure responses than men who were less likely to use this style of coping. Therefore, several personality factors distinguish people who are high from those who are low in reactivity.

Gender has also been a factor of substantial interest in reactivity. Because men develop cardiovascular disease at a younger age than women, researchers have expected to find gender differences, and such differences appear in connection with some stress tasks but not others. Stone, Dembroski, Costa, and MacDougall (1990) hypothesized that young men would show greater cardiac reactivity than young women. The researchers used both a physical stimulus (cigarette smoking) and a competitive challenge (playing a video game), but they failed to find a clear-cut pattern of responses. On some measures the women showed greater reactivity than the men; on other measures no differences appeared. On only one measure — systolic blood pressure as a response to the video game — the men showed greater reactivity than the women.

Subsequent research (Light, Turner, Hinderliter, & Sherwood, 1993a) also produced some variability in the tasks that elicit different cardiovascular reactions for women and men, but men showed greater overall blood pressure increases and slower recovery times than women. Blood pressure changes in the workplace are also related to reactivity (Light, Turner, Hinderliter, & Sherwood, 1993b). These gender differences appear during childhood (Treiber et al., 1993) and persist over time from childhood to adolescence (Murphy, Stoney, Alpert, & Walker, 1995). Therefore, boys and men seem to show higher reactivity than girls and women, and these gender-related differences may relate to the development of cardiovascular disease.

The higher rates of cardiovascular disease for African Americans compared to European Americans has led researchers to examine differences in reactivity between these two ethnic groups. The results generally confirm the differences in the expected direction: African Americans show higher cardiac reactivity than European Americans. Murphy et al. (1995) found that beginning during childhood and continuing to adolescence, African Americans showed greater reactivity than European

Americans. Treiber et al. (1993) found such differences among children as young as 6 years. These researchers also found that African American children with a family history of cardiovascular disease showed significantly greater reactivity than any other group of children in the study.

The ethnic and gender differences in reactivity are intriguing but not explanatory. The agreement between the demographics of cardiovascular disease and differences in reactivity among various groups suggests that reactivity plays a role in the development of disease. As Norman Anderson (1993) pointed out, the underlying nature of those differences remains to be explained. Knowing that African Americans are higher in reactivity and in rates of cardiovascular disease does not reveal the facet of membership in that group that leads to the development of cardiovascular problems.

Understanding both the reasons for ethnic and gender differences in reactivity and the mechanisms through which reactivity might produce cardiovascular disease will be necessary. The recent research is suggestive and promising.

Risky Behaviors.   In addition to affecting physiological responses in ways that promote disease, stress may alter health-related behaviors and produce an indirect effect on health (Herbert & Cohen, 1994). Epstein and Perkins (1988) hypothesized such an effect for smoking, noting that cigarette smoking doubles or triples a person's risk of developing cardiovascular disease but does not have the same impact on all smokers. Epstein and Perkins suggested three possible hypotheses for the variable effect of smoking, all relating stress and smoking to cardiovascular disease.

First, stress may increase the amount a person smokes. Many smokers report that they feel less tension after smoking and that they are more likely to smoke when experiencing stress. Second, Epstein and Perkins speculated that smoking may reduce subjective feelings of anxiety and stress, thereby increasing smokers' endurance to the stressor and changing the rate of habituation to that stressor. In other words, people may use smoking as means of coping with persistent stress rather than finding more beneficial ways of managing it. In time, a kind of tolerance or insensitivity builds up toward the stressful stimulus. Third, smoking and stress may have an additive or even synergistic effect on the cardiovascular system. This third hypothesis suggests that stressed smokers have a greater risk for cardiovascular disease than either nonstressed smokers or stressed nonsmokers.

These three hypotheses are not necessarily mutually exclusive, and each of them may have some validity. More research is needed to identify the specific mechanisms involved in the interaction among stress, smoking, and cardiovascular disease.

People may also increase their level of alcohol consumption, use illicit drugs, and change their eating habits when under stress. Berger and Adesso (1991) studied the expectation that drinking would change mood and found that those who experienced negative moods drank more than others and believed that drinking elevated their mood. Berger and Adesso also found that the tendency to drink as a way of coping with feeling bad is more common in men than in women. Tavris (1992) hypothesized that men are more likely than women to drink and use drugs as ways to manage stress and negative feelings. Women, however, are more likely to use food as a means of personal comfort, which can result in unhealthy eating habits.

Therefore, several risky behaviors are more common among people under stress. Those behaviors include increased smoking, drinking, illicit drug use, and unhealthy eating patterns. Men and women are not equally likely to use these behaviors as means to manage stress, with men more likely to drink heavily and use illicit drugs and women more likely to alter their eating patterns.

Other Physical Disorders

Besides headache, infectious illness, and cardiovascular disease, stress has been linked to several other physical disorders, including diabetes, premature delivery for pregnant women, asthma, and rheumatoid arthritis.

Diabetes mellitus is a chronic illness that may be related to stress. Two kinds of diabetes mellitus are Type I or insulin dependent diabetes mellitus (IDDM) and Type II or noninsulin dependent diabetes mellitus (NIDDM). IDDM is also called juvenile-onset diabetes, because it begins in childhood and requires insulin injections for its control. NIDDM usually ap-

pears during adulthood and can most often be controlled by dietary changes. (The lifestyle adjustments and behavioral management required by diabetes mellitus are discussed in Chapter 11.)

Cox and Gonder-Frederick (1991, 1992) listed reasons that stress may contribute to the development of both types of diabetes. First, stress may contribute directly to the *development* of insulin-dependent diabetes through the disruption of the immune system. In general, retrospective studies have found that insulin-dependent diabetics had somewhat more stressful life events than nondiabetics. However, prospective investigations of this issue are extremely difficult to conduct on humans. Second, stress may contribute directly to NIDDM through its effect on the sympathetic nervous system; and third, stress may contribute to NIDDM through its possible effects on obesity. Research on stress and noninsulin-dependent diabetics has shown that stress can be a triggering factor and thus play a role in the age at which people develop adult-onset diabetes.

In addition, stress may contribute to the *management* of diabetes mellitus through its direct effect of raising blood glucose. Also, stress may hinder people's compliance with routine self-care, thereby indirectly influencing both types of diabetes. Indeed, compliance is a major problem for this disorder, as discussed in Chapter 8.

Adler and Matthews (1994) reviewed studies showing that *stress during pregnancy* tends to make preterm deliveries more likely and to result in babies with lower birth weight, and both factors are related to a number of problems for the infants. Lobel, Dunkel-Schetter, and Scrimshaw (1992) conducted a prospective study of medical risks and prenatal stress as factors in premature delivery for low-income women, the majority of whom were Hispanic American or African American. These researchers found that stress during pregnancy was related to premature delivery as well as to medical risks. After controlling for the medical risks, stress during pregnancy was still a factor in premature delivery.

Asthma is a respiratory disorder characterized by difficulty in breathing due to reversible airway obstruction, airway inflammation, and increase in airway responsiveness to a variety of stimuli (Creer & Bender, 1993). Prevalence and mortality rate from

WOULD YOU BELIEVE . . . ?

Stress and Ulcers

Would you believe that stress is not a major factor in the development of ulcers? The notion that executives are at risk for stress-induced ulcers has two problems. First, executives who can control much of their own lives experience less stress than lower-level workers such as waiters and clerks. Second, and more important for our discussion here, stress is not the most important factor in the development of ulcers of the stomach or intestine.

During the 1980s, two Australian researchers, Barry Marshall and J. Robin Warren, proposed that ulcers were the result of a bacterial infection rather than stress (Alper, 1993). At the time, their hypothesis seemed somewhat unlikely because most physicians believed that bacteria could not live in the stomach environment with its extreme acidity. Researchers had searched for a bacterium that caused ulcers but had failed to find it, concluding that no bacteria could grow in the stomach.

The acceptance of stress as an underlying factor in ulcers was an additional problem with the search for an alternative cause, and Marshall (1995) reported that he had trouble receiving funding to research the possibility of a bacterial basis for ulcers. Marshall and Warren hypothesized that the *Helicobacter pylori* bacterium was responsible for ulcers. With no funding for his research and the belief that he was correct, Marshall infected himself with the bacterium to demonstrate its gastric effects. He developed severe gastritis and took antibiotics to cure himself, providing further evidence that this bacterium has gastric effects.

Beginning with the premise that the *Helicobacter pylori* bacterium was responsible for ulcers, Marshall and Warren set up a clinical trial in which half the patients received antibiotics and half received the traditional treatment — Tagamet, an acid suppressant (Alper, 1993). Results of this study revealed that stomach ulcers returned in 50%–95% of patients who received Tagamet, but only 29% of the patients treated with antibiotics experienced a recurrence of ulcers.

Heliocobacter pylori is also implicated in duodenal ulcers among children. Colin Macarthur, Norman Saunders, and William Feldman (1995) reviewed 45 studies dealing with this bacterium in children with gastroduodenal disease and found that for children under 18 with duodenal ulcer, an overwhelming majority also had the bacterium; and for children with gastric ulcer, a smaller but still substantial number had this bacterium.

Thus, *Heliocobacter pylori* does not explain all occurrences of ulcers. Some people with ulcers are not infected with the bacterium, and some people who are infected do not develop ulcers. *Heliocobacter pylori*, however, may also be a factor in gastric cancer, explaining the increased risk for stomach cancer among ulcer patients (Alper, 1993). What remains unexplained is the variability of response to people infected with the bacterium. Some infected people develop ulcers, some develop gastric cancer, and others apparently experience only a mild stomach irritation. These differences in response to infection suggest that other factors operate in the development of ulcers, but stress has not been implicated as this factor.

Even with the dramatic improvement from antibiotic treatment, many physicians were reluctant to accept the bacterial cause of ulcers (Alper, 1993; Marshall, 1995). Part of that reluctance was the continued belief that stress was involved in ulcer formation. In addition, pharmaceutical companies were slow to promote antibiotic treatment for ulcers and continued to advertise and promote the drugs that suppress stomach acid secretion. As a result, many physicians were reluctant to abandon their customary approach and to choose a new treatment. A 1993 editorial in the *New England Journal of Medicine* (Graham, 1993) recommended the antibiotic treatment, and pharmaceutical companies have recently begun to promote an antibiotic treatment for ulcers. Antibiotics may not be able to wipe out all ulcers, but this new means of treatment may reduce the prevalence of ulcers to a small fraction of their previous rate.

---

asthma have increased in recent years for both European American and African American women, men, and children, but poor African Americans living in urban environments are disproportionally affected.

Stress can be among the stimuli that are associated with precipitating an asthma attack, including emotional events, physical stressors such as pain, and the belief that an allergen is present (Bieliaus- kas, 1982; Elliott & Eisdorfer, 1982). Even though asthma's symptoms are physical, the events that trigger attacks can be emotional and may follow, either immediately or after a delay, from stressful events.

Rheumatoid arthritis, a chronic inflammatory disease of the joints, may also be related to stress. Rheumatoid arthritis is believed to be an autoimmune disorder in which a person's own immune system attacks itself (Young et al., 1993). The attack produces inflammation and damage to the tissue lining of the joints, resulting in pain and loss of flexibility and mobility.

Weiner's (1977) review of studies of the psychological characteristics of rheumatoid arthritis patients showed that stressful life events were associated with the disease. The evidence of a connection is completely correlational and will remain so until the cause of rheumatoid arthritis is discovered. Because the origin of the disorder is unknown, the role of stress in the development of this disorder remains unclear. However, rheumatoid arthritis brings about changes in people's lives that are frequently stressful and require extensive coping efforts.

Summary of the Stress and Illness Interaction

Much evidence points to a relationship between stress and illness, but claims that stressful life events and daily hassles cause various somatic disorders are still premature. Even those writers who accept the premise that stress and illness are causally linked qualify their claims. More than a decade ago, Lazarus and Folkman stated that the "evidence is less clear and less fully spelled out than is generally realized" (1984, p. 205). Today, that evidence is no more fully established. Just as most smokers will not die of lung cancer and most drinkers will not contract cirrhosis of the liver, most people who experience an abundance of stress in a given period of time will not develop an illness as a result. Nevertheless, enough evidence has accumulated to suggest that stress and the accompanying attempts at coping are likely to be two of the many factors implicated in the development of physical illness, especially viral disorders.

STRESS AND NEGATIVE MOOD

The relationship between stress and negative mood seems obvious—stress puts people in a bad mood. Being in a bad mood can change immune function, as research by Futterman, Kemeny, Shapiro, and Fahey (1994) demonstrated. They investigated the effect of mood change on immune function by inducing positive and negative mood states in a group of actors and measuring their immune function afterward. They found that mood changes of both types affected immune function. Therefore, even daily normal mood swings can influence the function of the immune system.

Negative mood, however, may refer to a stable way of looking at the world as well as to a temporary bad mood. The trait of *negative affectivity* is the tendency to "experience significant levels of distress and dissatisfaction in any given situation" (Watson & Pennebaker, 1991, p. 64). Individuals high in negative affectivity focus on the negative aspects of self, others, and situations, resulting in a pessimistic view of life.

Watson and Pennebaker (1989) argued that negative affectivity is a factor in the relationship between stress and health. They contended that self-reports of both life events and health complaints have a heavy component of negative affectivity but that the relationship to health status is less clear. That is, negative affectivity is more strongly related to health complaints than to health status. Thus, the existence of negative affectivity can act as a contaminant, complicating attempts to understand the extent of the relationship between stress and health.

The tendency to complain about health is also present in people who exhibit the trait of negative affectivity. Sheldon Cohen and his colleagues (1995) measured negative affectivity in people whom they infected with a respiratory virus. Those people high in negative affectivity who got sick complained more than those lower in negative affectivity, even though they were not objectively more sick.

Therefore, people with negative affectivity feel worse than other people when they are ill. In addition, the tendency for people high in negative affectivity to overreport stress and to see themselves as being in poor health makes them subject to depression and anxiety disorders.

Depression

The evidence that stressful life events cause depression is less than overwhelming. In general, research suggests a slight tendency for life events to be a factor in depressive symptoms. The ability to cope and coping resources, however, are more closely associated with depression, with those who can cope effectively being able to avoid depression. Again, the factor of negative affectivity may exacerbate stress, making people with this trait more prone to poor coping and to the tendency to ruminate over problems and experiences, which can increase depression (Nolen-Hoeksema, 1994).

The stress of major life events such as bereavement has been investigated in relation to depression. Early studies on the relationship between loss of a parent during childhood and adult depression indicated a positive relationship (Lloyd, 1980b), but a more recent review (Rabkin, 1993) concluded that no relationship exists between childhood bereavement and adult depression.

Stress is more likely to be an immediate precipitator of depression. Both earlier (Lloyd, 1980a) and later (Rabkin, 1993) reviews have found that depressed people were more likely than nondepressed individuals to have experienced major stressful life events preceding the onset of depression. Although the correlations between life events and depression are typically quite small, some life events have been shown to relate to depression. The experience of chronic illness, either as a person with the illness or as a caregiver, has been shown to relate to depression. Heart disease (Holahan, Moos, Holahan, & Brennan, 1995), cancer (Telch & Telch, 1985), AIDS (Fleishman & Fogel, 1994), and Alzheimer's disease (Rabins, 1989) have all been related to increased incidence of depression. In addition, some research (Bodnar & Kiecolt-Glaser, 1994) indicates that the depression of caring for an Alzheimer's patient persists even after the caregiving has ended with the patient's death. Therefore, major, continuing life stresses may be more strongly related to depression than stresses of lesser intensity or of shorter duration.

A more comprehensive approach to studying the relationship between stress and depression is to include people's appraisal of an event, their vulnerability, and their perceived ability to cope with stress. As mentioned earlier, Richard Lazarus and his colleagues (Kanner et al., 1981; Lazarus & DeLongis, 1983; Lazarus & Folkman, 1984) regard stress as the combination of an environmental stimulus and the person's appraisal, vulnerability, and perceived coping strength. According to this theory, people become ill not merely because they had too many stressful experiences but because they have evaluated these experiences as threatening or damaging, because they are physically or socially vulnerable at

that time, or because they lack the ability to cope with the stressful event.

Research has found some support for the hypothesis that depression results from a complex of interrelated factors. Persons and Rao (1985) found no significant relationship between depression and life events, but when they looked at the interaction between stressful events and such cognitive factors as irrational beliefs and attribution of personal responsibility, small but significant results began to emerge. In addition, they found some indication that depressed people are more likely to attribute positive life events to external factors; nondepressed people tend to attribute them to internal causes. For example, a depressed student might attribute good test performance to making lucky guesses whereas a nondepressed student might recognize a high grade as the result of long and hard study.

Revicki and May (1985) found evidence to support Lazarus's view that stressful events interact with vulnerability and perceived coping ability to bring about or worsen depression. They studied family physicians' occupational stress, their perceptions of family and peer social support, their views of control, and their levels of depression. As with studies that looked exclusively at life events, this study reported small but statistically significant relationships between stress and depression, but this relationship was moderated by family (but not peer) support and physicians' beliefs that they could control important aspects of their lives. This finding partially confirmed Lazarus's belief that the effects of stress are moderated both by social support and by the expectation that one can deal with the stressful event.

A study by Wise and Barnes (1986) also found that cognitive factors interact with stressful life events to mediate depression. This investigation used both clinically depressed and nondepressed college students to test the hypothesis that dysfunctional or irrational attitudes interact with negative life events either to lessen or to heighten depression. Normal students who did not have a large number of irrational views did not become depressed whereas those who thought in more catastrophic terms tended to become depressed. For the clinically depressed students, both life events and dysfunctional thinking predicted the level of depression, but the interaction between these two factors did not significantly increase the ability to predict depression. This study suggests that people may escape the harmful effects of negative life events by avoiding irrational or dysfunctional thoughts. Wise and Barnes concluded that psychological interventions might be directed at changing irrational beliefs so people could cope better with negative life events.

In a review of the literature, Brown and Harris (1989) found that although stress may be related to depressive symptoms, other factors also played an important role in the etiology of depression. Some of these psychosocial factors included low self-esteem, lack of social support, feelings of hopelessness, and loss of a sense of self-control—all common to those with negative affectivity. The results of these studies tend to support the hypothesis that stress may increase depression but that cognitive and other psychosocial factors interact with stressful events to affect subsequent levels of depression.

The relationship between stress and depression is complex, but depression has a relationship to immune function (Herbert & Cohen, 1993a). Depression that meets the diagnostic criteria for clinical depression (American Psychiatric Association, 1994) is associated with several measures of immune function, with larger effects for older and for hospitalized patients. In addition, the more severe the depression, the greater will be the alteration of immune function. However, this relationship may not be directly due to stress but may be mediated through changes in health-related behaviors that occur in depressed people. Research by Cover and Irwin (1994) suggested that sleep disturbances were more strongly related to the changes in immune function than to other behavioral changes among depressed patients.

Anxiety Disorders

Anxiety disorders include a variety of fears and phobias, often leading to avoidance behaviors. Included in this definition are such conditions as panic attack, **agoraphobia**, generalized anxiety, obsessive-compulsive disorders, and posttraumatic stress (American Psychiatric Association, 1994). This section looks at stress as a possible contributor to anxiety states.

One anxiety disorder that, by definition, is related to stress is **posttraumatic stress disorder (PTSD)**. The Diagnostic and Statistical Manual of Mental Disorders , Fourth Edition (DSM-IV) (American Psychiatric Association, 1994) defines PTSD as "the development of characteristic symptoms following exposure to an extreme traumatic stressor involving direct personal experience of an event that involves actual or threatened death or serious injury" (p. 424). PTSD can also stem from experiencing threats to one's physical integrity; witnessing another person's serious injury, death, or threatened physical integrity; and learning about death or injury to family members or friends. The traumatic events often include military combat, but sexual assault, physical attack, robbery, mugging, and other personal violent assaults can trigger posttraumatic stress disorder.

Symptoms of PTSD include recurrent and intrusive memories of the traumatic event, recurrent distressing dreams that replay the event, and extreme psychological and physiological distress. Events that resemble or symbolize the original traumatic event as well as anniversaries of that event may also trigger symptoms. People with posttraumatic stress disorder attempt to avoid thoughts, feelings, or conversations about the event and to avoid any person or place that might trigger acute distress.

Friedman, Clark, and Gershon (1992) reviewed several studies on PTSD and found support for the underlying assumption of the posttraumatic stress disorder; that is, PTSD symptoms are triggered by stressful events. Research has confirmed that exposure to crime and violence is related to the development of PTSD. Prevalence of PTSD in the general population is only around 1% (Helzer, Robins, & McEvoy, 1987), but 3.5% of civilians exposed to physical attack as well as Vietnam veterans who were not wounded showed symptoms of PTSD. In contrast, 20% of wounded veterans had PTSD symptoms. Resnick and her colleagues (Resnick, Kilpatrick, Best, & Kramer, 1992) investigated the relationship between crime victimization and PTSD in a sample of female crime victims and found that 35% of women involved in high crime stress (defined as life threats and physical injury) showed PTSD whereas only 13% of victims of low crime stress did so. Both figures are much higher than in the general population, and all these figures demonstrate the negative impact of stress produced by violence and victimization.

The relationship between stress and other anxiety disorders is less clear. In retrospective investigations in which phobic patients are asked whether they identify any stressful event as the trigger for their anxiety disorder, most patients implicate one or more stressful events. Rabkin (1993) found that about two-thirds of phobic patients reported some precipitating stressor. However, these subjective claims fall far short of proving that stress causes anxiety disorders. In her review of the literature, Rabkin (1993) reached a generally negative view of the possible connection between stress and anxiety or phobic reactions, concluding that "despite both clinical and lay expectations that phobic disorders are triggered, if not caused, by a particular stressor, investigators have not found a strong association" (p. 486). However, she noted that well-designed studies on the relationship between phobic disorders and stress remain to be conducted.

Summary of Stress and Negative Mood

Contrary to the commonsense belief that stress is a major contributor to psychological disorders, little evidence exists that a stressful life event, or even an accumulation of events, contributes significantly to the onset of depression or anxiety disorders, except, of course, posttraumatic stress disorder. One of the leading authorities on stressful life events, Bruce Dohrenwend, concluded that except for death of a loved one or severe physical illness or injury, "it is difficult to find consistent evidence that other types of single life events can produce psychopathology in previously normal adults in societies free from war and other natural disasters" (1979, p. 5). As for the link between multiple life events and psychological illness, Dohrenwend found that the correlations are usually modest (or lower) and that different studies report inconsistent findings.

The concept of negative affectivity relates both to a person's tendency to report negative life events and to a style of perceiving and dealing with stress that increases psychological problems. People with a pessimistic view of life and the tendency to ruminate over their problems increase their chances of becoming depressed, and the heightened sensitivity

to negative aspects of life can increase their anxiety. Furthermore, their pessimistic outlook decreases their ability to cope actively, heightening their vulnerability to stressful events.

CHAPTER SUMMARY

If stress causes physical illness, it must do so by affecting biological processes, and the most likely candidate is the immune system. The immune system consists of a number of tissues, organs, and processes that protect the body from invasion by foreign material such as bacteria, viruses, and fungi. It also offers protection by eliminating damaged body cells. Immune system responses may be nonspecific and capable of attacking any invader or specifically tailored to a specific invader. Immune system problems can stem from several sources, including organ transplants, allergies, and drugs used for cancer chemotherapy as well as immune deficiency. The most publicized type of immune deficiency is AIDS, a condition that destroys parts of the immune system and leaves the person subject to a wide range of viral and malignant diseases.

Psychoneuroimmunology is a relatively new multidisciplinary field that focuses on the interactions among behavior, the immune system, the central nervous system, and the endocrine system. Psychoneuroimmunology closely relates to health psychology because it is concerned with the role that behavior plays in provoking illness and promoting health. Research in this area has generally supported the notion that psychological factors can depress immune system function, and psychoneuroimmunologists have conducted a limited number of studies demonstrating a direct relationship between levels of immune depression and severity of physiological symptoms.

Current evidence indicates that stress is one of many factors that can produce disease, yet some people experience extreme stress and do not fall ill. Researchers have looked for personal variables that might account for these differential effects. One suggestion is the diathesis-stress model, which assumes that personal vulnerability interacts with stress to produce illness in people who are predisposed to that illness. If this model is valid, then even mild levels of stress would be sufficient to produce illness in diathetic individuals. A second possibility is that some people have a hardy personality that, despite the levels of stress, buffers their response to stress through their sense of control, commitment, and challenge. Despite nearly 2 decades of research on the hardy personality, investigators have found little consistent support for the notion that hardiness provides a buffer against stress. A third explanation comes from the identity disruption model, which suggests that positive life events have negative health effects only for people with low self-esteem. However, more research is needed before the identity disruption model can be used as an explanation for why different personalities are affected differently by stress.

In general, stress is a moderate risk factor for several physical disorders, including headache and infectious illness. The evidence for a relationship between stress and heart disease is complex, with the possibility that stress may be involved in hypertension. Differential reactivity to stress and gender differences in response to stress may also contribute. Stress is also a factor in other diseases, including diabetes, asthma, and rheumatoid arthritis, as well as some premature deliveries.

Evidence suggests that stress is one of many factors that contribute to negative mood and mood disorders. The concept of negative affectivity applies not only to bad mood but also to a stable trait describing a pessimistic life outlook that is related to high reports of stress and health problems. Negative affectivity may also be related to depression, but evidence is mixed concerning the effects of stress on the development of depression and anxiety disorders other than posttraumatic stress disorder.

SUGGESTED READINGS

Adler, N., & Matthews, K. (1994). Health psychology: Why do some people get sick and some stay well? *Annual Review of Psychology, 45,* 229–259. Two leaders in health psychology look at stress as a possible explanation for why some people get sick and others stay well.

Baum, A., Davidson, L. M., Singer, J. E., & Street, S. W. (1987). Stress as a psychophysiological process. In A. Baum & J. E. Singer (Eds.), *Handbook of psychology and health: Vol. 5. Stress* (pp. 1–24). Hillsdale, NJ: Erlbaum. In this review of the physiological responses to stress, the authors organize and present difficult material in a way that integrates the physiology and psychology of stress.

Kiecolt-Glaser, J. K., & Glaser, R. (1993). Mind and immunity. In D. Goleman & J. Gurin (Eds.), *Mind/body medicine: How to use your mind for better health* (pp. 39–61). Yonkers, NY: Consumer Reports Books. In this readable review, two important researchers discuss the growing field of psychoneuroimmunology, including an explanation of the immune system and the basic findings of the field.

Maier, S. F., Watkins, L. R., & Fleshner, M. (1994). Psychoneuroimmunology: The interface between behavior, brain, and immunity. *American Psychologist, 49,* 1004–1017. This review is oriented toward psychologists who may be unfamiliar with the field. In addition to a description of the field and some review of research, Maier and his colleagues explain the reciprocal relationship between nervous and immune systems and speculate on the adaptive advantages of such an arrangement.

Understanding Pain

Carl is a 23-year-old man who was suffering from almost constant pain and sought treatment from his physician. The physician diagnosed Carl's condition as *myofascial pain*—that is, aches and pain brought on by muscle tension. Carl's physician referred him to a health psychologist for biofeedback treatment. Carl was at a period in his life with a lot of changes. He had just finished a bachelor's degree in economics, had enrolled in a master's program in business administration, and was engaged to be married. He claimed that an injury from an automobile accident precipitated his pain, and he was suing the other driver's insurance company for a rather large amount of money.

The health psychologist made a psychophysiological profile that revealed moderate muscle tension in Carl's shoulders and lower back. After 12 sessions with *electromyograph biofeedback,* Carl's muscle tension was within normal limits. During some of his later sessions with the health psychologist, however, Carl complained about continuing pain in his shoulders, neck, and lower back, despite the electromyograph treatment and the muscle tension measurements within the normal range. He frequently went into detail about how each pain felt and described every pain he was currently feeling or had been feeling. Finally, the psychologist concluded that although there may have been some physical basis for the pain, Carl was (knowingly or unknowingly) exaggerating its severity. If Carl got better or learned how to live with and control his pain behaviors, he would not be eligible for the large amount of damages for which he had sued. The possibility of receiving a large amount of money was sustaining Carl in the role of a *chronic pain* patient.

Chronic pain is a serious health problem in the United States. Between 10% and 30% of the people in the U.S. suffer from some type of pain (Turk & Nash, 1993). Half to two-thirds of those with chronic pain are partially or completely disabled for days, weeks, months, or even the rest of their lives (Bonica, 1990b). More than 550 million workdays are lost each year because of chronic pain (Turk & Nash, 1993); the average worker misses more than 4 days a year (Bonica, 1990b). The expense of chronic pain has been placed at nearly $100 billion annually, including costs for surgery, loss of income, medication, hospitalization, disability payments, and litigation settlements (Turk & Nash, 1993). The costs in emotional distress and suffering are inestimable.

Although pain can affect people of any age, older people complain of more pain than younger ones. Mobily, Herr, Clark, and Wallace (1994) surveyed people 65 and older, living in rural areas, and found that 86% of them reported some type of pain in the year prior to the interview. In addition, 54% had multiple pain complaints. As might be expected with an older population, joint pain, leg pain, and back pain were the most frequently reported pains. Interestingly, respondents 85 and older were less likely to report pain than were younger ones.

PAIN AND THE NERVOUS SYSTEM

All sensory information begins with sense receptors on or near the surface of the body. These receptors change physical energy—such as light, sound, heat, and pressure—into neural impulses. We can feel pain through any of our senses, but most of what we think of as pain originates as stimulation to the skin and muscles.

Neural impulses that originate in the skin and muscles are part of the peripheral nervous system (PNS); all neurons outside the brain and spinal cord, the central nervous system (CNS), are part of the PNS. Neural impulses that originate in the PNS travel toward the spinal cord and brain. Therefore, it is possible to trace the path of neural impulses from the receptors to the brain. Tracing this path is a way to understand the physiology of pain.

THE SOMATOSENSORY SYSTEM

The **somatosensory system** conveys sensory information from the body to the brain. The word *soma* means body in Greek; the somatic division of the PNS exists in and serves the body. All the PNS neurons that reach the skin's surface and serve muscles are part of the somatic nervous system. The interpretation of this information results in a person's perception of sensations about his or her body and its movements. The somatosensory system consists of several senses, including touch, light and deep pressure, cold, warmth, tickling, movement, and body position.

Sensory input from the skin and muscles makes its way toward the spinal cord by way of the somatic nervous system. For example, a neural impulse that

originated in the right index finger would travel through the somatic nervous system to the spinal cord. At that point the impulse would be in the central nervous system. It would be relayed by the CNS to the brain, which is also in the CNS.

If the processing of information in the brain led to the decision to move that finger, a motor impulse would be initiated in the brain. That impulse would travel down the spinal cord. When it crossed into the body from the spinal cord, it would once again be in the somatic division of the PNS. That motor impulse would finally reach the muscles of the finger, and the finger would move.

A complex web of nerves carries sensations and motor impulses. The spinal cord gives rise to 31 pairs of spinal nerves, each nerve containing both sensory and motor neurons. These nerves branch into a finer and finer network covering the entire body below the neck. Sensory and motor functions of the head and neck are provided by the 12 cranial nerves emanating from the brain. The cranial nerves do not go through the spinal cord, but they carry the messages in the head and neck region that are equivalent to the information carried by the spinal nerves. The cranial nerves are also part of the somatic nervous system.

Afferent Neurons

Afferent neurons are one of the three types of neurons. *Afferent (sensory) neurons* relay information from the sense organs toward the brain. The action of *efferent (motor) neurons* results in the movement of muscles or the stimulation of organs or glands. *Interneurons* connect sensory to motor neurons.

The sense organs contain afferent neurons, called **primary afferents**, with specialized receptors that convert physical energy into neural impulses. By way of these receptors, we gain information about the world in the form of neural impulses. Afferent neurons convey this information to the spinal cord and then to the brain, where that information is processed and interpreted.

The action of neurons is partly electrical and partly chemical. An electrical impulse forms in the receptors when the sense organs are stimulated. Sufficient stimulation will result in the formation of an **action potential**, or electrical discharge, and the neuron will "fire." But the stimulation must exceed the neuron's threshold to create an action potential.

The action of each individual neuron is simple: Each neuron is sufficiently stimulated either to fire or not. However, the events that lead up to the firing (or failure to fire) are not simple. The number of afferent neurons and the pattern of their responses is what permits them to relay enormously complex information.

Involvement in Pain

The skin is the largest of the sense organs, and its numerous receptors provide sensation for the skin. Some are covered with **myelin**, a fatty substance that acts as insulation. Myelinated afferent neurons are called A fibers. A fibers conduct neural impulse faster than the unmyelinated **C fibers** do. In addition, neurons differ in size, and larger ones conduct impulses faster than smaller ones. Two types of A fibers are important in pain perception—the large **A-beta fibers** and the smaller **A-delta fibers**. The large, myelinated A-beta fibers conduct impulses over 100 times faster than small, unmyelinated C fibers (Melzack, 1973). A-beta fibers are easily stimulated to fire whereas C fibers require more stimulation. C fibers are much more common, however, with over 60% of all sensory afferents being C fibers (Melzack & Wall, 1982). Having two types of fibers involved with pain might account for some of the variations in people's experience of pain. The fast action of the A-delta fibers might account for the fast, sharp feeling of pain, whereas stimulation of the C fibers might result in slower, more diffuse aching.

The stimulation of A and C fibers creates neural impulses and starts the sensory message on its path to the brain. If the sensory information originates in the head and neck region, it will go to the brain by way of the cranial nerves. If the impulses originate in the rest of the body, the information will travel to the brain by way of the spinal cord.

THE SPINAL CORD

Protected by the vertebrae, the spinal cord is an avenue for sensory information traveling toward the brain and motor information coming from it. The spinal cord also produces the spinal reflexes. However, the most important role of the spinal cord is to provide a pathway for ascending sensory information and descending motor messages.

Damage to the spinal cord may interrupt the flow of sensory information or motor messages or both. The type and extent of the loss of function depends on the extent and location of damage. If the cord is completely cut, incoming sensory messages cannot reach the brain for interpretation. The region of the body below the break loses feeling. Motor impulses from the brain are also blocked when the cord is cut, resulting in paralysis from the point of injury downward, yet the function of the spinal cord above and below the injury may remain intact. For example, the spinal reflexes (such as the patellar reflex) still occur, but the same movements cannot be made voluntarily.

The afferent fibers group together after leaving the skin, and this grouping forms a nerve. Nerves may be entirely afferent, entirely efferent, or a mixture of both. Just outside the spinal cord, each nerve bundle divides into two branches (see Figure 5.1). The sensory tracts, which funnel information toward the brain, enter the dorsal (toward the back) side of the spinal cord. The motor tracts, which come from the brain, exit the ventral (toward the stomach) side of the cord. On each side of the spinal cord, the dorsal root swells into a dorsal root ganglion, which contains the cell bodies of the primary afferent neurons. The fiber of the neuron extends into the **dorsal horns** of the spinal cord. In the spinal cord, some afferent neurons connect to other neurons, called *secondary afferents* or **transmission cells**, and others continue to the lower part of the brain (Graham, 1990).

The dorsal horns contain several layers, or **laminae**. Each lamina receives incoming messages from afferent neurons. In general, the larger fibers penetrate more deeply into the laminae than the smaller fibers do (Melzack & Wall, 1982). The cells in laminae 1 and 2 receive information from the small A-delta and C fibers. These two laminae form the **substantia gelatinosa**; Melzack and Wall (1965) hypothesized that this structure modulates sensory input information. The substantia gelatinosa seems capable of such modulation because many afferent neurons from the skin terminate in it, and it receives projections from lower laminae. Other laminae also receive projections from A and C fibers as well as fibers descending from the brain and fibers from other laminae. Such reciprocal connec-

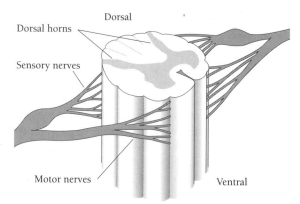

Figure 5.1 *Cross-section through the spinal cord.*
SOURCE: From *Biological Psychology* (2nd ed., p. 89) by
J. W. Kalat, 1984, Belmont, CA: Wadsworth. Copyright
1984 by Wadsworth Publishing Company. Reprinted by
permission.

tions would allow for elaborate interactions between
sensory input and the central processing of neural
information.

Information from the body is relayed toward the
brain through three spinal cord pathways that cross
from one side of the body to the opposite side of the
brain; few neurons carry information from one side
of the body to the same side of the brain. For the
majority of information, stimuli impinging on the
right hand would enter the spinal cord and cross
over to the left side of the brain for interpretation.
However, not all the neurons cross to the opposite
side of the brain at the same level. Some cross while
still in the spinal cord, and others do not cross until
they reach the brain. But most cross over at one or
the other level.

THE BRAIN

The **thalamus** receives information from all three of
the afferent systems in the spinal cord, although a
different part of the thalamus receives input from
each system. After making connections in the thalamus, the information is relayed to other parts of the
brain.

Neural impulses go to the **somatosensory cortex**
in the cerebral cortex, which is on the surface of the
brain. The *primary somatosensory cortex* receives information from the thalamus that allows the entire
surface of the skin to be mapped onto the so-

matosensory cortex. However, not all areas of the
skin are equally represented. Figure 5.2 shows the
area of the primary somatosensory cortex allotted
to various regions of the body. Areas that are particularly rich in receptors occupy more of the somatosensory cortex than those areas that are poorer
in receptors. For example, the hands take up more
of the somatosensory cortex than the back does.
Even though the back has more skin, the hands
have more receptors, and therefore more area of
the brain is devoted to interpreting the information
these receptors supply. This abundance of receptors also means that the hands are more sensitive;
hands are capable of sensing stimuli that the back
cannot.

The *secondary somatosensory cortex* is next to the
primary somatosensory cortex. This area also receives information from the thalamus, but it is not
mapped in the same well-organized way as the primary somatosensory cortex. Different body areas
are represented in roughly the same place and skin
areas are represented, but the organization does not
form a map of the entire skin's surface (Ludel,
1978). In addition, the neurons are not arranged by
the types of stimulation to which they are sensitive

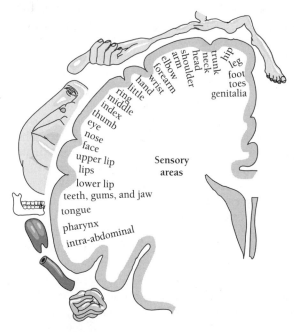

Figure 5.2 **Somatosensory areas of the cortex.**

because these neurons tend to be sensitive to various types of stimulation. The neurons in the secondary somatosensory cortex may not react to pressure on the skin but rather to active manipulation of an object (Graham, 1990). In short, the primary and secondary somatosensory cortices are different in terms of location, organization, and possibly function.

Not all sensory information enters the brain by way of the spinal cord. Sensory information from the head and neck regions enters the brain directly through the cranial nerves. These nerves serve a function similar to that of the afferent pathways that go through the spinal cord, but the cranial nerves enter the brain directly at the level of the **medulla,** a structure in the lower part of the brain. In the brain, the afferent impulses from the skin of the head and neck go to the thalamus, as do the tracts coming from the spinal cord.

The person's ability to localize pain on the skin's surface is more precise than it is for internal organs. The viscera are not mapped in the brain in the same way as the skin. Internal stimulation can also give rise to sensations, including pain, but localizing internal sensation is much harder. In fact, intense stimulation of internal organs can result in the spread of neural stimulation to the pathways serving skin senses. Thus, visceral pain may be perceived as originating on the skin's surface. For example, a person who feels pain in the upper arm may not associate this sensation with the heart, but that type of pain is commonly produced by a heart attack.

In summary, the activation of receptors in the skin results in neural impulses that move along afferent pathways to the spinal cord by way of the dorsal root. In the spinal cord, the afferent impulses proceed along one of three systems to the thalamus in the brain. Impulses from two of the three systems arrive in the somatosensory cortex in the cerebral cortex. Impulses from the third system also reach the cerebral cortex, but by a less direct route. The somatosensory cortex has two parts. The primary somatosensory cortex includes a map of the skin with more cortex devoted to areas of the body richer in skin receptors. The organization of the secondary somatosensory cortex is not so straightforward. Some types of nerve fibers, the A-delta and C fibers, are involved in pain, and the spinal cord is important in the perception of pain. However, pain perception is not specific to any one type of afferent neuron, nor is pain relayed to the brain by only one spinal system.

NEUROTRANSMITTERS AND PAIN

Neurotransmitters are chemicals that are synthesized and stored in neurons. The release of neurotransmitters carries neural impulses across the synaptic cleft, the space between neurons. The electrical action potential causes the release of neurotransmitters from the ends of neurons. After flowing across the synaptic cleft, neurotransmitters act on other neurons by occupying specialized receptor sites. Sufficient amounts of neurotransmitters will prompt the formation of an action potential in the stimulated neuron. Many different neurotransmitters exist, and each one is capable of causing an action. Each occupies a specialized receptor site like a key fits into a lock. Without the proper fit, the neurotransmitter will not affect the neuron.

In the 1970s, researchers demonstrated that the neurochemistry of the brain plays a role in the perception of pain. Pert and Snyder (1973; Snyder, 1977) discovered that receptors in the brain are sensitive to opiate drugs; they discovered that some neurons have receptor sites that opiate drugs are capable of occupying. This discovery explained how opiates reduce pain. Although the opiates are foreign substances, they apparently fit into receptors in the brain. There they stimulate neurons and produce pain relief.

The discovery of opiate receptors in the brain raised another question: Why does the brain respond to the resin of the opium poppy? In general, the brain is selective about the types of molecules that it allows to enter; only substances similar to naturally occurring neurochemicals can enter the brain. Researchers soon began to supply an answer to this question (Goldstein, 1976; Hughes, 1975). They found that a naturally occurring substance has properties similar to those of the opiate drugs. This discovery prompted a flurry of research that identified more neurochemicals with opiate-like effects, such as the **endorphins,** the *enkephalins,* and *dynorphin.*

Research has not yet revealed exactly how the body's own opiates affect pain perception. However, these neurochemicals seem to be one of the brain's mechanisms for relieving pain. One type of endorphin seems stronger than morphine in its ability to relieve pain. Whereas the enkephalins are weaker than morphine, dynorphin is 200 times more powerful. The pain-relieving properties of drugs like morphine may be coincidental. Perhaps they are effective only because the brain contains its own system for pain relief, which the opiates stimulate.

Neurochemicals also seem to be involved in producing pain. The neurotransmitters *serotonin* and *substance P* as well as the chemicals *brandykinin* and *prostaglandins* sensitize or excite the neurons that relay pain messages (Grunau & Craig, 1988). Brandykinin, a chemical composed of a string of amino acids, is released by body cells when damage occurs. If brandykinin is injected into an animal, the animal's experience of pain worsens. The prostaglandins share some properties of hormones (they are secreted by a variety of cells) and have some properties of neurotransmitters (they are released by neurons) (Creager, 1983). But the prostaglandins are classified as neither because they are not secreted by a gland and are secreted by cells that are not neurons. Prostaglandins are released in the case of injury and have a role in the inflammation response of the immune system.

THE MODULATION OF PAIN

Research directed toward finding the brain structures involved in pain led to the discovery that one area of the brain, the **periaqueductal gray**, is involved in modulating pain. This brain structure is in the midbrain, close to the center. If it is stimulated, pain is relieved, and the relief continues after stimulation of the area ceases (Graham, 1990). Neurons in the periaqueductal gray run down into the medulla, where they connect to neurons in the **nucleus raphe magnus**. These neurons descend into the spinal cord and make connections with neurons in the substantia gelatinosa. The result is that the dorsal horn neurons are kept from carrying pain information to the thalamus.

The inhibition of transmission also involves some familiar neurotransmitters. Endorphin acts in the periaqueductal gray where it initiates activity in this descending inhibitory system. The substantia gelatinosa contains synapses that use enkephalin as a transmitter. Indeed, neurons that contain enkephalin seem to be concentrated in the same parts of the brain that contain substance P, the transmitter that activates pain messages (McLean, Skirboll, & Pert, 1985).

These elaborate physical and chemical systems are the body's way to modulate the neural impulses of pain. They exist naturally in the brain, and drugs happen to produce pain relief by mimicking their action. Researchers have traditionally concentrated on developing more drugs that produce pain relief, believing that drugs (and surgery) were the only ways to relieve pain. Discovery of the body's own opiates and the brain structures that modulate pain have indicated that pain control may be possible without drugs. Researchers are now exploring the possibility of enlisting the brain's own mechanisms to relieve pain.

The circumstances that prompt the production of endorphins are not completely understood. Sherman and Liebeskind (1980) reviewed the evidence that the release of endorphins is influenced by expectation, length of pain stimulation, timing of painful stimuli, ability to cope with the pain, and previous pain experience. They also considered the possibility that nondrug methods of pain control may work because they prompt the release of endorphins. If environmental and psychological circumstances can cause the release of endorphins, voluntary control of pain seems within reach.

THE MEANING OF PAIN

Pain has been called "perhaps the most universal form of stress" (Turk, Meichenbaum, & Genest, 1983, p. 73). Yet pain differs from stress in that it is usually experienced as an unwanted physical stimulus located in a specific anatomical region. Like stress, it often has a strong psychological component.

Until about 100 years ago, pain was most frequently considered a direct consequence of physical injury, and its intensity was generally thought to be proportional to the degree of tissue damage. Near the end of the 19th century, Strong (1895) and others began to think of pain in a new light. Strong hypothesized that pain was due to two factors: the sensation and the person's reaction to that sensation. In other words, psychological factors and organic causes were of equal importance. This view received some support when Beecher (1946) reported that soldiers wounded at the Anzio beachhead during World War II reported very little pain despite serious battle injuries. These men had been removed from the front and thus from the threat of death or further injury. Under these conditions, the wounded soldiers were in a cheerful, optimistic state of mind.

Additional confirmation for the notion that a person's reaction to the physical sensation of pain strongly influences the degree of suffering came 10 years later from another study by Beecher (1956). In this report, injured civilians were found to have experienced more pain and requested more pain-killing drugs than did the wounded World War II soldiers, even though the civilians' injuries were less severe. These findings prompted Beecher (1956) to conclude that "the intensity of suffering is largely determined by what the pain means to the patient" (p. 1609) and that "the extent of wound bears only a slight relationship, if any (often none at all), to the pain experienced" (p. 1612). Finally, Beecher (1957), in a statement reminiscent of Strong, described pain as a two-dimensional experience consisting of both a sensory stimulus and an emotional component. Despite the methodological shortcomings of Beecher's studies, his view of pain as a psychological and physical phenomenon came to be accepted by others working in this field.

Most investigators now agree that personal perception mediates the experience of pain. Melzack (1973) listed such individual variables as anxiety, depression, suggestion, prior conditioning, attention, evaluation, and cultural learning as possible contributors to one's experience of pain. This multidimensional view has also been incorporated into the definition of pain offered by the International Association for the Study of Pain (IASP). The IASP Subcommittee on Taxonomy (1979, p. 250) defined pain as "an unpleasant sensory and emotional experience associated with actual or potential tissue damage, or described in terms of such damage."

John Loeser (1989) has proposed a model for understanding and evaluating pain that includes four components. The first level is *nociception,* which Loeser defined as the experience of tissue damage and the activation of A-delta and C fibers. *Pain* is the second level, which includes the perception of tissue damage. The third level is *suffering,* the negative

emotional response to tissue damage, and the fourth level is *pain behavior,* actions that reflect the presence of tissue damage.

This model's four levels highlight the separate processes of sensing and perceiving as well as the emotional and behavioral components of pain. A person can have nociception, tissue damage, without pain if something happens to block that perception. For example, anesthesia can block pain even in the presence of serious tissue damage. Suffering is connected to tissue damage but not necessarily proportional to it; that is, people may suffer a great deal with relatively minor tissue damage, as our case study Carl did, or very little even with a great deal of tissue damage, as Beecher's soldiers did. The behaviors that reflect the experience of pain and suffering vary according to many factors, but the stage of the pain experience is an important aspect.

THE STAGES OF PAIN

Pain is not a single entity but can be seen according to various stages or types. Keefe (1982) has identified three stages of pain: acute, prechronic, and chronic. **Acute pain** is ordinarily adaptive; it signals the person to avoid further injury. It usually lasts less than 6 months, and includes pains from cuts, burns, surgery, dental work, childbirth, and other injuries. **Prechronic pain** is experienced between the acute and the chronic stages. According to Keefe, this period is critical because the person either overcomes the pain at this time or develops the feelings of helplessness that lead to chronic pain. **Chronic pain** endures beyond the time of healing. It is more or less constant and is often self-perpetuating; that is, chronic pain frequently leads to behavior that is designed to elicit reward and comfort, which results in more pain behavior. Chronic pain is frequently experienced in the absence of any detectable tissue damage.

Although Keefe's classification is probably adequate for most practitioners working with pain patients, a more detailed scheme has been proposed by Turk, Meichenbaum, and Genest (1983). They categorize pain into five types: (1) acute pain; (2) chronic recurrent pain; (3) chronic intractable, benign pain; (4) chronic, progressive pain; and (5) experimentally induced pain. This last category usually

WOULD YOU BELIEVE . . . ?

Life Without Pain

Would you believe that a life with pain is preferable to one without pain? Although pain is always unpleasant, a person who feels no pain has anything but a pleasant life.

Some people might imagine that a life without pain would be pleasant, and that feeling no pain would be preferable to feeling pain. These people have not thought through the consequences of the inability to feel pain. Medical science has identified very few people who have been unable to feel pain, but studying those people shows that a life without pain is not enviable.

A young western Canadian woman, Miss C, was described by Melzack (1973) as unfamiliar with the experience of pain. The daughter of a physician, she was an intelligent young woman who attended college at McGill University in Montreal. Her father alerted his colleagues in Montreal about her condition, and these physicians studied her inability to feel pain.

Miss C was apparently normal in all respects except that she had never reported feeling pain. Once as a child she sustained third-degree burns because she had climbed on a hot radiator to look out of a window. Without the ability to feel pain, she was unaware of the damage that she was doing to her knees and legs. She could not remember ever sneezing or coughing. The gag reflex was difficult to elicit from her, and the corneal reflex that protects the eye was absent.

The physicians who tested her in Montreal subjected her to various stimuli that would have been horrible for a normal person. They administered electric shock to different parts of her body, applied hot water, immersed her limbs in cold water for prolonged periods, pinched tendons, and injected histamine under her skin. She felt no pain. In addition, her heart rate, blood pressure, and respiration remained normal throughout these tortures.

Without pain to alert her, Miss C sustained many injuries and failed to protect damaged tissues, thus making them worse. Her insensitivity to pain caused serious medical problems, especially in the joints and spine. Melzack and Wall (1982) explained that insensitivity to pain can lead people to remain in one position too long, causing inflammation of the joints. Even worse, the failure to feel pain leads one to neglect injuries and thus healing is obstructed. Injured tissue can easily become infected, and these infections are very difficult to treat if they extend into bone.

Miss C died when she was only 29 years old, and her death was from a failure to bring massive infections under control. During the last month of her life, Miss C finally complained of pain, which was relieved with aspirin. Although she felt practically no pain during her life, neither did she gain the benefits of feeling pain. Her insensitivity to pain directly contributed to the infections that killed her.

The story of Miss C provides ample evidence that a life without pain is not preferable to one with pain, and that pain provides us with a useful signal that we should take action to avoid potentially life-threatening damage to our bodies.

consists of electric shock, radiant heat, cold-water immersion, or pressure administered in a laboratory setting to voluntary participants with no previous pain problems. Experimentally induced pain is an important way to get valuable information about individual differences in the experience of pain and coping strategies that might be used to minimize pain.

Chronic recurrent pain is "characterized by intense episodes of pain interspersed with periods of no pain" (Turk et al., 1983, p. 120). Migraine headaches are perhaps the best example of chronic recurrent pain. Chronic intractable, benign pain is pain that is always present, although it is not always severe. Low back pain is a good example, always nagging but with varying degrees of intensity. Chronic progressive pain is omnipresent pain that gets stronger as the medical condition worsens. Chronic progressive pain is frequently associated with rheumatoid arthritis and cancer. These three types of chronic pain are most often the targets of pain management programs (see Chapter 6); acute pain frequently accompanies stressful medical procedures (see Chapter 7).

Chronic pain is often associated with some type of psychopathology. For example, Brewer and Karoly (1992) found that college students who suffered from recurrent pain were more depressed than those who did not and that pain intensity was positively correlated with depression among these students. Also, Kinney, Gatchel, Polatin, Fogarty, and Mayer (1993) found that patients suffering from chronic low back pain reported higher rates of psycho-pathology than those with acute low back pain and much higher rates than pain-free individuals. Compared with acute pain patients, those with chronic pain were more likely to be depressed, to abuse alcohol and other drugs, and to suffer from personality disorders. Although people who have chronic pain may develop psychopathological disorders as a result of their chronic pain, Kinney et al. found that their chronic pain patients had high rates of psychopathology prior to the inception of pain.

Bonica (1990a) contended that psychological or environmental factors play a central role in chronic pain but are rarely involved in acute pain. In other words, acute pain is due to tissue damage whereas chronic pain is a result of tissue damage plus one's experience of being rewarded for pain behaviors. Bonica agreed with most pain experts that acute pain is ordinarily beneficial because it warns that something is wrong and usually prompts the person to seek health care. But he disagreed with those who set 6 months as an arbitrary time to designate pain as chronic. To wait 6 months to term pain as chronic, he insisted, increases the chances that the pain will become irreversible. Instead he defined chronic pain as "pain that persists a month beyond the usual course of an acute disease or a reasonable time for an injury to heal or that is associated with a chronic pathologic process that causes continuous pain or the pain recurs at intervals for months or years" (Bonica, 1990a, p. 19). Chronic pain never has a biological benefit, and it "often imposes severe emotional, physical, economic, and social stresses on the patient and on the family" (p. 19).

PAIN SYNDROMES

Pain can also be categorized according to location, or syndrome. Headache and low back pain are the two most frequently treated types of pain but people also seek treatment for several other common pain syndromes.

Headache Pain

Bonica (1990b) estimated that 29 million Americans suffer from severe, disabling headache and that they spend $4 billion a year to alleviate it. Headaches account for an additional $12 billion annually in such indirect costs as lost workdays, compensation, litigation, and quackery.

Although many different kinds of headache have been identified, the most common are migraine and tension headaches. **Migraine headaches** are generally considered *vascular* in origin, although some authorities have questioned any distinction between migraine and tension headaches (Hatch, 1993). Migraine headaches are characterized by recurrent attacks of pain that vary widely in intensity, frequency, and duration. The attacks often are associated with loss of appetite, nausea, vomiting, and exaggerated sensitivity to light. Migraine headaches also often involve sensory, motor, or mood disturbances. The two most frequent kinds are migraine with aura and migraine without aura. The migraine with aura is characterized by identifiable sensory disturbances that precede the headache pain; migraine without aura has a sudden onset and an intense throbbing on one side of the head.

Women are more likely than men to have migraine headaches. Stewart, Lipton, Celentano, and Reed (1992) reported that about 18% of women but only about 7% of men in the United States suffered at least one migraine per year. For both men and women, migraine headaches occur most frequently between ages 35 and 45, with most migraine patients experiencing their first headache before age 30. However, no age group is exempt (Pearce, 1994). Children can have migraines, with a third of these patients below the age of 10. Few patients have a first migraine after age 40, but people who have migraines continue to do so, often throughout their lives.

The Stewart et al. (1992) survey also found that people in the lowest income group had 60% more migraines than did people in the two highest income brackets. They reported that women 30 to 49 from low-income households had the greatest risk for migraine headache. However, disability from migraines was not related to gender, age, income, or urban/rural background. Stewart et al. found that 8.7 million of the U.S. population suffer from migraine with moderate to severe disability and that 3.4 million women and 1.1 million men experience at least one attack each month.

Tension headaches are *muscular* in origin and are characterized by sustained contractions of the mus-

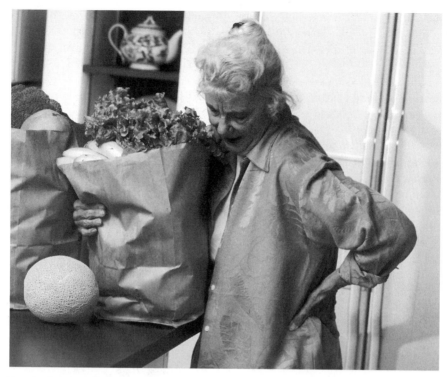

Low back pain extracts a cost in terms of personal suffering, limitation of activities, lost work days, and treatment expenditures.

cles of the neck, shoulders, scalp, and face. They are characterized by a gradual onset; sensations of tightness; constriction or pressure; highly variable intensity, frequency, and duration; and a dull, steady ache on both sides of the head (Blanchard & Andrasik, 1982).

A third type of headache is the **cluster headache,** a type of severe headache that occurs in daily clusters for 4 to 16 weeks (Pearce, 1994). Some symptoms are similar to migraine, including severe pain and vomiting, but cluster headaches are much briefer, rarely lasting longer than 2 hours. The headache is localized on one side of the head, and often the eye on the other side becomes bloodshot and waters. In addition, cluster headaches are much more common in men than women, with a ratio of 10:1. These headaches appear in a cluster and disappear, only to recur every year or two.

Low Back Pain

Compared with headache, only about half as many Americans suffer from low back pain, yet low back pain accounts for nearly twice as many lost work-days. Bonica (1990b) has estimated that 21 million people in the United States suffer from back pain and that 3.7 million of these are partially or totally disabled. He also estimated that workers lose 120 million workdays per year. The total annual cost attributable to low back pain is $20 billion.

Low back pain has many causes, including infections, degenerative diseases, and malignancies (Carron, 1984). But the most frequent cause is probably injury or stress resulting in musculoskeletal and neurological disorders in the lower back. Job-related activities account for more than 7 million cases of back pain per year in the United States. More than 2.6 million men and women incur back injuries at work and another 4.5 million develop low back pain from performing repeated job activities (Behrens, Seligman, Cameron, Mathias, & Fine, 1994).

Although many physiological factors have been implicated in low back pain, a good deal of mystery still surrounds this disorder. Loeser remarked that "there is considerable evidence that social and psychological factors play a major role in the symptom complex known as low back pain" (1980, p. 363). However, Loeser also cited evidence that improper posture and care may lead to spinal disk degeneration and thus to low back pain. Aging is another factor because the fluid content and elasticity of the intervertebral disks decrease as one grows older.

Loeser (1980) identified four common bases for low back pain. One, herniated disk (sometimes called *sciatica*), is caused by disc material compressing nerve roots, resulting in pain that radiates from the low back to the leg. Another, axial skeletal joint dysfunction, results from misalignments or stresses of the axial joint, located in the lower part of the spinal column. A third basis for low back pain is myofascial tension, or muscle spasm, which produces a continual dull ache. (Myofascial pain, a separate pain syndrome, is discussed in the next section.) The fourth basis for low back pain is environmental reinforcers, or "operant mechanisms." Pain behaviors can exempt people from unpleasant tasks and thus may encourage them to complain of pain constantly as a way to manipulate or control other people.

Myofascial Pain

Headache and low back pain are the two most common pain syndromes that psychologists treat, but the most common type of chronic pain is **myofascial pain.** Sola and Bonica (1990) defined myofascial pain syndromes as a large group of muscle disorders characterized by extremely sensitive trigger points within the muscles or connective tissue. Myofascial pain is experienced as a continual dull ache in nearly any part of the body, but the most common locations are the lower back, shoulders, neck, and head (Travell, 1976). Fricton (1982) commented that "virtually everyone at some point in life will develop 'muscle aches and pain' attributable to myofascial pain" (p. 24). Carl, the pain patient introduced at the beginning of this chapter, was diagnosed as suffering from myofascial pain.

Myofascial pain is one of the most overlooked diagnoses because it is frequently benign and results in only minor dysfunction. In past years, it has often been misdiagnosed as bursitis, arthritis, or visceral disease (Sola & Bonica, 1990). Myofascial pain can result from sustained muscle contraction, muscle

trauma, or muscle weakness. Some investigators believe that these muscle tensions can lead to a vicious, self-perpetuating cycle of pain, beginning with muscle tension (Fricton, 1982; Stroebel & Glueck, 1976). If prolonged, this tension produces pain, which in turn creates more muscle tension and even more pain. However, at least one team of investigators (Bush, Ditto, & Feuerstein, 1985) could find no consistent evidence to support this hypothesis.

Arthritis Pain

Another common pain syndrome is due to arthritis. The term *arthritis* literally means joint inflammation, but of the more than 100 arthritic conditions, only some involve inflamed joints (Achterberg-Lawlis, 1982). **Rheumatoid arthritis** is an autoimmune disorder characterized by swelling and inflammation of the joints as well as destruction of cartilage, bone, and tendons. These changes alter the joint, producing direct pain, and the changes in joint structure lead to change in movement, which may result in additional pain through this indirect route (Young et al., 1993). The symptoms of rheumatoid arthritis are extremely variable, with some people experiencing steady progression of increasing symptoms and most facing remissions and intensifications. In contrast, **osteoarthritis** is a progressive inflammation of the joints affecting mostly older people and characterized by a dull ache in the joint area, which is exacerbated by movement (Fricton, 1982).

Bonica (1990b) estimated that 24 million Americans suffer from arthritis, with 9 million being partially disabled and another 2.5 million totally disabled. According to Bonica, half of all Americans totally disabled by pain are disabled by arthritis.

Cancer Pain

Bonica (1980, p. 335) defined cancer pain as that "caused by any malignant neoplasm or as a consequence of therapeutic intervention for the disease or both." Cancer is the second leading cause of death in the United States (see Chapter 10), and studies have shown that pain is present in about 30% to 40% of all cancer cases and 60% to 90% of all terminal cancer cases (Fife, Irick, & Painter, 1993). Cancer pain afflicts about 1.1 million Americans annually (Bonica, Ventafridda, & Twycross, 1990). Some

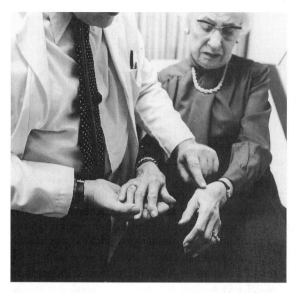

Arthritis is a source of pain and disability for over 20 million Americans.

cancers are much more likely than others to produce pain. Bonica (1980) estimated that about 85% of patients suffering from bone and cervix cancer experience pain, but only about 5% of leukemia patients experience pain. Compared with pain-free cancer patients, those who suffer pain are more likely to develop depression, anxiety, and hypochondriasis (Woodforde & Fielding, 1975).

Not infrequently, cancer patients suffer from two or more sources of pain at the same time. The tumor itself may cause pain, but such medical procedures as surgery, chemotherapy, and radiation can also be painful (Benedetti & Bonica, 1984). In addition, many cancer patients experience pain from arthritis, myofascial syndromes, low back pain, and other syndromes only partially related to their malignancy (Twycross, 1978).

Phantom Limb Pain

Just as injury can occur without producing pain, pain can occur in the absence of injury. One such type of pain is **phantom limb pain,** the experience of chronic pain in an absent body part (Loeser, 1990). Amputation removes the nerves that produce the impulses leading to the experience of pain. Despite removal of the physical basis for pain, phantom limb pain is not an unusual experience for amputees.

Estimates of the proportion of amputees who experience phantom limb pain have varied between 13% and 71% (Loeser, 1990). In a study reviewed by Melzack and Wall (1982), all amputees experienced phantom limb sensation, but not all experienced pain. Most commonly, amputees feel sensations from their amputated limbs soon after surgery. These sensations start as a tingling sensation and then develop into other sensations that resemble actual feelings in the missing limb. Nor are the sensations of a phantom limited to limbs (Loeser, 1990). Between 22% and 64% of women who have undergone breast removal also perceive sensations from the amputated breast, and some of these sensations are painful.

Loeser (1990) reported that age is a factor in the experience of phantom limb pain, claiming that infants and young children do not experience the phantom in the way that older children and adults do. Melzack (1992) disagreed, however, saying that even people born without a limb experience a phantom. For many amputees, the phantom limb seems to get smaller until the sensation of the phantom coincides with the size of the stump, but others experience phantom sensations for years.

Amputees who experience unpleasant sensations from their amputated limbs may feel that the phantom limb is of an abnormal size or in an uncomfortable position (Melzack & Wall, 1982). Phantom limbs can also produce painful feelings of cramping, shooting, burning, or crushing. These pains vary from mild and infrequent to severe and continuous. The pain may start shortly after amputation or not begin until years later. Melzack and Wall (1988) reported that 72% of amputees have pain in their phantom limb 8 days after their surgery, 65% have pain 6 months afterward, and 60% have pain 2 years later. The severity and frequency of the pain tend to decrease over time.

Loeser (1990) emphasized the distinction between phantom limb pain and stump pain. Phantom limb pain is experienced in the absent body part, but stump pain is perceived in the region of the amputation. Both types of pain can occur together or separately. Stump pain can be due to the surgery, to inflammation that persists afterward, or to a poorly fitted prosthesis. Treatments for stump pain involve treatments for these specific problems. Phantom limb pain is not well understood, however, and its treatment is controversial.

The underlying cause of phantom limb pain has been the subject of bitter controversy (Melzack, 1992; Melzack & Wall, 1982, 1988). Because surgery rarely relieves the pain, some have hypothesized that phantom limb pain has an emotional basis. Melzack (1992) argued that phantom limb sensation arises within the brain as a result of the generation of a characteristic pattern of neural activity, which he called a *neuromatrix*. Melzack contended that this brain activity constituted "a characteristic pattern of impulses indicating that the body is intact and unequivocally one's own" (p. 123). This neuromatrix pattern continues to operate, even if the neurons in the peripheral nervous system do not furnish input to the brain. Melzack believes that this brain activity is the basis for phantom limb sensations, which may include pain.

Relief from phantom limb pain can come from a variety of interventions, but in about half the cases, no therapy is successful in providing permanent relief (Melzack, 1992). One therapeutic approach is to use local anesthesia on peripheral nerves. The relief of pain can persist for days or months after the anesthesia has worn off. Relief from increased stimulation can come through massage or through the application of electrical stimulation to the skin, a technique called transcutaneous electrical neural stimulation (TENS). An experimental technique involving destruction of spinal cells that receive sensory messages from the stump has been more successful than other surgical interventions (Melzack, 1992).

THEORIES OF PAIN

Pain consists of several stages and a multitude of syndromes. How people experience pain, however, is the subject of a number of theories. Of the several models of pain, two capture the divergent ways of conceptualizing pain: the specificity theory and the gate control theory.

Specificity Theory

Specificity theory explains pain by hypothesizing that specific pain fibers and pain pathways exist, making the experience of pain virtually equal to the amount of tissue damage or injury. The view that

pain is the result of transmission of pain signals from the body to a "pain center" in the brain can be traced back to Descartes, who in the 1600s proposed that the body works mechanically. This mechanistic action of the body is consistent with the notion that transmission of pain signals is a relaying of information about body damage. Descartes hypothesized that the mind works by a different set of principles, and body and mind interact in a limited way. According to Ronald Melzack (1993), Descartes's view influenced not only the development of a science of physiology and medicine but also the view that pain is a physical experience largely uninfluenced by psychological factors.

Working under the assumption that pain was the transmission of one type of sensory information, researchers tried to determine which type of receptor conveyed what type of sensory information (Groves & Rebec, 1988; Melzack, 1973, 1992). Researchers tried to determine which type of receptor relayed information about heat, about cold, about pain, and so forth. The attempt to tie specific somatic sensations to specific types of receptors did not succeed. Researchers found that some parts of the body (like the cornea of the eye) contain only one type of receptor, yet those areas feel a full range of sensations. Some receptors seem specialized to react to specific types of stimulation, but these specialized receptors can also respond to other types of stimuli as well. The specificity of skin receptors is therefore limited, and any simple version of specificity theory is not valid.

Specificity does exist in the different types of receptors and nerve fibers. The different types of receptors in the skin allow us to sense light touch, pressure, itching, pricking, warmth, and cold. In addition, we can perceive texture, shape, and vibration and can localize the source of these stimuli on the surface of the skin. We can also sense pain, but pain can come through any of these stimuli rather than from another specific type of receptor.

The A and C fibers convey messages from the skin to the spinal cord, and other specific nerve tracts convey information to the brain. Melzack (1973) and Wall and Jones (1991) argued against the interpretation that these two fibers are exclusively pain fibers. Although these fibers relay messages that are interpreted as pain, not every neural impulse initiated in these fibers will receive this interpretation. Although Wall and Jones acknowl-

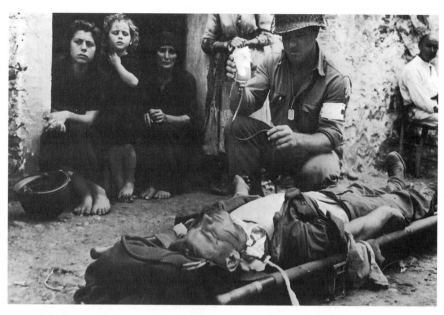

The experience of pain varies with the situation. Wounded soldiers removed from front lines may feel little pain despite extensive injuries.

edged that specific nerve fibers, such as the A and C fibers, play a role in the perception of pain, they argued against labeling any type of fiber as an exclusive pain fiber. Melzack (1993) argued against interpreting any nerve tract as exclusively devoted to pain and cited the failure of severing nerve tracts through surgery to control chronic pain as evidence supporting this point. Even when nerve tracts are surgically severed, pain relief is usually temporary, and the chronic pain that prompted the drastic measure of surgery typically returns within weeks or months.

Specificity theory fails to integrate the variability of the experience of pain with the physiology of the somatosensory system. The failure to find specific skin receptors devoted to relaying pain, the existence of pain without injury (phantom limb pain), injury without pain (as experienced by the soldiers at Anzio beach), and the failure of surgical treatments for pain make a simple, physiological theory of pain untenable.

The Gate Control Theory

In 1965, Ronald Melzack and Peter Wall formulated a new theory of pain. In their view, pain was not the result of a linear process that begins with sensory stimulation of pain pathways and ends with the ex-

perience of pain. Rather, pain perception is subject to a number of modulations that can influence the experience of pain. These modulations begin in the spinal cord.

Melzack and Wall hypothesized that structures in the spinal cord act as a gate for the sensory input that is interpreted as pain. Melzack and Wall's theory is thus known as the **gate control theory**. It is based on physiology but explains both sensory and psychological aspects of pain perception.

Melzack and Wall (1965, 1982, 1988) pointed out that the nervous system is never at rest, and the patterns of neural activation constantly change. When sensory information from the body reaches the dorsal horns of the spinal cord, that neural activation enters a system that is already active. The existing activity in the spinal cord and brain influences the fate of incoming sensory information, sometimes amplifying and sometimes decreasing the incoming neural signals. The gate control theory hypothesizes that these complex modulations in the spinal cord and in the brain affect the perception of pain.

According to the gate control theory, neural mechanisms in the spinal cord act like a gate that can either increase or decrease the flow of neural impulses. Figure 5.3 shows the results of opening

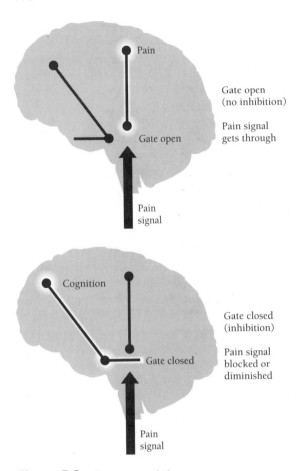

Figure 5.3   Gate-control theory.

travel through the substantia gelatinosa, which also receives projections from other laminae (Melzack & Wall, 1982, 1988). This arrangement of neurons provides the physiological basis for the modulation of incoming sensory impulses.

The gate control theory hypothesizes that information enters the dorsal horns of the spinal cord by way of primary afferent neurons. This information passes through the substantia gelatinosa, where the information is modulated by the activity of that structure, affecting the activity of the transmission cells. The transmission cells relay the modulated information toward the brain.

Melzack and Wall (1982) proposed that activity in the small A-delta and C fibers causes prolonged activity in the spinal cord. This type of activity would promote sensitivity, which produces pain. Activity of these small fibers would thus open the gate. On the other hand, activity of the large A-beta fibers produces an initial burst of activity in the spinal cord, followed by inhibition. Activity of these fibers closes the gate.

The gate may be closed by activity in the spinal cord and also by messages that descend from the brain. Melzack and Wall (1965, 1982, 1988) proposed the concept of a **central control trigger** consisting of nerve impulses that descend from the brain and influence the gating mechanism. They hypothesized that this system consists of large neurons that conduct impulses rapidly. These impulses from the brain affect the opening and closing of the gate in the spinal cord and are affected by cognitive processes. That is, Melzack and Wall proposed that the experience of pain is influenced by beliefs and prior experience, and they also hypothesized a physiological mechanism that would account for such factors in pain perception. According to the gate control theory, then, pain not only has sensory components but also motivational and emotional components.

The gate control theory explains the influence of cognitive aspects of pain by hypothesizing central control mechanisms that affect sensory input as well as being affected by it. Anxiety, worry, depression, and focusing on an injury can increase pain by affecting the central control trigger, thus opening the gate. Distraction, relaxation, and positive emotions can cause the gate to close, thereby decreasing pain.

and closing the gate. With the gate open, impulses flow through the spinal cord toward the brain, neural messages reach the brain, and the person feels pain. With the gate closed, impulses are inhibited from ascending through the spinal cord, messages do not reach the brain, and the person does not feel pain. Moreover, sensory input is subject to modulation, depending on the activity of the large A-beta fibers, the small A-delta fibers, and the small C fibers that enter the spinal cord and synapse in the dorsal horns.

The dorsal horns of the spinal cord are composed of several layers (laminae). Two of those laminae make up the substantia gelatinosa, and this structure is the hypothesized location of the gate (Melzack & Wall, 1965; Wall, 1980). Both the small A-delta and C fibers and the large A-beta fibers

The gate control theory seems to explain many personal experiences with pain. When you accidentally hit your finger with a hammer, many of the small fibers are activated, opening the gate. An emotional reaction accompanies your perception of acute pain. You may then grasp your injured finger and rub it. According to the gate control theory, rubbing stimulates the large fibers that close the gate, thus blocking stimulation from the small fibers and decreasing pain.

The gate control theory also explains how injuries can go virtually unnoticed. If sensory input is sent into a heavily activated nervous system, the stimulation may not be perceived as pain. A tennis player may turn an ankle during a game but not notice the acute pain because of excitement and concentration on the game. After the game is finished, however, the player may notice the pain because the nervous system is functioning at a different level of activation and the gate is more easily opened.

The gate control theory is perhaps the leading theory of pain. Although it has not been universally accepted, it is seen as an advance over simplistic sensory views of pain, including the view that pain is relayed by specific pain fibers. Melzack and Wall proposed the gate control theory before the discovery of the body's own opiates or discovery of the descending control mechanisms through the periaqueductal gray and the nucleus raphe magnus. These structures have been shown to modulate the experience of pain, much as the gate control theory proposed. The gate control theory has been and continues to be successful in spurring research and generating interest in the psychological and perceptual factors involved in pain.

Melzack (1993) has proposed an extension to the gate control theory, called the neuromatrix theory, that places a stronger emphasis on the brain's role in pain perception. He hypothesized a network of brain neurons that he called the neuromatrix, which is "distributed throughout many areas of the brain, comprises a widespread network of neurons which generates patterns, processes information that flows through it, and ultimately produces the pattern that is felt as a whole body" (p. 623). Normally, the neuromatrix acts to process incoming sensory information, including pain, but the neuromatrix acts even in the absence of sensory input, such as with phantom limbs. Melzack's neuromatrix theory extends gate control theory but maintains that pain perception is part of a complex process that is affected not only by sensory input but also by activity of the nervous system and by experience and expectation.

THE MEASUREMENT OF PAIN

We have seen that pain has physical and psychological elements, both of which can be quantified and measured. The measurement of pain is important because it allows researchers to evaluate different pain-reducing techniques. They can measure the level of pain both before and after treatment to see whether it has decreased during the course of therapy. Numerous techniques have been used to measure pain, but these can generally be categorized into three major approaches: (1) physiological measures, (2) behavioral assessment, and (3) self-reports (Syrjala & Chapman, 1984).

PHYSIOLOGICAL MEASURES

Because pain produces an emotional response and because strong emotional arousal affects the autonomic nervous system as well as other physiological conditions, one might assume that a number of organic states would be highly correlated with the experience of pain (Nigl, 1984). Research on this hypothesis, however, generally has not produced positive results.

Syrjala and Chapman (1984) identified three physiological variables that have been investigated as potential measures of pain: muscle tension, autonomic indices, and evoked potentials.

Muscle Tension

Electromyography (EMG) has been used by a number of researchers to measure the level of muscle tension experienced by patients suffering from low back pain (Basmajian, 1978; Goldstein, 1972). Although these researchers have found some evidence that EMG can reveal abnormal patterns of muscle activity, its level of activity does not consistently correlate with reported severity of the pain. In one study (Wolf, Nacht, & Kelly, 1982), researchers looked at a number of previous reports and found that EMG levels could either be elevated or reduced in patients with low back pain. The authors stated that "levels of paraspinal EMG activity can be at extreme ends of the spectrum even among patients who have allegedly identical diagnoses stemming from similar pathophysiological processes" (Wolf et al., 1982, p. 397).

Andrasik, Blanchard, Arena, Saunders, and Barron (1982) used a variety of physiological measures, including forehead and forearm EMGs, but found no support for the notion that muscle tension is a valid predictor of recurrent headaches. They compared participants suffering from migraine, tension, and combined migraine and tension headaches with a matched group of nonheadache participants during several experimental conditions, including rest, self-control, and stress. Andrasik et al. found no consistent results to suggest that level of muscle tension is an accurate predictor of headache pain. These studies failed to support the notion that muscle tension, as measured by electromyography, is a reliable and valid index of pain.

Autonomic Indices

Researchers have also attempted to assess pain through several autonomic indices—such involuntary processes as hyperventilation, blood flow in the temporal artery, heart rate, hand surface temperature, finger pulse volume, and skin resistance level. Again, most of these attempts have met with only limited success. Glynn, Lloyd, and Folkard (1981) found evidence that chronic pain patients exhibited more hyperventilation (uncontrolled rapid and deep respiration) than did a group of patients who were no longer suffering from pain. Also, Andrasik et al. (1982) found no difference between people with and without headache on measures of temporal artery blood flow, hand surface temperature, heart rate, and skin resistance level. These findings cast doubt on the validity of using certain autonomic nervous system functions to measure pain.

One exception to these generally negative results has been the use of thermography to measure skin temperature (LeRoy & Filasky, 1990). Thermographic instruments measure minute changes in skin temperature and provide an estimate of autonomic nervous system functioning. This procedure has demonstrated some success in measuring some

types of pain, but more research is needed before thermography can be accepted as a useful tool. As Nigl (1984) pointed out, pain is only one of many factors contributing to changes in skin temperature; others include alcohol, diet, infection, tone or thickness of skin, and environmental temperature. In conclusion, although intense pain may affect autonomic functions, the devices used to measure these changes have not yet yielded satisfactory results.

Evoked Potentials

Electrical signals generated by the brain in response to sensory stimuli are called **evoked potentials.** Measurements of evoked potentials are similar to electroencephalograms. Instead of measuring the entire electrical activity of the brain, the measurement of evoked potentials concentrates on areas of the brain that receive input from the various senses. Initially used with visual and auditory input, evoked potentials seem to be the brain's response to all sensory stimulation, including pain.

Syrjala and Chapman (1984) reviewed research on evoked potentials in response to pain and concluded that the technique has some capacity to differentiate between the responses of patients with chronic pain and responses of people in a control group who did not suffer pain. Evoked potentials correlate with subjective reports of pain, but they are limited in their ability to measure pain. Syrjala and Chapman (1984) cited research showing that evoked potentials may increase while subjective reports of pain remain constant, thus indicating that this technique is not a precise measure of pain.

BEHAVIORAL ASSESSMENT

A second major approach to pain measurement is observation of patients' behavior. People in pain often groan, grimace, rub, sigh, limp, miss work, remain in bed, or engage in other behaviors that signify to observers that they may be suffering from pain (Fordyce, 1976). Other observable behaviors include lowered levels of activity, use of pain medication, body posture, and facial expressions (Keefe & Block, 1982). Each of these behaviors has potential reward value; that is, pain patients are frequently reinforced by some sort of disability compensation, avoidance of responsibility, and sympathy and attention from other people. Fordyce (1976, 1990b) has pointed out that these types of environmental reinforcers increase the tendency for pain behaviors to recur and for their prominence to increase.

The use of operant conditioning techniques to decrease these learned behaviors is discussed in Chapter 6. As for behavioral methods of assessing pain, methods can be divided into (1) observations made by significant others and (2) observations made by trained personnel in either a clinic or a laboratory setting.

Observations by Significant Others

Spouses and others close to the pain patient can be trained to make careful observations of pain behaviors without further reinforcing these behaviors. For example, Fordyce (1976) has trained significant others by first asking them to list 5 to 10 items indicating that the patient is in pain. This list might include such behaviors as requesting medication, moaning, or verbalizing pain. Fordyce recommends a list of this length because more than 10 items might prompt too much attention to pain behaviors and fewer than 5 items would probably not be enough to make reliable observations. Once the list is complete, the significant other is asked to record the amount of time the patient spends exhibiting each of these behaviors. Next, the significant other records his or her own behaviors immediately following the patient's pain behaviors.

This system has been modified and refined by others, notably Turk, Meichenbaum, and Genest (1983), who developed both a spouse diary and a significant-other pain questionnaire. The spouse diary asks the husband or wife to note the time, date, and location of behaviors that express unusually severe pain. Next, the spouse's subsequent feelings and actions are recorded. Then the spouse estimates the effectiveness of such actions along a 6-point scale from "did not help at all" to "seemed to stop the pain completely." The significant-other pain questionnaire is made up of 30 items inquiring about the patient's severity of pain and its effect on such areas as work, recreation, and family relations. Some questions deal with the significant other's feelings and responses toward the patient and the pain situation. These two assessment devices can be com-

pared with the patient's own diary and pain questionnaire over the same period.

Clinical and Laboratory Observations

A number of investigators have relied on trained observers to assess pain behaviors in clinic and laboratory settings (Follick, Ahern, & Aberger, 1985; Fordyce, 1990a; Keefe, 1982; Keefe & Block, 1982; LeResche, 1982; Philips & Hunter, 1982). Observer ratings of patient behaviors can be reliably scored (Kerner & Alexander, 1981), especially when the behaviors are broken down into specific components, such as rubbing, bracing, or moaning. Investigators have used both direct observations (carried out surreptitiously) and videotape recordings, and both techniques have demonstrated acceptable reliability and validity.

A study by Keefe and Block (1982) used two trained observers to independently view and record videotapes of patients with low back pain. They tallied five nonverbal pain behaviors: sighing, grimacing, rubbing, bracing, and guarding. The percentage of agreement between observers for these five categories ranged from 93% to 99%, indicating strong reliability for this technique. Patients also rated their intensity of pain, thus allowing a validity check of the observers' ratings. For all behaviors except grimacing, the correlation was significant, a result suggesting that the ratings of trained observers have some validity. Keefe and Block also found that the frequency of pain behaviors tended to decrease with behaviorally oriented treatment and that changes in behavior correlated with changes in pain ratings. In addition, Keefe and Block found that the five behaviors differentiated pain patients from normal people and also from pain-free depressed patients.

Another team of researchers (Follick et al., 1985; Kulich, Follick, & Conger, 1983) has taken a somewhat different approach to developing a system for observing pain behaviors. Instead of predetermining the behaviors to be observed, they developed a taxonomy of pain behaviors by asking a group of raters to view videotapes of patients with chronic low back pain as the patients engaged in different activities and to nominate the behaviors they believed displayed pain. In all, the raters nominated more than 2,000 behaviors, which were eventually grouped into 16 categories. Unlike the Keefe and Block study, this investigation included some verbal behaviors such as limitations statements—comments that the pain was limiting movement. Only 7 of the 16 categories had acceptable reliabilities, and of these, only four (partial movement, limitation statements, sounds, and position shifts) accurately differentiated pain patients from normal controls.

Combining these results with those of Keefe and Block, it appears that a number of pain behaviors can be reliably measured. Raters independently agree when pain patients are guarding their movements, bracing, rubbing, grimacing, emitting pain sounds, and restricting their movements. Moreover, a number of these behaviors can distinguish between patients known to be in pain and those who are pain free.

SELF-REPORTS

The third approach to pain measurement is the use of self-reports. Self-reports include simple rating scales, standardized pain inventories, and standardized personality tests.

Rating Scales

One of the oldest pain measures, the self-report scale, is still widely used. On the simplest rating scales, the patients are asked to rate their intensity of pain on a scale from 1 to 10 or 1 to 100, with 100 being the most excruciating pain possible, and 1 being the least amount of pain detectable. A similar technique is the Visual Analog Scale (VAS), which is simply a line anchored on the left by a phrase like "no pain" and on the right by a phrase like "worst pain imaginable."

The VAS and the numerical rating scales are both easy to use, and both have acceptable reliability ratings (Kremer, Atkinson, & Ignelzi, 1981). However, they have been criticized as sometimes being confusing to older patients and for not taking into account the multidimensional nature of pain (Syrjala & Chapman, 1984). Pain experts have long recognized that pain has several dimensions and that valuable information is lost when measurement is limited to intensity alone.

Pain Questionnaires

Melzack (1975b, p. 278) was referring to the multidimensional nature of pain when he stated that "the word 'pain' refers to an endless variety of qualities that are categorized under a simple linguistic label, not to a specific, single sensation that varies only in intensity." He contended that describing pain on a single dimension was "like specifying the visual world only in terms of light flux without regard to pattern, color, texture, and the many other dimensions of visual experience" (p. 278). In an attempt to rectify this weakness in single-dimensional measurement scales, Melzack (1975b) developed the McGill Pain Questionnaire (MPQ).

The McGill Pain Questionnaire, which grew out of earlier work by Melzack and Torgerson (1971), provides a subjective report of pain and categorizes it in three dimensions: sensory, affective, and evaluative. *Sensory* qualities of pain are its temporal, spatial, pressure, and thermal properties; *affective* qualities are its fear, tension, and autonomic properties; *evaluative* qualities are the subjective overall intensity of the pain experience.

The MPQ has four parts. Part 1 consists of front and back drawings of the human body. Patients mark on these drawings the areas where they feel pain. Part 2 consists of 20 sets of words describing pain, and patients draw a circle around the one word in each set that most accurately describes their pain. These adjectives are ordered from least to most painful—for example, *nagging, nauseating, agonizing, dreadful,* and *torturing.* Part 3 asks how patients' pain has changed with time. Part 4 measures the intensity of pain on a 5-point scale from *mild* to *excruciating.* This fourth part yields a Present Pain Intensity (PPI) score. As might be expected, the PPI has been found to correlate highly with the Visual Analog Scale (Walsh & Leber, 1983).

The MPQ is the most frequently used multidimensional measure of pain (Bradley, 1993). It has been used to assess pain relief in a variety of treatment programs (Rybstein-Blinchik, 1979) and has demonstrated some validity in assessing cancer pain (Dudgeon, Raubertas, & Rosenthal, 1993), headache (Hunter & Philips, 1981), and several other pain syndromes (Chapman & Syrjala, 1990; Dubuisson & Melzack, 1976; Melzack, 1975b). Syrjala and Chapman (1984) reviewed the MPQ and found that it showed considerable promise as a multidimensional pain assessment inventory. On the negative side, they were critical of its difficult vocabulary and its lack of a standard scoring format. In 1990, Chapman and Syrjala reported that the MPQ was useful in defining the quality of a patient's pain, but they cautioned that the oral and written responses to the inventory are not necessarily equivalent.

In 1987, Melzack developed a short-form of the McGill Pain Questionnaire (SF-MFQ), which has 11 sensory and 4 affective descriptors that patients rate for intensity on a scale of 0 to 3. Like the full-length MPQ, the short form has a Present Pain Intensity index. Melzack (1987) reported that SF-MFQ scores correlate consistently high with scores on the standard MPQ. Dudgeon et al. (1993) confirmed the value of the SF-MFQ's sensory, affective, and total scores to predict scores on the long form of the MFQ. Cancer pain patients filled out both the long and short forms three times, 3 to 4 weeks apart. Scores on the two inventories changed in the same manner over a period of time, suggesting that the short form measures the same expressions of pain as the long form.

In 1985, Kerns, Turk, and Rudy developed the West Haven-Yale Multidimensional Pain Inventory (WHYMPI), another assessment tool specifically designed for pain patients. The 52-item WHYMPI is divided into three sections. The first rates (1) pain severity, (2) pain's interference with patients' lives, (3) patients' dissatisfaction with their present functioning, (4) patients' view of the support they receive from others, (5) patients' perceived life control, and (6) patients' negative mood states. The second section rates the patients' perceptions of the responses of significant others, and the third measures how often patients engage in each of 30 different daily activities.

Kerns et al. analyzed data from 120 participants who completed the WHYMPI and developed 13 different scales that capture different dimensions of the lives of pain patients. Further studies (Turk & Rudy, 1988; Rudy, Turk, Zaki, & Curtin, 1989) have used the statistical technique of cluster analysis to group pain patients according to the pattern of their responses on the WHYMPI. The pain patients fell into three clusters. The researchers called one cluster *dysfunctional* because the patients in this cluster tended to report higher levels of pain, greater psychological distress, lower perceived control, greater interference with their lives, lower levels of activity, and lower levels of perceived control over their lives. These patients experienced many problems attributable to their pain. The second cluster of patients perceived that their families and significant others did not support them, so this group was called *interpersonally distressed*. The people in this profile had problems because they perceived that those around them were failing to provide necessary support. The researchers called people in the third cluster *adaptive copers*. These individuals reported lower levels of pain severity, lower interference with their lives, lower personal distress, and higher levels of activity and control. These patients were less troubled by their pain and appeared to be coping with it.

The WHYMPI assesses many aspects of psychological and physical functioning and could provide a comprehensive assessment of the lives of pain patients. The researchers involved with the development of the MPI have validated it against many standardized tests, including the McGill Pain Questionnaire and the Minnesota Multiphasic Personality Inventory.

Rudy et al. (1989) have also attempted to validate the WHYMPI by conducting cluster analyses on patients suffering from temporomandibular joint syndrome, a disorder that may involve pain in the head, neck, and face. Although these patients differed from the sample of Turk and Rudy's (1988) study, they fell into the same three clusters. Walter and Brannon (1991) tested a sample of headache patients and obtained similar clusters. These studies suggest that the characteristics measured by the WHYMPI are similar in chronic pain patients and that the three clusters represent common approaches to coping with chronic pain. If these three configurations can be found in all chronic pain patients, scores from the WHYMPI may be useful in devising and administering therapy programs.

In addition to the West Haven-Yale Multidimensional Pain Inventory, Kerns and his associates (Kerns et al., 1991) have developed the Pain Behavior Check List (PBCL) to assess the multidimensional nature of chronic pain. The PBCL is based on the earlier work of Turk, Wack, and Kerns (1985), who had clustered 20 pain behaviors into four major groups. Kerns et al. (1991) combined two of these items and added six new ones, for a total of 25 items. Pain patients rate on a 7-point scale how often they do each of the 25 pain behaviors. Kerns et al. conducted a factor analysis of the responses of

126 chronic pain patients and found nearly the same four factors identified earlier by Turk et al. (1985) — namely, Distorted Ambulation, Affect Distress, Facial/Audible Expressions, and Seeking Help. Although Kerns et al. found satisfactory reliability for the PBCL, little additional research has been reported on this scale.

Another promising pain inventory is the Pain Anxiety Symptoms Scale (PASS) developed by Lance McCracken and his co-workers (McCracken, Zayfert, & Gross, 1992, 1993). The PASS is a 40-item self-report assessment of fear and anxiety symptoms associated with pain. Rather than tapping pain itself, the PASS attempts to measure fear of pain. It yields four subscale scores — (1) cognitive, (2) fear, (3) escape/avoidance, and (4) physiological — as well as a total score. McCracken et al. (1992) claimed the PASS has sufficient validity because it significantly correlates with measures of anxiety and depression and adequately predicts level of disability due to pain.

Osman, Barrios, Osman, Schneekloth, and Troutman (1994) confirmed the potential usefulness of the PASS with a group of nonclinical participants. They administered the PASS, along with a battery of other scales, to 224 community-dwelling adults and found support for both the one-factor and the four-factor structures identified by McCracken et al. in pain patients. In addition, Osman et al. found the PASS to have good internal consistency and moderate correlations with measures of anxiety, depression, and health locus of control. Despite its promising beginning, much more research is needed on the Pain Anxiety Symptoms Scale.

Standardized Psychological Tests

Another approach to pain measurement is the use of standardized psychological tests, especially the Minnesota Multiphasic Personality Inventory (MMPI). This instrument was not originally designed to assess pain but to measure such clinical diagnoses as hypochrondriasis, depression, paranoia, schizophrenia, and other psychopathologies. From the time that Hanvik (1951) first found that different types of pain patients could be differentiated on several MMPI scales, other researchers have used this inventory for pain measurement. Research has indicated that high scores on the hypochondriasis scale

(a measure of preoccupation with body functions) correlate with pain (Sternbach, 1978). Other researchers have found that clusters of three or four MMPI scales reliably predict pain in clinical populations (Bradley, Prokop, Gentry, Van der Heide, & Prieto, 1981; Bradley, Prokop, Margolis, & Gentry, 1978; Bradley & Van der Heide, 1984; Prokop, Bradley, Margolis, & Gentry, 1980). The so-called neurotic triad — a cluster of elevated scores on hypochondriasis, depression, and hysteria — consistently relate to reports of pain.

The MMPI has been used with mixed results to predict treatment outcomes. Two studies (Long, 1981; Turner, Herron, & Pheasant, 1981) found that some MMPI clusters successfully predicted patients' response to surgical treatment for low back pain. Patients with no elevated MMPI scores responded better to treatment than those with high scores on certain clusters. Other studies (McGill, Lawlis, Selby, Mooney, & McCoy, 1983; Moore, Armentrout, Parker, & Kivlahan, 1986) reported no differences among MMPI subgroups in their response to multimodal pain treatment. Turner and Romano (1990) concluded that although the MMPI has had some success in measuring chronic back pain, its most effective use is in predicting which patients will respond to medical treatments for pain.

Mikail, DuBreuil, and D'Eon (1993) conducted a comparative analysis of nine commonly used self-report measures of chronic pain and found five core dimensions tapped by these inventories. These factors were (1) General Affective Distress, (2) Coping, (3) Support, (4) Pain Description, and (5) Functional Capacity. Mikail et al. reported that the McGill Pain Questionnaire, the West Haven-Yale Multidimensional Pain Inventory, and the Beck Depression Inventory (Beck, Ward, Mendelson, Mock, & Erbaugh, 1961) measured the pain experience with very little overlap, a result suggesting that each of these three has something unique to offer.

PREVENTING PAIN

Pain can be prevented by avoiding injury or by medical or psychological treatment for pain. The next section looks at medical treatments for pain, and Chapter 6 discusses psychological treatments. Physicians and psychologists would agree that preventing pain in the first place is preferable to treating it once it occurs. This section briefly addresses some attempts to prevent pain.

Because low back pain is a frequent cause of lost work days, several programs target the prevention of this type of pain. C. Stuart Donaldson and his associates (Donaldson, Stanger, Donaldson, Cram, & Skubick, 1993) reported on the results of an educational program called Back to Balance. Participants of this study were nursing aides, orderlies, and other employees at a health care facility who had a very high rate of lost work time due to chronic repetitive lifting injuries to the back. Donaldson et al. randomly assigned half the employees to an educational group who were instructed in the Back to Balance program and half to a control group. The Back to Balance procedure consists of an easy-to-read booklet that contains information on the anatomy of the back and guidelines on how to keep the back balanced while engaging in repetitive lifting. After 3 months, the employees in the control also participated in the educational program.

Results from this study indicated that the treatment group reported significantly less pain (as measured by the McGill Pain Questionnaire) than the controls at 3- and 12-month follow-up periods. Moreover, participants generalized their knowledge to the home. Most important for the facility, wages and relief costs were reduced to less than 25% of previous rates. The Donaldson et al. study is one of very few that indicate the effectiveness of educational programs in pain prevention. Lahad, Malter, Berg, and Deyo (1994) searched all articles in English from 1966 to 1993 in an effort to evaluate the effectiveness of different interventions for back pain prevention. From the 64 studies with original data, they noted four principal interventions: (1) back and aerobic exercise; (2) education; (3) mechanical supports such as corsets; and (4) risk factor modification—for example, smoking cessation and weight loss. For people with no pre-existing back pain, only exercise showed much promise in decreasing the incidence and duration of low back pain. Lahad et al. found very little evidence to support education as a pain prevention measure, insufficient evidence to recommend back supports, and no evidence that weight loss or other risk factor modifications could prevent low back pain. These authors concluded that there is some limited evidence to recommend exercise, but no evidence to recommend any of the other three interventions. However, the Donaldson et al. study shows that some educational programs can work to prevent pain.

MEDICAL TREATMENTS FOR PAIN

For centuries, physicians have used a variety of means for alleviating pain. Presently, many of these procedures are supplemented by psychological or behavioral procedures. Eisenberg et al. (1993) reported that a substantial number of patients receive both medical and nonmedical treatments for the same disorder at the same time. Most of these nonmedical therapies are behavioral, and these are discussed in the next chapter. This section looks at traditional medical treatments for pain.

A study by Krokosky and Reardon (1989) highlights an important problem in the medical treatment of pain: agreement between patients and health care professionals about the experience of pain. These researchers administered a shortened form of the McGill Pain Questionnaire to 50 inpatients, most of whom were recuperating from surgery. The researchers also administered the questionnaire to the nurses and physicians who were caring for these patients, asking the nurses, physicians, and patients to rate each patient's pain. In comparing the three sets of pain scores for each patient, the researchers found many discrepancies. The correlations between the patients' ratings of their pain and the nurses' ratings of the patients' pain failed to show a statistically significant relationship, as did the correlation between physicians' and patients' ratings. The lack of correlation shows that neither type of health care professional perceived the amount and duration of their patients' pain. In general, nurses and physicians underestimated the pain their patients experienced.

These results indicate that patients who are in pain may not be perceived to be in pain by those who are caring for them or that patients' pain may be perceived as less severe by professionals than by the patients themselves. These differing perceptions of pain may cause problems in the treatment of acute pain and the management of chronic pain.

Medical treatments have traditionally been chosen according to the type and source of pain. Acute pain is usually treated with drugs. Both acute and chronic pain have been treated by stimulation to the skin, either electrical impulses (transcutaneous electrical neural stimulation) or needles (acupuncture). Chronic pain that has not responded to other methods of management is sometimes treated by surgery.

DRUGS

Analgesic drugs relieve pain without causing loss of consciousness. Hundreds of different analgesic drugs are available, but almost all fall into two major groups: the aspirin type and the opium type (Melzack & Wall, 1982). Both types exist naturally as derivatives of plants, and both have many synthetic variations. Of the two, the opium type is stronger and has a longer history of use.

Aspirin comes from an extract of willow bark. The active component is salicin, a compound isolated in 1827 (Melzack & Wall, 1982). The Bayer Company used the name aspirin as a trade name beginning in 1899. In addition to having analgesic properties, aspirin acts against inflammation and fever, making it one of the nonsteroidal anti-inflammatory drugs (NSAIDs). Ibuprofen and naproxen sodium are also in this class of drugs, and all are available without prescription in the United States.

NSAIDs appears to block the synthesis of prostaglandins (Winter, 1994), a class of chemicals released by damaged tissue and involved in inflammation and the sensitization of neurons that increase pain. These drugs act at the site of injury instead of crossing into the brain and changing neurochemical activity in the nervous system. As a result, NSAIDs do not alter pain perception when no injury is present, as in laboratory situations with people who receive experimental pain stimuli.

Aspirin and the other NSAIDs have many uses in pain relief. Because these drugs appear to work by influencing the effects of injury, they are especially useful for pain in which injury has occurred. This description takes in a wide variety of pain, including minor cuts and scratches as well as more severe injuries such as broken bones. But pain that occurs without inflammation is not so readily relieved by

NSAIDs, and some gastric problems are worsened by the irritation that these drugs cause.

Another of aspirin's side effects is the alteration of blood clotting time, a condition that can be either an advantage (as in patients who are at risk for forming internal blood clots) or a disadvantage (as in patients who are candidates for surgery). This side effect makes aspirin unsuitable for some people who are in pain. Aspirin and other NSAIDs are also toxic in large doses and can cause damage to the liver and kidneys. People who take an overdose of these drugs may do so by taking a combination of over-the-counter analgesics without recognizing the similarity of many of them (Winter, 1994).

Acetaminophen, another over-the-counter analgesic, is not one of the NSAIDs. It has no anti-inflammatory properties but has a pain-relieving capability that is similar to aspirin but somewhat weaker. Under brand names like Tylenol, acetaminophen has become the most frequently used drug for pain relief (DeNitto, 1993). Acetaminophen does not have the gastric side effects of aspirin, so people who cannot tolerate aspirin find it a good substitute. Nor does acetaminophen have anti-inflammatory properties, making it less appropriate for conditions involving inflammation. Large quantities of acetaminophen can be fatal, but even nonlethal doses can do serious damage to the liver, especially when combined with alcohol (Winter, 1994).

The most powerful analgesics are of the opium type. The extract of the opium poppy has been in use for at least 5,000 years, and its analgesic properties were known to the ancient Romans (Melzack & Wall, 1982). In 1803, morphine was isolated. Many synthetic compounds have structures and actions similar to morphine, and several neurotransmitters produce analgesia in the same way that the opiates do (Pert & Snyder, 1973). This mechanism is responsible for the pain-relieving effect of opiates and explains why even strong pain can be alleviated by these drugs.

Because morphine is so powerful, many physicians are reluctant to prescribe it in amounts strong enough to reduce intense pain. Thus, many acute pain patients and people with chronic pain due to cancer do not receive sufficient relief. Fife, Irick, and Painter (1993) discovered that physicians and nurses see the problem of undermedication as common but also believe that patients should have more control over their level of medication. Similarly, C. Stanton Hill (1995) contended that all types of pain are inadequately treated and that patients should begin to demand adequate pain relief. Hill also condemned health care workers for overtly or covertly conveying the message that patients who request pain medication are drug abusers.

One procedure that has overcome the undermedication problem is a system of self-paced administration. Patients can activate a pump attached to their intravenous lines and deliver a dose of medication whenever they wish (Moyer, 1989). Such systems began to appear in the late 1970s and have since gained wide acceptance. The initial fears that patients would overmedicate if allowed free access to self-administered opiate analgesics has proven unfounded. In fact, the average amount of medication consumed is often lower than with the traditional type of delivery. Because an intravenous line is necessary for this system of drug delivery, it is most common in postsurgical patients. The system has also been used with success for burn patients (Moyer, 1989) and cancer patients (Sheidler, 1987).

How realistic are the fears of drug abuse as a consequence of prescribed opiate drugs? Do patients become addicted while recovering from surgery? What about the dangers to patients with terminal illnesses? According to a study by Porter and Jick (1980), the risk of addiction is less than 1%. Several authorities have even questioned the risk of problems due to tolerance in cancer patients, contending that tolerance occurs for only the first few days of administration and does not continue to escalate (Catalano, 1987; Elliott & Elliott, 1992; Foley, 1989; Melzack & Wall, 1982).

Like all drugs, the opiates have side effects. They alter a person's perception, usually by decreasing anxiety or clouding judgment. They affect the digestive system, producing constipation and sometimes nausea. They also depress the respiratory system and can cause death by respiratory failure.

The advantages of opiate drugs outweigh their dangers. No other type of drug produces more complete pain relief. However, their potential for abuse and their side effects make them more suitable for treating acute pain than for managing chronic pain. The opiate drugs remain an essential part of pain management for the most severe, acute injuries, for recovery from surgery, and for terminal illnesses.

TRANSCUTANEOUS ELECTRICAL NEURAL STIMULATION (TENS)

As Melzack and Wall (1982) pointed out, the electrical stimulation of nerves is only one form of cutaneous stimulation that has been used to control pain. Other forms include massage and the application of heat and cold. Manipulations of the skin to relieve pain have a long and successful history.

Transcutaneous electrical neural stimulation (TENS), however, has a short history, dating only to the early 1970s (McCaffery, 1979). Electrical stimulation, which affects all nerves within about 4 centimeters of the skin's surface, can be accomplished by placing an electrode on the surface of the skin. The TENS system typically consists of electrodes that attach to the skin and are connected to a unit that supplies electrical stimulation. Many of these units are portable, and run on rechargeable batteries (McCaffery, 1979). Patients can vary the strength of the stimulation to suit their needs. Usually, pain decreases during the stimulation (Melzack & Wall, 1982), and the relief can persist for hours after the stimulation has ceased. Patients with both chronic and acute pain can use TENS units to achieve pain relief.

Nelson and Planchock (1989) reported on patients' pain and drug use as they recovered from surgery with TENS as analgesia. In this study, the TENS patients were comparable to the other patients recovering from surgery. The TENS patients, however, requested fewer doses of drugs to control their pain and were discharged from the hospital significantly sooner than the patients who received standard postsurgical care.

Melzack and Wall (1982) reviewed the use of TENS with arthritis patients and found that TENS produced significant pain relief. They also pointed out that this approach seems to work with patients who have not obtained adequate relief from other methods, including surgery. TENS, therefore, provides relief from a great variety of pains, even those that have been resistant to medical treatment.

ACUPUNCTURE

Acupuncture is an ancient Chinese form of analgesia that consists of inserting needles into specific points on the skin and continuously stimulating the needles (Melzack & Wall, 1982). The stimulation can be accomplished electrically or by twirling the needles. Inherent in the use of acupuncture is a philosophy of the body and illness not accepted by many Westerners. Hence, many physicians and laypeople in the United States are skeptical about acupuncture.

Acupuncture has been used as an anesthetic for surgery, and some patients in China have undergone surgery with acupuncture as their only anesthetic (Melzack & Wall, 1982). However, even in countries where the technique is well accepted, only about 10% of all patients experience sufficient analgesia from acupuncture during surgery. Its effects are not instantaneous, and the needles must be stimulated for about 20 minutes to produce analgesia. Furthermore, the stimulation must be fairly intense and continuous. But the analgesia can last for hours after the stimulation has ceased.

According to both Melzack (1975a) and Melzack and Wall (1982), acupuncture is more effective than a placebo in producing pain relief. Nor are acupuncture's effects due to the placebo effect because the technique can also produce analgesia in dogs and monkeys.

Although acupuncture is an interesting phenomenon, it is not a major approach to the control of pain in Western countries. Chapman and Gunn (1990) concluded that after 10 years of research, the literature does not permit firm conclusions concerning the effectiveness of acupuncture. Thus, this treatment for pain relief remains an experimental therapy. More optimistically, they stated that properly practiced, acupuncture is quite safe and "offers an alternative to the conventional, often ineffectual, prescription of analgesic medication for patients with persisting pain" (Chapman & Gunn, 1990, p. 1819).

SURGERY

Surgery is the most extreme form of treatment for pain and is usually used only when other treatments have failed. The most common use of surgery is to alleviate chronic low back pain. Not all patients experience analgesia from surgery, and of course, surgery has its own dangers and possibilities for complications.

Surgery to control pain can occur at any level of the nervous system. The least radical surgery involves destroying the peripheral nerves close to the site of the pain (Carson, 1987). This type of surgery is recommended only if the pain is localized well enough to allow limited destruction of nerves and if this destruction is likely to produce relief. The best approach is to first use a local anesthetic on the nerves so the patient can experience the effects of nerve destruction. Some patients prefer the pain to the complete loss of sensation that surgery confers. Another consideration is that, in most cases, the peripheral nerves include both sensory and motor fibers. Thus, surgery will cause not only loss of sensation but also loss of movement. Because nerves in the peripheral nervous system regenerate, the entire nerve section must be destroyed; otherwise, the pain will recur when the nerves regenerate.

Another possible site for surgery is the dorsal root ganglion, just outside the spinal cord. Nerves split into the dorsal and ventral branches before entering the spinal cord. Because the dorsal branch is entirely sensory, severing it will produce only sensory loss and leave motor functioning unaffected. Carson (1987) pointed out that some patients experience distress at the complete loss of sensation, and some even develop phantom limb-type sensation and even pain as a result of this surgery.

Other possible sites for surgical intervention to control pain include the spinal cord and the brain itself. The most common of the surgeries to the spinal cord involve severing the spinothalamic tract (Schürmann, 1975; Melzack & Wall, 1982). This surgery initially produces a complete loss of sensation for the area of the body below the damage. However, patients often experience a return of an unpleasant sensation. This recurrent sensation typically starts as a tingling and often progresses to a serious pain. Therefore, spinal cord surgery is usually performed on people with terminal conditions who would benefit from a relief of pain for the remainder of their lives.

Pain control through surgery to the brain is possible but rare. Brain surgery, of course, is very serious, because lesions to the brain can produce many effects in addition to pain relief. Interestingly, prefrontal lobotomies produce pain relief in the form of a decreased concern with pain, but this surgery produces no sensory deficit; it merely causes patients to be so little concerned with the sensation that they do not report pain. Surgery to the thalamus and the somatosensory cortex are dangerous and have not proven to be effective in relieving pain.

In summary, neurosurgery for pain control involves the implantation of devices that stimulate the brain and produce pain relief. Stimulating a small electrode in the periaqueductal gray has been somewhat successful in controlling pain (Carson, 1987). A similar approach is to introduce an opiate drug directly into the brain, usually by way of the ventricles. The drug spreads throughout the brain and affects the opiate receptors, thus relieving pain by a more direct route than oral, intramuscular, or intravenous administration.

LIMITATIONS OF MEDICAL TREATMENTS

Medical treatments are usually the first choice for the treatment of acute pain and are frequently used to manage chronic pain. Analgesic drugs, especially the NSAIDs, acetaminophen, or the opiate group, are the most common of the medical treatments. Surgery is another common prescription for relief from chronic low back pain. All medical treatments for pain have limitations, and doctors are not always aware of these limitations.

One limitation of opiate drugs is the tolerance and dependence they produce in patients. *Tolerance* occurs when a larger and larger dose of a drug is required to bring about the same effect. *Dependence* occurs when the drug's removal produces withdrawal symptoms. Because opiates produce both tolerance and dependence, they are potentially dangerous and subject to abuse. As a result, health care professionals are reluctant to prescribe these drugs, and the public is afraid to use them, even when they could relieve intractable pain (Donovan, 1989; McCaffery, 1979; Melzack & Wall, 1982).

Donovan (1989) pointed out that because of these concerns, patients are often undermedicated and do not receive sufficiently large or frequent doses of medication to produce relief. She reported that the average dose of opiate drugs was below the therapeutic level and that patients took only a fourth to a third of the medication that their physicians had ordered. Unfortunately, such patients can suffer needlessly as a result.

Similarly, Elliott and Elliott (1992) found that physicians embraced several misconceptions about the use of morphine for cancer pain. More than one-half of physicians who worked directly with cancer pain patients misunderstood the concept of morphine tolerance, nearly 40% held misconceptions about morphine's side effects, and despite evidence to the contrary, 20% believed that morphine addiction was a potentially serious problem to cancer pain patients. Elliott and Elliott found significant levels of misunderstanding in physicians of all ages, indicating that recently trained physicians embrace traditional attitudes toward opioid use. Fife et al. (1993) found that the nurses and physicians in their study were more accurate in understanding the problem of undermedication for cancer patients and in believing that addiction is not a problem.

Whereas undermedication may be a problem for cancer pain patients, overmedication is often a problem for patients suffering from low back pain. Von Korff, Barlow, Cherkin, and Deyo (1994) grouped primary care physicians into low, moderate, and high frequency of prescribing pain medication and bed rest for back pain patients. A 1- and 2-year follow-up found that patients who took less medication and who remained active did just as well as back pain patients who were told to take more medication and to rest. In addition, patients with the least amount of medication were the most satisfied with their treatment. Moreover, patients whose physicians rated low in prescription of medication and bed rest spent only about half as much money on treatment as patients whose doctors rated high on medication and bed rest.

A recent study in Finland indicated that physicians and nurses were unable to predict which back pain treatment would be most effective. Malmivaara et al. (1995) randomly assigned Helsinki city employees with acute nonspecific low back pain to three groups: (1) complete bed rest for 2 days, (2) slow back-mobilizing exercises every second hour, and (3) a control group who continued ordinary activities as tolerated. Prior to the study, both physicians and nurses predicted that the exercise group would do best. After 3- and 12-weeks of treatment, the group with the best recovery was the control group. That is, people who continued their ordinary activities had significantly less pain intensity and duration and were more able to work than people who had complete bed rest or who had done back exercises. Malmivaara et al. reasoned that these differences in favor of the control group were not due to the placebo effect, which ordinarily would favor the experimental groups. Instead, this study demonstrates the limitation of medical treatment in dealing with this common type of pain.

CHAPTER SUMMARY

Pain stems from both physiological and psychological factors. The physiology of pain involves the somatosensory system, the part of the nervous system that handles sensing, relaying, and interpreting information throughout the body. Receptors near the skin's surface react to several different types of stimulation, all of which may be interpreted as pain if the stimulation is sufficiently intense. The nerve impulses generated by these receptors relay the message to the spinal cord, where some modulation of the neural impulse takes place in the laminae of the dorsal horn of the spinal cord.

Information that goes to the somatosensory cortex in the cerebral cortex first travels through the thalamus. A map of the skin's surface lies in the primary somatosensory cortex, but the secondary somatosensory cortex is not mapped in the same way. Both areas of the brain receive projections from the skin.

The brain also contains mechanisms for modulating sensory input and thereby affecting the perception of pain. One mechanism is through the naturally occurring neurochemicals that relieve pain and mimic the action of opiate drugs. These neurochemicals exist in many places in the central and peripheral nervous systems. The second mechanism is a system of descending control through the periaqueductal gray and the nucleus raphe magnus. This system affects the activity of the spinal cord and provides a descending modulation of activity in the spinal cord.

The degree of tissue damage may contribute to one's experience of pain, but personal perceptions are frequently more crucial. The two types of pain most central to health psychology are acute and chronic pain. Acute pain is usually adaptive and lasts for less than 6 months; chronic pain continues beyond the time of healing and is often experienced in the absence of detectable tissue damage.

Pain syndromes include headache pain, low back pain, myofascial pain, arthritic pain, cancer pain, and phantom limb pain. Health psychologists have worked mostly with headache and low back pain, two common and troublesome pain syndromes.

Several models have been proposed to explain pain. The experience of pain has no clear relationship to the stimulation of neurons, making untenable simple theories, such as the specificity theory. The gate control theory is currently the most influential; its hypothesis is that the perception of pain can be increased or diminished by mechanisms in the spinal cord and the brain. A revision of the gate control theory, neuromatrix theory, places even more emphasis on brain-level processes in pain perception.

A variety of measures have been used to assess pain, and these can be grouped into three broad categories: physiological measures, behavioral assessment, and self-reports. Physiological measures, including muscle tension, autonomic indices, and evoked potentials, have been used with only limited success. Many psychologists have preferred to observe pain-related behavior, and research indicates that many behavioral assessment techniques have at least some reliability and validity. Self-reports used to assess pain include (1) rating scales; (2) pain questionnaires, such as the McGill Pain Questionnaire and the West Haven-Yale Multidimensional Pain Inventory; and (3) standardized objective tests, such as the Minnesota Multiphasic Personality Inventory.

Medical approaches to controlling pain have had a long history and some success. Although health psychologists do not use these methods, patients undergoing behavioral treatment for pain control often receive medical treatments as well. These medical treatments include surgery, drugs, transcutaneous electrical neural stimulation (TENS), and acupuncture. Surgical methods for pain control are used when other methods have failed and are most successful for pain associated with terminal illnesses. Drugs can control severe pain, but because of fears about abuse, their use is limited mostly to acute pain. TENS, a recent advance, can be used to control chronic and acute pain. Acupuncture can control pain but remains experimental and rare in Western society. Limitations of medical treatments include undermedication for some pain, especially cancer pain, and overmedication for other types, especially low back pain. Also, many doctors and nurses hold several misconceptions about medical treatments, including lack of understanding of pa-tients' tolerance and dependency, and the addictive properties of some drugs. Recent evidence has suggested that the continuation of ordinary activities may be a more effective treatment for back pain than either bed rest or back exercise.

SUGGESTED READINGS

Bonica, J. J. (1990). History of pain concepts and therapies. In J. J. Bonica (Ed.), *The management of pain* (2nd ed., pp. 2–17). Malvern, PA: Lea & Febiger. Bonica presents an interesting historical account of pain perspectives and also includes an examination of various pain theories, including ones discussed in this chapter.

Fordyce, W. E. (1990). Learned pain: Pain as behavior. In J. J. Bonica (Ed.), *The management of pain* (2nd ed., pp. 291–299). Malvern, PA: Lea & Febiger. One of the foremost authorities on pain discusses the influence of learning on pain behavior. Fordyce points out that the consequences of pain behaviors are often reinforcing to the pain patient.

Melzack, R. (1992, April). Phantom limbs. *Scientific American, 266,* 120–126. This article includes a review of the gate control theory and a description of Melzack's neuromatrix theory, which he formulated as a result of the failure of the gate control theory to explain phantom limb sensation and pain.

Morris, D. B. (1994, Autumn). Pain's dominion: What we make of pain. *Wilson Quarterly*, pp. 8–33. Morris concentrates on the cultural meaning of pain in the historical context. His review is easy to read and provides current information on the personal difficulties of dealing with pain in a medical establishment that tends to find the concept troublesome.

6 Coping with Stress and Pain

In Chapter 3 we met Rick, the college student who had lost his job, experienced a divorce and the loss of his father and close friend, and faced financial problems. Rick was feeling an unusually high level of stress as a result of the myriad life events that befell him. We learned that Rick tried to cope with his stress by isolating himself and working two and sometimes three jobs. These strategies, of course, were not beneficial to his overall health. He also decided to begin college and to become more involved in church activities. Were any of these choices good alternatives for managing his problems? What other methods were available to Rick? Would those alternatives have been more helpful?

In Chapter 5 we considered the case of Carl, a young man suffering from chronic pain. Carl seemed to be making the most out of his pain by trying to secure monetary compensation for his distress. He was also being rewarded by his family and friends for his pain behaviors. What did biofeedback treatment accomplish for Carl? Was biofeedback the best choice of treatment for him? In this chapter, we reconsider the problems of Rick, Carl, and the mil-

lions of other Americans who suffer from elevated stress and chronic pain.

PERSONAL RESOURCES THAT INFLUENCE COPING

Stress and chronic pain are common conditions for humans—common but not normal. The normal tendency is toward health, and any inclination away from health sets up a state of "dis-ease." People fight against distress and disease in a variety of ways. One way is through the immune system, the body's natural protection from invasion by foreign material, as discussed in Chapter 4. People sometimes adjust to pain through medical treatments, such as drugs and surgery, which were discussed in Chapter 5. Still other ways of seeking relief from stress and chronic pain are such practices as taking recreational drugs, overeating, abusing alcohol, smoking, or exercising. Exercising usually promotes health, but the other behaviors are ultimately unhealthy, and exercising can be done to an unhealthy extreme. The health-related effects of smoking, eating, drinking, and exercising are discussed in Chapters 13 through 16.

This chapter looks at several psychological strategies for coping with stress and chronic pain. A person's ability to cope depends in part on personal resources, especially social support and a feeling of personal control.

SOCIAL SUPPORT

Some people react better than others to stress and chronic pain. They are the ones who have greater personal resources for coping. One of the most beneficial personal resources appears to be social support from family members, friends, and health care providers. This section discusses the meaning of social support and suggests possible reasons why social support seems to protect against disease and death.

The Meaning of Social Support

What is social support? Although social support has been widely researched, no single definition of the concept has emerged (Sarason & Sarason, 1994; Veiel & Baumann, 1992). Unfortunately, various researchers have used dozens of inventories to measure social support, and most of them have questionable reliability and validity (Heitzmann & Kaplan, 1988; Kaplan, 1994). Social support includes such things as perceived emotional concern from others, health-related advice and information, material aid, self-enhancing words and behaviors received from others, and many other factors. If social support buffers stress (as both health professionals and the general public seem to believe), researchers must find the protective agent or agents from the myriad components of social support.

A general definition of **social support** refers to a variety of material and emotional supports a person receives from others. The related concepts of **social contacts** and **social network** are sometimes used interchangeably, and both refer to the number and kinds of people with whom one associates. On the opposite side of the ledger is **social isolation**, which refers to an absence of specific meaningful interpersonal relations. People with a high level of social support ordinarily have a broad social network and many social contacts; socially isolated people have neither.

The Link between Social Support and Health

Stress researchers generally agree that a link exists between social support and health; people who receive high levels of social support are usually healthier than those who do not. Evidence from the Alameda County Study (Berkman & Syme, 1979) and from the Tecumseh Community Health Study (House, Robbins, & Metzner, 1982) revealed the health benefits of social support and the health risks of social isolation.

The Alameda County Study was the first to establish a strong link between social support and longevity. Berkman and Syme found that lack of social support was as strongly linked to mortality as cigarette smoking and a sedentary lifestyle. Figure 6.1 shows that women in all age groups had lower mortality rates than men (as indicated by the height of the bar in the graph). However, for both men and women, as the number of social ties decreased, the death rate increased. In general, participants with the fewest social ties were two to four times more likely to die than participants with the most social ties. This trend was most pronounced from age 30 to 49 for women and 50 to 59 for men.

Marriage, Gender, Ethnicity, and Social Support

Both the Alameda County Study and the Tecumseh Community Study found that marriage benefited men's health: Married men received more social support than unmarried men, and this social support helped them live longer. Other studies have confirmed this finding. For example, Kaplan et al. (1988) studied over 13,000 men and women from eastern Finland and found that men who had few social connections, compared to those who had many, were 1.5 to 2.0 times more likely to die. More specifically, men were at an elevated risk for death from both cardiovascular disease and ischemic heart disease. For women, however, Kaplan and his associates found no strong or consistent relationship between absence of social connections and subsequent death. The authors concluded that, for men at least, these findings presented the "strongest evidence to date that reduced social connections are related to mortality from cardiovascular disease" (Kaplan et al., 1988, p. 377).

Death of a spouse typically results in loss of an important source of social support, but men and women are not equally affected. Helsing, Szklo, and Comstock (1981) found that widowed men had a higher mortality rate than married men but that widowed women were no more in danger of death than married women. Helsing et al. also found that widowed men who remarried lived longer than those who did not, but widowed women who remarried had no such advantage. In a review of the literature, Schwarzer and Leppin (1992) investigated the possibility that loss of a spouse could result in premature death for the survivor, finding that both men and women were at an increased risk for

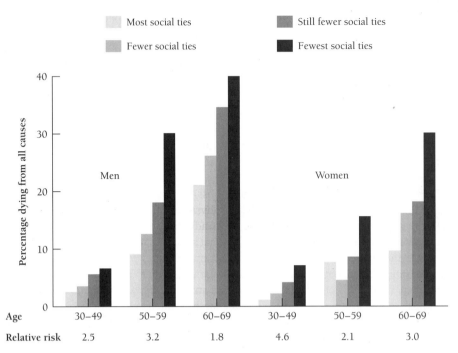

Figure 6.1   *Social isolation and 9-year mortality in Alameda County, California, 1965–1974.*
SOURCE: From "Social Networks, Host Resistance, and Mortality: A Nine-Year Follow-up of Alameda County Residents" by L. F. Berkman & S. L. Syme, 1979, *American Journal of Epidemiology, 109*, p. 190. Copyright 1979 by the Johns Hopkins University School of Hygiene and Public Health. Reprinted by permission of the publisher and the senior author.

mortality during bereavement. Men, however, were at the greatest danger during the first 6 months following the death of their wives. Schwarzer and Leppin suggested two reasons for the gender difference. First, women cultivate a larger social network of family members and friends than do men and are thus more likely to receive support after the death of a husband; men tend to rely on their wives for social support. Second, women are likely to be younger than men at the time a spouse dies, and this younger age places them at a decreased risk for death.

Schwarzer and Leppin suggested that the first 6 months of bereavement may be dangerous to men for several reasons. Lacking a broad social network, men frequently develop severe loneliness and depression, and these psychological conditions may increase their risk of suicide, poor eating habits, and alcohol abuse. Also, loneliness and depression may suppress the immune system and challenge the cardiovascular system.

Although men gain more from marriage, women gain more from social support. In the Alameda County Study (Berkman & Syme, 1979), women age 30 to 49 with few social ties had a relative risk for mortality of 4.6 whereas men of the same age with few social ties had a relative risk of only 2.5. From ages 60 to 69, the risk for women with few social ties was 3.0, but for men it was only 1.8 (see Figure 6.1). A meta-analysis by Schwarzer and Leppin (1989) confirmed this finding, revealing that for women the overall correlation between social support and good health was about .20, but for men the correlation was only .08.

Why do women profit more from social support than men? Perhaps it is because women have larger social networks that include many other women. Argyle (1992) suggested that the social styles of men and women are different. "Women seek close, supportive relationships, are warm and trusting, send more positive nonverbal signals and other rewards, and are more cooperative than men" (p. 28). Argyle stated that both men and women prefer to have women as confidants, but women are more likely than men to fulfill this preference. As a consequence, women tend to have more emotionally intimate friendships, and this supportive social network may contribute to better psychological and physical health for women.

For older people, marriage may not be as important as having a confidant. Lisa Berkman and her associates (Oxman, Berkman, Kasl, Freeman, & Barrett, 1992) surveyed nearly 2,000 community men and women 65 and older. They found that the more social support these elderly people experienced, the lower were their levels of depression. The researchers also found that perceived emotional support provided more protection against depression than tangible support, such as a visit from a friend. But more important to our discussion is their finding that the older people who never had a confidant were more likely to become depressed than were those who had never been married. In addition, they found that long-standing confidants were more protective than those gained in more recent years.

Does ethnic background play a role in social support? In 1986, Berkman looked at previous studies on social support and concluded that social support clearly helps White men cope with the stress that might be related to mortality, especially death from heart disease. The data on nonwhites in these studies, however, showed much weaker effects. One of the studies reviewed by Berkman was essentially a replication of the Alameda County Study, conducted in Evans County, Georgia, by Schoenbach, Kaplan, Fredman, and Kleinbaum (1986). These investigators found a strong positive relationship for European American men between lack of social ties and mortality. However, for European American women, African American men, and African American women, no consistent relationship emerged. The reason for the lack of a relationship among African Americans is not clear. But Berkman (1986) suggested that for African American women at least, social support is usually quite strong, and thus any sample of African American women would be too homogeneous for significant differences to emerge.

How Does Social Support Contribute to Health?

If stress causes illness, then social support may offer some buffer against stress-related illnesses. Evidence suggests, at least for European American men, that social support seems to lessen or eliminate the harmful effects of stress and therefore provides some protection against disease and death. What does social support provide that is helpful? What is stressful, even life-threatening, about social isolation? Answers to these questions are still not clear, but one possibility is that people who are isolated live in physically different circumstances and that those conditions affect their health. Another possibility is that social support provides a buffer that can protect against stress. This buffering hypothesis assumes that some of the people who experience high levels of stress are protected or buffered against its damaging physiological consequences by the social support they receive from friends and family members (Cassel, 1976; Kaplan, Cassel, & Gore, 1977).

Some people not only receive more social support than others but are more likely to profit from the support they receive. One study, for example, found that married men recovered more quickly from coronary bypass surgery than unmarried men (Kulik & Mahler, 1989). Other studies have suggested that personality variables account for the relationship between social support and physical health. Connell and D'Augelli (1990) proposed a model that included the personality factors of affiliation, succorance (receiving help), and nurturance (giving help). These three personality variables contribute directly not only to perceived social support but also to network size and supportive behaviors, both of which are related to perceived social support. In other words, liking people and wanting to give and receive help from them broadens one's network of friends and increases one's friendly and supportive behaviors. Friendliness, network size, and supportive behaviors all enable a person to feel that social support is available when needed. Although Connell and D'Augelli presented some evidence from a study they conducted in support of their theoretical model, more research is needed to validate the interactions among personality factors, network size, supportive behaviors, perceived support, and perceived health.

If friendly, helpful people receive adequate social support, then hostile people should receive less support. Hardy and Smith (1988) found some supporting evidence. Participants in this study who were high in hostility received less social support than those low in hostility and reported more negative life events and daily hassles. Can people increase their social support by becoming less hostile and more friendly and helpful? Results of these studies suggest an affirmative answer. However, simply visiting more often with one's friends or joining social organizations will probably not increase one's social support. As some researchers have pointed out, it would be misleading to suggest that the more one socializes, the better off one will be (Reis, Wheeler, Kernis, Spiegel, & Nezlek, 1985). The source of emotional support is probably more crucial to health than the frequency of social contact.

Besides personality, what else might contribute to social support? One possibility is that socially isolated people are less likely to have friends and acquaintances who encourage them to protect their health or go to the doctor when they are sick. Langlie (1977) and Broman (1993) found evidence that social contacts influence a person's preventive health practices. For example, Broman found that married people were less likely than unmarried participants to smoke or to abuse alcohol. Also, people who were members of a voluntary organization were more likely to use seatbelts and less likely to smoke or abuse alcohol. Broman also found that loss of social relationships was related to poorer health behaviors.

However, an increased number of healthy practices is not the only explanation for the link between social contacts and good health. In both the Alameda County study and the Tecumseh study, for instance, health practices were taken into account, and lack of social support still had an independent association with mortality. Suggestions and encouragement from friends may enhance healthy behaviors, but they are not the only answer.

Perhaps the most frequently suggested explanation is that social support lessens or eliminates the harmful effects of stress and therefore protects against disease and death. This buffering hypothesis assumes, of course, some physiological consequences of stress. John Cassel and his associates (Cassel, 1976; Kaplan, Cassel, & Gore, 1977) are among those who have suggested that the absence of social support interacts with stressful life events to produce illness. People who have strong social support are protected against the normally deleterious effects of ordinary daily hassles and life events. Some evidence exists to support this buffering hypothesis. In one study (Brown, Bhrolcháin, & Harris, 1975), women who had a close, intimate relationship were largely unaffected by severely stressful events whereas those with no strong social supports experienced a substantial increase in psychiatric disturbance when faced with a stressful life event.

Cohen and McKay (1984) accepted some aspects of the buffering hypothesis but suggested that its basic assumptions are too general. Instead, they proposed a multidimensional model that takes into account both the specific sources of support and the specific nature of the stressful experience. Cohen and McKay hypothesized that some relationships are more supportive than others and that only those providing appropriate forms of social support act as effective buffers against stress. Dunkel-Schetter (1984) found some confirmation for this hypothesis in a study on social support with cancer patients. Not only did the cancer patients rate social support as helpful in dealing with their illness, but the types of support seen as most helpful varied depending on the person providing the support, with emotional support from physicians rated as especially helpful.

In summary, low social support is likely to be associated with increased mortality rates, although the exact cause of this association is open to speculation (Cohen, 1988; Coyne & DeLongis, 1986; Hazuda, 1994; Wallston, Alagna, DeVellis, & DeVellis, 1983). People with adequate social support probably receive more encouragement and advice regarding good health practices, have a greater sense of personal control (Satariano & Syme, 1981), and are buffered against the harmful effects of stress.

Losing his father, his friend, and his family resulted in Rick's social support system "falling apart." In addition, he began to have trouble in getting along with his colleagues at work. Being isolated and feeling alone was one of the aspects of the situation that Rick found most distressing. This lack of a social support system added to his stress. Rick managed to construct another support system through beginning college and becoming more involved in church activities, and this strategy was wise and probably beneficial.

PERSONAL CONTROL

A second factor that may affect a person's ability to cope with the strain of stressful life events is a feeling of personal control. Many investigators believe that people who feel that they have some control over the events of their lives are better able to cope with stress than are people who feel that their lives are determined by forces outside themselves. Rick felt that the events that happened to him were beyond his control, and he was accustomed to feeling in control.

Research in the area of personal control was given an impetus in 1966 when Julian Rotter published a scale for measuring internal and external control of reinforcement. Rotter hypothesized that people could be placed along a continuum according to the extent to which they believe they are in control of the important events in their lives. Those who believe they control their own lives score in the direction of *internal locus of control* whereas those people who believe that luck, fate, or the acts of others are the determinants of their lives score high on *external locus of control*.

In 1976, Langer and Rodin reported on a study in which older nursing home residents were encouraged to assume more responsibility and control over their daily lives. Residents on the fourth floor of the nursing home were told that they could change their daily routine if they wished. They could rearrange their furniture, decide how to spend their time, choose to visit with other people in the home, decide whether or not to attend a movie, and so on. In addition, these residents were given a small plant, which they were free to accept or reject. They were told they could care for it in any manner they wished. All accepted the plant. A comparison group of residents on the second floor of the home received a parallel communication, but this communication emphasized the responsibility of the nursing staff. Each of these residents also received a plant, a

gift she or he was not free to reject. Although the plant would belong to the resident, the nurses were responsible for taking care of it.

The two groups of residents were approximately equal in age, gender, physical and psychological health, and prior socioeconomic status. Also, throughout the experiment, residents on the two floors received equal attention by the staff. Thus, the two groups were quite comparable except that the fourth-floor residents had more control and responsibility over their daily lives, including the responsibility of caring for the plant. The second-floor residents seemingly had a more comfortable and care-free existence. Their daily decisions were made for them, thus relieving them of the necessity of having to make choices in their lives. However, Langer and Rodin found that residents in the responsibility-induced group were happier, more active, and more alert; they had a higher level of general well-being. In just 3 weeks, most of the comparison group (71%) had become more debilitated whereas nearly all the responsibility-induced group (93%) showed some overall mental and physical improvement.

Rodin and Langer (1977) conducted an 18-month follow-up of these same residents, excluding those who had died or had been discharged. Although nearly all participants at that time lived in different rooms and had received no additional communication about personal control and responsibility, residents in the original responsibility-induced group retained their advantage. They were more healthy, active, sociable, vigorous, and self-initiating than residents in the original comparison group. In addition, the mortality rate in the original responsibility-induced group was lower than expected and also lower than that for the original comparison group. Interestingly, no differences were found in causes of death between the two groups.

The significance of Rodin and Langer's findings is obvious. Older people (and perhaps others as well) probably thrive on personal control and responsibility. Taking care of a plant, of course, was just one aspect of the responsibility encouraged in these residents, but this study seems to indicate that older people do better when they have something to nurture such as another person, a pet, a garden, or

WOULD YOU BELIEVE . . . ?

Can Cheerfulness Kill You?

Would you believe that coping through cheerfulness and an optimistic sense of humor may *decrease* your life expectancy? Strange as this may seem, research by Howard Friedman and his associates (Friedman et al., 1993; Friedman, Tucker, Schwartz, Martin, et al., 1995; Friedman, Tucker, Schwartz, Tomlinson-Keasey, et al., 1995) suggests that cheerfulness and an optimistic sense of humor during childhood are negatively related to longevity. Although coping through the use of humor and optimism may be beneficial in the short run, archival research by Friedman and his associates suggests that in the long run, optimism may shorten people's lives.

Friedman's data come from perhaps the most famous longitudinal study in the history of American psychology — Lewis M. Terman's study of gifted children. Soon after Terman published the 1916 edition of the Stanford-Binet, he began thinking about ways to investigate his genetic theories of intelligence. In 1921–1922, he recruited more than 1,500 very bright California

youngsters, 8 to 12 years old. Nearly all these children had IQs above 140, and their average IQ was slightly over 150.

Terman carefully followed his gifted sample, collecting extensive data on their physical size, emotional stability, eyesight, family background, parents' and teachers' ratings, and dozens of other bits of information (Terman & Oden, 1947). After Terman died in 1956, other investigators continued to gather data on these people, including information on their children and grandchildren. This extraordinary longitudinal study, originally called the Genetic Studies of Genius, is now called the Terman Life-Cycle Study, and its participants are sometimes called "Termites," a nickname they gave to themselves.

Friedman (1990, 1991) hypothesized that childhood personality relates to physical health across the life span. With access to the Terman Life-Cycle data, he had a unique opportunity to test this hypothesis. Friedman et al. (1993) studied the "Termites" born between 1904 and

1915 to discover what, if any, psychosocial factors would predict longevity 7 decades later. Somewhat more than half the participants were still living in 1986, and information concerning time and cause of death was available for most of those who had died. ("Termites" who had died prior to 1930 were excluded from the analysis.) Friedman et al. had sufficient data on the childhood of these gifted people to construct six predictor dimensions that they surmised might relate to longevity: (1) Sociability — for example, fondness for large groups; (2) High Self-Esteem Motivation, such as self-confidence and will power; (3) Conscientiousness, such as prudence and truthfulness; (4) Cheerfulness, or an optimistic sense of humor; (5) High Energy — that is, high physical energy; and (6) Permanency of Moods, or emotional stability.

Only two of these predictor variables related to longevity: Conscientiousness, which was positively related, and Cheerfulness, which was negatively related to length of life.

even a small plant. When individual choice and personal control are taken away, elderly people are more likely to lose assertiveness, become less alert and active, develop more illnesses — and die. Rodin and Langer (1977, p. 197) concluded that "the negative consequences of aging may be retarded, reversed, or possibly prevented by returning to the aged the right to make decisions and a feeling of competence."

How much control is necessary for a person to feel in control? The Langer and Rodin study suggests that control over relatively minor matters is sufficient to have major consequences in the life of the individual. Deciding where to move furniture, when to water a plant, and whether to attend a movie are hardly major events in the history of the world or even in most people's lives, but in the history of an

individual who had previously been stripped of personal control, such events are apparently very important. People need to be able to make choices and to assume responsibility for these choices.

TECHNIQUES FOR COPING WITH STRESS AND PAIN

Both social support and personal control seem to enhance one's ability to cope with stress and pain. Other than these two personal resources, what strategies are available to help people deal with stress and pain?

In recent years, an increasing number of nonmedical interventions have been used by health pro-

The finding that children who cope through cheerfulness and an optimistic sense of humor die earlier than those who scored low on this dimension may seem somewhat surprising in view of other research indicating that optimism and humor can help speed recovery from disease and injury. Friedman et al. hypothesized that optimism and a sense of humor are adaptive adult coping mechanisms that help people recover from surgery, traumatic injuries, and disease. However, optimism may also result in what Neil Weinstein (1984) called an **optimistic bias**; that is, an unrealistic belief that everything will turn out all right regardless of personal behavior. People with an optimistic bias may underestimate the risks of certain activities, such as smoking or driving after drinking.

Friedman et al. (1993) defined Conscientiousness as prudence, truthfulness, social dependability, and freedom from vanity. When they compared people in the top quartile with those in the bottom quartile on Conscientiousness,

Friedman et al. found a significant difference. Highly conscientious participants had a relative risk of .77, meaning that their risk of dying in any given year was only 77% as high as that of less conscientious participants. Such a relative risk indicates that the psychosocial factor of childhood conscientiousness predicts life span about as well as systolic blood pressure, serum cholesterol, diet, and exercise. The authors hypothesized that conscientious people are likely to take better care of themselves and to engage in fewer risky behaviors. They concluded that the "will to behave in a healthy manner may be more important than 'will to live' " (Friedman et al., 1993, p. 184).

In 1995, Friedman and his associates (Friedman, Tucker, Schwartz, Martin et al., 1995; Friedman, Tucker, Schwartz, Tomlinson-Keasey et al, 1995) examined other factors in the Terman participants, including their specific causes of death, divorce of their parents, and instability of the their own marriages. Like the general population, the leading cause of death of these highly intelligent

people was cardiovascular disease, followed by cancer. Although people high in conscientiousness had lower mortality rates than those low in conscientiousness, their rates of death from specific causes were similar. Instability of parents' marriage, however, was significantly and negatively related to longevity. Children of divorced parents had a one-third greater risk of death than those whose parents remained married at least until the participant was 21 years old. Also, "Termites" who had several marriages and divorces had a higher mortality rate than those in stable marriages.

Conscientiousness embraces several positive characteristics, such as dependability, trust, prudence, achievement, and competence. Because the Terman children with these traits lived longer than others, Friedman, Tucker, Schwartz, Tomlinson-Keasey et al. (1995, p. 76) stated: "In terms of the rush toward death, the encouraging news may be that good guys finish last."

fessionals to help people cope with pain and stress. Among these are hypnosis, relaxation training, biofeedback, behavior modification, and cognitive therapy.

HYPNOSIS

Except for relaxation and acupuncture, hypnosis is the oldest nonmedical treatment for pain. Early in the 19th century, physicians were using hypnosis as an analgesia during surgery (Hilgard & Hilgard, 1975). The history of hypnosis, however, reveals a cycle of acceptance and rejection, and some controversy still surrounds its effectiveness as a treatment for pain relief (Hilgard & Hilgard, 1975).

Although trancelike conditions are as old as human history, modern hypnosis is usually thought to have had its beginnings in the last part of the 18th century when Franz Anton Mesmer, an Austrian physician, conducted elaborate demonstrations in Paris. Mesmer's work was discredited by a committee of "scientific experts," but modifications of his technique, known as *mesmerism,* soon spread to other parts of the world. By the 1830s, mesmerism was being used by some surgeons as an anesthetic during major operations (Hilgard & Hilgard, 1975). With the discovery of chemical anesthetics, the popularity of hypnosis waned, but during the late 19th century, many European physicians, including Sigmund Freud, employed hypnotic procedures in the treatment of mental illness. Since the beginning of the 20th century, the popularity of hypnosis as a medical and psychological tool has continued to wax and wane. Its present position is still somewhat controversial, but a significant number of practitioners within medicine and psychology are taking advantage of the positive aspects of this procedure to treat health-related problems, especially the management of pain.

What Is Hypnosis?

Not only is the use of hypnosis still controversial, but its precise nature is also a debatable issue. Some authorities, such as Ernest Hilgard (1975, 1978, 1979; Hilgard & Hilgard, 1975), regard hypnosis as an altered *state* of consciousness in which the person's stream of consciousness is divided or dissociated. Others, such as Theodore X. Barber (1980, 1982, 1984), view it as a more generalized *trait,* or a relatively permanent characteristic of people who respond well to suggestion. To Hilgard, the process of **induction**—that is, being placed into a hypnotic state—is central to hypnosis. After induction, the responsive person enters a state of divided or dissociated consciousness that is essentially different from the normal state. This altered state of consciousness allows people to respond to suggestion and to control physiological processes that they cannot in the normal state of consciousness. Barber, however, rejects the notion that induction is necessary and holds that the suggestive procedures can be just as effective without the person's entering a trancelike state. Other authorities, such as Karen Olness (1993, p. 278), regard hypnosis as "simply a form of self-induced, focused attention" that makes it easier for people to relax and to learn to control their body functions. Like most current hypnotherapists, Olness believes that all hypnosis is self-hypnosis.

How Effective Is Hypnosis?

Despite their debate over the nature of the hypnotic state and the necessity of induction, Hilgard and Barber agree that hypnosis, or the hypnosuggestive procedure, is an important clinical tool, especially for the control of pain. Both also believe that not all patients will profit equally from these procedures. Some people are more suggestible than others, and these "good subjects" are better able to use hypnosis to cope with pain.

What percentage of people are suggestible? Barber and Hilgard agree that suggestibility is widely distributed among the population, almost following a normal, bell-shaped curve. For this reason, clinicians need to determine the level of suggestibility of their patients prior to employing hypnosis as an analgesic. Barber (1982) contended that although every professional who treats pain should be able to use hypnosuggestive procedures, not every patient nor every type of pain is amenable to this treatment. The list of pain that is responsive to hypnotic procedures is extensive, including childbirth, headache, cancer pain, low back pain, myofascial pain, and laboratory-induced pain. The important variable is not the type of pain but the type of patient.

Hilgard (1978) found that for some highly suggestible people, laboratory-induced pain can be completely eliminated through hypnosis and the suggestion that they will feel no pain. The suggestion is critically important, and people hypnotized without an analgesia suggestion reported nearly as much pain as did unhypnotized people (Miller, Barabasz, & Barabasz, 1991). Hypnosis with a suggestion of analgesia is superior to a placebo (Spanos, Perlini, & Robertson, 1989), waking suggestions of analgesia (Jacobs, Kurtz, & Strube, 1995), and acupuncture (Moret et al., 1991) in controlling laboratory-induced pain. Hypnotizability as well as the suggestion during induction is an important factor in hypnotic analgesia, and people who are low in hypnotizability tend to respond to hypnotic suggestions of analgesia at rates comparable to response to placebos.

But does suggestion actually block pain or does it merely lower reports of pain? Hilgard's (1979) concept of dissociated consciousness allows for the possibility that hypnotized people given a suggestion of analgesia still experience the physical sensations of pain, but if the hypnotist has suggested that they will not feel any pain, they may report that they do not. Hilgard and Hilgard (1975) demonstrated that highly hypnotizable people given the suggestion that they feel no pain could still rate their pain as substantial if they were given instructions to report all their sensations. Even though they showed few behavioral signs of pain and verbalized little or no discomfort, these hypnotized people still rated their pain as substantial. Another researcher (Orne, 1980), however, reported that hypnosis does not totally suppress behavioral signs of pain and that physiological reactions such as changes in respiration, heart rate, and blood pressure accompany increases in pain for people who have been hypnotized.

Other investigators, led by Barber (1969, 1982), minimized the dissociated consciousness view and emphasized the notion that hypnotized individuals are willing to accept suggestion and to expect that "hypnosuggestive" procedures will be effective. Despite similarities between this view and the placebo effect (Evans, 1988; Turner & Chapman, 1982b), several studies (McGlashan, Evans, & Orne, 1969; Orne, 1976) have shown that people high in susceptibility to hypnosis experienced much greater pain tolerance during hypnosis than did people low in susceptibility, even though there was little difference in pain tolerance between the two groups when both groups expected a pain-killing drug. These results suggest that for those people who are easily hypnotized, the placebo or expectancy effect is not nearly as effective as hypnosis in controlling pain, thus refuting the contention that the placebo effect underlies all hypnotic analgesia.

For individuals who are not easily hypnotized, the effects of hypnotic analgesic suggestions seem similar to placebo effects, and these individuals experience comparable analgesia from hypnotic suggestions of analgesia and placebo medication. Orne (1980, p. 165) concluded that "the dramatic effect of hypnosis on pain cannot be explained in terms of subjects' expectations, but rather . . . turns out to be directly related to hypnotizability." In other words, the pain-controlling effects of hypnosis are real and do not depend on one's expectations. Individual differences in susceptibility prevent the widespread use of hypnosis as an analgesic, but some people can receive substantial analgesic benefits.

Although authorities differ in their opinions concerning the nature of the mechanisms for hypnotic analgesia, few doubt that hypnosis works, at least with some patients. Barber (1982) reviewed the research and found evidence that hypnosis has been used as an effective analgesia for surgical pain, postsurgical discomfort, low back pain, and childbirth.

Van der Does and Van Dyck (1989) examined 28 studies that used hypnosis with burn patients. They found consistent evidence that hypnosis is an effective analgesia for alleviating burn pain but no evidence that hypnosis could speed the healing of burn

Table 6.1 Effectiveness of hypnosis

Problem	Effectiveness
Experimentally induced pain	Hypnosis can completely eliminate in hypnotizable people; acts as a placebo in less hypnotizable people
Childbirth pain	Hypnosis reduces pain and anxiety
Dental pain	Hypnosis reduces pain and anxiety
Burn pain	Hypnosis reduces pain but does not speed healing

wounds. Moreover, they concluded that pain treatment is the most promising area of application for hypnosis.

Despite strong evidence that hypnosis can be used effectively to decrease acute pain and manage chronic pain, many health care providers have gross misunderstanding of this form of analgesia. Richard Bryant (1993) surveyed a large number of burn therapists and rehabilitation therapists concerning their beliefs about hypnosis as a means of coping with pain and found that many of them were not aware of recent research on the efficacy of hypnosis. Some of these therapists expressed many of the same misconceptions of hypnosis that nonprofessionals have; for example, hypnosis is an altered state of consciousness in which patients are not aware of their surroundings and possess an enhanced ability to recall past events. Such misconceptions discourage the use of hypnosis.

As Table 6.1 shows, hypnosis can be an effective tool for coping with pain. Nevertheless, more research is needed to identify those people who will respond favorably to hypnosis, under what conditions they will respond, and for what types of pain problems.

RELAXATION TRAINING

Relaxation training is perhaps the simplest and easiest to use of all psychological interventions (Blanchard & Andrasik, 1985). Like hypnosis, the therapeutic uses of relaxation methods predate modern psychology, with ancient Egyptians, Hebrews, Tibetans, and others using some form of rhythmic breathing or chanting for the purpose of healing (Lavey &

Taylor, 1985). Modern uses of relaxation training are usually traced to Edmond Jacobson (1934, 1938) who termed this method *progressive relaxation.* In progressive muscle relaxation, people learn to relax one muscle group at a time, progressing through the body's entire range of muscle groups until the whole body is relaxed.

What Is Relaxation Training?

Progressive muscle relaxation is only one of several types of relaxation techniques; others include meditative relaxation and guided imagery. With *progressive muscle relaxation,* patients are first given a rationale for the procedure, including an explanation that their present tension is mostly a physical state resulting from tense muscles. While reclining in a comfortable chair with no distracting lights or sounds, patients first breathe deeply and exhale slowly. After this, the series of deep muscle relaxation exercises begins. Because patients must have some sense of how relaxation feels, they are instructed to tense a particular muscle group (for example, the hand) and to hold the tension for about 10 seconds (Jacobson, 1938). Then they are asked to slowly release the tension, concentrating on the relaxing, soothing sensations in their hand as tension gradually drains. Once the hand is relaxed, patients go through the same tensing and relaxing sequence progressively with other muscle groups, including the arms, shoulders, neck, mouth, tongue, forehead, eyes, toes, feet, calves, thighs, back, stomach, and other muscle groups. Patients may repeat the breathing exercises until they achieve a deep feeling of relaxation. Frequently, patients are also encouraged to focus on the pleasant feeling of relaxation, a condition that restricts attention to internal events and away from external sources of anxiety and stress. Level of relaxation can be rated on a scale of 1 to 10, or patients can signal by raising an index finger when tension begins to increase.

Once patients learn the relaxation technique, they may practice independently at home. If independent practice is too difficult, prerecorded audiotapes are available that allow patients to listen to the soothing voice of a professional instructor without returning to the clinic. Length of relaxation training programs varies, but 6 to 8 weeks and about 10 sessions with an instructor are usually sufficient to allow patients to easily and independently enter a state of deep relaxation (Bernstein & Borkovec, 1973; Blanchard & Andrasik, 1985).

Another frequently used relaxation technique is *meditative relaxation,* developed by Herbert Benson and his colleagues (Benson, 1974; Benson, Beary, & Carol, 1974). This approach derives from various religious meditative practices, but as used by psychologists, it has no religious connotations. Bensonian relaxation combines muscle relaxation with a quiet environment, comfortable position, a repetitive sound, and a passive attitude. Participants usually sit with eyes closed and muscles relaxed. They then focus attention on their breathing and repeat silently a sound, such as "om" or "one" with each breath for about 20 minutes. Repetition of the single word prevents distracting thoughts and sustains muscle relaxation. Meditation involves conscious intention to focus attention on a single thought or image along with effort not to be distracted by other thoughts.

Jon Kabat-Zinn (Kabat-Zinn, 1991, 1993; Kabat-Zinn, Lipworth, & Burney, 1985) has taught a different form of meditation called *mindfulness meditation,* which has its roots in ancient Buddhist practice but has implications for anyone suffering from stress, anxiety, or pain. With mindfulness meditation, people do not try to ignore unpleasant thoughts or sensations by focusing on their breathing or on a single sound. Rather, they take the opposite approach, focusing on any thoughts or sensations as they occur. However, they are asked to observe these thoughts nonjudgmentally. By noting thoughts objectively as they occur, people can gain insight into how they see the world and what motivates them. Kabat-Zinn (1993) explained the process in this way: "Observing without judging, moment by moment, helps you see what is on your mind without editing or censoring it, without intellectualizing it or getting lost in your own incessant thinking" (p. 263).

Guided imagery has some elements in common with meditative relaxation, but it also has important differences. With guided imagery, patients conjure up a calm, peaceful image such as the repetitive rhythmic roar of an ocean or the quiet beauty of a pastoral scene. Patients then concentrate on that image for the duration of a painful or anxiety-filled situation. The assumption underlying guided imagery is that a person cannot concentrate on more than

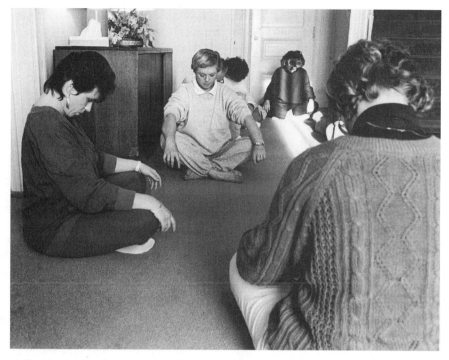

Meditation is one relaxation technique that can help people cope with a variety of stress-related problems.

one thing at a time. Therefore, the patient must imagine an especially powerful or delightful scene — one so pleasant or powerful that it averts attention from the painful experience.

Some forms of guided imagery do not involve pleasant images. For example, patients can imagine extremely *unpleasant* situations, such as an embarrassing childhood experience, an argument with a spouse, or the death of a friend. Whether pleasant or unpleasant, the image must be sufficiently intense to block any feelings of pain. Another variation of guided imagery is to ask patients to concentrate on real-life situations, a procedure called *in vivo* imagery (Horan, 1973). With in vivo imagery, patients are urged to recall experiences that have contributed to their feelings of pride, self-assertion, or self-esteem. Again, by concentrating on these images, patients are able to cope with pain by inhibiting most of its unpleasant effects.

How Effective Is Relaxation Training?

Progressive relaxation, meditative relaxation, mindfulness meditation, and guided imagery are all techniques to help patients cope with a number of stress-related problems, including headache pain, anxiety, chronic pain, and hypertension. Lehrer, Carr, Sargunaraj, and Woolfolk (1994) reviewed studies on the effectiveness of relaxation therapy and found this approach to be associated with improvements for a variety of problems.

In examining the studies dealing with the effect of relaxation treatment on hypertension, Lehrer et al. found that relaxation training can be effective in lowering blood pressure in hypertensive patients, especially those with less serious hypertension. Such treatment does not seem to be as effective as drug treatment, but relaxation can add to the benefits of drug treatment, allowing lower dosages of medication.

Relaxation techniques have also been used to treat several types of chronic pain, with tension-type headaches responding most successfully. Turner and Chapman (1982a) reviewed the research on relaxation training and chronic clinical pain syndromes, including tension headache. Of the studies reviewed, all reported at least some benefit for relaxation training, but half these studies lacked adequate control groups. One well-controlled study (Cox, Freundlich, & Meyer, 1975) compared progressive relaxation with EMG biofeedback and also with a medication placebo. The results were typical of other studies (Chesney & Shelton, 1976; Haynes, Griffin, Mooney, & Parise, 1975) that compared relaxation training with EMG biofeedback in treating tension headache pain. All these studies indicated that both treatment interventions were superior to a placebo, but they showed no significant differences between the effects of relaxation and biofeedback. (Later discussions examine the effectiveness of biofeedback as well as the combination of relaxation with other psychological procedures.)

In a later review of the effectiveness of various stress management techniques, Lehrer et al. (1994) concluded that several varieties of relaxation training were effective in treating tension headache. Indeed, despite its use for a wide variety of chronic pain treatment, relaxation training is most effective in the relief of tension headache. Several reviews (Blanchard & Andrasik, 1985; Lavey & Taylor, 1985; Lehrer et al., 1994; Syrjala & Chapman, 1984) have reported that relaxation training alone (1) significantly reduces a substantial number of chronic headaches, (2) is more effective than a placebo, and (3) is at least equal to biofeedback in decreasing tension headache pain.

However, progressive relaxation training is no panacea for pain reduction. Perhaps as many as 50% of tension headache patients do not experience significant relief through relaxation. For this reason, Blanchard and Andrasik (1985) viewed relaxation as a necessary first step in a pain management program, and one that may not be effective for all pain sufferers.

Can meditative relaxation be used to cope with pain, stress, and anxiety? Shapiro (1985) reviewed the research on meditation and found consistent and positive results. Meditation has been shown to be effective in reducing stress, anxiety, phobias, and hypertension. Despite these impressive findings, Shapiro insisted that meditation has not been proven to produce physiological changes that are different from those produced by other relaxation strategies. In summary, although meditation is an

effective therapy for some stress-related disorders, it is probably no more powerful than progressive muscle relaxation.

Kabat-Zinn, Lipworth, and Burney (1985) studied the effectiveness of mindfulness meditation on chronic pain patients and found it to be more effective than a traditional intervention that included physical therapy, analgesics, and antidepressants. Patients trained to use mindfulness meditation reported less present pain, negative body image, depression, anxiety, and mood disturbance, and fewer psychological symptoms. Moreover, they decreased their use of pain medications, improved their activity levels, and increased their feelings of self-esteem. In a later study, Kabat-Zinn et al. (1992) studied a meditation-based stress-reduction program for treating anxiety disorders and found it effective in over 90% of the participants. In this study, patients with generalized anxiety disorder, panic disorder, or panic disorder with agoraphobia learned meditation techniques and then participated in one of several different therapy groups. Group facilitators did not know the clinical diagnosis of their patients nor which of them were study participants. Patients taught meditation techniques had significant reductions in anxiety and depression and maintained these gains at the 3-month follow-up.

The effectiveness of guided imagery is also about the same as that of meditation and progressive relaxation. For example, Horan, Layng, and Pursell (1976) found that in vivo imagery reduced reported dental discomfort, although patients did not reduce their heart rate. Earlier, Horan (1973) cited evidence that guided imagery could reduce childbirth anxiety and discomfort, and Horan and Dellinger (1974) found that experimentally induced pain could be alleviated through guided imagery. In 1982, Lyles, Burish, Krozely, and Oldham reported on a study they had conducted with cancer patients receiving chemotherapy. A combination of progressive muscle relaxation training and guided imagery was more effective than either a therapist-attention group or a no-treatment control group in reducing anxiety and nausea both during and after chemotherapy.

Achterberg, Kenner, and Lawlis (1988) examined the effects of guided imagery, relaxation, and thermal biofeedback on pain management. Achterberg

Table 6.2 Effectiveness of relaxation techniques

Problem	Relaxation Technique	Effectiveness
Hypertension	Several types of relaxation training	Effective for mild hypertension Not as effective as drugs
Tension headache	Progressive relaxation	More effective than placebo As effective as biofeedback
Anxiety	Meditative relaxation	As effective as relaxation training
Chronic pain	Mindfulness meditation	Better than physical therapy or medication
Anxiety	Mindfulness meditation	Effective for 90% of people
Nausea and anxiety from chemotherapy	Guided imagery plus progressive relaxation	More effective than no treatment
Burn pain	Guided imagery plus relaxation	More effective than other combinations of relaxation therapy

et al. divided 149 severely burned patients into four groups according to the treatment they received: (1) relaxation only, (2) relaxation plus guided imagery, (3) relaxation plus guided imagery plus thermal biofeedback, and (4) a control group that received the usual wound care. All three experimental groups improved more than did the control group in their ability to cope with severe burn pain. Imagery added significantly to relaxation alone, and biofeedback added some benefit over the combination of relaxation and guided imagery. However, because biofeedback is expensive and did not add appreciably to the other two procedures, the authors concluded that the gains from it were not sufficient to compensate for its costs. They suggested that relaxation plus imagery was the preferred treatment for burn pain.

Later, Ilacqua (1994) compared the effectiveness of guided imagery with biofeedback in treating migraine headache. He found that neither approach nor a combination of the two was effective in reducing the *frequency* of migraines, but participants who received guided imagery reported greater ability to cope with their pain than those who received either biofeedback or a combination of biofeedback and guided imagery. Table 6.2 summarizes a number of relaxation techniques and their effectiveness.

The findings from Ilacqua's study cast doubt on the ability of biofeedback to help people cope with pain. Is this study representative of the research on biofeedback? Is biofeedback the preferred treatment

for stress or pain of any sort? These questions are examined next.

BIOFEEDBACK

Until the 1960s, most people in the Western world assumed that conscious control of such physiological processes as heart rate, the secretion of digestive juices, and the constriction of blood vessels was impossible. These biological functions do not require conscious attention for their regulation, and conscious attempts at regulation seem to have little effect on these functions controlled by the autonomic nervous system.

Then, during the late 1960s, a number of researchers began to explore the possibility of controlling biological processes traditionally believed to be beyond conscious control (Nigl, 1984). Their efforts culminated in the development of **biofeedback**, the process of providing feedback information about the status of biological systems. Early experiments indicated that biofeedback made possible the control of some otherwise automatic functions. In 1969, Neal E. Miller reported a series of experiments in which he and his colleagues had altered the levels of animals' visceral response through reinforcement. Some subjects received rewards for raising their heart rate and others for lowering it. Within a few hours, significant differences in heart rate appeared. Salivation, kidney function, intestinal contractions, and blood pressure also changed as a response to training. Miller, who used rats and dogs as subjects, expressed the belief that humans too could learn to control visceral responses.

Experiments by other investigators soon proved Miller correct. Joseph Kamiya (1969) and Barbara Brown (1970) both reported that humans are capable of learning to control their brain waves using electroencephalogram (EEG) biofeedback. A variety of biofeedback machines soon appeared on the market. Muscle tension, skin temperature, blood pressure, heart rate, gastric motility, skin conductance, and many other physiological measures have the potential to be affected by biofeedback training.

What Is Biofeedback?

In biofeedback, biological responses are measured by electronic instruments, and the status of those responses is immediately available to the person being tested. In other words, a person gains information about changes in biological responses as they are taking place. This feedback allows the person to alter physiological responses that cannot be voluntarily controlled without the biofeedback information.

The feedback can be supplied by way of auditory, tactile, or visual signals, and all three types are commonly used. For example, if biofeedback is directed toward lowering heart rate, the machine that is monitoring the heart will give a signal when heart rate decreases. The signal is often a tone that decreases in pitch as heart rate decreases and rises as heart rate accelerates. In this way, people being monitored know whether their heart rate is changing in the desired direction. With such information, people can gain some degree of voluntary control over their heart rate.

The type of biofeedback most commonly found in clinical use is **electromyograph (EMG) biofeedback**. EMG biofeedback reflects the activity of the skeletal muscles by measuring the electrical discharge in muscle fibers. The measurement is taken by attaching electrodes to the surface of the skin over the muscles to be monitored. The level of electrical activity reflects the degree of tension or relaxation of the muscles. The machine responds with a signal that varies in accordance to the electrical activity of the muscle. The electrodes may be placed over any muscle group, and the choice of placement depends on the type of problem. Biofeedback can be used to increase muscle tension in rehabilitation or to decrease muscle tension in stress management.

EMG biofeedback to decrease muscle tension has a wide variety of clinical applications. Spasmodic disorders, facial tics, and other disorders involving muscle spasm have responded to EMG biofeedback (Blanchard & Epstein, 1977; Nigl, 1984). EMG biofeedback has also been used to control the two most commonly treated sources of pain: low back pain and headaches.

Temperature biofeedback, which is also frequently used to help people cope with stress and pain, is based on the principle that skin temperature varies in relation to levels of stress. High stress tends to constrict blood vessels whereas relaxation opens them. Therefore, cool surface skin temperature may indicate stress and tension; warm skin temperature suggests calm and relaxation.

Temperature biofeedback involves placing a **thermister**—a temperature-sensitive resistor—on the skin's surface. The thermister signals changes in skin temperature, thereby furnishing the information that allows control. The feedback signal, as with EMG biofeedback, may be auditory, visual, or both. The thermister is most often placed on fingers and less often on toes. These sites represent the most distal points in the circulatory system and are the most subject to temperature variations. However, temperature measurements taken from fingers or toes do not directly relate to any pathological condition. Skin temperature may be an indirect measurement of tension and relaxation, or the fingers may represent vasoconstriction for the entire body. But in neither case can temperature biofeedback be seen as a direct intervention in the physiology that underlies any disorder.

The goal of temperature biofeedback is almost always to raise skin temperature. The vasodilation that causes warming accompanies relaxation. Migraine headache and **Raynaud's disease** are the disorders most commonly treated with temperature biofeedback. The review by Lehrer et al. (1994) indicated that temperature biofeedback is superior to relaxation training or EMG biofeedback for migraine headache.

Raynaud's disease is a vasoconstrictive disorder in which the fingers (and less often the toes) suffer from restricted blood flow. The digits become numb,

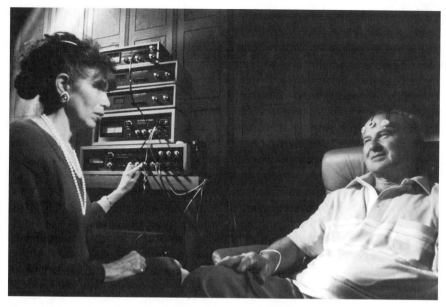

Electromyograph (EMG) biofeedback can help people lower muscle tension.

and attacks are often accompanied by pain. The phase of vasoconstriction is usually followed by vasodilation, and that too may be painful. The cause of Raynaud's disease is not known and no cure is available. Medical treatment may involve surgery or drugs that dilate blood vessels, but both treatments have unwanted side effects. Biofeedback offers an alternative treatment.

Early reviews of biofeedback studies (Blanchard & Epstein, 1977; Nigl, 1984; Turner & Chapman, 1982a) showed no advantage for temperature biofeedback over relaxation, but a later review (Lehrer et al., 1994) indicated that finger temperature biofeedback was more effective. Adding the component of cold stress to the training procedure boosts the effectiveness of temperature biofeedback in the treatment of Raynaud's disease.

How Effective Is Biofeedback?

In an evaluation of the effectiveness of biofeedback techniques, two points must be considered. First, biofeedback requires expensive technology and trained personnel and must justify its expense through benefits; second, any benefits derived from biofeedback must result specifically from that treatment and not some other component of the treatment, such as relaxation, suggestion, and the placebo effect.

When biofeedback first appeared, researchers thought that it might allow patients to intervene in the physiological processes that underlie the development of certain disorders. As research proliferated, evidence began to mount that the effects of biofeedback were more general than had been originally believed (Blanchard & Andrasik, 1982; Nigl, 1984; Schuman, 1982). More recently, Lehrer et al. (1994) evaluated the question of specific versus general effects for biofeedback and other stress management techniques and concluded that the therapies oriented toward changing autonomic processes have specific effects on those processes.

The question of specificity is important. If all modes of biofeedback decrease sympathetic nervous system arousal, then they should be comparable to relaxation training, a nonspecific technique. The effectiveness of the various modes of biofeedback should, therefore, be evaluated in comparison to relaxation training or other types of nonspecific behavioral therapy. To attempt to answer the question about specific advantages for biofeedback, Blanchard and his colleagues (Blanchard et al., 1982) conducted a study on headache pain that used both relaxation training and temperature biofeedback. They examined patients with tension, migraine, and mixed (both tension and migraine symptoms) headache complaints. After a 4-week baseline, patients received 10 weeks of relaxation training. All groups, especially the tension headache group, showed significant improvement. Those patients who had not individually improved after relaxation training received 12 weeks of thermal biofeedback therapy. The biofeedback training led to further significant reductions of headache pain, especially for patients with either migraine headache or the combined migraine and tension headache. In another study, McGrady, Wauquier, McNeil, and Gerard (1994) also tested a combination of biofeedback and relaxation training and found that biofeedback was more effective for migraine headache patients than relaxation alone. These findings suggest that although relaxation alone is sufficient to reduce headache pain, patients who are not helped by relaxation can be successfully treated by thermal biofeedback.

The study by Blanchard et al. also suggests that headache patients might be best treated by tailored treatment programs rather than by initial use of all components of a complex pain management program. Relaxation training may be sufficient for many patients, and the less expensive techniques should be tried first and given a chance to work. However, temperature biofeedback can be effective for some patients, including those for whom other techniques have failed. Therefore, biofeedback seems to have specific effects and therapeutic benefits for some patients.

Does biofeedback aid in coping with stress? EMG is frequently used for lowering muscle tension levels, one indicator of stress. A review by Andrasik et al. (1985) indicated that research in this area has been quite consistent in finding that people are able to produce significant reduction in muscle tension during EMG biofeedback training. The Lehrer et al. (1994) review indicated that although biofeedback can produce specific changes in autonomic responses, biofeedback treatment showed no benefit over other types of behavioral therapy for reducing anxiety, insomnia, and tension headache pain. Biofeedback therapy can be an effective mode of stress management for certain patients, but because several forms of biofeedback promote relaxation, some of its positive effects may be attributable to increases in relaxation rather than to the precise control of the physiology involved with responses to stress.

Does biofeedback help in coping with pain? Although earlier reports (Nigl, 1984) indicated no additional benefits for this procedure over other techniques, several more recent studies have shown some advantage for biofeedback. For example, Elton (1993) divided pain and stress patients into two groups: (1) those using EMG biofeedback combined with hypnosis and (2) those receiving hypnosis alone. After treatment, both groups improved on such measures as anxiety levels, self-esteem, intensity and duration of pain, and levels of stress. However, the combination of biofeedback with hypnosis was more effective than hypnosis alone.

In spite of the prevalence of low back pain, biofeedback has not been a frequent treatment for this pain syndrome. When used, it rarely has been the only mode of treatment. Other behavioral techniques and drugs are frequently used in a comprehensive program of pain management. In addition, many biofeedback studies on low back pain have included few patients, often with varying pain symptoms. Two studies (Bush, Ditto, & Feuerstein, 1985; Sargent et al., 1986) failed to find an advantage for EMG biofeedback over nonspecific treatment and a placebo treatment, but in a more recent study Flor and Birbaumer (1993) compared the effectiveness of EMG biofeedback, cognitive-behavioral therapy, and conservative medical interventions in the treatment of chronic back pain and chronic temporomandibular pain. They randomly assigned patients to one of the three treatment groups. At the end of treatment, patients in all three groups showed improvement, but the biofeedback group reported the greatest decrease in pain severity. Moreover, after 6- and 24-month follow-ups, only the biofeedback group maintained significant reductions in pain, suggesting that biofeedback may be of some use in pain management for low back and temporomandibular joint pain.

Lehrer et al. (1994) reviewed the effectiveness and specific effects of biofeedback for headaches and other pain syndromes. Their conclusions were that biofeedback can have specific effects in addition to relaxation and offers some benefits for some pain syndromes, especially migraine headache. Table 6.3 summarizes the effectiveness of various types of

Table 6.3   Effectiveness of biofeedback techniques

Problem	Type of Biofeedback	Effectiveness
Hypertension	Blood pressure	Comparable to relaxation
Raynaud's disease	Temperature	Superior to relaxation
Tension headache	Electromyograph (EMG)	Comparable to relaxation
Migraine headache	EMG	Comparable to relaxation
Migraine headache	Temperature	Superior to relaxation
Anxiety	EMG	Comparable to relaxation
Low back pain	EMG	Superior to cognitive-behavioral therapy and placebo
Temporomandibular pain	EMG	Superior to cognitive-behavioral therapy and placebo

biofeedback for stress and pain. Whether biofeedback is a good choice for any particular pain patient depends not only on the effectiveness of biofeedback treatment for that patient's pain problem but also the level of training of the therapist and the availability of the biofeedback equipment.

BEHAVIOR MODIFICATION

A fourth coping procedure used by health psychologists is **behavior modification,** a process for changing behavior through the application of operant conditioning principles. The goal of behavior modification is to shape *behavior,* not to alleviate *feelings* of stress or *sensations* of pain. Because stress is difficult to define in terms of specific behaviors, behavior modification is not frequently used for coping with stress. However, pain behaviors can be more clearly identified and thus lend themselves more easily to modification by operant conditioning techniques.

What Is Behavior Modification?

People in pain usually communicate their discomfort to others. They complain, moan, sigh, limp, rub, grimace, miss work, or behave in a variety of other ways that indicate to other people that they are suffering. Many of these behaviors have been reinforced by the surroundings—that is, other people have in some manner rewarded these verbal and nonverbal expressions of pain.

Behavior modification strategies for coping with stress and pain are based on B. F. Skinner's (1953) notion that positive and negative reinforcers are central to operant conditioning. A **positive reinforcer** is any stimulus that, when added to a situation, increases the probability that the behavior it follows will recur. Positive reinforcers are also known as rewards. An example might be the attention and sympathy a person receives from family and friends when exhibiting pain behaviors. A **negative reinforcer** is any aversive or painful stimulus that, when removed from a situation, increases the probability that the behavior it follows will recur. Examples are the relief from pain one experiences after taking pain medication and the avoidance of work or school responsibilities that can occur when a person shows pain.

Wilbert E. Fordyce (1974) was among the first to emphasize the role of operant conditioning in the perpetuation of pain behaviors. He recognized the *reward* value of increased attention and sympathy, financial compensation, relief from work and social obligations, and other positive reinforcers that frequently follow the various pain behaviors. Carl, the pain patient introduced in Chapter 5, has a long history of drawing reinforcement from his environment. He has not worked full time since his accident because he has been in too much pain. His parents allowed him to escape from chores at home because they are afraid he would aggravate his injuries. Then too, Carl would decrease his chances of losing a large reinforcement—the money involved in his legal suit—if his pain decreased. Having much to gain from pain behaviors, Carl learned to use them to his advantage. To say that Carl had been reinforced for pain behaviors does not imply that he deliberately intended to deceive anyone. However, because his pain behaviors were acquired largely through operant conditioning principles and his circumstances supported his pain behaviors, the psychologist who treated Carl with biofeedback techniques might have had more success with a behavior modification program.

Behavior modification techniques of pain management assume that pain behaviors are observable and can be reliably measured. Indeed, good evidence exists for these assumptions (Keefe & Block, 1982; Keefe & Williams, 1992; Turk, Wack, & Kerns, 1985). Once pain behaviors and their reinforcers have been identified, the process of behavior modification can begin. Nursing staff and patients' spouses have been trained (Fordyce et al., 1973) to use praise and attention to reinforce more desirable behaviors and to withhold reinforcement when patients exhibit less desired pain behaviors. In other words, the inappropriate groans and complaints are now ignored while efforts toward greater physical activity and other positive behaviors are reinforced. Progress is noted by such criteria as amount of medication taken, absences from work, time in bed or off one's feet, number of pain complaints, physical activity, range of motion, and length of sitting tolerance.

How Effective Is Behavior Modification?

Fordyce and his colleagues have successfully used behavior modification to improve mobility in pain patients. Using a single-subject design, Fordyce, Shelton, and Dundore (1982) used behavior modification treatment for a young man suffering abdominal pain, dizziness, and disturbances in walking. As part of his therapy, the young man was given his choice of either walking the assigned distance at a predetermined speed or walking twice that distance at his own pace. The young man's mother was instructed to ignore him when he failed to walk and to encourage him when he showed progress in walking. The treatment intervention, which also included vocational counseling, was successful. At the end of treatment, the young man was walking more freely and complaining less of severe pain. Twenty-seven months later, the patient had maintained his gains despite no further treatment. Single-subject studies such as this show that behavior modification can work in individual cases, but

they do not demonstrate the treatment's general efficacy.

The success of behavior modification for the control of pain is difficult to judge because many of the studies have lacked adequate controls and have employed a variety of treatment interventions along with behavior modification. However, Turner and Chapman (1982b) found some consistent trends when they reviewed more than a dozen studies that used behavior modification to control pain (largely low back pain or a combination of pain syndromes). Treatment programs based on operant conditioning seem to increase patients' level of physical activity and decrease their use of medication, two important targets in any pain treatment regimen.

Turner and Romano (1984) looked at the research published since this earlier review and found only four subsequent studies that had used operant conditioning techniques to control pain. Of these, three had no control groups, but all four found tentative evidence to support the effectiveness of behavior modification. Brownell (1984b) also reviewed the research and reached the same conclusion: Operant conditioning approaches appear to be effective in increasing patients' levels of physical activity and decreasing their use of analgesic drugs.

How do behavior modification methods compare with traditional medical treatments in treating chronic low back pain? One report (Heinrich, Cohen, Naliboff, Collins, & Bonebakker, 1985) compared a behavior modification program with a traditional physical therapy regimen that used instructions on drug management, proper posture and exercise, and methods of simplifying work and conserving energy during work. The behavior therapy group received a complex package of behavior modification techniques, including training in stress and pain management, cognitive therapy, group discussion, and social reinforcement for decreases in pain behavior. The emphasis was on self-responsibility, setting up appropriate goals, and monitoring progress toward these goals. Both the physical therapy and the behavioral therapy groups showed general improvement during treatment, and both tended to maintain that improvement during follow-up. No overall differences appeared between the two groups, indicating that multimodal behavior therapy is as effective as physical therapy, but no more so.

Fordyce and his associates (Fordyce, Brockway, Bergman, & Spengler, 1986) also compared traditional management and behavior therapy methods with back pain patients and found some evidence to support the superiority of behavioral methods. Patients in the traditional management group received medication on an "as needed" basis and with the possibility of prescription renewal while patients in the behavior therapy group were given medication on a time-contingent basis and with no renewal of the original prescription. In addition, the traditional treatment patients could stop their activity and exercises whenever they wished. For the behavior treatment patients, activity and exercises were completed on a predetermined basis. A 6-week follow-up revealed no differences between the two groups, but at 9 to 12 months, the behavior management group scored lower on several measures of "sickness"— that is, they were doing better than patients treated with traditional procedures. The Heinrich et al. (1985) and Fordyce et al. (1986) studies both suggest that behavior-based programs of pain management are at least comparable in effectiveness to the more traditional physical therapy programs. However, both studies used small groups and followed somewhat different definitions of traditional and behavioral therapy. Much more research is needed comparing behavior modification programs, not only with traditional medical therapies but also with hypnosis, relaxation training, biofeedback, and cognitive therapies.

One study did compare behavior modification with cognitive therapy in treating low back pain. Turner and Clancy (1988) randomly assigned 81 mildly dysfunctional chronic low back pain patients to one of three groups by type of treatment: (1) operant behavior treatment, (2) cognitive-behavior therapy, and (3) waiting-list control. The operant behavior treatment was based on principles discussed by Fordyce (1976) and included training spouses to ignore patients' pain behaviors and to reinforce their well behaviors. Patients worked toward goals and kept daily records to chart their progress. In addition, they were placed on an aerobic exercise program that was gradually increased in time and intensity. The cognitive-behavioral group was trained in progressive muscle relaxation and guided imagery as suggested by Turk, Meichenbaum, and Gen-

Table 6.4 Effectiveness of behavior modification

Problem	Effectiveness
Low back pain	Allows increased physical activity
	Allows decreased intake of analgesic drugs
	Is comparable to physical and medical therapies
	Provides longer-lasting effects than medical therapies
Myofascial pain	Is comparable to electromyograph (EMG) biofeedback

est (1983). These patients also kept records of their negative emotions and negative life events. Both experimental groups reported decreased physical and psychosocial disability compared to the control group. The behavior modification group showed the greatest gains during treatment, but their performance leveled off at the 6- and 12-month follow-up periods. The cognitive-behavior group improved more slowly at first, but they continued their gains over the 12-month follow-up and eventually caught up with the operant behavior group. These findings suggest that cognitive therapy methods may bring about more permanent improvement for pain patients. Table 6.4 shows the effectiveness of behavior modification.

COGNITIVE THERAPY

Cognitive therapy also utilizes reinforcement but places more emphasis on intrinsic or self-reinforcers than on those from therapists or other external sources. Cognitive therapy is based on the principle that a person's beliefs, personal standards, and feelings of self-efficacy strongly affect his or her behavior (Bandura, 1977, 1986; Beck, 1976; Ellis, 1962). Cognitive therapies concentrate on techniques designed to change cognitions rather than on the immediate reinforcement of overt behavior.

Although he did not originally use the term *cognitive*, Albert Ellis (1962) evolved an approach called *rational emotive therapy* that became the precursor of modern cognitive therapies. According to Ellis, an analysis of a person's problem behavior will reveal a pattern of irrational or catastrophic thoughts that underlie such behavior. In other words, thoughts are the root of behavior problems. Once irrational cognitions have been identified, the therapist actively attacks these beliefs, with the goal of eliminating or changing them into more rational beliefs. Ellis believes that humans have the ability to use logic and to deal rationally with their problems. His therapy, then, is based on the assumption that people possess the ability to examine their belief systems logically and to alter those systems when necessary.

Ellis contends that irrational beliefs form the basis for a variety of problems. All these problems are self-reinforced by an internal monologue in which people perpetuate their misery with continued self-statements of irrational beliefs and unreasonable expectations. Ellis has proposed that the most effective way to alleviate stressful problems is to change the irrational beliefs. Escaping an overbearing boss may not be possible, but a suffering employee may learn to manage the situation with less stress. The cognitive management occurs through the application of rational self-statements that lead to a realistic perception of the stressful situation and a more effective way to deal with the boss. Another employee working for the same overbearing boss may "catastrophize" this experience with such irrational self-statements as "Because my boss is a tyrant, I am miserable in my job, and it is ruining my life." The therapist would teach this person to substitute rational self-statements for this irrational one. A rational statement might be "Even though my boss often behaves in an overbearing manner, I am not forced to react to her behavior with negative emotions because I have the resources to cope with these episodes constructively." Thus, the emotional element of the stress response is averted or minimized, and the person has a greater opportunity to cope rationally and positively with stress.

The experience of pain is one that can easily be turned into a catastrophe, and any exaggeration of feelings of pain can lead to maladaptive behaviors and further exacerbation of irrational beliefs. A study by Chaves and Brown (1987) found that 44% of dental pain patients spontaneously used cognitive strategies to cope with pain and stress while 37% of the patients "catastrophized" their pain experiences. When the "copers" and the "catastrophizers" were

compared, the researchers found that people who spontaneously coped with dental pain reported less stress but no less pain than did those who made a catastrophe of the situation. On the other hand, a later study (Keefe, Brown, Wallston, & Caldwell, 1989) showed that catastrophizing pain led to long-term exaggerations of pain. In this study, rheumatoid arthritis pain sufferers completed a coping strategies questionnaire on two occasions 6 months apart. Those who catastrophized their pain at the first occasion tended to report more intense pain, more functional impairments, and greater depression 6 months later. This finding supports Ellis's contention that magnifying an event into a catastrophe will lead to increased emotional distress and elevated levels of pain.

What Is Cognitive Therapy?

Cognitive therapy rests on the assumption that a change in the interpretation of an event can change people's emotional and physiological reaction to that event. Although this approach typically utilizes operant conditioning techniques, it adds an emphasis on patients' ability to think about and evaluate their own behaviors. Because both behavior modification and cognitive therapy usually use multiple procedures, the two overlap a good bit, making accurate labeling of any multimodal package quite difficult.

As applied to pain management, cognitive therapy assumes that patients frequently exaggerate their pain-engendering thoughts, thus exacerbating their subjective feelings of pain and ultimately adding a psychological component to the physical experience of pain. Albert Bandura (1986) proposed that perceived self-efficacy can bring relief from pain by decreasing stress and bodily tension. For this reason, many cognitive therapists attempt in various ways to increase pain patients' feelings of **self-efficacy** — that is, their confidence that they can perform the behaviors necessary to produce the desired outcomes.

Bandura hypothesized that cognitive therapy may block pain sensations at either the level of physiological transmission or the level of psychological awareness. He cited evidence suggesting that one's *belief* in the effectiveness of a placebo seems to release endorphins, the body's natural pain fighters (Bandura, 1986; Bandura, O'Leary, Taylor, Gauthier,

& Gossard, 1987) These findings may explain why about one-third of all pain patients achieve relief from placebos. Because endorphins produce a biochemical reaction to placebos, at least some of the pain relief stemming from cognitive therapy or any other type of psychological treatment is just as physically based as that attained through medication. Cognitive therapy also works to reduce pain on another level. Increased self-efficacy allows pain patients to return their attention to matters other than their pain. When people are confident that they can cope with impending increases in pain, they are less likely to dwell on the pain, thus decreasing their perceived suffering.

A variety of cognitive strategies have been devised for coping with pain and/or stress. Two of these are the inoculation techniques and the overt expression of strong negative emotions and unpleasant experiences.

Inoculation Techniques.   Dennis Turk, Donald Meichenbaum, and their associates (Meichenbaum & Jaremko, 1982, 1983; Meichenbaum & Turk, 1976; Turk, 1978; Turk, Meichenbaum, & Genest, 1983; Turk & Rudy, 1992) have devised a cognitive program for pain management, and Meichenbaum and Roy Cameron (1983) have developed a parallel strategy for stress management. Both procedures rely on inoculation techniques; that is, they work in a manner analogous to vaccination. By introducing a weakened dose of a pathogen (in this case, the pathogen is a stressor) the therapist attempts to build some immunity against high levels of pain and stress.

Because pain is at least partially due to psychological factors, therapists who use inoculation techniques work first at getting patients to think differently about the source of their pain experience. During this *reconceptualization* stage, patients are encouraged to accept a psychological explanation for at least some of their pain and to come to an understanding of how behavior therapy can help. Once patients accept the potential effectiveness of psychologically based treatment, they are ready to enter the second stage—*acquisition and rehearsal of skills*. During this phase of treatment, patients are taught relaxation and controlled breathing skills. Because physical and mental relaxation is incompatible with tension and anxiety, learning to relax can be a valuable tool in managing pain. Patients may also be taught to direct their attention away from the pain experience by concentrating on a pleasant scene, such as a cool waterfall, or by focusing their attention outside themselves—for example, by counting spots on ceiling tiles or by thinking about a funny movie they have seen recently.

After patients have acquired and consolidated these various skills, they are ready to enter the final, or *follow-through,* phase of treatment. During this stage, patients apply their coping skills to their natural environment. Physical activity and exercise are encouraged to give patients a greater feeling of self-efficacy and a quantifiable means of evaluating their progress. Also during this stage, pain patients receive medication on the basis of time rather than on their reports of pain. They are also encouraged to gradually increase the time between doses while decreasing their level of medication. During this follow-through stage, therapists give instructions to spouses and other family members in methods of ignoring patients' pain behaviors and of reinforcing such healthy behaviors as greater levels of physical activity, decreased use of medication, fewer visits to the pain clinic, or an increased number of days at work. Finally, patients construct, with the help of their therapists, a posttreatment plan for coping with future pain. They must accept the reality that pain may return, sometimes more severe than ever, and that such a "relapse" is not a sign that the treatment was ineffective. Instead, the patients, no longer in need of a therapist, approach these pain episodes armed with a variety of self-help skills and with the confidence that they can cope with these experiences.

The **stress inoculation** program of Meichenbaum and Cameron is quite similar to Turk and Meichenbaum's method for coping with pain. Stress inoculation includes three stages: conceptualization, skills acquisition and rehearsal, and follow-through or application.

The *conceptualization* stage is a cognitive intervention in which the therapist works with clients to identify and clarify their problems. During this overtly educational stage, patients learn about stress inoculation and become aware of how this technique can reduce their stress. The *skills acquisition and rehearsal* stage involves both educational and behavioral components to enhance patients' repertoire of coping skills. At this time, patients learn and practice new ways of coping with stress. One of the goals of this stage is to improve self-instruction by changing cognitions, a process that includes monitoring one's internal monologue — that is, self-talk. During the *application and follow-through* stage, patients put into practice the cognitive changes they achieved in the two previous stages.

Stress inoculation has been effective in a variety of stressful situations, ranging from math anxiety among college students (Schneider & Nevid, 1993) to hypertension in people of all ages (Amigo, Buceta, Becona, & Bueno, 1991). Some researchers have combined a stress inoculation technique with other interventions to alleviate stress. For example, Kiselica, Baker, Thomas, and Reedy (1994) used a combination of stress inoculation, progressive muscle relaxation, cognitive restructuring, and assertiveness training to significantly reduce trait anxiety and stress-related symptoms among adolescents. However, the effects of this training did not extend to academic performance. In other words, although students became less anxious and felt less stress, their grades did not improve. Similarly, Hains and Ellman (1994) found that a stress inoculation training program that included a variety of other cognitive behavioral strategies reduced depression, anxiety, and anger in high school students but did not improve their grade point averages. Wilcox and Dowrick (1992) found that stress inoculation in combination with other cognitive behavioral interventions reduced anger in adolescents with substance abuse problems.

Although these studies all combined stress inoculation training with other techniques, some evidence exists that stress inoculation by itself can be an effective procedure for managing stress. Keyes and Dean (1988) used stress inoculation training with people who worked with mentally retarded individuals. The training not only reduced the staff members' stress and anger, but most of them felt that it increased their ability to work with clients. Finally, Lopez and Silber (1991) found that elderly people who received a stress inoculation intervention showed greater reduction in stress than either a no-treatment control group or an information/attention control group. These studies suggest that stress inoculation training, either alone or in combination with other procedures, can be an effective intervention for stress management.

Expressing Emotions. During the past decade, James Pennebaker and his associates have studied the notion that talking or writing about negative events allows people to work toward a cognitive resolution of traumatic experiences. The therapeutic value of **catharsis**, or the venting of unpleasant emotions, goes back at least as far as Breuer and Freud (1895/1955), but Pennebaker has recently been able to demonstrate the physical health benefits of talking or writing about traumatic events. In one study, survivors of the Holocaust talked for 1 to 2 hours about their experiences during World War II while being measured for skin conductance level and heart rate. Fourteen months later, Pennebaker, Barger, and Tiebout (1989) collected data on health problems of the participants and found that the more survivors disclosed personally traumatic experiences, the better their subsequent health became.

Writing about negative experiences also seems to produce positive health results. Pennebaker, Colder, and Sharp (1990) divided college freshmen into an experimental group who wrote about their anxieties of going to college and a control group who wrote about superficial topics. Regardless of the week during the school year that students wrote, those who ventilated feelings about entering college had fewer illnesses than those who merely wrote about superficial topics. Similarly, Francis and Pennebaker (1992) looked at the health effects of writing about personal traumatic experiences of university employees age 22 to 70 and found that those who wrote about traumatic experiences had more health benefits than those who wrote about nontraumatic experiences.

More recently, Pennebaker and his associates have examined several variables that may contribute to the health benefits of catharsis. They found that in general, people who use negative emotion words improve more than those who use positive emotion words (Pennebaker, 1993); nonverbal expression of traumatic experiences through art and music may be therapeutic (Berry & Pennebaker, 1993); and writing about a particular topic (such as intimacy or school) helps people gain some cognitive resolution of that topic (Mancuso & Pennebaker, 1994). Pennebaker's research has added an effective and easily assessable tool in the arsenal of coping strategies. Expressing rather than denying negative experiences may benefit both psychological and physiological health.

How Effective Is Cognitive Therapy?

Evaluations of the effectiveness of cognitive therapy programs are difficult because widely diverse procedures have been placed under the rubric of cognitive therapy. As with behavioral therapies, cognitive programs often use a broad range of strategies, including relaxation training, biofeedback, behavior modification, systematic desensitization, and other techniques that are not strictly cognitive. Also, cognitive strategies themselves are not always used in the same way. For example, Blanchard and Andrasik (1985) reviewed 12 studies that had investigated the effectiveness of cognitive-behavioral treatments for headache and found that no one cognitive procedure was employed in the same manner across different research settings.

Early reviews (Turner & Chapman, 1982b; Turner & Romano, 1984) indicated that many studies lacked adequate controls and most included few participants, but findings concerning the effectiveness of cognitive therapy for pain were generally positive. In a later, well-designed study, Turner and Jensen (1993) evaluated the effectiveness of three programs: (1) cognitive therapy, (2) relaxation training, and (3) cognitive therapy combined with relaxation training. Participants on a waiting list served a control group. Patients with mild disability from chronic low back pain were measured for severity of pain and assigned to one of these groups. At the end of treatment, patients in all three experimental groups significantly decreased their pain, but those in the control group did not. The investigators also assessed levels of depressive symptoms and found that depression diminished in all groups, including the control group.

Combined cognitive and behavioral approaches have been shown to be effective with a variety of pain syndromes. Sanders, Shepherd, Cleghorn, and Woolford (1994) worked with children suffering recurrent abdominal pain and compared a cognitive-behavioral intervention with a standard pediatric care program. This cognitive-behavioral intervention included teaching the children relaxation and coping techniques and teaching parents to encourage nonpain behaviors in their children. Parents of children in the standard pediatric care were told not to overreact to the child's pain behaviors, that the child would eventually outgrow the pain, and that the child should learn self-coping skills. Both conditions resulted in some lessening of pain intensity, but children who received the cognitive-behavioral intervention had higher rates of pain alleviation and lower rates of pain relapse at 6- and 12-month follow-up.

Cognitive behavioral and relaxation strategies may produce differential effects, depending on the location of pain. Bru, Mykletun, Berge, and Svebak (1994) compared the effectiveness of a cognitive-behavioral approach, a relaxation intervention, and the combination of cognitive-behavioral and relaxation treatments. Although only the cognitive-behavioral approach was effective in shortening the duration of pain, each of the three interventions was able to reduce some pain. The relaxation technique was most successful in reducing low back pain, the cognitive-behavioral approach combined with relaxation was effective in reducing neck pain, and all three interventions were successful in alleviating shoulder pain. More research on the differential effectiveness of pain interventions is needed, but these results suggest that different types and locations of pain may call for different treatments.

Keefe and Van Horn (1993) reviewed several studies to determine the long-term effects of cognitive-behavioral interventions with rheumatoid arthritis pain. They found that cognitive-behavioral strategies were generally successful, at least for some arthritis patients. They also suggested that the cognitive-behavioral approach could be an effective means of preventing pain relapse.

Lehrer et al. (1994) reviewed a number of relaxation and biofeedback techniques for a variety of problems, and their evaluation of cognitive therapy was generally positive. This component was typically valuable for both pain and stress control. Although cognitive therapy did not add to the effectiveness of thermal biofeedback in managing migraine headache pain, it was effective in tension headache, back pain, and anxiety.

In summary, cognitively oriented treatment for stress and pain seems to be at least as effective as either relaxation training or biofeedback, but an important part of cognitive therapy programs may be the relaxation aspect. One possible advantage of cognitive approaches is their ability to change patients' self-perceived efficacy to cope with a variety of stresses and pains and to reduce depression, emotionality, and irritability (Blanchard & Andrasik, 1985). Cognitive therapy appears to be an appropriate tool for a variety of health-related behaviors. Its focus is broader than any of the other four psychological interventions we have discussed, all of which are primarily symptom oriented. Instead of concentrating on a specific behavior or behaviors, cognitive therapies take into account cognitive, affective, sensory, and behavioral components of a particular disorder. In other words, the goal of cognitive therapy is not limited to a specific target behavior such as stress reduction or pain management. Meichenbaum (1977) and Ellis (1986) have both emphasized the need for *general* therapies that look at antecedent stressors such as depression, anxiety, feelings of self-confidence, and other global aspects of personal life. Cognitive therapies rate higher on this criterion than do hypnosis, relaxation training, biofeedback, or behavior modification. Table 6.5 summarizes the effectiveness of cognitive therapy and the problems it can be used to treat.

MULTIMODAL APPROACHES

One difficulty in evaluating psychological approaches for treating pain and stress is that they frequently combine several treatment strategies in a multimodal program. Such an approach will usually result in lower levels of pain or stress, but sifting out the effectiveness of one treatment mode from the others is often problematic. Eisenberg et al. (1993) suggested that evaluation of traditional medical programs may be difficult because more than one-third of patients seek nontraditional therapies but do not disclose that fact to their physician. When participants in a study designed to test the efficacy of traditional pain reduction procedures are simultaneously seeking other treatments, no valid conclusions are possible concerning the effectiveness of the experimental treatment.

Evaluation of multimodal and other pain treatments is also complicated by the placebo effect. In 1994, Turner and her associates (Turner, Deyo, Loeser, Von Korff, & Fordyce, 1994) reviewed more than 200 studies on pain treatment to evaluate the importance of the placebo effect. They defined placebo as "an intervention designed to simulate medical therapy, but not believed . . . to be specific therapy for the target condition" (Turner et al., 1994, p. 1610). In other words, a placebo effect is any nonspecific effect, such as that resulting from patients' expectations, decreases in their anxiety, or other conditions not produced by traditional medical treatment. Turner et al. reported that traditional treatments such as surgery can produce strong placebo effects and that those effects are frequently much higher than the often-quoted 33% effectiveness.

Turner et al. suggested that pain patients usually improve for one or more of three possible reasons. First, pain is cyclical. People will seek help and be enrolled in treatment studies when their pain is at its most intense. As the study continues, one would expect a reduction in pain even without treatment or without the placebo effect. For this reason, any treatment will likely produce significant results because people simply return to their typical level of pain. Second, the intervention may actually help. Third, the program may produce nonspecific effects attributable to factors other than the specific treatment. Included in these nonspecific or "placebo effects" are the physician's attention, interest, concern, and expectations of positive results. Nonspecific effects also include the physician's reputation, the expense of the treatment, and the clinical setting. Turner et al. suggested that most physicians underestimate the placebo effect, an effect that "may explain some or all of the benefits attributed to treatment" (p. 1613).

Despite these difficulties, Edward Blanchard and his associates attempted to evaluate two multimodal approaches for pain. Blanchard et al. (1990a) assigned tension headache patients to one of four groups: (1) a progressive muscle relaxation group, (2) a progressive muscle relaxation plus cognitive therapy group, (3) an attention placebo control group that received pseudomeditation, and (4) a headache monitoring control group. Both experimental groups reported significant improvement

Table 6.5 **Effectiveness of cognitive therapy**

Problem	Effectiveness
Stress, anxiety, and anger	Stress inoculation training is effective either alone or in combination with other cognitive behavioral strategies.
Traumatic events	Writing or talking about negative events reduces stress and the likelihood of subsequent health problems.
Tension headache	Cognitive therapy is as effective as electromyograph (EMG) biofeedback.
Migraine headache	Cognitive therapy is not as effective as temperature biofeedback.
Low back pain	Cognitive therapy has benefits but is not as effective as relaxation.
Abdominal pain in children	Cognitive therapy is more effective than standard pediatric care.
Arthritis pain	Cognitive therapy is generally successful and may prevent relapse.

over the two control groups on a headache index. In addition, the two experimental groups significantly decreased their pain medication. However, the addition of cognitive therapy to progressive muscle relaxation resulted in only a minimal gain, thus indicating once again that relaxation alone may be the salient ingredient in any pain management program.

In a second study, Blanchard et al. (1990b) used a combination of thermal biofeedback, relaxation training, and cognitive therapy to treat headache pain. They randomly assigned vascular headache pain patients to one of four groups: (1) a biofeedback plus relaxation training group, (2) a biofeedback, plus relaxation training plus cognitive therapy group, (3) an attention placebo group that received instruction in body awareness training and mental relaxation, and (4) a headache monitoring group. The first three groups received 16 treatment sessions over 8 weeks while the fourth group continued to monitor their headaches. The two experimental groups and the placebo group all improved significantly more than did the headache monitoring group, but there was no difference in headache pain among the first three groups. In this study, cognitive therapy added no significant gain to the combination of thermal biofeedback and relaxation training. Moreover, neither experimental group was superior to the attention placebo group, a finding that led the authors to believe that the body awareness training and mental relaxation received by the placebo group became, in time, an active relaxation condition.

More recently, some pain researchers have simply combined several programs with no attempt to evaluate their individual contributions. Such approaches will usually result in pain reduction, but they leave unanswered the question of which specific technique is most effective. Scharff and Marcus (1994) evaluated a headache pain coping program that included education, information about medication management, physical therapy, and pain and stress management skills. Patients who declined treatment served as a comparison group. During follow-up, more than 70% of the treatment patients experienced significant pain reduction and were able to reduce their medication by 50% or more. On the other hand, only about one-fourth of the patients in the comparison group experienced a significant reduction in headache pain. Also, treatment patients who continued to comply with their program continued to maintain their improvement. In another study, Nicholson and Blanchard (1993) evaluated a multimodal program that combined relaxation training, cognitive therapy, and biofeedback. Elderly chronic headache patients who received the combined program were able to reduce their medication significantly after a 12-session treatment. At a 1-month follow-up, they were less depressed and less anxious than they were at the beginning of treatment.

Results from these and other multimodal programs suggest that various psychologically oriented treatments for pain and stress are generally effective. Moreover, their parallel treatments for pain almost always result in reductions in pain medication, increases in patients' physical activity, and decreases in their lost work time. Indeed, psychological treatments for pain are probably more effective than traditional medical treatments.

CHAPTER SUMMARY

We humans have a natural tendency toward health and away from distress, disease, and pain. When "dis-eases" become part of our lives, we attempt to cope with them in order to restore our health. Some attempts at coping, such as self-medication with alcohol and drugs, have long-term disadvantages rather than benefits, but other methods of coping provide ways to manage these problems.

Some people cope successfully with stress and chronic pain because they possess sufficient personal resources such as social support and a strong feeling of being in control of their lives. Social support, defined as the emotional quality of one's social contacts, is inversely related to disease and death. In general, people with high levels of social support, compared to those with low levels, are only about half as likely to die within a designated period of time. These findings are most pronounced for European American men, but other groups also show some benefit from a network of quality relationships. Several hypotheses have been advanced concerning the reasons for the benefits of social support. The two most likely of these are that (1) people with adequate social support receive more encouragement and advice to seek medical care and (2) social support itself acts as a buffer against disease.

Adequate feelings of personal control also seem to enable people to cope better with stress and illness. A study by Langer and Rodin (1976) provided evidence that when people are allowed to assume even small amounts of personal control and responsibility, they live longer and healthier lives. This study, conducted in a nursing home, has implications for people of all ages.

Health psychologists have used a variety of techniques to help people cope with stress and chronic pain. Among these are hypnosis, relaxation training, biofeedback, behavior modification, and cognitive therapy. Some debate still exists over the exact nature of hypnosis, but there is little disagreement that hypnosis can be a powerful analgesic for managing pain. The benefits of hypnosis vary individually, but the technique has some effectiveness for many people.

A second psychological technique for coping with stress and pain is relaxation training. Four types of relaxation are discussed in this chapter: (1) progressive muscle relaxation, (2) meditative relaxation, (3) mindfulness meditation, and (4) guided imagery. All four approaches have demonstrated some success in helping patients cope with such stress-related problems such as headache pain, asthma, insomnia, and hypertension. For several problems, relaxation is more effective than a placebo and about as effective as biofeedback, which requires specialized machinery and therapists trained in its use.

Biofeedback techniques provide immediate information to people concerning the status of their biological systems. Some evidence exists that biofeedback can be an effective procedure—either alone or in combination with other techniques—for lessening some kinds of pain. Temperature biofeedback is effective in alleviating migraine headache, and EMG biofeedback has demonstrated some effectiveness in reducing tension and migraine headache, anxiety, low back pain, and temporomandibular joint pain.

Health psychologists have also used behavior modification, a technique based on the principles of operant conditioning, to help people cope with pain. Behavior modification techniques are directed at altering pain behaviors, not lessening the sensations of pain. They are based on the assumption that withholding reinforcement for pain behaviors will decrease the likelihood that those behaviors will recur. When people are no longer rewarded for moaning, limping, missing work, or complaining, they tend to stop doing these things and begin to exhibit more nonpain behaviors. Behavior modification principles are frequently included in a multimodal package of pain and stress management that also includes cognitive therapy.

Cognitive therapy programs often rely on reinforcement techniques, but add a multitude of other strategies, including self-talk, self-efficacy, and self-evaluation of behavior. Because pain is at least partially due to psychological factors, cognitive therapists attempt to get patients to think differently about their pain experiences. One goal of cognitive treatment for pain is to increase patients' confidence that they can cope with increases in pain. Increased self-efficacy permits patients to concentrate on non-pain experiences. Cognitive therapists have developed a program for dealing with stress called stress inoculation, a procedure analogous to vaccination. Patients learn to cope with mild doses of stress and then to use these same strategies to cope with more stressful life experiences. Another successful procedure for coping with stress calls for patients to overtly express strong negative emotions through writing or talking.

An evaluation of psychological strategies for dealing with stress and pain is difficult because such strategies typically involve a multimodal program that includes some combination of hypnosis, relaxation training, biofeedback, operant conditioning techniques, cognitive therapy, and a strong placebo effect, which can be especially powerful in pain treatment programs.

SUGGESTED READINGS

Fordyce, W. E. (1990a) Contingency management. In J. J. Bonica (Ed.), *The management of pain* (2nd ed., pp. 1702–1710). Philadelphia: Lea & Febiger. Fordyce discusses terminology and principles of behavioral management of pain. Contingency management procedures typically target some combination of problem behaviors that include overmedication, reduced activity levels, excessive pain behaviors, deficits in well behavior, and inappropriate responses to pain behavior.

Schwartz, M. S., & Schwartz, N. M. (1993). Biofeedback: Using the body's signals. In E. Goleman & J. Gurin (Eds.), *Mind/body medicine: How to use your mind for better health* (pp. 301–313). Yonkers, NY: Consumer Reports Books. This article describes the background of biofeedback and provides information on the types most common in clinical practice.

Schwarzer, R., & Leppin, A. (1992). Possible impact of social ties and support on morbidity and mortality. In H. O. E. Veiel & U. Baumann (Eds.), *The meaning and measurement of social support* (pp. 65–83). New York: Hemisphere. Although this chapter is somewhat technical, it provides a solid background on the rationale and research on social support and its relationship to morbidity and mortality.

Turner, J. A., Deyo, R. A., Loeser, J. D., Von Korff, M., & Fordyce, W. E. (1994). The importance of placebo effects in pain treatment and research. *Journal of the American Medical Association, 271,* 1609–1614. An excellent review of the placebo in pain treatment, this article presents a broad definition of the placebo effect.

7

Seeking Health Care

While playing a game of half-court basketball, Jeff jabbed his right hand on the backboard and felt an immediate pain. However, he continued playing, as minor injuries were merely "part of the game." For the rest of the day, his hand continued to hurt, and he had difficulty writing, eating, or using the hand for other tasks. The next day, Jeff's hand was somewhat discolored and quite swollen. To reduce the swelling, he wrapped an ice pack around the hand for 20 to 30 minutes two or three times that day. Still, Jeff continued with his daily activities as well as he could, believing that the swelling would soon disappear. On the third day, however, his hand was no better, so he decided to seek advice. But the advice he sought was not from a physician or other health practitioner; rather, it was from two colleagues at his law office, neither of whom had any medical training. Both colleagues advised Jeff to have his hand X-rayed to learn whether it was broken. Still, Jeff hesitated. He did not want to miss

work, and he knew that being X-rayed and seeing a doctor would be time-consuming.

When he finally decided that an X-ray was warranted, Jeff went to a local imaging center that specialized in X-rays. The person at the imaging center informed Jeff that his hand could not be X-rayed there unless he was referred by a physician. Indeed, she seemed shocked that anyone would come to the imaging center without a physician's referral. So Jeff called his internist and asked her to order an X-ray, which she did. The internist also referred him to an orthopedic specialist, whom he saw the next day. Results of the X-ray revealed a broken metacarpal — that is, the part of the hand between the wrist and the fingers. Jeff's hand was put into a cast, and six weeks passed before he played any more basketball or used his right hand for nearly anything else.

Why was Jeff reluctant to seek medical care? Why was the pain he experienced not sufficient to prompt him go to the doctor? Why did he ask the opinion of people with no medical training prior to getting advice from a trained professional?

ADOPTING HEALTH-RELATED BEHAVIORS

Most people in the world value health and want to avoid illness and disability. Nevertheless, many people do not behave in ways that maximize health and minimize disease and disability. Why do some people, such as Jeff, seem to behave unwisely on issues of personal health? Why do others seek medical treatment when they are not ill? What explains people's reluctance to believe that their own risky behaviors are unsafe and their willingness to believe that those same behaviors place other people in jeopardy? No final answers to these questions are possible at this point, but psychologists have formulated several theories or models in the attempt to make sense of and to predict behaviors related to health. This chapter looks briefly at some of these theories as they relate to health-seeking behavior, Chapter 8 examines theory-driven research that relates to people's adherence to medical advice, and Chapter 12 discusses several theories that deal with behaviors directed at staying healthy.

THEORIES OF HEALTH-PROTECTIVE BEHAVIORS

Health psychologists frequently use theoretical models to explain and predict health-enhancing behaviors. These models include the health belief model, which originally grew out of the work of Geoffrey Hochbaum (1958) and his colleagues at the Public Health Service; the theory of reasoned action by Martin Fishbein and Icek Ajzen (Ajzen & Fishbein, 1980; Fishbein & Ajzen, 1975); the concept of planned behavior, which Ajzen developed as an alternative to the theory of reasoned action (Ajzen, 1985, 1991); the self-regulation theory of Albert Bandura (1986, 1991); the stages of change theory of James Prochaska and his colleagues (Prochaska, DiClemente, & Norcross, 1992); and the precaution adoption process of Neil Weinstein (Weinstein, 1988; Weinstein & Nicolich, 1993; Weinstein & Sandman, 1992).

The Health Belief Model

Since the early work of Hochbaum (1958), several versions of the *health belief model* (HBM) have been devised. The one that has attracted the most attention and generated the most research is that of Marshall Becker and Irwin Rosenstock (Becker, 1979; Becker & Rosenstock, 1984; Rosenstock, 1986; Rosenstock, Strecher, & Becker, 1988).

Like all health belief models, the one developed by Becker and Rosenstock assumes that beliefs are important contributors to health-seeking behavior. This model includes four beliefs or perceptions that should combine to predict health-related behaviors, such as Jeff's eventual decision to seek the aid of an orthopedic physician when he broke his hand: (1) perceived *susceptibility* to disease or disability, (2) perceived *severity* of the disease or disability, (3) perceived *bene-*

fits of health-enhancing behaviors, and (4) perceived *barriers* to health-enhancing behaviors. After first hurting his hand, Jeff did not believe that his injury was serious or that he was vulnerable to disability. Thus, he saw little benefit in going to a doctor, an action that would have been costly in terms of money and time. After two of his colleagues expressed their belief that his injury might be serious and after two days of eating, driving, writing, and dressing with his left hand, Jeff changed his beliefs and subsequently sought medical attention.

The health belief model corresponds with common sense, but does it predict health-related behavior? Research on the utility of the health belief model has been extensive, but the results have been inconsistent. If the health belief model is useful, then interventions to change beliefs should be effective. Beginning with this assumption, Champion (1994) used the HBM to inform women with no family history of breast cancer about the benefits of **mammography**. Women who received an intervention aimed at enhancing their knowledge and changing their beliefs were nearly four times more likely to seek mammography testing than an equivalent group of women in a control group. However, a prospective study by Hyman, Baker, Ephraim, Moadel, and Philip (1994) indicated that perceived susceptibility to breast cancer did not predict a woman's mammography utilization, although both perceived benefits and perceived barriers did. Moreover, ethnicity was a better predictor than either benefits or barriers, with African American women being more likely to utilize mammography than European Americans. Aiken, West, Woodward, and Reno (1994) found some predictive value for the health belief model, but they also found that having a regular place to go for health care and a physician who recommended a mammogram were better predictors than the combined factors of the health belief model. Incidentally, none of these studies included the factor of perceived severity in the prediction of mammography utilization because they assumed that nearly all women view breast cancer as a severe disease.

The health belief model, of course, has been used to predict health-related behaviors other than mammography utilization. Several recent studies have found some ability of the HBM to predict safe sex behaviors (Abraham & Sheeran, 1994; Lux & Petosa,

1994; Rimberg & Lewis, 1994; Yep, 1993; Zimmerman & Olson, 1994). However, studies that showed the strongest predictive value of the HBM generally used an expanded version of the model, including cues to action, self-efficacy, intentions to behave, and perceived social norms. For this reason, some researchers have begun to combine aspects of the health belief model with concepts from other models, including the theory of reasoned action.

The Theory of Reasoned Action

The theory of reasoned action (Ajzen & Fishbein, 1980; Fishbein & Ajzen, 1975) assumes that people are quite reasonable and make systematic use of information when deciding how to behave. Moreover, they "consider the implications of their actions before they decide to engage or not engage in a given behavior" (Ajzen, 1985, p. 5). In addition, the theory of reasoned action assumes that behavior is directed toward a goal or outcome and that people freely choose those actions that they believe will move them in the direction of that goal. They can also choose not to act, if they believe that such an action would move them away from their goal, as when Jeff decided not to seek immediate medical attention because he believed that a cast on his hand would hamper his regular work routine.

The immediate determinant of behavior is the *intention* to act or not to act. Intentions, in turn, are shaped by two factors. The first is a personal evaluation of the behavior—that is, one's *attitude toward the behavior.* The second is one's perception of the social pressure to perform or not perform the action—that is, one's *subjective norm.* One's attitude toward the behavior is determined by beliefs that the behavior will lead to positively or negatively valued outcomes. One's subjective norm is shaped by one's perception of the evaluation that a particular individual (or group of individuals) places on that behavior and one's *motivation* to comply with the norms set by that individual (or group of individuals). In predicting behavior, the theory of reasoned action also considers the relative weight of personal attitudes measured against subjective norms (see Figure 7.1).

In predicting whether Jeff, with a painful, discolored, and swollen hand, will seek medical attention, the theory of reasoned action relies on several pieces of information. First, does he believe that going to the doctor's office is related to his goal of a healthy hand? Second, how strong are his beliefs that other people expect him to seek medical attention balanced against his need to comply with others' expectations? The answer to the first question reveals Jeff's attitude toward seeking medical assistance, and the answer to the second question suggests the level of social pressure on him to seek assistance. These two answers reflect his attitude toward seeking medical care and his subjective norm about seeking care. Because Jeff's attitudes and his subjective norms were initially in conflict, his early intention was somewhat mixed, making prediction of his behavior difficult. Nevertheless, the theory of reasoned action has the potential to make valid predictions when investigators accurately measure both the strength of a person's attitude toward a behavior and the person's need to conform to social norms.

Does the theory of reasoned action predict health-seeking behavior? In general, researchers have found the theory to be useful for predicting certain health-related behaviors. Montano and Taplin (1991) found that the theory of reasoned action accurately predicted mammogram utilization in women past age 40, and Lierman, Kasprzyk, and Benoliel (1991) reported that a modified theory of reasoned action explained much of the difference between women who frequently performed breast self-examination and those who only infrequently examined themselves. In this second study, intention to perform breast self-examination was a strong predictor of who would perform breast self-examination and who would not. Intention to perform contributes heavily to the usefulness of the theory of reasoned action. Michie, Marteau, and Kidd (1992) found that pregnant women's intention to attend health-information classes after delivery was the most important predictor of subsequent attendance, but other factors also contributed, including social norms and the attitude of the baby's father.

Although these studies did not directly compare the usefulness of the theory of reasoned action with the health belief model, the results indicate that the theory of reasoned action is at least as adequate as the health belief model in explaining and predicting health-seeking behaviors. A key element in the the-

BELIEFS ⟶ ATTITUDES ⟶ INTENTION ⟶ BEHAVIOR

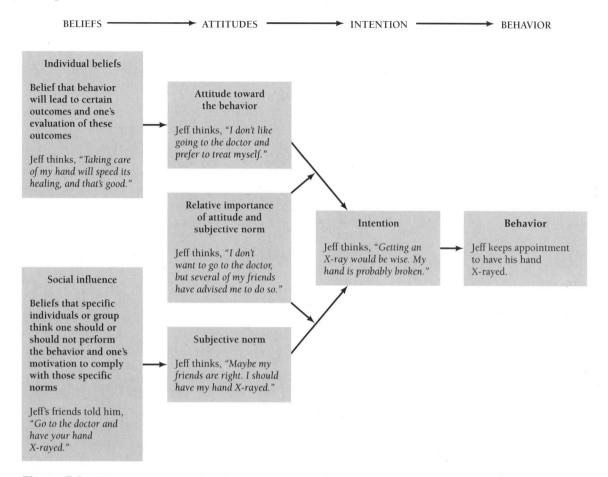

Figure 7.1 Theory of reasoned action applied to health-seeking behavior. SOURCE: Adapted from Ajzen/Fishbein, *Understanding Attitudes and Predicting Social Behavior* © 1980, p. 8. Adapted by permission of Prentice Hall, Upper Saddle River, New Jersey.

ory of reasoned action seems to be the intention to perform a behavior.

The Theory of Planned Behavior

Ajzen has extended the theory of reasoned action to include the concept of perceived behavioral control, an extension he calls the theory of planned behavior. The primary difference between the theory of reasoned action and the theory of planned behavior is the latter's inclusion of the *perception of how much control* people have over their behavior (Ajzen, 1985, 1988, 1991; Doll & Ajzen, 1992; Madden, Ellen, & Ajzen, 1992). The more resources and opportunities people believe they have, the stronger are their beliefs that they can control their behavior. Figure 7.2

shows that predictions of behavior can be made from knowledge of (1) people's attitude toward the behavior, (2) their subjective norm, and (3) their perceived behavioral control. All three components interact to shape people's intentions to behave. In addition, perceived behavioral control may have a direct influence on people's behavior (Ajzen, 1991). Perceived behavioral control is the ease or difficulty one has in achieving desired behavioral outcomes; it reflects both past behaviors and perceived ability to overcome obstacles. Perceived behavioral control operates both directly and indirectly to influence behavior. The direct path is the actual control a person has over performing the behavior. This direct path may occur when people perform behaviors almost

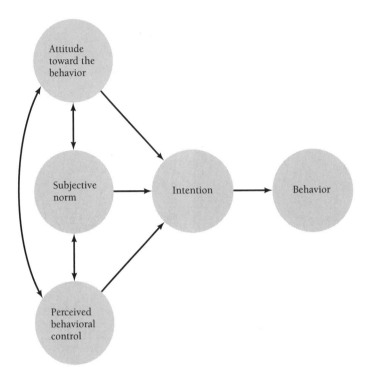

Figure 7.2 **Theory of planned behavior.** SOURCE: From I. Ajzen, 1991, "The Theory of Planned Behavior," *Organizational Behavior and Human Decision Processes, 50,* p. 182. Reprinted by permission of Academic Press.

automatically, such as brushing their teeth. In addition, perceived personal control operates indirectly to shape behavior by influencing people's intention to behave. The theory assumes that people who believe they can easily perform a behavior are more likely to *intend* to perform that behavior than people who believe they have little control over performing that behavior (Madden, Ellen, & Ajzen, 1992).

The theory of planned behavior has not yet produced the quantity of health-related research that the health belief model has generated, but a few studies have provided some confirmation of the theory. Norman and Conner (1993) found that both the health belief model and the theory of planned behavior were useful in predicting attendance in a health check program, and consistent with the theory of planned behavior, intention and perceived behavior control were strong and independent predictors of attendance. Earlier, Ronis and Kaiser (1989) had combined elements of the theory of planned behavior and the health belief model and found that this combination was able to predict frequency of breast self-

examination of college women. Also, McCaul, Sandgren, O'Neill, and Hinsz (1993) looked at factors that might predict undergraduate students' health-related behaviors such as breast self-examination, testicular self-examination, or dental flossing. They found that attitudes toward the behavior and subjective norms predicted intentions to perform these behaviors. In addition, perceived control added significantly to the prediction of these health-protective behaviors.

Self-Regulation Theory

Like the theory of reasoned action and the theory of planned behavior, Albert Bandura's social cognitive theory of self-regulation is a general theory of behavior and not limited to predicting health-seeking behaviors. Bandura's theory of self-regulation stresses the interaction of behavior, environment, and person factors, especially cognition. Bandura (1986) referred to this interactive triadic model as **reciprocal determinism.** An important component of the person variable is self-efficacy.

Self-efficacy refers to "people's beliefs about their capabilities to exercise control over events that affect their lives" (Bandura, 1989, p. 1175). Self-efficacy is a specific rather than a global concept; that is, it refers to people's beliefs that they can perform those behaviors that will produce desired outcomes in any *particular* situation. Bandura (1986) suggested that self-efficacy can be acquired, enhanced, or decreased through one of four sources: (1) performance, or enacting a behavior; (2) vicarious experience, or seeing another person with similar skills perform a behavior; (3) verbal persuasion, or listening to the encouraging words of a trusted person; and (4) physiological arousal states such as anxiety, which ordinarily decrease feelings of self-efficacy. Bandura believes that the combination of self-efficacy and specific goals is an important predictor of behavior.

Although self-efficacy has attracted a great deal of research attention, it is but one aspect of Bandura's self-regulation theory. Bandura (1991) contended that our behavior is motivated and regulated by the continual exercise of self-influence, including (1) monitoring the determinants and the effects of our behavior, (2) judging our behavior in terms of personal standards and environmental circumstances, and (3) responding positively or negatively to our behavior depending on how it measures up to our personal standards.

Research on self-regulation and self-efficacy theories generally shows a positive relationship between levels of self-efficacy and health-seeking behaviors. For example, Winkleby, Flora, and Kraemer (1994) found that participants in the Stanford Five-City Project who had most difficulty changing behaviors related to cardiovascular disease also had low self-efficacy concerning their ability to make such changes. In another study, Borrelli and Mermelstein (1994) examined the role of self-efficacy and goal setting among participants in a smoking cessation program and found that self-efficacy, or the confidence in being able to quit smoking and maintain abstinence, accurately predicted who would reach their subgoals and who would attain abstinence.

Despite some success of self-efficacy theory to predict health-seeking behaviors, research concerning its added advantage over the theories of reasoned action and planned behavior has produced inconsistent results. For example, McCaul et al. (1993)

found the theory of planned behavior to be a better predictor of breast self-examination than a self-efficacy model. However, Tedesco, Keffer, Davis, and Christersson (1993) found that self-efficacy added significantly to the theory of reasoned action in predicting self-reports of brushing and flossing of people suffering from dental disease.

Stages of Change Theory

Another theory that attempts to explain and predict changes in health-seeking behavior is the stages of change theory developed by James Prochaska and his colleagues (Prochaska, DiClemente, & Norcross, 1992). The stages of change theory assumes that people progress through five stages in making changes in behavior: precontemplation, contemplation, preparation, action, and maintenance.

Those people in the precontemplation stage have no intention of changing their behavior and may fail to see that they have a problem. The contemplation stage involves awareness of the problem and thoughts about changing behavior within 6 months, but people in this stage have not yet made an effort to change. The preparation stage includes both thoughts and action, and people in this stage make specific plans about change. The modification of behavior comes in the action stage, when people make overt changes in their behavior. During the maintenance stage people try to sustain the changes they have made and to resist temptation to relapse. Prochaska et al. maintained that people move from one stage to another in a spiral rather than a linear fashion, with relapses that recycle people into a previous stage from which they again progress through the stages until they have completed their behavioral change. Thus, relapses are to be expected and can serve as learning experiences that help people recycle back through the stages.

Prochaska et al. suggested that people in each of these stages need different types of assistance in making changes. For example, change efforts aimed at people in the precontemplation stage will be unsuccessful because these people do not believe they have a problem. Information about their increased risks, however, may help them move from the precontemplation to the contemplation stage. On the other hand, people in the preparation stage do not need to be convinced to change their behavior; they need specific suggestions about how to change. Those in the maintenance stage need help or information oriented toward preserving their changes.

Does the stages of change theory apply equally to different problem behaviors? Prochaska and his colleagues (Prochaska, 1994; Prochaska, Velicer, et al., 1994) have looked at the theory across 12 problem behaviors, including quitting smoking, controlling weight, practicing safe sex, and utilizing mammography screening. They found clear commonalities among the 12 problem areas in that people progress from precontemplation to action in each of these areas by weighing the pros and cons of behavior change.

Research on the stages of change model has demonstrated some limited value for this approach. Glanz et al. (1994) applied the model to adopting healthy diets and found, as one would expect, that people in the precontemplation, contemplation, and preparation stages tended to eat high-fat diets whereas those in the action and maintenance stage ate less fat and more vegetables. Although the stages of change variables predicted dietary intake better than demographic variables and a measure of body mass, its ability to predict changes in eating habits was quite modest. Prochaska, Redding, Harlow, Rossi, and Velicer (1994) reviewed earlier studies on the stages of change theory applied to HIV prevention. Cross-sectional studies generally have found that the theory differentiates people who are effectively reducing their risk of HIV infection from those who are not. The authors acknowledge that longitudinal studies should be the next step in determining the value of the theory.

The Precaution Adoption Process Model

Neil Weinstein (Weinstein, 1988; Weinstein & Nicolich, 1993; Weinstein & Sandman, 1992) has formulated a precaution adoption process that serves as a model to explain why some people find difficulty in changing health-related behaviors. The precaution adoption process model assumes that when people begin new and relatively complex behaviors aimed at protecting themselves from harm, they go through as many as seven stages of belief about their personal susceptibility.

In Stage 1, people have not heard of the hazard and thus are unaware of any personal risk. In Stage 2, they are aware of the hazard and believe that others are at risk, but they hold an optimistic bias regarding their own level of risk. Stage 3 people acknowledge their personal susceptibility and accept the notion that precaution would be personally effective, but they have not yet decided to take action. In Stage 4, people decide to take action, whereas in the parallel Stage 5, people decide that action is unnecessary. In Stage 6, people have already taken the precautions aimed at reducing risks. Stage 7 involves maintaining the precaution, if needed. Maintenance would be unnecessary in the case of a lifetime vaccination, but it is essential for smoking cessation or dietary changes. Before people take action, they must first perceive that the relative benefits of the precaution outweigh its costs. The variables that influence action fluctuate, so that people who do not act at one point in time may do so at another time.

Although Weinstein's notion of optimistic bias has generated substantial research, his more global concept of the precaution adoption process model is just beginning to attract the attention of researchers. In one study, Boney McCoy et al. (1992) tested the model by investigating the relationship between smoking status and perceptions of smoking risk. These researchers looked at current smokers, former smokers, nonsmokers, and current smokers in a cessation clinic. As expected, smokers in the cessation clinic reported the highest perceived risk for smoking and the greatest perceived benefit of not smoking whereas current smokers reported the lowest risk and the least benefit of quitting. Also, current smokers were the only group to show an optimistic bias. Boney McCoy et al. asked participants to estimate their own risks and the risks of the "typical smoker" for developing coronary heart disease, emphysema, and lung cancer in two circumstances: (1) if they continued to smoke and (2) if they did not smoke. Most participants (84%) were aware of the risk of smoking for all three diseases. Consistent with the precaution adoption model, however, differences appeared among smokers in various stages of quitting. Current smokers who were not trying to quit saw that smoking was dangerous, but they retained an optimistic bias that harm would not come to them. Thus, these smokers had not advanced to Stage 3 of Weinstein's model. However, Stage 5 smokers — those in the cessation clinic — saw their risks as very high and had already made a decision to quit. Former smokers — those who had actually quit — perceived that smoking was a health hazard. This study supported Weinstein's contentions that people adopt a precaution only after they perceive personal susceptibility, see that the hazard is detrimental to them, evaluate the precaution as personally effective, and appraise the benefits of the precautions over the risk of taking them.

CRITIQUE OF HEALTH-RELATED THEORIES

In Chapter 2 we said that a useful theory should (1) generate significant research, (2) organize and explain observations, and (3) help the practitioner predict and change behaviors. How well do these health-related theories meet the three criteria? First, the older theories — namely, the health belief model, the theory of reasoned action, and self-efficacy theory — have all produced substantial amounts of research, and the newer models show promise of stimulating additional research. In addition, all these models are able to do better than chance in explaining and predicting behavior, and they generally are more accurate than demographic factors in predicting health-related behaviors.

Despite some modest success of health-related theories, a need still exists for better models that will more accurately differentiate between people who will seek medical attention and those who will not in a variety of health-related situations. Fleury (1992) reviewed studies that tested the health belief model, the theory of reasoned action, the theory of planned behavior, and self-efficacy theory as they applied to cardiovascular disease risk reduction. None of the theories received high marks. In her review, Fleury looked at 10 studies that used the health belief model and concluded that, at best, this model has yielded inconsistent results when attempting to predict or explain behavior of people diagnosed with heart disease. Fleury's review found somewhat more support for the theory of reasoned action and the theory of planned behavior, largely because both these theories include the concept of intention, which is a strong factor in predicting health-related behaviors. However, the subjective norm factor was only a weak predictor of behavior.

Fleury reviewed 14 studies on self-efficacy and concluded that efficacy expectations can be important in a person's decision to initiate health-related behaviors, but its role in maintaining change is much less clear. Also, people may feel confident that they can change a behavior, such as quitting drinking alcohol, but they may place more value on secondary benefits of drinking, such as visiting a favorite bar or drinking with friends. Self-efficacy theory does not weigh the differential values of drinking cessation and maintaining a risk-producing lifestyle.

Why are these theories somewhat less than adequate in explaining and predicting health-related behaviors? Several reasons exist. First, health-seeking behavior is determined by factors other than an individual's beliefs or perceptions. Rosenstock (1990) pointed out that interpersonal processes, institutional factors, community factors, and public policy (including law) all affect health-seeking behaviors. Rosenstock further commented that some health-related behaviors, such as cigarette smoking and dental care, can develop into habits that become so automatic that they are largely beyond the personal decision-making process. In addition, other health-producing behaviors, such as dietary changes, may be undertaken for the sake of personal appearance rather than health.

Another reason for the failure of theories to better predict health-seeking behaviors is that they must rely on consistent and accurate instruments to assess their various components, and such measures have not yet been developed. The health belief model, for example, might more accurately predict health-seeking behavior if valid measurements existed for each of its components. If a person feels susceptible to an illness, perceives his or her symptoms to be severe, believes that treatment will be effective, and sees few barriers, then, logically, that person should seek health care. But each of these four factors is difficult to assess.

Also, a model may have some value for predicting health-seeking behaviors related to one disorder but not to another. Similarly, a theory may relate to health-seeking behavior but not to prevention behavior or to adherence to medical advice. No current theory is sufficiently comprehensive to encompass all these areas. Also, the theories seldom consider that many people, such as children and some elderly persons, are often sent to health care professionals by someone else and have only limited choice in seeking care.

Finally, most of the models postulate some type of barrier or obstacle to seeking health care, and an almost unlimited number of barriers are possible. Often these barriers are beyond the life experience of researchers. For example, barriers for affluent European Americans may be quite different from those of poor Hispanic or African Americans. Cochran and Mays (1993) discussed some of the difficulties in applying the health belief model, the theory of reasoned action, and self-efficacy theory to African Americans. They pointed out that these models tend to emphasize the importance of direct and personal control of behavioral choices. Little allowance is made for such barriers as racism and poverty. These and other barriers are seldom considered, much less accurately measured by researchers testing the efficacy of health-related models.

In summary, if and how people go about seeking medical attention when they feel unwell depends on several factors, many of which are included in one or more of the theories of health-seeking behaviors. Some of these determinants are (1) the characteristics of the symptoms being experienced, (2) the cost/benefit ratio of seeking help, (3) the perceived severity of the illness, (4) a person's intention to act, and (5) multiple social and demographic factors. The balance of this chapter discusses issues involved in seeking medical attention, the problems of being in the hospital, and the preparations necessary to cope with stressful medical procedures.

SEEKING MEDICAL ATTENTION

How do people know when to seek medical attention? How do they know whether they are ill? When Jeff injured his hand, he experienced pain that persisted for hours, yet he tried several alternatives before he sought medical attention. Those alternatives included home care and consulting nonexperts about his injury. Was Jeff unusually reluctant to seek medical care or was his behavior typical? Deciding when formal medical care is necessary is a difficult problem, compounded by personal, social, and economic factors. These issues come up later, but first a consideration of health and illness is in order.

Perhaps the definition of illness should be straightforward, but such is not the case. Indeed, the definitions of both *illness* and *health* have been elusive. Is health the absence of illness, or is it the attainment of some positive state? Is disease due to pathogens that have invaded the organism, or is it due to degenerative processes? Experts in the field of health psychology (Stone, 1979) have considered the difficulties with the definitions of health and illness, yet they have produced no universally accepted definition. In the first chapter, health was defined as positive physical, mental, and social well-being, and not merely as the absence of disease or infirmity. This definition was adopted by the World Health Organization (WHO), but it provides little practical information to people trying to make decisions about their state of health or illness.

People frequently experience physical symptoms, but these symptoms may or may not indicate serious illness. Symptoms such as sniffles and sneezing would probably not prompt a person to seek medical care, but an intense and persistent stomach pain probably would. At what point should a person decide to seek health care? Errors in both directions are possible. People who decide to go to the doctor when they are not really ill feel foolish, must pay the bill for an office visit, and lose credibility with people who know about the error, including the physician. If they choose not to seek health care, they may get better, but they may remain uncomfortable from symptoms and become even more ill, thus making the illness more difficult to treat. In some cases, this behavior can seriously endanger their health or increase their risk of death. A prudent action would seem to be to chance the unnecessary visit, but research indicates that people are often reluctant to go to the doctor (Feldman, 1966).

Without a visit to a physician, one is not "officially" ill because in our culture, the physician is the gatekeeper to further health care; physicians not only *determine* illness by their diagnoses but also *sanction* it by giving a diagnosis. Hence, the person with symptoms is not the one who officially determines his or her health status. Instead, the practitioner makes the diagnosis that determines illness.

Jeff's case illustrates this process. The imaging center would not provide him with an X-ray of his hand without a physician's referral—the gate to medical care was closed without a physician's permission to receive these services.

Kasl and Cobb (1966a, 1966b) made a distinction between two stages of dealing with symptoms of poor health, which they called illness behavior and sick role behavior. **Illness behavior** consists of the activities undertaken by people who experience symptoms of illness but have not received a diagnosis. That is, illness behavior occurs *before* diagnosis. These activities are oriented toward determining one's state of health and discovering suitable remedies. **Sick role behavior,** on the other hand, is the term applied to the behavior of people after a diagnosis, either from a health care provider or a self-diagnosis. The activities of sick role behavior are oriented toward getting well. Jeff was engaging in illness behavior when he sought the opinion of his colleagues, when he went to the imaging center, and when he called his internist for a referral. All these actions took place before his diagnosis and were oriented toward receiving a diagnosis. He was exhibiting sick role behavior when he got his broken hand put in a cast, kept his appointments to have his hand checked, stopped playing basketball for 6 weeks, and took care not to reinjure his hand. All these activities occurred after diagnosis and were oriented toward getting well. Therefore, the diagnosis is the event that separates illness behavior from sick role behavior.

ILLNESS BEHAVIOR

Illness behavior takes place before one is officially diagnosed. It is directed toward determining health status in the presence of symptoms. People routinely experience symptoms that may signal illness. Symptoms are a critical element in seeking medical care, but the presence of symptoms is not sufficient to prompt a visit to the doctor (Cameron, Leventhal, & Leventhal, 1993). Some people seek help for these symptoms whereas others do not. What factors affect to the decision to determine health status or to seek professional care? Four factors may shape people's response to symptoms: (1) personal reluctance to seek care, (2) certain social and demo-graphic factors, (3) the characteristics of the symptoms, and (4) one's personal view of illness.

Personal Reluctance

A discrepancy exists between what people recommend to others and what they report that they themselves would do about seeking health care. A national survey found that most people were willing to advise other people to see a doctor, but, with the same symptoms, they were less likely to go to the doctor themselves (Feldman, 1966). Indeed, many people said they would take care of even serious health problems without professional aid. This attitude is consistent with a general reluctance among many people to seek professional health care and a tendency to interpret any symptoms in a way that indicates the lowest level of threat.

Personal reluctance to seek health care may not be consistent for all disorders and for all people. Klonoff and Landrine (1993) investigated the possibility that people think of different body parts in terms that affect their willingness to seek help when these body parts develop problems. They asked college students to rate different body parts along several dimensions, and they analyzed the responses to determine the effects on willingness to seek care. They found that people viewed some body parts, such as the anus, as stigmatized and other body parts, such as the genitalia, as private. People were more reluctant to seek medical care for such body parts than those lower in stigma and privacy. In addition, people were more likely to seek help for body parts perceived as important and vulnerable, such as the heart and blood.

This reluctance may be especially strong for screening procedures, which are often oriented toward disease detection. Some evidence exists that thinking about disease detection may be more distressing than considering the adoption of health-promoting behaviors (Millar & Millar, 1995). Such distress can contribute to personal reluctance and can provide a barrier for health screening for a variety of conditions.

Screening procedures include mammograms for the detection of breast cancer, Pap smear tests for the detection of cervical cancer, blood sugar tests for the detection of diabetes, and blood pressure measurements for the detection of hypertension. Although breast cancer screening programs that include mammography can reduce breast cancer deaths, women are reluctant to get these tests. Lerman and her colleagues (1991) studied the emotional impact of having a mammogram and found that receiving the news of an abnormal mammogram, even for the women whose subsequent testing ruled out cancer, produced emotional problems and continued cancer anxiety. For many people, avoiding screening tests prevents the anxiety. This type of personal reluctance puts people at risk for the diseases that these screening procedures can identify.

Social and Demographic Factors

Aside from a general personal reluctance to go to the doctor, the tendency to seek professional care differs with several social and demographic variables. One is gender. Although women are more likely to use health care than men, the reasons for this difference are somewhat complex. Pennebaker (1982) found that women report more symptoms than men. He hypothesized that women are more sensitive to their internal body signals than men, and this condition is responsible for their greater number of symptom reports. This gender-related difference does not indicate that women are sicker than men, only that they are more sensitive to the symptoms they experience.

Verbrugge (1989) stated that the reported differences between frequency of health care for men and women are due almost exclusively to social factors. Whereas men are more likely to need health care because of such risks as alcohol consumption and job hazards, women are at greater risk through physical inactivity, nonemployment, and stress. Also, men feel more mastery of their lives and have a more fixed weekly routine than women. On the other hand, women are more likely to have a regular physician but less likely to have health insurance. Verbrugge claimed that when all risk factors are controlled, the illness gap between men and women is quite narrow. In fact, she said, men have worse general and chronic health than women. Similarly, the female gender role allows women to seek many sorts of assistance whereas the male gender role teaches men to act strong and to deny pain and discomfort. In addition, men's social role permits them to take more risks (Waldron, 1988), and failure to seek health care is among these risks.

In addition to gender differences, socioeconomic factors relate to people's frequency of seeking medical care. People in higher socioeconomic groups experience fewer symptoms and report a higher level of health than do people at lower socioeconomic levels (Pennebaker, 1982). Yet when higher income people are sick, they are more likely to seek health care. Nevertheless, poor people are overrepresented among the hospitalized, an indication that they are much more likely than middle- and upper-class people to become seriously ill. In addition, people in lower socioeconomic groups tend to wait longer before seeking health care, thus making treatment more difficult and hospitalization more likely. The poor also have less access to medical care, have to travel longer to reach health care facilities, and must wait longer once they arrive at those facilities.

Cultural and social factors also affect how people respond to symptoms. In some cultures, people are socialized not to react with strong emotion to illness whereas in other cultures, a strong reaction is expected. David Mechanic (1978) reviewed several studies that reported varying attitudes toward illness in different ethnic groups. Jewish Americans, for example, were more likely to seek professional help, accept the sick role, and engage in preventive medical behavior; Mexican Americans tended to ignore some symptoms that physicians felt were serious and to inflate others that doctors regarded as minor; Irish Americans tended to deny pain stoically. These differences demonstrate the powerful effects of socialization on illness and sick role behavior.

Age is yet another factor that influences people's willingness to seek medical care, with young and middle-aged adults showing the greatest reluctance. Garland and Zigler (1994) studied children and adolescents and found that children were more willing to seek help than adolescents, especially male adolescents. As people age, they must make distinctions between symptoms of aging and illness, discriminating between what is normal and symptoms that signal problems. This distinction is not always easy, but people tend to interpret problems with a gradual onset and mild symptoms as resulting from age compared to those with sudden onset and severe symptoms (Leventhal & Diefenbach, 1991).

People who are able to attribute their symptoms to age tend to delay in seeking medical care, but older adults are not as strongly influenced by this tendency as the middle-aged (Leventhal & Diefenbach, 1991). Although older and middle-aged people did not differ in type of complaint or ease of access to health care, older people were quicker to seek medical care for symptoms that they could not identify. Leventhal and Diefenbach interpreted this difference as a lack of tolerance for uncertainty in older adults and a desire to deny or minimize the severity of illness in the middle-aged adults the authors studied.

The amount of stress in people's lives is also a factor in their readiness to seek care. People who experience a great deal of stress are more likely to seek health care than those under less stress, even when the symptoms are equal. Research by Cameron, Leventhal, and Leventhal (1995) examined people's readiness to seek health care in response to the appearance of symptoms. Those who experienced concurrent and prolonged stress were more likely to seek care when the symptoms were ambiguous. When symptoms were clearly health threats, stress was not a factor. Many symptoms are unclear, presenting the possibility that stress sensitizes people to their symptoms and makes them more likely to seek health care.

Ironically, people under stress are less credible when they claim that they are ill. Skelton (1991) found that patients who report physical and psychological distress compromise their credibility. When people complain to their friends and family about stress and pain, they are less likely to be judged to have a "real" illness than when their complaints center around physical symptoms. In addition, this lowered credibility extends to health care professionals, with nurses and physicians tending to discount the distress of patients who have many complaints. Skelton explained these tendencies to discount symptom reports for people under stress as the distinction between the physical and the psychological, with physical complaints having an organic basis and stress-related problems being psychological and thus not "real." The more psychological complaints people report, the less "real" physicians consider patients' reports of physiological symptoms.

In summary, the demographic factors of gender, socioeconomic level, and age influence the seeking of professional health care in the United States. In addition, cultural factors play a role in the experience of illness and also in the likelihood and timing of seeking health care. People whose cultural backgrounds teach the value of promptly seeking professional health care tend go to the doctor sooner than do people from cultures that do not hold this value. Life stress is also a factor in seeking help, with stress increasing the likelihood of seeking health care but decreasing the credibility of illness reports.

Symptom Characteristics

In addition to personal and demographic factors, several symptom characteristics influence when and how people look for help. Symptoms themselves do not inevitably lead people to seek care, but certain characteristics are important in their response to symptoms. Mechanic (1978) listed four characteristics of the symptoms that determine one's response to illness.

First is the *visibility of the symptom* — that is, how readily apparent the symptom is to the person and to others. Klohn and Rogers (1991) presented information on intentions to adopt osteoporosis prevention that confirmed the importance of the visibility of symptoms. Young women who received messages about osteoporosis as a disfiguring condition were significantly more likely to say that they intended to adopt precautions against osteoporosis than young women who were not alerted to the disfiguring aspects of osteoporosis.

Mechanic's second symptom characteristic was *perceived severity of the symptom*. He contended that symptoms seen as severe would be more likely to prompt action than less severe symptoms. Mechanic acknowledged the importance of personal perception and recognized that a difference exists between the perceived severity of a symptom and the judgment of severity by medical authorities. Mechanic cited a study by Suchman (1965) on symptom severity and the likelihood of reporting to a physician. Suchman found that symptoms perceived as more serious brought greater concern and were also more likely to be interpreted as indicating illness. Cameron et al. (1993) confirmed that perceived severity of symptoms rather than the presence of symptoms was critical in the decision to seek care.

The third symptom characteristic mentioned by Mechanic was the *extent to which the symptom interferes with a person's life*. Again, Suchman's (1965) research found that the degree of incapacitation affected the person's action. That is, the more incapacitated the person is, the more likely he or she is to seek medical care.

Suchman also provided support for Mechanic's fourth hypothesized determinant of illness behavior; the *frequency and persistence of the symptoms*. Conditions that people view as requiring care tend to be those that are both severe and continuous. Intermittent symptoms are less likely than persistent ones to generate illness behavior. Prohaska, Keller, Leventhal, and Leventhal (1987) provided support for the idea that the persistence and severity of symptoms are factors in seeking health care. They found that severe symptoms prompted people to seek health care from friends and family as well as from a physician. Even mild symptoms prompted people to seek help if those symptoms persisted.

In Mechanic's description, symptom characteristics alone are not sufficient to prompt illness behavior. Research by Cameron et al. (1993) confirmed Mechanic's view that symptoms are not sufficient to prompt people to seek formal medical care. However, if symptoms persist or are perceived as severe, people are more likely to evaluate them as indicating a need for care. Thus, people are prompted to seek care when they interpret their symptoms as indicative of a serious problem. This interpretation relates to each person's view of illness.

Personal View of Illness

Despite a vast amount of knowledge in the fields of physiology and medicine, most people are largely ignorant of how their bodies work and how they become ill. Even well-educated people and those who have had their illness fully explained to them tend to conceptualize their illness inaccurately and incompletely, partly because when people gain information, they integrate it into their existing knowledge structure. If the new information seems incompatible with what they already "know," they may modify this new information to make it fit their preexisting knowledge rather than changing their knowledge to conform to the new information. This process may, of course, lead to substantial distortions.

One's personal view of illness depends on both knowledge of the illness and the structure of one's cognitions. An interest in how these cognitions develop has prompted a number of studies on how people conceptualize illness. For example, Burbach and Peterson (1986) summarized findings from studies indicating that children often have unrealistic beliefs about why people get sick and how they get well. One study by Bibace and Walsh (1979) organized children's early concepts of disease by developmental stage. These researchers found that childhood concepts of illness include a magical possibility of getting sick for no discernible reason. Later, children develop the concept of contagion, and even later they come to understand the mechanisms of how infectious diseases spread. With additional cognitive development, children begin to comprehend that they can do things to control their health. Finally, they form the idea that both psychological and physiological factors can influence health. Burbach and Peterson concluded that a person probably needs a high level of cognitive development to integrate psychological and physiological factors into his or her concepts of illness.

Surprisingly, Bibace and Walsh (1979) also found that a group of college biology majors gave the same sort of explanations of illness as another group of college students who had taken no biology courses. Indeed, both groups gave explanations for catching a cold that were quite similar to those given by 7-year-old children. All three groups attributed their colds to such factors as cold weather, insufficient sleep, or not dressing warmly, even though the biology students knew that viruses cause colds. Although biology majors have been exposed to more accurate information about disease than most people, their inclusion of environmental and personal factors in the list of things that cause colds seems to reflect acceptance of the idea that illness has several causes—a personal version of the biopsychosocial model of health and illness.

Landrine and Klonoff (1994) found that many people hold beliefs in supernatural causes for illness, such as punishment from God, sinful thoughts, bad blood, and the evil eye. Landrine and Klonoff's focus was cultural and ethnic differences, and they found that people from ethnic minorities were more likely than Whites to hold beliefs in the supernatural as a cause for illness. However, Whites too held beliefs in supernatural causes of illness. For example, 30% of the White college students in this study reported that a lack of faith was at least somewhat important in getting sick. The overall belief in supernatural causes of illness was low for all ethnic groups, but this study demonstrated the discrepancy between knowledge and beliefs.

Nemeroff (1995), too, pointed out that although anthropologists have identified magical thinking in many traditional societies, people in contemporary U.S. society also tend to hold some magical beliefs about infectious illness. For example, she found that college students rated their lover's "germs" as less infectious than a disliked peer's "germs."

Even disorders that are well understood medically may not be well understood by patients. Several studies by psychologist Howard Leventhal and his colleagues (Leventhal & Diefenbach, 1991; Leventhal, Meyer, & Nerenz, 1980; Leventhal, Nerenz, & Steele, 1984; Meyer, Leventhal, & Gutman, 1985) have explored how people conceptualize various illnesses. They have studied four components in the conceptualization of illness: (1) identity of the disease, (2) time line (the time course of both disease and treatment), (3) consequences of the disease, and (4) cause of the disease. Studies by Lau and Hartman (1983) and Lau, Bernard, and Hartman (1989) have confirmed the factors identified by Leventhal and his colleagues. These results indicate that people construct their concepts of illness around personally relevant factors rather than medically important factors.

The *identity of the disease,* the first component identified by Leventhal and his associates, is very important to illness behavior. A man who has identified his symptoms as a "heart attack" should react quite differently from one who labels the same symptoms as "heartburn." The presence of symptoms is not sufficient to initiate help seeking, but the labeling that occurs in conjunction with symptoms may be critical in a person's either seeking help or ignoring symptoms.

Baumann, Cameron, Zimmerman, and Leventhal (1989) demonstrated how important labeling can be in the interpretation of symptoms. To determine how information about high blood pressure would affect the cognitive process, they provided partici-

pants in their study with either false information that indicated high blood pressure readings or correct information that indicated normal blood pressure. Participants who were told that their blood pressure was high then reported symptoms commonly associated with high blood pressure. This study demonstrated that people actively try to construct a representation of their symptoms and that they follow the symmetry rule (Leventhal & Diefenbach, 1991), trying not only to find a label consistent with their symptoms but also to make their symptoms consistent with the label they have found.

Labels provide a framework within which symptoms can be interpreted. People experience less emotional arousal when they find a label that indicates a minor problem (heartburn rather than heart attack). Initially, they will probably adopt the least serious label that fits their symptoms. For example, Jeff initially interpreted his broken hand as a bruise. To a large extent, a label carries with it some prediction about the time course of the illness, so if the time course does not correspond to the expectation implicit in the label, the person has to relabel the symptoms. When Jeff's hand failed to respond to the ice packs and the pain continued, he began to doubt the label he had applied. His friends told him he was foolish to ignore the swelling and pain, believing that these symptoms would disappear. However, the tendency to interpret symptoms as indicating minor rather than major problems is the source of many optimistic self-diagnoses, and Jeff was no exception.

The second component in conceptualizing an illness is the *time line.* Even though the time course of an illness is usually implicit within the diagnosis, people's understanding of the time involved is not necessarily accurate. Meyer et al. (1985) presented evidence that people with hypertension, a chronic disease, tend to conceptualize their illness as acute. That is, these patients saw their disease as corresponding to the pattern of most temporary illnesses, with the onset of symptoms followed by treatment, a remission of symptoms, and then a cure. This belief was frequent among patients who had been recently diagnosed as hypertensive, with 40% expressing a belief that they would be cured. It was much less common among those who had stayed in treatment for at least 3 months, with only 12% of these patients holding an acute concept of their illness.

The *consequences of a disease* are the third component in Leventhal's description of illness conceptualizations. Again, the consequences of a disease are implied by the diagnosis. However, an incorrect understanding of the consequences can have a profound effect on illness behavior. Many people view a diagnosis of cancer as a death sentence. Some neglect health care because they believe themselves to be in a hopeless situation. Women who find a lump in their breast sometimes delay in making an appointment with a doctor (Stillman, 1977), not because they fail to recognize this symptom of cancer but because they fear the possible consequences—surgery and the loss of a breast.

The last component of the personal view of illness is the *determination of cause*. For the most part, determining causality is more a facet of the sick role than of illness behavior because it usually occurs after a diagnosis has been made. But the attribution of causality for symptoms is an important factor in illness behavior. For example, if a person can attribute the pain in his hand to a blow received on the day before, he will not have to consider the possibility of bone cancer as the cause of the pain.

Attribution of causality, however, is often faulty. People may attribute a cold to "germs" or to the weather, and they may see cancer as caused by microwave ovens or by the will of God. Klonoff and Landrine (1994) found that some college students believe God's will and sin play a role in the development of some illnesses, such as AIDS. These students expressed the belief that other illnesses, such as headaches and hypertension, have an emotional cause, and yet others, such as colds, are the results of natural causes.

Klonoff and Landrine speculated that if such beliefs are common among well-educated college students, the general population may endorse supernatural causes for illness even more strongly. Furthermore, these beliefs have important implications. People are less likely to seek professional treatment for conditions they consider as having emotional and natural causes. A study by Swartzman and McDermid (1993) also confirmed the contribution of emotional factors to people's reluctance to accept physical symptoms as indicative of illness. Thus, even specific physical symptoms may not lead to the interpretation of a physical illness, and people are likely to ignore or use self-treatments for problems they do not consider physical.

Being able to attribute illness to a cause is apparently very important. Although medical research has found no one cause of cancer, cancer patients try very hard to arrive at a causal explanation. The result, as Taylor (1983) found, is that many cancer patients accept explanations of their illness that do not agree with medical science. Patients who encounter disconfirming evidence reject their explanation and find another, which too may be medically unsound. Indeed, Taylor found that the motivation to find the cause is strong enough to persist despite the irrationality of the search for a single cause.

Summary of Illness Behavior

We have seen that people's concepts of illness have a substantial effect on their likelihood of seeking medical care. Of the four components of illness that Leventhal proposed, the assignment of a label is probably the most important because a label carries with it two of the other three components. If an illness has been officially labeled or diagnosed, then its time course and its consequences are implicit. However, research indicates that people who know the name of their illness do not always have an accurate concept of its time course and consequences. Instead, many people see chronic illnesses as having a short time course, even for a disease such as hypertension. Finally, the factor of causality bears more on sick role behavior (postdiagnosis) than on illness behavior (prediagnosis), but the attribution of causes for symptoms may be a significant force in a person's seeking medical care.

THE SICK ROLE

Kasl and Cobb (1966b) defined sick role behavior as the activities engaged in by those who believe themselves ill for the purpose of getting well. In other words, sick role behavior occurs after a person has been diagnosed. The concept of the sick role is not original to Kasl and Cobb but can be traced back to sociologist Talcott Parsons (1951, 1978). In Parsons's view, the sick role is based on three assumptions: (1) being sick is not the sick person's fault, (2) being sick relieves the sick person of normal responsibilities, and (3) a sick person will take steps to get

WOULD YOU BELIEVE . . . ?

Learning to Be Sick

Would you believe that people learn how to be sick? Most people imagine that because illness is due to biological factors, being sick is a physical response to these biological factors. However, research by William Whitehead and his colleagues (1994) demonstrated that being sick is influenced by reinforcement and modeling of the sick role during childhood.

Whitehead et al. asked women between the ages of 20 and 40 how their parents responded to their childhood health complaints and also how their parents dealt with their own illnesses. These researchers reasoned that the measurement of parental responses to their children's illness would reflect reinforcement and that the parents' own behavior when they were sick would reflect modeling. They measured the women's frequency of symptoms, disability days, and number of health care visits over a 12-month period.

Whitehead et al. hypothesized that both reinforcement and modeling would influence adult sick role behavior, and their results confirmed these predictions. Furthermore, they found that illness behavior was disease-specific. That is, the reinforcement that participants received and the modeling they saw as children predicted the types of disorders they experienced as adults. In addition, the predictive power of these childhood experiences was independent of adulthood stress or neuroticism, both of which could have influenced the tendency to report symptoms and seek health care. Therefore, it seems that learning during childhood is an important factor in how we deal with sickness as adults.

well. As Arluke (1988) pointed out, this conception includes both rights and privileges. The lack of blame and relief from responsibilities are privileges that the sick person maintains as long as he or she also makes the best possible effort to get well.

Lack of Blame

The first of Parsons's assumptions is that being sick is not the sick person's fault, but research has revealed that people tend to blame the victim for his or her misfortune (Lerner & Simmons, 1966; Ryan, 1971). In the case of chronic illness such as heart disease and some cancers, this tendency may be somewhat justified; these diseases have strong behavioral components.

Although personal behavior may contribute to the development of such chronic illnesses as cardiovascular disease and cancer, it is seldom totally responsible. In other words, a person with heart disease or cancer is usually not completely to blame for that illness. Nevertheless, Lau and Hartman (1983) found a tendency for people to blame *themselves* for many common illnesses. For example, about 20% of the reasons that college students gave for their last illness involved personal behavior. Many reported that they got a cold because they did not take care of themselves or did not dress properly. Attributing illness to behavior may be one way for people to feel that they have some control over illness. As Lau (1988) pointed out, this feeling may be comforting for several reasons. Control guarantees predictability, and predictability allows people to cope better with illness. Also, control reduces stress and alleviates feelings that one's illness will become too terrible to endure.

This tendency toward self-blame also applies to those who have been involved in life-threatening events such as accidents. Bulman and Wortman (1977) found that over half the accident victims they studied held themselves responsible for their injuries. Whether their personal behavior had really contributed to the accident had no relationship to self-blame. Patients who blamed themselves adjusted better to their injuries than those who blamed others. Again, by taking responsibility for their accident, these patients also assumed personal control over the situation. Both responsibility and feelings of control have profound implications for the feelings that sick people experience in our society.

Parsons's main point was that society relieves sick people from responsibility for their illness, a situation that helps people assume sick role behaviors. This hypothesis may be true, but the assumption that people attribute disease to forces beyond their control is not well grounded. Research has indicated that people tend to blame sick people and they tend to blame themselves for their illness, whether they were responsible or not. Other research (Janis & Rodin, 1979) indicated that health care workers shared this tendency to blame sick people for being sick. This finding demonstrates that health care workers are susceptible to the same erroneous health beliefs as other people.

Relief from Normal Responsibilities

The second feature of the sick role in our society, according to Parsons, is the exemption of the sick person from normal social, occupational, and family duties. Sick people are usually not expected to go to work, school, or meetings; to cook, clean house, or care for children; to do homework or mow the lawn. Sick people are frequently allowed, and often expected, to stay home and act sick.

Some sick people, however, have trouble acting sick, even when they are. This reluctance may be situational, as when someone has recently started a new job and is therefore reluctant to be absent even for justified reasons. The reluctance to assume the sick role may also arise from a personal disinclination to become passive and cared for. Parsons (1978) jokingly referred to those who are unwilling to assume the sick role as "*hyper*chondriacs" but contended that such people are rare.

Richard Lazarus (1984b) agreed that the sick role allows for relief from certain responsibilities, but he pointed out that other obligations are incurred by sick people. For example, they are expected to be optimistic and cheerful and are not allowed to appear miserable or depressed. Although most people are distressed by illness, Lazarus emphasized that sick people are frequently discouraged from displaying distress. Instead, they are encouraged to be brave and cheerful, even when they do not feel like it. Lazarus maintained that our society trivializes distress. Healthy people encourage sick people to be optimistic, even when they know there is little basis for optimism. We admire stories about those who face catastrophic illness bravely, and such admiration conveys the expectation that courage is a requirement in the face of adversity. Lazarus contended that this attitude is unfair to sick people, adding stress to their already stressful state of illness. Although Lazarus's hypothesis concerning optimism and cheerfulness may be valid, and sick people are burdened with alternative expectations, they are generally exempt from normal responsibilities. This exemption supports Parsons's second assumption.

Desire to Get Well

Parsons's third component of the sick role concerns the sick person's desire to get well. Our society tends to assume that sickness is a temporary state and that sick people should be actively involved in getting better. Research has confirmed the notion that most people believe illness is a temporary state (Lau & Hartman, 1983; Leventhal et al., 1984). For many diseases, this belief is true. But for chronic diseases like hypertension, cancer, and diabetes, this view is not only invalid but can also have harmful implications for treatment. When people with hypertension believe they can discontinue treatment because they feel better, these beliefs threaten the treatment outcome.

Arluke (1988) criticized aspects of Parsons's sick role concept, pointing out that the concept of the sick role applies to acute illnesses but not to chronic diseases. People with chronic illnesses like hypertension and asthma are not exempt from normal responsibilities and must carry out their daily activities with little realistic hope of full recovery. Arluke also pointed out that the sick role concept is based on a middle-class view of illness and that other social groups have different conceptualizations of how sick people should behave.

CHOOSING A PRACTITIONER

As part of their attempts to get well, sick people usually consult a health care practitioner. For most middle-class people in industrialized nations, the health care practitioner is a physician, but other types of health care practitioners exist. For example, midwives, nurses, physical therapists, psychologists, osteopaths, chiropractors, dentists, nutritionists, and herbal healers all provide various types of health care. Some of these sources of health care are considered "alternative" because they provide alternatives to traditional medicine. Almost a third of U.S. residents seek some form of alternative health care (Cowley, King, Hager, & Rosenberg, 1995). These alternative forms of health care are growing in acceptability to the point that insurance companies cover some of the expenses for these treatments, which can be less expensive than traditional medical care.

The growing acceptability of alternative health care is but one of the changes taking place in the provision of health care. The traditional setting for health care has been the physician's private office, and the patient has paid the practitioner directly for services received. Greenley and Davidson (1988) discussed changes that are occurring in this system, suggesting that the era of the solo practitioner is coming to an end and the transition to corporate medicine will force changes in choice of health care providers. Changes are also taking place in the traditional authoritarian role of various health care providers and in the types of providers patients want. Haug (1988) reported that the authority and power of physicians has diminished in recent years and that over half the public now doubts that physicians are sufficiently competent and concerned to provide the type of health care patients want. Haug indicated that people under age 35 were more likely than those over 65 to challenge the authority of physicians. Younger people are also more likely to view patients as consumers of health care who, like any consumers, have choices in their selection of services and service providers.

Adolescents' fear of HIV infection may play a crucial role in their selection of a health care provider. Ginsburg et al. (1995) surveyed ninth graders in Philadelphia public schools and found that most of these adolescents' decisions to seek health care related to cleanliness and control of infection. Their top two considerations were that health care providers wash their hands and use clean instruments. Further, they wanted to *see* the providers wash their hands or use gloves or both. Interestingly, gender, ethnicity, and socioeconomic status made little difference in the list of characteristics that most concerned the adolescents. Their concentration on the issue of cleanliness might be specific to young adolescents, but younger people are becoming more demanding in what they want from health care providers.

Satisfaction with medical encounters is most strongly related to the amount of information provided by the physician, and patients are most satisfied with physicians who are willing to interact with them regarding their health problems; talk about nonmedical topics; and display immediate, positive nonverbal behavior. In contrast, patients are most displeased with physicians who seem uninterested, who use an angry tone of voice, who act through power and authority, or who display anger in any way (Roter, 1988).

After questioning patients about their views of the ideal physician, Feletti, Firman, and Sanson-Fisher (1986) compared these expectations to patients' impressions after their initial appointment. Patients had high expectations before consultation, and they were generally satisfied after seeing the physician. The biggest factor in patient satisfaction was the care, communication, and reassurance that the physician provided. Other important factors were patient perception of the physician's professional conduct, respect for patients, and technical competence.

To sum up, many patients have begun to treat medical care as another type of service and have started to challenge the traditional authority of physicians. One aspect of this challenge has been the growth of alternate types of health care practitioners, and another has been a different attitude about physicians and their interactions with their patients. Patients have high expectations of their health care providers and want them to be caring and reassuring as well as very communicative. Patients expect professional behavior and competence, and they want physicians to treat them with respect and to refrain from expressing anger in their questions or responses.

BEING IN THE HOSPITAL

Although the majority of health care takes place on an outpatient basis, sometimes a person requires hospitalization. The decision to be hospitalized is almost never a patient's decision. Greenley and Davidson (1988) reported that patients initiate only 2% of hospitalizations; physicians initiate the other 98%. Because few people want to be hospitalized, the physician frequently must make this decision from a position of authority rather than one of cooperation.

Even if the decision is made jointly, the patient may have little voice in the hospital's procedure.

Chapter 4 discussed how stress may act to produce illness, but being ill can also cause stress, and being hospitalized is frequently an acutely distressing experience. Hospitalization can be an irritating experience for a number of reasons. First, the conditions that require hospitalization are usually quite serious. Also, simply being in the hospital and facing various medical procedures can be distressing. This section examines the latter group of factors.

THE HOSPITAL PATIENT ROLE

The role of hospital patient is not the same as the sick role because the health care organization that cares for the patient defines the hospital patient role. The sick role consists of those behaviors oriented toward getting well. Part of the sick role is to be a patient, and being a patient means conforming to the rules of the health care institution and complying with medical advice. But an outpatient has a significantly different role from that of the person treated in a hospital, whose role may involve being a "nonperson."

Nonperson Treatment

When a person is hospitalized, all but his or her illness becomes invisible; frequently the person loses the status of being human. Goffman (1961) described this "nonperson" treatment as a process "whereby the patient is greeted with what passes as civility and said farewell to in the same fashion with everything in between going on as if the patient weren't there as a social person at all but only as some possession someone has left behind" (pp. 341–342). Although this statement is more than 30 years old, it still applies in many hospitals.

Being referred to as "the multiple fracture in Room 458" may be both startling and annoying, but impersonal reference is not the extent of nonperson treatment. Not only are patients' identities ignored but their comments and questions may also be overlooked. During examinations or treatment, the depersonalization of patients is so blatant that they often are not spoken to directly (Zimbardo, 1969), and their comments may be totally ignored (Tay-

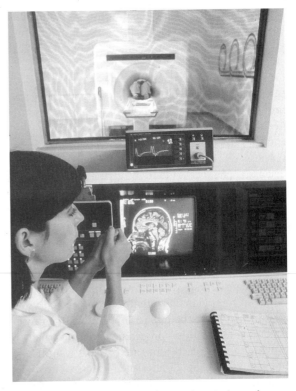

The increasing level of technology in hospitals can be a factor in "nonperson" treatment.

lor, 1982). Practitioners frequently converse among themselves in the patient's presence, using technical jargon that the patient is unable to comprehend. As Bennett and Disbrow (1993) pointed out, this manner of conversing allows practitioners to convey a great deal of information to each other but leaves patients feeling anxious and helpless. The hospital procedure focuses on the technical aspects of medical procedures but usually ignores patients' emotional needs. Indeed, patients' comments are usually neither solicited nor welcomed. Patients are expected to respond if questioned and to follow directions but otherwise to be verbally and physically passive.

The extent to which the hospital staff ignores the person extends to the experience of pain: Nurses and physicians seem to perceive the pain of patients quite differently from the way patients view their own pain. In a study with hospitalized patients, Krokosky and Reardon (1989) found that patients' ratings of their pain were not significantly correlated with nurses' ratings of the patients' pain. The correlations between the pain ratings of physicians and patients were even lower. The patients' ratings revealed more severe pain than did the ratings of nurses and doctors. Perhaps this depreciation of patients' pain is part of their depersonalized treatment: Nonpersons should not feel much pain.

Lack of Information

Being in the hospital should include an open exchange of information between patient and practitioner. Ideally, the practitioner should listen to the patient, ask questions, and inform the patient about diagnoses and instructions for treatment. Although it is somewhat more likely to occur in a practitioner's private office, this ideal communication is not always typical in hospitals.

Patients may lack information because health providers lack knowledge about patients' condition — that is, people may be admitted to the hospital for elaborate testing in order to receive a diagnosis. Patients in this situation have usually experienced distressing symptoms, and their health care providers have been unable to make a diagnosis. If no cause for the symptoms is found despite extensive and sometimes painful diagnostic testing, these patients are likely to suffer anxiety, uncertainty, and fear because of a lack of information about their condition. On the other hand, receiving a diagnosis may produce even more anxiety. Also, diagnosed patients are not exempt from undergoing additional tests, the purpose of which they may not understand. Therefore, lack of information and the accompanying fear and anxiety frequently characterize both patients who have been diagnosed and those who have not.

Recently, however, hospital patients have been receiving more complete information about their diagnosis and prognosis. Many physicians now adhere to the philosophy that patients should be fully and honestly informed about the nature of their illness. However, the hospital staff may fail to inform patients of their condition because they believe (or hospital policy dictates) that physicians have that responsibility. Thus, patients may still lack information, but their plight is not likely to be the result of the outdated philosophy that patients have neither a need for nor a right to complete and accurate information about their illness.

Loss of Control

Hospitalized patients are expected to conform submissively to the rules of the hospital and the orders of their doctor, thus relinquishing much control over their lives. In her account of the impact of health organizations, Taylor (1979) argued that loss of control is patients' major complaint, and it can apply to three aspects of illness and hospitalization: (1) loss of normal control of one's body, (2) loss of typical activities such as work and leisure activities, and (3) loss of ability to predict what will happen.

First, illness and hospitalization can upset the control over one's body functions that people ordinarily perform with little conscious effort. Second, the loss of control also extends to normal, everyday activities, such as working, being with one's family, or enjoying leisure pursuits. Being in the hospital may mean that people lose control over decisions about what to wear, what and when to eat, when to sleep, who may touch (and even hurt) them, and when they can see their family and friends. Third, not being allowed to make decisions about even the simplest aspects of their lives is a psychological loss of control that reduces people's ability to take effective action concerning their health. This loss of control reduces people's ability to forecast the course of their illness or to predict what will happen to them. Once admitted to the hospital, patients relinquish much personal control and can do very little to restore it. Even leaving the hospital without another's consent is difficult.

The loss of control over those aspects of life that are usually under one's control can be very stressful. Several experts (Bennett & Disbrow, 1993; Taylor, 1982) have proposed that research findings concerning loss of control can readily be applied to patients in hospital settings, including the finding (Glass & Singer, 1972) that when exposed to uncontrollable, unpleasant stimulation, people experience more discomfort than they do when the situation is equally unpleasant but under their control. In addition, people in uncontrollable situations tend to manifest heightened physiological responses. They

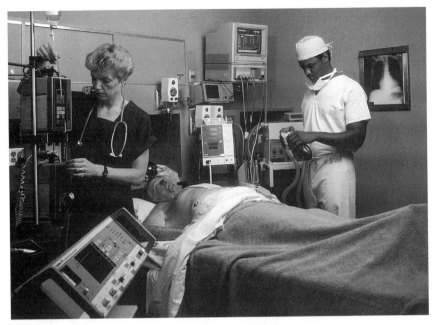

Hospitalized patients lack control of their lives and information about their condition, resulting in increased distress.

react on a physical level to uncontrollable stimulation more strongly than they do when they can exert some control over the condition. Lack of control can decrease people's capacity to concentrate and can increase their tendency to report physical symptoms. These findings suggest that hospitalization can be a negative experience for both the staff and the patients.

"GOOD" PATIENTS VERSUS "BAD" PATIENTS

To be a "good" patient from the viewpoint of hospital personnel, one must conform to a "nonperson" role. Good patients do not ask questions; they do as instructed and cooperate with requests. Above all, being a good patient means not making trouble for the staff. Conversely, "bad" patients make trouble; they ask questions and demand answers. They behave like consumers who have rights. Bad patients demand attention, and they complain.

In 1975, Lorber described these two patient roles and concluded that about 25% of patients exhibit "problem patient" behavior and about 75% conform to the "good patient" role. What are the consequences of each type of role? Which type of behavior is more conducive to a patient's recovery?

Consequences of Being a "Bad" Patient

Taylor (1979) explained the behavior of "bad" patients as an attempt to restore control. She analyzed patients' problem behavior as an angry reaction to nonperson treatment and the loss of freedom associated with hospitalization. To assert control, patients may exhibit petty violations of hospital procedures, such as smoking, drinking, or flirting with the nurses, or they may fail to comply in more major ways that could endanger their health, such as failing to take medication or prematurely leaving the hospital. Taylor termed these angry behaviors **reactance**, borrowing the term from Brehm's (1966) theory of psychological reactance. According to Brehm, people who are deprived of personal freedom or threatened with loss of freedom react angrily and try to restore their control.

Physiologically, the anger and frustration experienced by the reactant patient stimulate the same physiological responses that other stressors do. Abundant anger may therefore have negative effects on the patient's health, but is it always bad for the patient?

Some possibility exists that being a bad patient may be healthier than being a good one, at least when being bad includes a questioning of medical care and developing an understanding of the treatment regimen.

Consequences of Being a "Good" Patient

Will a sick person benefit by being a good, compliant patient? Good patients receive more attention from the hospital staff, but Taylor (1979) argued that good patient behavior may not reflect a peaceful acceptance of the situation. Although good patients by definition are compliant and noncomplaining, they too may experience turmoil about their situation. What passes for acceptance of the patient role may actually be an expression of feelings of helplessness. These feelings are quite different from the anger experienced by the reactant patient, but both may result from extreme frustration over the patient role.

Seligman (1975) investigated the notion that extreme frustration can produce **learned helplessness**. He reported on studies demonstrating that some animal species learn to do nothing when put into stressful situations in which no control is possible. Because these animals have learned that nothing they did worked, they did nothing. They also failed to make appropriate responses when put into similar situations; that is, they generalized their learned helplessness. Seligman and his colleagues (Abramson, Garber, & Seligman, 1980) reviewed the research on learned helplessness as it applies to humans and found that the same sort of behavior observed in laboratory animals also occurs in humans in a variety of situations in which they experience (or perceive) loss of control.

Taylor (1979) used the learned helplessness model to explain the cognitive and emotional process of some "good" patients: They express helplessness as passivity, which is consistent with the good patient role. Taylor argued that this passivity extends beyond the lack of response expected by the hospital staff and includes the withholding of information that may be important to treatment. This passivity is actually another form of "getting even" with the staff but may be indistinguishable from ideal patient behavior.

Abramson et al. (1980) and Alloy and Abramson (1980) hypothesized that depression is a result of learned helplessness. This analysis is also relevant to the evidence about hospitalization. Depressed people are passive and uncommunicative. However, depression can lead to a depletion of norepinephrine and a suppressed immune system, reactions that make recovery more difficult.

Implications

Loss of control, lack of information, and nonperson treatment may cause reactance or helplessness in hospitalized patients. Both these response patterns may be troublesome to the hospital staff, but both are patients' ways of coping with the stresses of hospitalization. Patients can react to stress in more constructive ways, but most people have no specific training or assistance in constructively coping with hospitalization. They also lack the extensive experience with hospitalization that might help them to develop effective coping strategies.

How can these problems be solved? The hospital staff could treat patients as people rather than as nonpersons. This solution would be ideal for the patients but perhaps not for the staff. Too much personal involvement on the part of health care workers can make the job of providing health care more stressful and can contribute to occupational "burn-out" (Maslach, 1976). Providing personal care without personal involvement would, of course, be difficult.

Also, hospitalized patients cannot be given a great deal of control. For the efficiency of the organization, uniform treatment and conformity to hospital routine are desirable. Although hospitals have no insidious plot to deprive patients of their freedom, that is the result when hospitals impose their routine on patients. Restoring control to patients in any significant way would further complicate an already complex organization, but the restoration of small types of control may be effective. For example, many hospitals can allow patients some choice of foods and provide TV remote controls to give patients the power to select a program to watch (or not watch). These aspects of control are small, but a little control may go a long way toward combating feelings of helplessness.

Cotanch (1984) recommended a number of changes hospitals could make to improve health care. She suggested that, along with treatment, hospitals should offer health education and try to persuade patients to change their health habits. Individual responsibility is not easy in the hospital, but Cotanch contended that it should be encouraged. She also suggested that hospitals offer such treatment alternatives as relaxing massages instead of tranquilizers and a selection of appetizing food on hospital menus. The changes that Cotanch envisioned might make hospitalization somewhat less stressful.

PREPARING FOR STRESSFUL MEDICAL PROCEDURES

Simply being in the hospital can be a stressful experience, but some patients encounter additional stress because they must undergo unpleasant medical procedures. Even some outpatient procedures, such as dental visits and blood donation, can be stressful. Patient anxiety ordinarily increases in anticipation of such painful medical procedures as surgery, **gastrointestinal endoscopy** (examining the gastrointestinal tract by inserting a tube through the esophagus or the rectum), and **cardiac catheterization** (inserting a tube into a vein and directing it to the heart where dye is then injected to make a clear X-ray possible). Chemotherapy for cancer is another stressful medical procedure, and most cancer patients anticipate this treatment with apprehension and anxiety. In all these cases, the anticipation may exaggerate the pain of the procedure, which becomes a serious problem for the patient and for the hospital staff.

Most patients cope with preparations for stressful and potentially painful medical procedures as well as they can, but health care providers, including psychologists, have devised support programs and specific training to help patients prepare. Psychological efforts to prepare patients can be traced back to work done by Irving Janis. In 1958, he reported a study in which he compared a group of patients who

were psychologically prepared for surgery with a group given only the usual information provided by physicians and hospital staff. The preparation consisted of information about what would happen before, during, and after surgery. Janis found that the patients in the preparation group requested less medication for pain, made fewer demands on the staff, and were discharged earlier than those who received the usual information. These results were both promising and intriguing and have prompted many additional studies, most of which have confirmed the benefits of preparation.

One such study was conducted by Shipley, Butt, Horwitz, and Farbry in 1978 and involved patients waiting for a stressful endoscopy procedure. They either viewed a videotape of the endoscopy procedure three times, saw it once, or did not see the endoscopy tape but watched an irrelevant tape. In addition, all participants received extensive verbal information about the procedure. As predicted, Shipley et al. found that patients who viewed the endoscopy tape three times were the least distressed and those who did not see the tape were the most distressed.

In addition, the Shipley et al. study revealed different coping styles; the researchers labeled the patients Sensitizers and Repressors. Sensitizers tend to deal with stress by constant vigilance, overt anxiety, and sensitivity to cues of distress whereas Repressors are overtly nonanxious, repress distressful thoughts, and deny potential stress. Shipley et al. found that the Sensitizers showed a consistent negative relationship between the number of times they viewed the endoscopy tape and their level of distress; that is, those who watched the tape three times manifested the least stress, followed in order by those who saw it once and finally by those who did not see it. In contrast, the Repressors showed an inverted V-shaped relationship, with participants who viewed the tape once having much more distress than either the patients who never saw it or those who viewed it three times. The latter finding supported the investigators' hypothesis that Repressors would be low in distress at first, and although one viewing of the tape would greatly increase their fears, three exposures would provide sufficient information to buffer these patients against anticipatory distress.

TECHNIQUES FOR COPING

The study of Shipley et al. (1978) suggested that modeling (watching others undergoing an endoscopic procedure), receiving accurate information, and having repeated exposure to a film were three possible means by which patients could reduce the distress of preparing for stressful medical procedures. In addition, the researchers found that people have different styles of coping with those procedures. Other investigators supported the findings of Janis and Shipley et al. in examining different techniques as well as different styles of coping. These researchers have tended to use any one or a combination of three procedures: giving patients information, training them in relaxation techniques, and modeling appropriate behaviors for them.

Information

The sort of information that Janis provided was procedural; that is, patients received specific information about the procedures they would undergo. Another possible type of information deals with the sensations that patients will experience during medical procedures. An early review of studies with these types of information (Kendall & Watson, 1981) indicated that sensory information is generally more valuable. In a later meta-analysis, Johnson and Vögele (1993) considered a variety of outcome measures as well as studies that have used sensory and procedural information as preparations for surgery. Various studies have used definitions of improvement that include reduced length of hospital stay, reduced pain or requests for pain medication, increased speed of recovery, and improvements in physical measures related to recovery. This meta-analysis considered not only the different types of interventions before surgery but also these different outcome measures. In general, the results substantiated the overall advantage for procedural information but showed that both types of preparation can provide advantages.

Although most of the interventions with surgical patients have focused on preparing them for surgery or helping them cope with the experience of surgery, one study (Kulik & Mahler, 1987) provided surgical patients with information about the roommates they would have after their surgery. Telling patients about their postsurgical roommates helped to relieve their presurgical anxiety, regardless of the type of surgery they faced.

The research by Shipley et al. revealed two distinct coping styles that interact with the information provided in preparation for stressful medical procedures, and other research has confirmed these differences. Sensitizers, or vigilant copers, acknowledge the negative emotions that accompany such procedures whereas Repressors, or avoidance copers, deny thoughts about the negative aspects of the situation. Other studies (Andrew, 1970; DeLong, 1971) have shown that people using the active coping and the avoidance coping style were affected differently by preparatory information about surgery. The avoiders generally did not do as well postsurgically as the active copers, who had acknowledged their negative feelings. In fact, when given specific information about the procedures, the avoiders did worse than when they were given no information or only general information. The results for the active copers were the opposite: They did better when given specific information. The results indicate that coping style and type of information about the procedure interact.

Research has confirmed the effectiveness of both avoidant and active coping styles. Anderson (1987) found that preparation for surgery that included information increased patients' feelings of control and produced better physical and psychological adjustments postsurgically. In contrast, a study by Kiyak, Vitaliano, and Crinean (1988) demonstrated that avoidance coping could also be an effective strategy for dealing with surgery. They found that expectations predicted postsurgical adjustment and that people who expected fewer problems experienced fewer problems.

Different coping styles may each be effective with different medical procedures as well as for different patients. Wong and Kaloupek (1986) found that avoidance coping through distraction was the most effective strategy for lowering anxiety during dental surgery. They speculated that more active, vigilant coping might be maladaptive in medical situations requiring passivity whereas more active coping might be better in situations requiring action on the patient's part. Therefore, perhaps not only personal but also situational coping differences have an influence.

Apparently, specific information about a stressful medical procedure may help some patients cope. The success of the coping strategy depends partly on the type of information given to patients, with information about *sensations* being more helpful than information about *procedures*. In addition, patients' styles of coping interact with the information conveyed, so that only some patients do better when given information as a preparation for stressful medical procedures. Whereas some patients want and use information to help them cope, others prefer to avoid thoughts about the procedure, and this avoidance style helps them cope. An additional factor that predicts the success of information as a way of coping is the type of stressful medical procedure performed. Patients might be advised to adopt an avoidance coping style for procedures that require passivity and a vigilant style for procedures that require patient activity.

Relaxation Training

A second technique for coping with stressful medical procedures is relaxation training. Kendall and Watson (1981) reviewed several studies on relaxation training as an adjunct to surgery and reported that the effects of relaxation are significant and positive for relatively minor medical procedures, such as dental surgery. However, with more serious procedures, the results of relaxation training are less dramatic but generally positive. The review led Kendall and Watson to conclude that relaxation training is warranted in aiding patients' overall hospital adjustment.

Active coping efforts can improve patients' ability to cope with serious medical procedures. Manyande et al. (1995) tested the effectiveness of an imagery intervention for patients undergoing abdominal surgery. Those patients who increased their feelings of being able to cope experienced less pain and distress, requested less analgesia, and had lower levels of stress hormones. This study demonstrated that active coping can be effective in helping people deal with serious medical procedures.

Johnson and Vögele's (1993) meta-analysis of the effectiveness of surgical preparation also indicated that behavioral instructions such as information about relaxation and cognitive coping instructions can be effective in preparing people for surgery, but they concluded that hypnosis was less effective. In the studies they examined, all techniques showed some effectiveness, but none were effective for all measures of improvement or in all studies.

Modeling

Finally, modeling — learning by watching others perform — is an effective technique for coping with unpleasant medical procedures. Modeling is often used with children who are facing surgery. The model appears on film in the same situation that the patient will soon encounter. Melamed (1984) found that the most effective models appear anxious at first, even fearful, but in the end they successfully cope with the stress of the procedure. A necessary component of the filmed modeling seems to be the display of some initial anxiety, which the model then successfully overcomes. Melamed's research also indicated that viewing the film more than once may be useful. In addition, timing of the filmed presentation is important. A person's anxiety tends to increase immediately after viewing a filmed model coping with a stressful situation, but the anxiety decreases with time. Therefore, enough time must elapse between the presentation of the model and the procedure in order for the patient to make full use of the effect.

Modeling has also been a component in a program to reduce dental anxiety in adults. Law, Logan, and Baron (1994) showed dental patients a film of an anxious patient who learns to cope through relaxing and communicating with the dentist. Not all patients benefited from this technique. Those who wanted a high degree of control but felt little control experienced decreased pain and stress whereas other patients did not. Therefore, patients' style of coping interacts with the type of preparation, making modeling and other preparations for stressful procedures good choices for some patients. To be effective, preparations must allow for individual differences in coping style.

CHILDREN AND HOSPITALIZATION

Hospitalization is a common experience for children as well as for adults. Few children negotiate childhood without some injury, illness, or condition that requires hospitalization, and the commonalities of the hospitalization experience are sources of stress and anxiety — separation from parents, an unfamiliar environment, diagnostic tests, administration of anesthesia, surgery, and postoperative pain (Routh & Sanfilippo, 1991).

Training children to cope with their fear of treatment presents special problems to health psychologists. First, young children's understanding of illness may not allow them to understand the reason for their illness or the necessity for the treatment (Bibace & Walsh, 1979). Although kindergarten-age children show signs of understanding the same dimensions that adults do (Goldman, Whitney-Saltiel, Granger, & Rodin, 1991), many adults fail to understand the tests and treatments that occur in hospitals.

Second, many lifelong treatment phobias are learned in childhood (Lautch, 1971), making early prevention of unrealistic fears a critical goal for pediatric health psychology. A child's first experience with medical treatment should not be a traumatic one because early unpleasant experiences tend to generalize. One study (Dahlquist et al., 1986) indicated that children 3 to 12 years old whose previous medical experiences had been negative demonstrated more distress during routine medical examinations than did children whose previous experiences had been either neutral or positive. Liddell (1990) found parallel results with dental anxiety in children; previous aversive dental experiences related more closely to dental anxiety than did the children's general fearfulness.

A third special problem in helping children prepare for stressful medical procedures comes from parents. Some interventions have trained parents to be less anxious and more informative. Several studies (Bush, Melamed, Sheras, & Greenbaum, 1986; Dahlquist et al., 1986; Zastowny, Kirschenbaum, & Meng, 1986) have shown that training parents to help their children learn various coping skills is an effective method of reducing children's anxiety.

Parents' presence can either help or hurt their children's coping with stressful medical procedures, depending on the parents' behavior (Manne et al., 1992). The time-honored parental technique of persistently reassuring a child facing medical treatment is not only ineffective but also tends to increase the child's feelings of distress (Bush et al., 1986). Distraction can be effective in helping children deal with a distressing medical procedure, but, interestingly, adults are not necessarily helped by distrac-

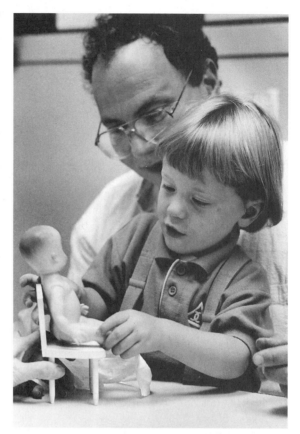

An effective technique to prepare children for hospitalization involves using dolls in play situations so children can express their fears.

tion (McCaul, Monson, & Maki, 1992). Like adults, children respond with less obvious distress when they are given some control over the medical procedures they must endure (Manne et al., 1992).

A fourth problem for children is their tendency to interpret their illness as a form of punishment for real or imagined misconduct (Long & Cope, 1961). Guilt and anxiety often combine with hostility toward and fear of nurses and doctors to produce a complex of negative emotions in children. These problems are more prominent for children receiving treatment for chronic conditions such as cancer or burns.

A variety of psychological interventions, including some not used with adults, have been tried with children who are anticipating fear-provoking medical procedures. Elkins and Roberts (1983) examined the literature from the perspective of five themes or approaches. The first approach involves giving information to the child. A review of informational studies revealed that some reported positive results, but others found that preschool-age children may not always understand the information presented. A later study by Manne et al. (1992) found that this strategy was not effective in reducing children's distress.

A second approach encourages emotional expression in children who are anxious about hospitalization. Children are given a chance to express their fears and anxieties by playing with puppets, doctors' kits, and other play materials and games. The Elkins and Roberts review found mixed results with this type of play therapy. One study even suggested that play techniques may actually increase rather than ameliorate children's fears.

A third theme centers on helping children establish a relationship of trust and confidence with members of the medical staff. This trust is typically achieved by using films, hospital tours, and books and by allowing parents to stay with the child in the hospital. Elkins and Roberts found evidence that building a supportive relationship can be helpful, but by itself it is not sufficient to alleviate children's feelings of distress.

The fourth theme discussed by Elkins and Roberts involves the psychological preparation of parents whose children are facing hospitalization or other stressful medical procedures. Children of psychologically prepared parents are generally less anxious and better able to handle distressing hospital procedures. Pinto and Hollandsworth (1989) tried to reduce emotional arousal in pediatric patients facing first-time elective surgery by showing them an informational videotape in the presence of their parents. A third of the children viewed an adult-narrated tape, a third saw a peer-narrated presentation, and a third were assigned to a control group who saw no videotape. Half the children in each group remained with their parents during the treatment and half were separated from their parents. Children who viewed the videotape with their parents and children who viewed the tape alone showed less preoperative arousal than children who did not view the tape. In general, children who were with their parents during psychological preparation experienced less emotional arousal than children who

were separated from their parents. Moreover, the videotape also decreased parents' anxiety. Contrary to expectations, the researchers found no differences between adult-narrated and child-narrated videotapes; both were equally effective. The results of this study indicate an advantage for both the videotape presentation and the presence of parents during psychological preparation.

The fifth approach includes providing children with various coping strategies such as relaxation training, peer models, distraction, and instruction on self-talk techniques. Films and videotapes are commonly used for teaching all these techniques, and each has been used with some success. Jay, Elliott, Katy, and Siegel (1987) employed a cognitive-behavioral intervention that included modeling, breathing exercises, and imagery distraction. Using children who were receiving painful treatments for leukemia, these researchers compared this cognitive-behavioral intervention to the administration of valium and to a no-treatment control group. They found that children receiving cognitive-behavioral therapy experienced less distress, lower pain ratings, and lower pulse rates during treatment than did children in the control group and in the valium group.

An advantage for cognitive-behavioral preparation techniques also appeared in a study by Jay, Elliott, Woody, and Siegel (1991). These researchers compared a cognitive-behavioral intervention including filmed modeling, breathing exercises, behavioral rehearsal, imagery/distraction, and positive incentives for positive behavior to the same intervention with valium as a relaxant. They were interested in comparing the effectiveness of the two interventions because drugs are often considered an easier way to promote relaxation during stressful medical procedures. They found that the drug treatment offered no advantages over the cognitive-behavioral intervention but that this intervention was effective.

Most of this research has demonstrated the effectiveness of one or another technique, but few investigations have tried to compare the various types of interventions. Elkins and Roberts concluded that empirical research is needed to evaluate one preparation procedure against another before any one approach can be recommended with confidence.

CHAPTER SUMMARY

Although most people value good health and wish to avoid illness, many fail to seek health care when necessary. This chapter looked at several theories of health-related behavior, discussed other factors related to seeking medical attention, examined problems of being in the hospital, and considered psychological issues of preparing for stressful medical procedures.

The *health belief model* was developed specifically to predict and explain health-related behaviors and includes the concepts of perceived severity of the illness, personal susceptibility, and perceived benefits and barriers of health-enhancing behaviors. Although recent research has demonstrated some utility for the health belief model, other studies have introduced questions about its usefulness in changing health-seeking behaviors. *The theory of reasoned action* and *the theory of planned behavior* are general behavior theories that have also been applied to health-related situations. Both theories include attitudes, subjective norms, and intention; in addition, the theory of planned behavior includes the person's perceived behavioral control. These two theories have not yet produced the volume of research generated by the health belief model, but some research suggests that the concepts of intention and perceived behavioral control add to the predictive ability of theories of reasoned action and planned behavior. Bandura's concept of *self-efficacy,* a component of his *self-regulation theory* and similar to perceived behavioral control, has been found to relate positively to a number of health-related behaviors. However, research also suggests that some people may have confidence to change health-related behaviors (high self-efficacy) but lack motivation to do so (low outcome expectancies). Prochaska's *stages of change* theory assumes that people progress through five stages in making changes in behavior—precontemplation, contemplation, preparation, action, and maintenance. Although cross-sectional studies show some promise for the stages of change model, more research is needed to establish its utility. Finally, Weinstein's *precaution adoption process model* assumes that when people are faced with adopting health protective behaviors, they go through seven possible stages of belief about their personal susceptibility. Built into one stage is optimistic bias, a topic that has been heavily researched. However, most research on the total precaution adoption model has been limited to Weinstein and his colleagues. A limitation of each of these models is their inability to accurately assess various social, ethnic, and other demographic factors that also affect people's health-seeking behavior.

How people determine their health status when they don't feel well depends not only on social, ethnic, and demographic factors but also on the characteristics of their symptoms and their concept of illness. In deciding whether they are ill, people consider at least four characteristics of their symptoms: (1) the obvious visibility of the symptoms, (2) the perceived severity of the illness, (3) the degree to which the symptoms interfere with their lives, and (4) the frequency and persistence of the symptoms.

Once people are convinced they are ill, they adopt the sick role. In our society, the sick role involves relief from normal social and occupational responsibilities and the duty to try to get better.

A major aspect of receiving health care is being hospitalized. Most patients conform to hospital routine and are considered "good" patients. A significant minority, however, complain, ask questions, and demand answers; they are therefore regarded as "bad" patients. "Problem" patients insist on exercising control in their daily lives, and their nonconforming behavior while in the hospital can be seen as an attempt to restore control. Even though these patients may not receive as much positive attention from the hospital staff as "good" patients, some evidence shows that such attitudes and behaviors may be helpful to them in restoring their health.

Health psychology has a role to play in preparing patients for hospitalization and stressful medical procedures. Information, relaxation training, and modeling have helped adults whereas interventions with children have also included play therapy and procedures designed to prepare parents to help their child cope. Psychological techniques can help children, parents, and adult patients cope with stressful and painful medical procedures by lowering their anxiety, enhancing their feelings of control, and even lowering their need for medication and shortening hospital stays.

SUGGESTED READINGS

Bennett, H. L., & Disbrow, E. A. (1993). Preparing for surgery and medical procedures. In D. Goleman & J. Gurin (Eds.), *Mind/body medicine: How to use your mind for better health* (pp. 401–427). Yonkers, NY: Consumer Reports Books. Bennett and Disbrow discuss techniques and situations that help patients cope with surgery and stressful medical procedures and give practical advice on how such patients can design their own presurgical program.

Fleury, J. (1992). The application of motivational theory to cardiovascular risk reduction. *Image: Journal of Nursing Scholarship, 24,* 229–239. In a review of studies using the health belief model, the theory of reasoned action, the theory of planned behavior, and self-efficacy theory as they have been applied to cardiovascular risk reduction, Fleury finds both strengths and weaknesses for each theory.

Rosenstock, I. M., & Kirscht, J. P. (1979). Why people seek health care. In G. C. Stone, F. Cohen, & N. E. Adler (Eds.), *Health psychology: A handbook* (pp. 161–188). San Francisco: Jossey-Bass. This is a concise review of the demographic and situational factors that affect those seeking health care for prevention as well as in response to symptoms of illness.

Taylor, S. E. (1982). The impact of health organizations on recipients of services. In A. W. Johnson, O. Grusky, & B. H. Raven (Eds.), *Contemporary health services: Social science perspectives* (pp. 103–137). Boston: Auburn House. This article is an excellent analysis of the effects of being in the hospital, along with an interpretation of the psychological reactions that guide the behavior of hospitalized patients.

Adhering to Medical Advice

Two years ago, Paul, a 47-year-old European American, suffered a heart attack (myocardial infarction), and since that time he has been under treatment for coronary heart disease. After spending 3 weeks in a hospital, Paul felt well enough to go home, and soon afterward he returned to his job as a college professor. After his heart attack, Paul visited his physician on a regular basis and never missed a scheduled appointment. In addition, he strictly followed his doctor's orders concerning his prescribed medication. Despite these dutiful deeds, Paul was not a compliant patient. He continued to smoke a pack and a half of cigarettes a day, allowed himself to remain 60 to 70 pounds overweight, and refused to follow a regular exercise regimen. Paul knew that smoking, improper eating, and a sedentary lifestyle were associated with increased risk of a second heart attack, yet he continued to engage in these unhealthy behaviors. Why?

No completely satisfactory answer to this question is possible. However, some additional information may be illuminating. First, Paul had been smoking for 30 years and had never seriously tried to quit. Second, he had had a weight problem since he was about 25 and had tried several diets in years past, but none had been successful. Third, Paul had not exercised regularly since he played football in high school and college. For Paul, therefore, nonadherence to known healthy behaviors was simply a matter of continuing a lifestyle of long duration. There was a fourth factor involved in his nonadherence as well: His physician was himself a model for unhealthy behaviors. He smoked heavily, was considerably overweight, and did not exercise regularly. Moreover, he had never made clear to Paul what he should do to lower his risk of future coronary problems. Paul, who was divorced and lived alone, had little support or encouragement from family or physician to change his lifestyle.

THE PROBLEM OF ADHERENCE

For medical advice to affect the health of patients beneficially, two contingencies must be met. First, the advice must be accurate. Second, patients must follow this good advice. Both conditions are essential. Ill-founded advice that patients strictly follow may introduce new health problems, which lead to disastrous outcomes for the compliant patient. On the other hand, excellent advice is essentially worthless if patients do not follow it.

Interestingly, inadequate treatment recommendations combined with low levels of patient adherence to that advice are probably less harmful than either adequate recommendations not followed or invalid advice closely heeded. Irving Janis (1983, 1984) suggested that as long as health care providers make mistakes, people are better off not adhering to certain aspects of their advice. Determining which advice is valid and which is not is an important health care problem but largely within the province of medicine; understanding why people adhere or fail to adhere to recommendations and finding ways to improve adherence entails behaviors that are mostly within the realm of psychology.

Paul had gone to considerable effort and expense to seek medical care only to undermine his own progress by neglecting to follow recommended medical regimens. Why do people engage in such self-defeating behavior? What theoretical models explain noncompliant behavior? Is nonadherence a matter of situational factors, such as money, convenience, and time, or do certain personality traits relate to adherence? How pervasive is the problem? How can adherence be measured? How can it be predicted? Does adherence pay off in better health? How can it be improved? This chapter addresses each of these questions, but first we ask a more basic question: What is adherence?

Traditionally, people in the medical profession have used the term *compliance* to refer to patient behaviors that conform to physicians' orders. But because the term compliance connotes reluctant obedience, many health psychologists and some physicians advocate the use of other words, and the terms *adherence, cooperation, obedience,* and *collaboration* have all been suggested as substitutes for compliance. Perhaps the most accurate term to describe the ideal relationship between physician and patient would be *cooperation,* a word that implies a relationship in which both the health care provider and the consumer are actively involved in the restoration and maintenance of the patient's health. However, because cooperation is not yet the accepted label for this relationship, the terms *compliance* and *adherence* are still the most frequently used words, and many researchers employ these two words interchangeably to describe the patient's ability and willingness to follow recommended health practices (Turk & Meichenbaum, 1991).

What does it mean to be compliant? Haynes (1979b) took a broad view of compliance, defining it as "the extent to which a person's behavior (in terms of taking medications, following diets, or executing lifestyle changes) coincides with medical or health advice" (pp. 1–2). This definition expands the concept of compliance beyond merely taking medications to include maintaining healthy lifestyle practices, such as abstaining from smoking cigarettes, eating properly, getting sufficient exercise, avoiding undue stress, and not abusing alcohol. In addition, the concept of compliance or adherence includes making and keeping periodic medical and dental appointments, using seatbelts, and engaging in other behaviors that coincide with the best health advice available.

THEORIES OF ADHERENCE

Why do some people comply with medical advice while others fail to comply? Several theoretical models that apply to behavior in general have also been applied to the problem of adherence and nonadherence. Some of the most frequently used models include the biomedical model, the behavioral model, and various cognitive learning theories, including self-efficacy theory, the theory of reasoned action, and the health belief model.

THE BIOMEDICAL MODEL

The *biomedical model* does not explain why individuals are noncompliant; it simply identifies demographic factors that are related to compliance, such as age, gender, ethnic background, income, and so forth (Fisher, 1992). It also looks at other variables, such as complexity of the treatment regimen, side effects of the medication, and severity of the illness to determine the extent that each of these affects adherence or nonadherence. This model assumes that these various personal characteristics and disease characteristics can be used to predict who will be and who will not be compliant. R. Brian Haynes and associates (Haynes, 1979a; Haynes, Wang, & da Mota Gomes, 1987; Macharia, Leon, Rowe, Stephenson, & Haynes, 1992; Sackett & Haynes, 1976) have used this approach to identify those characteristics of the patient, the illness, and the practitioner that predict nonadherence. Haynes and his associates also used such information in an attempt to improve patient compliance (Macharia et al., 1992).

THE BEHAVIORAL MODEL

The *behavioral model* of adherence is based on the principles of operant conditioning proposed by B. F. Skinner (1938, 1953). The key to operant conditioning is the immediate *reinforcement* of any response that moves the organism (person) toward the target behavior—in this case better compliance with medical recommendations. Psychologists have used reinforcement to strengthen compliant behavior. An example might be a monetary payment to a patient contingent on his or her keeping a doctor's appointment. Whereas reinforcers strengthen behavior, the effects of **punishment** are limited and difficult to predict. At best, punishment will merely inhibit or suppress a behavior. At worst, it conditions strong negative feelings toward any persons or environmental conditions associated with it. Punishment, including threats of harm, are seldom useful in improving a person's compliance with medical advice.

Advocates of the behavioral model use cues, rewards, and contracts to reinforce compliant behaviors. Cues include written reminders of appointments, telephone calls from the practitioner's office, and a variety of self-reminders. Rewards can be extrinsic (money and compliments) or intrinsic (feeling healthier). Contracts can be verbal, but they are more often written agreements between practitioner and patient. Most adherence models recognize the importance of incentives in improving compliance.

Some evidence exists demonstrating that relatively simple behavioral strategies may be at least as potent as more complex cognitive approaches in improving adherence. Hegel, Ayllon, Thiel, and Oulton (1992) compared the relative effectiveness of behavioral and cognitive interventions to increase adherence in adult male hemodialysis patients. The behavioral strategy included incentives such as lottery tickets and private use of television and videotapes to reinforce compliant behaviors. The cognitive regimen was based on the health belief model and included both counseling and information designed to modify health beliefs. Although the cognitive intervention provided immediate help to hemodialysis

patients in controlling their weight, this approach was no more effective than the behavioral program that relied on incentives and a behavioral contract. Moreover, the behavioral intervention was superior to the health belief intervention in maintaining weight control. We review additional studies on the effectiveness of behavioral techniques in a later section on improving adherence.

COGNITIVE LEARNING THEORIES

Cognitive learning theories are based on many of the same learning principles that underlie behavioral models, but they include additional concepts, such as people's interpretation and evaluation of their situation, their emotional response, and their perceived ability to cope with illness symptoms. Many cognitive learning models exist, including self-efficacy theory, the theory of reasoned action, and the health belief model.

Self-Efficacy Theory

Several researchers have used Albert Bandura's (1977, 1986) notion of *self-efficacy* as an explanation for adherence or nonadherence. Bandura has contended that people's beliefs concerning their ability to initiate difficult behaviors (such as an exercise program) predict their accomplishment of those behaviors. Self-efficacy is a situation-specific concept that refers to people's confidence that they can perform necessary behaviors to produce desired outcomes in any particular situation.

Self-efficacy theory has been used to predict adherence to a variety of health recommendations. In a study of the relationship between self-efficacy and the maintenance of an aerobic exercise program, McAuley (1992, 1993) assessed the self-efficacy of sedentary, middle-aged participants with poor cardiorespiratory fitness and high percentages of body fat who had begun an exercise program. McAuley (1993) found that self-efficacy was a strong predictor of which participants would maintain the exercise regimen over a 4-month follow-up: People who believed they could successfully complete the behaviors necessary to maintain an aerobic exercise program had an increased likelihood of adhering to such a program. In addition, Duncan and McAuley (1993) found that self-efficacy interacted with social support to improve people's adherence to an exercise program.

In another study, Borrelli and Mermelstein (1994) examined the role of self-efficacy and goal setting among participants' adhering to a smoking cessation program and found that self-efficacy, or confidence in being able to quit smoking, accurately predicted which participants would be able to attain abstinence. Also, some evidence suggests that self-efficacy predicts compliance with dental regimens. For example, Tedesco, Keffer, and Fleck-Kandath (1991) found that adult dental patients with high self-efficacy were more likely to brush and floss than were those patients low in self-efficacy. Therefore, self-efficacy shows a relationship to adherence to a variety of treatment programs.

The Theory of Reasoned Action

The *theory of reasoned action* (Ajzen & Fishbein, 1980; Fishbein & Ajzen, 1975) assumes that the immediate determinant of behavior is people's *intention* to perform that behavior. Behavioral intentions, in turn, are a function of (1) people's *attitudes* toward the behavior, which are determined by their beliefs that the behavior will lead to positively or negatively valued outcomes, and (2) their *subjective norm,* which is shaped by their perception of the value that significant others place on that behavior and by their motivation to comply with those norms (see Figure 7.1).

Miller, Wikoff, and Hiatt (1992) used the theory of reasoned action in an attempt to predict how well recently diagnosed hypertensive patients would comply with recommendations concerning diet, smoking, physical activity, stress reduction, and medication. They found solid support for the model with regard to compliant behaviors toward dieting, quitting smoking, increasing physical activity, and coping with stress. For diet, physical activity, and stress, compliant behaviors were directly influenced by intentions, which in turn were influenced directly by patients' attitudes and their motivation to comply. For smoking cessation, interestingly, motivation to comply was negatively related to intention to quit. In other words, some people were strongly motivated to quit smoking, but they had no intention of doing so. With regard to taking medication, Miller

et al. found that the model did not support intentions as the immediate predictor of correctly taking medications, although motivation to comply, which was strongly influenced by perceived beliefs of others, had a direct influence on taking medications. This study suggests that the theory of reasoned action has at least some value in predicting adherence to medical recommendations.

The Health Belief Model

The *health belief model* (Becker, 1979; Becker & Maiman, 1975; Rosenstock, 1974) assumes that four interactive belief states influence compliance as well as health-seeking behaviors. These belief states, which have a cumulative effect for either increasing or decreasing compliant behavior, include (1) perceived susceptibility to the negative consequences of nonadherence, (2) perceived severity of these consequences, (3) the perceived costs/benefits ratio of performing compliant behaviors, and (4) the perceived barriers to incorporating adherence behaviors into one's lifestyle.

Evaluation of the health belief model is complicated by the number of different concepts in the model and the different ways the model has been tested. For example, Bond, Aiken, and Somerville (1992) found some support for a three-construct model of health beliefs applied to predicting diabetic adolescents' adherence to their treatment regimen. The three variables were *Threat* (a combination of perceived susceptibility and perceived severity), *Benefits/Costs,* and *Cues* (a willingness to seek treatment whenever the adolescents experienced severe symptoms). Consistent with the health belief model, Benefits/Costs and Cues predicted adherence in the expected direction. However, Bond et al. found some evidence that Threat might predict poor compliance, a finding that led the authors to hypothesize that people with a chronic disease such as diabetes might be less likely to comply with a complex regimen under conditions of high threat. Rather than rationally adhering to their treatment program, people with severe chronic illnesses may be more strongly motivated to reduce their emotional reactions to the threatening aspects of that disease. In other words, these adolescents could reduce Threat—perceived susceptibility and perceived severity of the disease—

through such negatively reinforcing behaviors as thinking of something else or keeping occupied with distracting activities.

For whatever reason, a high percentage of people do not comply with the best health advice. Although psychologists have yet to develop a model that can account for all noncompliant behaviors, they have made some contribution toward a better understanding of reasons for adherence and nonadherence.

ASSESSING ADHERENCE

The assessment of adherence raises at least two questions. First, how do researchers know the percentage of patients who fail to comply with their practitioner's recommendations? Second, how can noncompliant behaviors be identified? The answer to the first question is that compliance rates are not known with certainty, and that any reported percentage is usually only an estimate.

Second, at least five basic means of measuring patient compliance are available: (1) ask the clinician, (2) ask the patient, (3) ask other people, (4) count pills, and (5) examine biochemical evidence. The first of these methods, asking the clinician, may well be the poorest choice. Physicians generally overestimate their patients' compliance rates, and even when their guesses are not overly optimistic, they are usually wrong. One early study (Caron & Roth, 1968) reported a correlation of only .01 between physicians' estimates of compliance and an objective pill count. Although other studies have found somewhat higher correlations (after all, they couldn't be lower), the overall accuracy of estimates by physicians and other practitioners is poor.

Asking patients themselves is a more valid procedure, but it is fraught with many difficulties. Self-reports are inaccurate for at least two reasons: First, patients may lie to avoid the displeasure of their health care provider; second, they may simply not know their own rate of compliance. Patients not only underreport poor adherence, but they also overreport good compliance. Roth and Caron (1978), for example, reported that about 30% of the patients claimed that they were 100% compliant, but a pill count for these people indicated that they were us-

ing from 2% to as much as 130% of the prescribed pills. Thus, whereas some patients took more medication than recommended, others took far less. Dunbar (1979) suggested that trained interviewers could help improve the accuracy of self-reports and, at the same time, identify the types of errors typically made by patients. Obviously, self-report measures have questionable validity and should be supplemented by other assessment techniques.

One other technique is to ask hospital personnel and family members to monitor the patient, but this procedure also has at least two inherent problems. First, constant observation may be physically impossible, especially with regard to such regimens as diet and alcohol consumption. Second, persistent monitoring creates an artificial situation and frequently results in higher rates of compliance than would otherwise occur. This outcome, of course, is desirable, but as a means of assessing compliance, it contains a built-in error that makes observation by others inaccurate.

A fourth method of assessing compliance is to count pills. This procedure may seem ideal because very few errors would be made in counting the number of pills absent from a bottle or a drug dispenser. Unfortunately, this method also may be inaccurate. Even if the required number of pills are gone, the patient may not have been compliant. Once again, there are at least two possible problems with pill counts. First, the patient, for a wide variety of reasons, may have simply discarded some of the medication. Second, the patient may have taken all the pills, but in a manner other than the prescribed one.

Several investigators have developed automated devices that facilitate pill counting and determine whether patients take their medication at the prescribed time. Cramer, Mattson, Prevey, Scheyer, and Ouellette (1989) reported on a novel assessment technique in which a microprocessor in the pill cap recorded every bottle opening and closing. They assumed that each bottle opening equaled one dose of medication, and the pill cap microprocessor yielded information concerning the time of day that the bottle was opened. This procedure did not detect the number of pills removed with each opening, and although this procedure represents an improvement over the pill-counting technique, it too cannot ascertain whether patients are taking medication according to their doctor's recommendations.

Examination of biochemical evidence is a fifth method of measuring compliance. This procedure looks at the outcome of compliant behavior to find some biochemical evidence, such as analysis of blood or urine samples, to determine whether the patient has behaved in a compliant fashion. Roth (1987) reviewed the data on this method and concluded that blood and urine levels are more reliable measures of medicine intake than pill counts, but these measures are also more expensive and often not worth the cost. Other problems arise with using biochemical evidence as a means of assessing compliance. First, some drugs are not easily detected in blood or urine samples. Second, individual differences in absorption and metabolism of drugs can lead to wide variations among people who are equally compliant. Third, biochemical checks must be carried out frequently and regularly to assess compliance rates accurately. Fourth, biochemical methods do not measure the degree of compliance; the presence of a drug or drug marker merely reveals that the patient ingested some amount of the drug at some time and does not indicate that the patient took the proper amount at the proper time.

Computerized recording devices can also assess biochemical outcomes of adherence. One such automatic recording procedure is a *glucometer,* a device used with diabetic patients to record automatically both the occurrence and the results of each blood glucose test. The date and time of day for each test become part of the information stored in memory, so patients cannot alter it. Several studies (Gonder-Frederick, Julian, Cox, Clarke, & Carter, 1988; Mazze et al., 1984; Wysocki, Green, & Huxtable, 1989) have reported on the usefulness of such procedures as a check on the reliability of self-reports of compliance and as a measure of the effectiveness of blood glucose self-monitoring. However, use of the glucometer alone does not appear to increase the frequency of self-monitoring of blood glucose levels or to improve diabetic control. Wysocki et al. (1989) found that over a relatively short period of time, the glucometer by itself was about as effective as the meter plus a behavioral contract in maintaining acceptable levels of compliance with self-monitoring of

blood glucose. After 8 weeks, however, patients who used only the meter showed a marked decline in testing frequency, whereas patients using the meter plus a behavioral contract continued an acceptable level of blood glucose testing. Thus, biochemical techniques alone do not appear to be adequate for assessing rates of compliance with medical recommendations.

In summary, no one of the five basic means of assessing compliance is both reliable and valid. However, with the exception of clinician judgment, most have some limited validity and usefulness. Therefore, when accuracy is crucial, it seems appropriate to use two or more of these basic measures for assessing patient compliance, a procedure that yields greater accuracy than reliance on a single assessment technique.

HOW FREQUENT IS NONADHERENCE?

How pervasive is the problem of nonadherence? The answer to this question depends in part on how nonadherence is defined, the nature of the illness under consideration, the demographic features of the population, and the methods used to assess compliance. In general the rate of noncompliance with medical or health advice is approximately 50%. DiMatteo (1994) reported that at least 38% of patients do not follow short-term treatment plans, and more than 45% fail to adhere to recommendations for long-term treatment. Moreover, as many as three-fourths of all people are unwilling or unable to stick to recommended healthy lifestyles, such as eating a low-fat diet, avoiding cigarette smoking, or exercising regularly. These figures agree with Sackett (1976), who estimated that about half the patients who had been prescribed medication for an illness failed to take that medication in accordance with instructions.

In the late 1970s, Sackett and Snow (1979) reviewed more than 500 studies that dealt with the frequency of compliance and noncompliance. They eliminated studies with serious methodological flaws and summarized the results from the remainder. At that time about 75% of the patients kept their scheduled appointments when they had initiated them, but only about 50% kept appointments that had been scheduled by the health care professional. As expected, compliance rates were higher when treatment was to cure an illness than when it was to prevent an illness. For example, with reference to taking medication for a short time, 77% were compliant when the treatment was designed to cure a disease; only 63% complied when treatment was aimed at prevention. According to Sackett and Snow, when medication must be taken over a long period, compliance is around 50% for either prevention or cure. Compliance rates for dietary regimens ranged from 30% to 70%, again with a mean of about 50%.

Have compliance rates risen since this early review? Macharia et al. (1992) found that compliance rates for keeping appointments ranged from 8% to 94%, with a mean rate of 58%. Rates of adherence to physical activity programs are also only about 50% after 6 months (Dishman, 1982; Oldridge & Steiner, 1990; Ward & Morgan, 1984). Indeed, Lynch et al. (1992) found only 36% adherence for participants advised to exercise to control their cholesterol levels. These results indicate that compliance rates have remained quite constant, with about half of all patients failing to comply with recommended medical programs. What factors determine who will be compliant and who will be noncompliant?

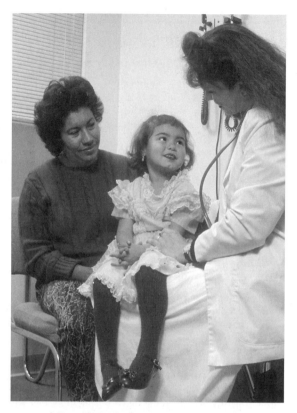

Parents follow medical advice for their sick children at a similar rate as for themselves—about 50%.

WHAT FACTORS PREDICT ADHERENCE?

If we assume that people always act in their own best interests, we may be at a loss to explain the factors that do and do not relate to adherence. For example, it may seem intuitively obvious that the amount of money invested in the treatment procedure would predict compliance. Intuition, however, does not always agree with the evidence. Jamison and Akiskal (1983) found that a third to half of the patients suffering from bipolar (manic-depressive) disorder stopped taking lithium, despite the very low cost of that drug and the potential disadvantages of noncompliance. Also, Becker, Drachman, and Kirscht (1972) found that more than half the mothers who were giving penicillin to their children for middle ear infection stopped prematurely even though the medication was given to them at no cost. These mothers did what many noncompliant patients do—they simply stopped the medication when the symptoms disappeared.

Other than the disappearance of symptoms, what factors do or do not predict compliance? Possible predictors can be divided into three categories: characteristics of the disease, characteristics of the person, and characteristics of the relationship between the health care provider and the patient.

ILLNESS CHARACTERISTICS

Characteristics of the disease include the unpleasantness of the medication's side effects, the duration of treatment, the complexity of treatment, and the severity of the disease (see box—Would You Believe . . . ?).

Side Effects of the Medication

One might guess that a drug with few or no unpleasant side effects will produce greater patient

WOULD YOU BELIEVE . . . ?

Compliance and Severity of Illness

Would you believe that people with a serious illness are no more likely than people with a mild illness to seek medical treatment or to comply with medical advice? Common wisdom might suggest that people with severe, potentially crippling or life-threatening illnesses will be highly motivated to adhere to regimens that will protect them against such major catastrophes.

Interestingly, little evidence exists to support this logical hypothesis. Indeed, people sometimes seek health care not because they have a serious medical problem but because someone might casually mention that they looked bad. For example, Robin DiMatteo and Dante DiNicola (1982) reported a case study concerning a woman who had been hit by a baseball bat and had suffered some loss of vision in her left eye. The loss of vision, however, did not prompt her to go to a doctor. She sought treatment only after a friend casually commented that her eyelid drooped!

Research indicates that compliance with regimens designed to treat or prevent major illnesses tends to be no higher than those aimed at treating or preventing minor disorders. For example, Pauline Vincent (1971) reported that among patients diagnosed for glaucoma and told either to use eyedrops three times a day or risk blindness, only 42% adhered to these instructions. Even when people became legally blind in one eye, the rate of compliance rose to only 59%! This finding suggests that about half the people will remain noncompliant, even at the risk of a devastating disorder.

R. Brian Haynes (1979a) reviewed many studies on compliance and disease severity and found no consistent evidence that people are more likely to comply with treatment regimens for a serious illness than they are when the disorder is minor.

Of the 13 studies he examined, only 6 reported any relationship between severity of illness and compliance, and 4 of these indicated that people with serious medical problems were less likely to comply. Haynes summed up these studies by noting that "counter to common wisdom, not a single study has found that increasing severity of symptoms encourages compliance" (p. 51).

Although the severity of the illness as judged by the physician or by some external criterion fails to predict compliance, Marshall Becker and Lois Maiman (1980) suggested that the severity of the illness as viewed by the patient could make some difference. Earlier, Becker (1979) had found several studies that reported a positive relationship between the patient's judgment of illness severity and his or her compliance with treatment regimens. In these studies, the diagnosis had already been made, and the patients

---

compliance, but the evidence in support of this position is not overwhelming. Some studies (Caldwell, Cobb, Dowling, & DeJongh, 1970; Kirscht & Rosenstock, 1977) have found that increasingly unpleasant side effects are associated with a greater likelihood of noncompliance. However, Masur (1981) cited several studies indicating that unpleasant side effects are not a major reason for discontinuing a drug or dropping out of a treatment program. This evidence does not mean that side effects are completely unrelated to noncompliance but simply that most noncompliant people do not consider them a very important factor.

Duration of the Treatment

A second illness characteristic is the duration of the treatment. In general, the longer people must submit to treatment or preventive regimens, the more likely they are to drop out of treatment. Haynes (1976a) reviewed several studies that compared compliance rates to the length of treatment and concluded that in most cases, noncompliance increases as duration of therapy increases. However, as Masur (1981) pointed out, most long-term treatment programs are for illnesses that have no symptoms, such as hypertension. Understandably, people are less motivated to continue a lengthy therapeutic regimen in the absence of unpleasant symptoms. Masur argued that it is this asymptomatic feature of the disease and not the duration of treatment that leads to noncompliance.

Complexity of the Treatment

Another illness characteristic is the complexity of the treatment. Are people less likely to comply as the treatment procedures become increasingly more

were already experiencing pain and discomfort from the illness. Becker concluded that "it may therefore be that the presence of physical symptoms produces an elevating or 'realistic' effect on perceived severity, motivating the patient to follow the physician's instructions as long as indications of illness persist" (p. 10).

Results of research on compliance and the severity of illness suggest two general conclusions. First, no direct relationship exists between the severity of an illness (as perceived by physicians) and a patient's probability of complying with recommended medical regimens, especially those prescriptions aimed at prevention. Second, if patients have experienced pain from a disorder that has already been diagnosed, they are more likely to comply with their physician's recommendations. Pain by itself, of course, is not a true indicator of the severity of an illness, but it may be one of several factors that help

convince patients to cooperate in protecting their own health.

Why do people undermine their own health by not adhering to sound medical advice? One possible answer can be found in the *parallel response model* suggested by Howard Leventhal (Leventhal, 1970, 1971; Leventhal, Diefenbach, & Leventhal, 1992). The parallel response model assumes that when people perceive a dangerous situation, such as a severe illness, their appraisal of that threat produces two relatively independent processes — Danger Control and Fear Control. People primarily motivated by Danger Control ignore or overcome their fear by behaving adaptively — for example, they seek medical care when symptoms first appear. On the other hand, people motivated largely by Fear Control behave in a manner aimed mostly at reducing their fear. Behaviors that reduce fear are negatively reinforcing, even those that are

maladaptive — for example, drinking alcohol, using drugs, or ignoring illness symptoms. Leventhal believes that level of fear interacts with the perceived adequacy of a preventive measure to predict compliance. For example, if people believe that tetanus shots are completely reliable, that belief combined with a high level of fear should produce a high rate of compliance. Conversely, if people believe that a preventive program (such as dental hygiene) is less than adequate, that belief combined with a high level of fear should produce a low level of compliance.

Leventhal's parallel response model suggests that at times, people are more strongly motivated to reduce their fear than to avoid the danger that accompanies a devastating and chronic disease. This may account for the poor relationship between severity of an illness and rate of adherence to treatment.

complex? In general, the greater the variety of medications a person must take, the greater is the likelihood of that person's noncompliance. However, evidence regarding the number of daily doses is not clear. Haynes's (1979a) review included five studies in which compliance and increasing daily doses were investigated. Two of these studies showed that compliance decreased as the number of daily doses increased from one to four, but three studies found no relationship between compliance and number of daily doses.

Other studies have generally found that the greater the number of daily doses required, the lower will be the likelihood that patients will take pills in the prescribed manner. For example, Cramer et al. (1989) found that patients with seizures who were required to take only one pill a day achieved 88% adherence; those who were required to take two

pills a day were 81% compliant; and patients who were required to take three pills daily complied 77% of the time. However, patients who were prescribed four doses per day achieved only a 39% compliance rate. These data indicate that compliance drops dramatically when pills are to be taken more than three times a day.

The reason seems obvious. For most people, a day has one, two, or three prominent periods, and medicine can be cued to each. For example, pills prescribed once a day can be taken early in the morning; those prescribed twice a day can be cued to early morning and late night; and those prescribed three times a day can be taken after each meal. Adherence to any of these three schedules is quite high. Schedules calling for medication to be taken four or more times a day create an unnatural division of the day for most people, resulting in low compliance rates.

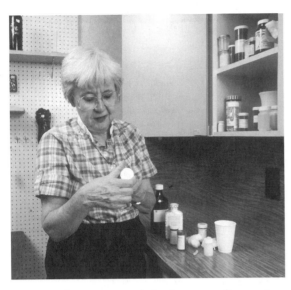

More complex treatments tend to lower compliance rates.

PERSONAL CHARACTERISTICS

Researchers have investigated such individual characteristics as age, gender, social support, personality traits, and personal beliefs about health to determine their association with people's adherence to medical advice. Do any of these variables predict compliance?

Age

The relationship between adherence and age is complicated by several factors. Depending on the specific illness, the time frame, and the adherence regimen, studies show that compliance either increases or decreases with age. Lynch et al. (1992) studied adherence to an exercise program for adults with high cholesterol who were 26 to 68 years old. At the 8- and 16-week points in the intervention, these investigators observed a positive correlation between age and adherence, suggesting that as people get older they become more concerned with their health and are more likely to comply with an exercise program designed to reduce cholesterol. However, after 26 months of the program, age was not significantly related to adherence, a finding that prompted the authors to suggest that older participants may have suffered some minor physical discomfort that interfered with exercise. A study by Thomas et al. (1995) added a further complication to this issue. These in-

vestigators found a curvilinear relationship between age and compliance with colorectal cancer screening. In this large-scale, longitudinal study of both men and women, the best compliers were around 70 years old; the worst were below 55 or over 80. Perhaps after age 80 people simply do not regard screening for colorectal cancer to be important. Among adults, adherence to regimens for diabetes, hypertension, or heart disease tends to increase as people get older. Sherbourne, Hays, Ordway, DiMatteo, and Kravitz (1992) investigated several predictors of compliance among a large number of patients with these disorders who ranged in age from 19 to 97. Sherbourne et al. found a consistent positive relationship between age and adherence, with patients 45 and older being more likely to comply with their doctor's specific recommendations. However, with young diabetic patients, age may be inversely related to compliance. Bond et al. (1992) studied 10- to 19-year-old diabetics and found that as the patients' age increased, their compliance with their exercise program and insulin self-injection decreased. That is, as young diabetics grow into adolescence, they tend show greater noncompliance with an inconvenient health-protective regimen.

Gender

With regard to gender, researchers have found few differences between the overall adherence rates of women and men but some differences in specific recommendations. Several studies (Emery, Hauck, & Blumenthal, 1992; Lynch et al., 1992; Ward & Morgan, 1984) found that men and women were about equal in their tendency to drop out of or stay with an exercise program. However, women seem to be better at adhering to healthy diets and taking some types of medication. For example, Laforge, Greene, and Prochaska (1994) found that women were more likely than men to eat at least two servings of fruit and vegetables daily, and Sellwood and Tarrier (1994) reported that men were more likely than women to be extremely resistant to taking medication for a mental disorder.

Social Support

The introduction to this chapter presented the case of Paul, the coronary heart patient who faithfully adhered to his physician's prescriptions concerning medication but who was less compliant with regard to good health practices. Paul was divorced, lived alone, and enjoyed no close personal relationships. His case suggests an association between compliance and the support a patient receives from family and friends.

One of the strongest predictors of adherence is the level of social support one receives from friends and family, but even this factor is not invariably related to compliance. In general, people who are isolated from others are likely to be noncompliant; those whose lives are filled with close interpersonal relationships are more likely to follow medical advice. For example, Sherwood (1983) found that compliance by hemodialysis patients increased with the family's understanding of kidney disease, medical regimens, and the emotional effects of the illness. Significantly, Sherwood found that the highest compliance occurred when families were neither emotionally distant nor emotionally overinvolved. Similarly, Christensen et al. (1992) found that hemodialysis patients who saw their family as cohesive and expressive of feelings were more likely to adhere to fluid-intake restrictions than patients who perceived conflict within their family. This study also found that severity of impairment was inversely related to compliance; that is, more severely impaired patients did not adhere to diet restrictions as well as less severely impaired patients.

Living with another person who is part of the same compliance procedure seems to increase an individual's adherence. In a longitudinal study of compliance, Thomas et al. (1995) found that the people who lived with another person who was also a participant in the study were more likely to comply with a cancer screening regimen than those who lived in a household where they were the only participant. This study also found that receiving news that one's screening examination showed no evidence of colorectal cancer tended to lower subsequent rate of compliance.

Some evidence suggests that *quality* rather than *quantity* of social support predicts diabetics adherence to complex medical recommendations. Sherbourne et al. (1992) found that the number of friends a diabetic patient had was unrelated to the patient's compliance, but that quality of interpersonal relations was a significant predictor of adherence. Inci-

dentally, Sherbourne et al. found no relationship between social support and adherence for patients with hypertension or heart disease.

Other studies, however, have found that support of family and friends relates to adherence in heart patients. For example, Doherty, Schrott, Metcalf, and Iasiello-Vailas (1983) determined the effects of spousal support on adherence to coronary treatment through an intensive personal interview. Men whose wives were highly supportive had significantly greater compliance with coronary preventive measures than men whose wives offered less support. Also, Stanton (1987) found that strong social support was positively related to the likelihood that hypertensive patients would adhere to medical advice, including keeping medical appointments. In Stanton's study, social support included tangible and affective support provided by people other than medical personnel — that is, family members and friends who were actively involved in helping hypertensive patients follow treatment instructions for their disorder. More recently, Bovbjerg et al. (1995) found that spousal support was related to dietary compliance in men with high cholesterol. Compared with men whose wives offered little support, those whose wives were highly supportive were more likely to have maintained their dietary goals at 3, 12, and 24 months after attending a series of dietary classes.

Emotional support may be a better predictor of compliance than marriage for men who have undergone artery bypass surgery. Kulik and Mahler (1993) followed 85 male heart patients for more than a year after they had received bypass surgery and found that married men were more likely than unmarried men to have complied with a doctor's advice to smoke less and walk more. However, when equated for emotional support, married and unmarried patients showed no difference in levels of compliance.

Personality Traits

Are certain personality types more likely than others to be noncompliant? If so, no one seems to know what they are. Several studies (Caron & Roth, 1968; Davis, 1966; Mushlin & Appel, 1977) have shown that physicians not only seriously overestimate patient compliance but that they are notoriously inept at predicting which patients are most likely to be noncompliant. In the Davis study, 65% of the physicians responded that a patient's "uncooperative personality" was the primary cause of noncompliance. Despite the widespread belief among doctors that patient personality is the most likely explanation for nonadherence to medical advice, little research evidence supports this supposition. Some research (Davis, 1968; Hammel & Williams, 1964; Jacobs, 1972) has reported an association between noncompliance and such personality factors as authoritarianism, neuroticism, and impulsivity. However, most of these early studies did not use standardized personality inventories; rather, they relied on clinical judgments made by interviewers who were looking for and expecting to find stereotyped personal characteristics in noncompliant individuals.

In one study that used a standardized psychological test, Kabat-Zinn and Chapman-Waldrop (1988) administered the Symptoms Checklist-90-R to nearly 800 patients referred to an 8-week stress-reduction program. Of all the scales on the test, only scores on the obsessive-compulsive scale predicted adherence; obsessive-compulsive people, as one might guess, were more likely to complete the stress-reduction program. Another study that used a standardized psychological inventory (Pfohl, Barrash, True, & Alexander, 1989) involved administration of the Personality Diagnostic Questionnaire (PDQ) to male hypertensive outpatients. Although more than a fifth of the patients met the criteria for at least one personality disorder, the PDQ was *not* useful in identifying people who were at risk for noncompliance.

After reviewing the issue of noncompliance and personality traits, DiMatteo and DiNicola (1982, p. 120) concluded that "little evidence exists to implicate personality factors (in the sense of traits as unchangeable psychological characteristics) as causal agents in patient compliance." Since that date, little evidence has been reported to contradict this conclusion. Situational variables are much better predictors of compliance and noncompliance than are stable personality traits.

If personality traits did predict noncompliance, the same people should be noncompliant in a variety of situations. Again, little evidence supports this conclusion. On the contrary, some indications exist that noncompliance is specific to the situation. Lutz, Silbret, and Olshan (1983), for example, exposed a group of people experiencing intense pain to five different pain relief regimens and found that compli-

ance with one program was unrelated to compliance with the others. Orme and Binik (1989) obtained similar results, finding that adherence to one diabetic treatment regimen was independent of adherence to others. These researchers looked at diabetic patients' adherence to five different regimen demands: (1) weight control, (2) urine/blood testing, (3) medication taking, (4) symptom reporting, and (5) safety. They assessed adherence using several different measures, including reports by significant others, nurses, and physicians. Even though all regimens related to diabetic treatment, Orme and Binik found only a weak relationship among the different demands. They concluded that adherence was a function of the specific regimen and that no general personality characteristic exists that affects responses to different treatment demands. Thus, the evidence suggests that noncompliance is not a global personality trait and that the "noncompliant personality" is a myth.

Personal Beliefs

Although personality traits do not predict who will adhere to medical recommendations, some evidence suggests that patients' beliefs are related to compliance. We have seen that perceived self-efficacy, the theory of reasoned action, the precaution adoption process, and the health belief model all have some ability both to predict and to explain adherence and nonadherence. In general, when patients believe that adherence to treatment recommendations will result in health benefits, they are likely to comply with those recommendations. Data from Sackett and Haynes's 1976 review suggested that health beliefs might be a promising alternative to traditional personality traits in explaining adherence. Since that time, some evidence has pointed to personal beliefs as a strong predictor of compliance.

Brownlee-Duffeck et al. (1987) examined health beliefs and their effects on adherence to diabetic treatment regimens for both adults and adolescents. For adults, the belief that compliance will benefit one's health predicted adherence. For adolescents, however, the perceived health benefits of compliance were not important. Young diabetic patients have notoriously low levels of compliance, and this study suggested that even when they see the long-range value of following treatment recommendations they are not very likely to comply. Factors that did predict adolescents' rate of adherence were financial costs, perceived severity of the illness, and their belief that they were susceptible to diabetic complications if they did not follow their treatment regimen. Brownlee-Duffeck et al. concluded that older diabetics are able to see the long-range benefits of adherence whereas adolescent patients are more likely to adhere to their treatment regimen when they are experiencing immediate discomfort.

Some people cope with illness by denying personal vulnerability or by avoiding personal responsibility for taking actions that might restore health. These people use **avoidance coping** strategies to reduce the stress of being sick. They may smoke more, overeat, abuse alcohol or other drugs, or simply hope for a miracle. Such strategies are often effective for a short time, but in the long run they are usually hazardous to health. Sherbourne et al. (1992) found that, as might be expected, the best predictor of nonadherence to medical advice for hypertension, diabetes, and heart disease 2 years later was nonadherence at the beginning of the study. However, the next strongest predictor was an avoidance coping style. People who used avoidance coping were less likely than others to adhere to their doctor's advice, perhaps because they either denied the efficacy of such advice or because they rejected responsibility for their own health care.

Studies indicate that people are more likely to adhere to medical advice when they believe they are personally responsible for their own health. Helby, Gafarian, and McCann (1989) investigated situational and behavioral correlates of compliance with a diabetic regimen and found that patients who assumed responsibility for their health care were more likely to adhere to their treatment program. Similarly, Stanton (1987) found that one of the determinants of adherence to medical regimens by hypertensive patients was the belief that they exercised some personal control over both their blood pressure and their health. These studies suggest that adherence is enhanced when patients believe that their own actions will bring about a health benefit.

CULTURAL NORMS

One factor that definitely relates to compliance is the patient's cultural beliefs and attitudes. DiNicola and DiMatteo (1984) suggested that people fail to comply not because they have basically uncooperative personalities, but because they live within a culture that holds beliefs and attitudes, which the patients share, that are not conducive to adherence to health regimens. A number of studies have found that cultural norms are important factors in determining who is likely to comply. If one's family or tribal traditions include strong beliefs in the efficacy of witch doctors, for example, it seems reasonable that the individual's compliance with modern medical recommendations might be low. Zyazema (1984) interviewed people in Zimbabwe who were suffering from hypertension and diabetes and who were not adhering to their recommended therapies. As might be expected, many of these patients still believed in traditional healers, and they had little faith in modern medical procedures. Another example of the way cultural norms may affect treatment compliance was reported by Ruiz and Ruiz (1983), who found that Latino patients were more likely comply with medical advice when their physicians demonstrated some understanding of Hispanic cultural norms and practices. These findings have important implications for physicians and other health care providers whose clientele consists largely of people from many different cultural backgrounds.

THE PRACTITIONER-PATIENT INTERACTION

We have seen that both illness characteristics and personal characteristics are only minimally successful at predicting compliance with medical regimens. A more satisfactory group of predictors are those subsumed under the category of patient-practitioner interaction. Within this category are such factors as the verbal communication between health care provider and patient, the practitioner's perceived level of competence, the amount of time between referral and treatment, and the length of time patients must spend in the practitioner's waiting room.

Verbal Communication

Perhaps the most crucial factor in patient noncompliance is the insufficiency of verbal communication between the practitioner and the patient. Again, Paul's case illustrates this point. Because Paul recalled only vague and general information regarding diet and smoking, either his physician was remiss in detailing the precise healthful practices that Paul

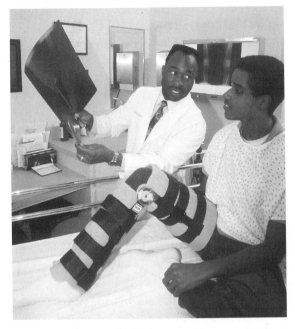

Patient compliance is high when practitioners convey information about the condition and the reasons for treatment.

was to follow, or Paul was less than receptive to the information—or perhaps both.

The miscommunication can start when physicians ask patients to report on their symptoms and fail to listen to patients' concerns. What constitutes a concern for the patient may not be essential to the diagnostic process, and practitioners can seem unconcerned when they are, in fact, trying to elicit information relevant to making a diagnosis. However, patients may misinterpret the physician's focus as a lack of personal concern or as overlooking what patients consider important symptoms. After practitioners come to a diagnosis, they typically tell patients about that diagnosis. If the diagnosis is minor, patients are relieved and not highly motivated to adhere to (or even listen to) any instructions that may follow. If the verdict is grave, patients are likely to become anxious, and this anxiety may then interfere with their concentration on subsequent medical advice.

As already noted, physicians tend to overestimate the level of patient compliance and to assume that their directions will be heard, understood, and acted on. Little evidence exists, however, to support this assumption, and research indicates that misunderstanding and miscommunication in conveying information and instructions can adversely affect compliance. For example, Fincham and Wertheimer (1986) found that noncompliant patients tended to blame their physician for not telling them specifically how to take their newly prescribed drug.

Even when patients are both highly motivated and reasonably relaxed, they may not understand the information they hear. For a variety of reasons, physicians and patients frequently do not speak the same language. First, physicians operate in familiar territory. They know the subject matter, are comfortable with the physical surroundings, and are ordinarily calm and relaxed with procedures that have become routine to them. Patients, in contrast, may be unfamiliar with medical terminology; distracted by the strange environs; and distressed by anxiety, fear, or pain. Differences in native language, educational level, or social class may also contribute to problems in communication.

How great is the problem of patient misunderstanding? Research indicates that patients either fail to remember or misunderstand about half the information given to them by their doctors. Svarstad (1976) reported that 52% of patients could not correctly report what their physician expected of them, and Ley and Spelman (1967) found that outpatients could not recall approximately 40% of what their physicians had told them 10 to 80 minutes earlier. Also, Boyd, Covington, Stanaszek, and Coussons (1974) reported that over 60% of the patients interviewed immediately after the visit with their doctors had misunderstood the directions concerning prescribed medications. Directions given orally, however, are not the only kind that are misunderstood. Williams et al. (1995) found that 42% of all patients and more than 80% of elderly patients at two public hospitals were unable to read and understand written basic medical instructions.

What types of verbal communication improve patient adherence? Research suggests that patients are most likely to comply when they are given information about their illness and reasons for their particular treatment regimen. Helby et al. (1989) found that diabetic patients were more compliant when they had sufficient information on diabetes. Similarly, Stanton (1987) found that one of the determinants of adherence by hypertensive patients was their knowledge of the hypertensive treatment program.

Rorer, Tucker, and Blake (1988) investigated long-term nurse-patient interactions and their effects on hemodialysis patients' compliance or noncompliance with their dietary regimen. As one would expect, emotionally negative responses by the nurses were significantly related to patient noncompliance. An emotionally negative response was defined as one that tended to make the nurse-patient relationship less cohesive or attractive to both nurse and patient. Interestingly, Rorer et al. found that emotionally positive verbal responses — those that made the nurse-patient relationship more cohesive — increased noncompliance! The researchers also found that more experienced nurses spent less time addressing the problem of patient noncompliance. Possibly more experienced health care providers have seen the futility of providing information on treatment regimens and thus spend less time talking to patients about compliance.

Evidence also exists that physicians either fail to recommend good health practices or their patients fail to understand their communication. For example, data from the Stanford Five-City Project (Frank, Winkleby, Altman, Rockhill, & Fortmann, 1991) indicated that only 50% of smokers said that their doctors had ever advised them either to stop smoking or to smoke less. Moreover, fewer than 4% of ex-smokers reported that their physicians had helped them to quit, which indicates that the overwhelming proportion of people who stop smoking do so without the aid of their physicians.

Russell and Roter (1993) studied health promotion advice from physicians during visits with patients who had a variety of chronic illnesses. They found that in 53% of the visits, physicians provided information or made suggestions about changes in patients' lifestyle and health behaviors. The most frequent suggestions were about diet and weight control, but physicians also mentioned exercise, stress, smoking, and alcohol. Unfortunately, physicians tended not to use the most effective behavioral strategies for getting their patients to adopt the suggested changes, leading Russell and Roter to conclude that physicians miss important opportunities to urge their patients to change unhealthy behaviors.

The Practitioner's Personal Characteristics

A second aspect of the practitioner-patient interaction is the perceived personal characteristics of the physician. As might be expected, patients' compliance improves as confidence in their physician's technical ability increases (Becker, Drachman, & Kirscht, 1972; Gilbar, 1989). In addition, several physician personality variables — as perceived by the patient — are related to compliance. DiNicola and DiMatteo (1984) reported that people were more likely to follow the advice of doctors who were seen as warm, caring, friendly, and interested in the welfare of patients. When physicians display a good bedside manner such as making eye contact, smiling, leaning forward, and even joking and laughing, patient compliance improves.

Although patients are more likely to adhere to recommendations from competent and knowledgeable physicians, they become less eager to comply when the physician's expertise is expressed in an authoritarian fashion. Gastorf and Galanos (1983) found that patients were more likely to remain noncompliant when they saw their doctors as authoritarian and when they felt as though they were treated as inferiors in the decision-making process. Also, Heszen-Klemens (1987) reported that doctors who take noncompliance personally and react defensively are more likely to have patients with low compliance rates. These studies suggest that compliance could be enhanced by warm and caring physicians who take an interest in their patients' health and who regard patients as partners in the treatment and prevention processes.

Research by Hall, Irish, Roter, Ehrlich, and Miller (1994) indicated that physicians' gender may play a role in the exchange of information between doctor and patient. They studied both female and male physicians during patient visits and found that female physicians made more partnership statements, made more positive statements, and asked more questions than male physicians. In addition, patients talked to female physicians more than to male physicians, and the gender of both physician and patient contributed to the communication pattern during the visit.

Effective patient-physician interaction also encourages the patient to volunteer information. Although many patients merely respond to their physicians' questions, research by Rost, Carter, and Innui (1989) found that compliance improved when patients both initiated information and provided it in answer to questions. Rost et al. referred to this interaction as *bidirectional* information and concluded that the physician's willingness to allow bidirectional information may contribute to a patient-doctor partnership that can arrive at meaningful treatment decisions.

Time Spent Waiting

Two final predictors of compliance are the length of time patients must wait to secure an appointment and the amount of time they must spend in the practitioner's waiting room. In both cases, the longer the wait, the greater is the probability of a patient's noncompliance. Davidson and Schrag (1969) found that compliance rates were not greatly affected by waiting-room delays up to 30 minutes. However, when patients are detained more than one hour, compliance rates dropped to 40% below those of patients who waited less than 30 minutes.

SUMMARY OF FACTORS THAT PREDICT ADHERENCE

In summary, disease characteristics are an unreliable predictor of adherence to medical recommendations. *Severity of the treatment's side effects* is a poor predictor of noncompliance because most people who discontinue medication do so for reasons other than unpleasant side effects. Also, *severity of the illness* is not a determinant of compliance, but severity as viewed by the patient—particularly with the boost of some personal pain or discomfort—is directly related to the probability of the patient's complying with medical regimens. *Duration of treatment* seems to be directly related to noncompliance, although some evidence suggests that people discontinue a lengthy treatment not so much because of its duration but because they experience no uncomfortable symptoms. *Complexity of treatment* is inversely related to compliance, particularly when noncompliance is measured in terms of the number of errors a patient makes in taking prescribed medication. Table 8.1 shows the inconsistency of the relationship between disease characteristics and rate of patients' adherence.

On the whole, *personal characteristics* are only marginally satisfactory predictors of adherence. Age

has an inconsistent relationship with compliance. Young and very old adults are least likely to adhere to a regular schedule for cancer screening tests, and young diabetics become less compliant with their prescribed treatment as they advance through adolescence. As for *gender,* men and women are about equal in adherence to exercise programs, but women are more likely to eat vegetables and less likely to resist taking medication. *Social support*—defined as quality of emotional support—predicts compliance, but quantity or number of friends is not a reliable predictor. People who lack emotional support have higher rates of nonadherence than people with adequate social support. Currently, no evidence exists that certain *personality traits* are more likely to be noncompliers, but *personal beliefs* that one's own behavior can produce a health benefit is positively related to adherence. *Cultural norms,* as they influence a person's beliefs about illness and treatment, are positively related to compliance.

Table 8.1 also summarizes the findings concerning compliance and *patient-practitioner interaction.* Lack of accurate *verbal communication* between physician and patient is probably the most serious problem in patient compliance; many patients fail to understand or fail to remember instructions. *Personal qualities of the physician,* as seen by the patient, are also related to noncompliance. Unfriendly, uninterested, and authoritarian doctors are not heeded as well as warm and caring ones, and female physicians are usually better at eliciting compliance than male physicians. Finally, *delays* in getting an appointment or in waiting in the office or clinic are both negatively related to good adherence. Delayed attention may well be seen as indicating the doctor's lack of interest in and low personal regard for the patient.

REASONS FOR NONADHERENCE

After his heart attack, Paul's physician told him, "Well, I guess we're going to have to get you off those damned weeds." This statement may have been meant as a requirement to quit smoking, but Paul interpreted it as a mere comment. Unfortunately, many patients leave the doctor's office still unclear about their instructions and with no specific plan for carrying out their medical regimen. Vagueness of physician advice is one of the communication problems

Table 8.1   Predictors of patient adherence

	Findings	Studies
I. *Disease Characteristics*		
A. *Severity of side effects*	No relationship	Masur, 1981
B. *Severity of illness*		
(As seen by the physician)	No relationship	Haynes, 1979a; Vincent 1971
(As seen by the patient)	Positive relationship	Becker & Maiman, 1980
C. *Duration of treatment*	Negative relationship	Haynes, 1976a
D. *Complexity of treatment*	Complexity leads to nonadherence, as does number of doses over 3	Cramer, et al., 1989; Haynes, 1979a
II. *Personal Characteristics*		
A. *Age*		
Adults		
(exercise up to 6 months)	Positive relationship	Lynch et al., 1992
(exercise after 6 months)	No relationship	Lynch et al., 1992
(cancer screening)	Curvilinear relationship	Thomas et al., 1995
(diabetes)	Positive relationship	Sherbourne et al., 1992
(heart disease)	Positive relationship	Sherbourne et al., 1992
Adolescents		
(diabetes)	Negative relationship	Bond et al., 1992
B. *Gender*		
(exercise)	Men and women equal	Ward & Morgan, 1984
(diet)	Women more compliant	Laforge et al., 1994
(medication)	Women more compliant	Sellwood & Tarrier, 1994
C. *Social support*	Positive relationship	Bovbjerg et al., 1995; Christensen et al., 1992; Sherwood, 1983; Thomas et al., 1995
D. *Emotional support*	Positive relationship	Kulik & Mahler, 1993; Sherbourne et al., 1992
E. *Personality traits*	No relationship	Kabat-Zinn & Chapman-Waldrop, 1988; Pfohl et al., 1989
F. *Patients' beliefs*		
Avoidance coping	Negative relationship	Sherbourne et al., 1992
Personal control	Positive relationship	Helby et al., 1989; Stanton, 1987
III. *Cultural Norms*	Patients' cultural beliefs predict compliance	Ruiz & Ruiz, 1983; Zyazema, 1984
IV. *Practitioner/Patient Interaction*		
A. *Verbal communication*	Positive relationship	Fincham & Wertheimer, 1986; Frank et al., 1991; Russell & Roter, 1993
B. *Practitioner's personal qualities*		
Friendliness	Predicts compliance	DiNicola & DiMatteo, 1984
Gender	Women provide more information	Hall et al., 1994
Communication skills	Positive relationship	Rost et al., 1989
C. *Delays*		
Getting an appointment	Negative relationship	Davidson & Schrag, 1969
In the waiting room	Negative relationship	Davidson & Schrag, 1969

between patient and physician, but it is only one of several reasons people fail to follow medical advice.

One reason for high rates of nonadherence is that the current definition of adherence demands certain difficult lifestyle changes. At the beginning of the 20th century, when the leading causes of illness and death were infectious disease, compliance was simpler. Patients were compliant when they followed the doctor's advice with regard to medication, rest, diet, and so on. With health restored, patients could return to their former way of living. Adherence is no longer a matter of taking the proper pills and following short-term advice. The three leading causes of death in the United States—cardiovascular disease, cancer, and chronic obstructive lung disease—are all affected by unhealthy lifestyles. Thus compliance, broadly defined, currently includes adherence to healthy and safe behaviors as part of an ongoing lifestyle. To be compliant, people must now avoid cigarette smoking, use alcohol wisely or not at all, eat properly, and exercise regularly. In addition, of course, they must also make and keep medical and dental appointments, listen with understanding to the advice of health care providers, and finally, follow that advice. These requirements present a complex array of requirements that are difficult to fulfill.

The second category of reasons for nonadherence includes all those problems inherent in hearing and heeding physicians' advice. Patients may reject the prescribed regimen as being too difficult, time-consuming, or expensive, or they may reject the practitioner as being incompetent, arrogant, or unfriendly. Also, many patients stop taking their medication when their symptoms disappear. Paradoxically, others stop because they begin to feel worse and thus believe the medication is useless. Still others, in squirrel-like fashion, save a few pills for the next time they get sick.

Responsibility for adherence rests with both the patient and the health care professional, and both contribute to patients' noncompliant behavior. Faberow (1986) suggested that some noncompliance can be seen as patients' indirect self-destructive behavior. Orme and Binik (1989) found that many patients had no clue about their physician's criteria for specific adherence. Fincham and Wertheimer (1986) reported that noncompliant patients frequently felt that doctors prescribed too many drugs. Hunt, Jor-

dan, Irwin, and Browner (1989) found that three-fourths of their patients who sought treatment for nondebilitating complaints stopped taking their medication after 4 months, because adherence was too much trouble and did not fit into the routine of their daily lives. Brock and Wartman (1990) suggested that normally competent patients often make irrational choices about adherence because they have an *optimistic bias* that they will be spared the grave consequences of noncompliance. Similarly, Sherbourne et al. (1992) suggested that some patients fail to follow medical advice because they hope for a miracle.

Other patients may be noncompliant because prescription labels are too difficult to read. Mustard and Harris (1989) found that fewer than half the college students they studied were able to correctly understand prescription labels that had been randomly selected from a pharmacist's records. Millard, Waranch, and McEntee (1992) found that nearly 80% of the noncompliers who refused to chew nicotine gum simply did not like its taste. Table 8.2 summarizes some of the reasons given by patients for nonadherence to medical advice.

DOES ADHERENCE PAY OFF?

We have seen that at least half of all patients do not fully follow their health care practitioner's advice and that patients give a variety of reasons for nonadherence. In addition, most health care providers view noncompliance as a serious problem and an obstacle to the prevention of disease and the restoration of health. Is such concern justified? Does adherence pay off?

Evidence for the efficacy of adherence is not clearcut; some studies have shown that compliance pays off whereas others have suggested that it does not. Results of studies from the National Heart, Lung, and Blood Institute's Beta-Blocker Heart Attack Trial indicated that heart patients who took their prescribed medication were less likely to have died from all causes than those patients who did not. Gallagher, Viscoli, and Horwitz (1993) followed female heart patients who were good adherers and those who were poor adherers, examining their rates of death from all causes. The researchers randomly

Table 8.2   Reasons given by patients for not complying with medical advice

"It's too much trouble."

"I won't get sick. God will save me."

"I just didn't get the prescription filled."

"The medication was too expensive."

"The medication didn't work very well. I was still sick, so I stopped taking it."

"The medication worked after only one week, so I stopped taking it."

"I have too many pills to take."

"I forgot."

"I want to remain sick."

"I don't want to become addicted to pills."

"If one pill is good, then two pills should be twice as good."

"I saved some pills for the next time I get sick."

"I gave some of my pills to my husband so he won't get sick."

"They're trying to poison me."

"This doctor doesn't know as much as my other doctor."

"The medication makes me sick."

"The medication tastes bad."

"Taking medication is just another bad habit."

"I was hoping for a miracle."

"I don't see any reason to take something to prevent illness."

"My doctor prescribes too many pills. I don't need all of them."

"I don't like my doctor. She thinks she knows everything."

"I didn't understand my doctor's instructions and was too embarrassed to ask him to repeat them."

"I don't like the taste of nicotine chewing gum."

"I won' t get very sick anyway, so I don't need to take anything."

"I didn't understand the directions on the label."

assigned more than 600 women who had suffered a heart attack to either a heart medication group or a placebo group. After 26 months, women who were poor adherers were nearly two and a half times more likely to have died than women who were good adherers. The effect of compliance was independent of age, severity of the heart attack, congestive heart failure, marital status, smoking history, and other factors. Earlier, Horwitz et al. (1990) had reported much the same findings for over 2,000 men who were part of the same study. Men low in compliance were more than 2.6 times as likely to have died than men high in adherence.

These two studies demonstrate a significant relationship between adherence and survival following a heart attack, but they do not prove that good ad-

herence to the medical regimen prevented death from heart disease. Interestingly, the poor adherers in both studies had a greater risk of death whether they were in the heart medication group or in the placebo group. Women who took no heart medication but who were poor adherers to the placebo were 2.8 times more likely to have died than women in the placebo group who were good adherers. Noncompliant men in the placebo group were 2.5 times as likely to have died than compliant men in the placebo group. These findings suggest that noncompliance itself may contribute to all-cause mortality. Perhaps noncompliant people are not conscientious and have little regard for their own health. As noted earlier, researchers have not yet detected any global personality trait that reliably predicts compliance or noncompliance, but the Gallagher et al. (1993) and the Horwitz et al. (1990) studies suggest that either the power of the placebo is much stronger than earlier studies indicated or that some heart patients do not protect themselves well from a variety of potentially fatal conditions.

Other studies have failed to show any strong positive association between faithful adherence and improved health. For example, in a study of social support, compliance, and cardiac health, Kulik and Mahler (1993) found that although social support predicted compliance, it was not related to subsequent cardiac health of male heart patients.

In a larger study, Hays et al. (1994) followed over 2,000 adult patients with hypertension, diabetes, myocardial infarction, congestive heart failure, depression, or some combination of these conditions. They found that after 4 years, patients' ratings of their health improvements were only minimally related to their adherence to medical advice. Of the 132 comparisons these researchers examined, only 11 showed a significant positive association between adherence and health outcome. (Chance alone would yield about seven significant findings.) The relationships among health and adherence were complex and not always consistent with what the researchers hypothesized. The strongest positive relationship was between adherence to diet in insulin-using diabetics and subsequent ratings of positive health, but some negative relationships appeared between adherence and health. That is, the higher the compliance to their medication schedule, the lower the ratings of health for insulin-using diabetics and for depressed patients. Hays et al. hypothesized that people with these disorders might have rated their health as worsening because of the side effects they experienced when they took their medication as prescribed.

Hays et al. suggested four possible explanations for their finding of a generally poor relationship between adherence and improved health. First, their study relied on patient self-reports of adherence, so some errors may have existed in the assessment of compliance; second, physician advice may have been quite vague, a condition we discussed earlier; third, 4 years may not have been enough time to observe the results of continual noncompliance; and fourth, other factors, such as heredity or environ-

mental conditions, may have affected the course of the illnesses. Somewhat pessimistically, Hays et al. (1994, p. 356) stated: "We cannot conclude from these data that assisting patients with these conditions to adhere to their physicians' recommendations will necessarily lead to better health over time." They added that adherence to unproved medical recommendations may be a questionable practice and concluded that "it may be time to turn the focus toward documenting what really works in medicine rather than spotlighting the failure of patients to follow recommendations that may or may not be therapeutic" (p. 357).

IMPROVING ADHERENCE

Although faithful adherence may not pay off in terms of better health, psychologists and physicians are still interested in improving compliance. Haynes (1976b) divided the methods for improving compliance into educational and behavioral strategies. Educational procedures are those that impart information, sometimes in an emotion-arousing manner designed to frighten the noncompliant patient into becoming compliant. Included with educational strategies are such procedures as health education messages, individual patient counseling with various professional health care providers, programmed instruction, lectures, demonstrations, and individual counseling accompanied by written instructions. Behavioral strategies, on the other hand, focus more directly on changing the person's behaviors involved in compliance. They include a wide variety of techniques, such as reducing economic barriers to compliance, using reward to reinforce compliance, notifying patients of upcoming appointments, simplifying medical schedules, making home visits, and persistently monitoring and rewarding the patients' compliant behaviors.

In 1976, when Haynes reviewed the literature on educational, behavioral, and combined educational-behavioral strategies for improving compliance, he found educational techniques to be relatively ineffective. Of 16 studies reviewed, only 7 reported significant results. Interventions that threaten patients with disastrous consequences for noncompliance are only marginally effective in bringing about a meaningful change in their personal behavior.

Behavioral techniques proved to be more effective in improving patient compliance. Haynes (1976b) reviewed 20 studies that had employed various behavioral strategies and found that 16 of them had reported a significant and positive effect on compliance. When he examined studies that had combined educational and behavioral approaches, Haynes found that all eight had reported significant results. According to Haynes's review, therefore, both behavioral strategies and combination approaches have an advantage over educational procedures. Although Haynes's definition of behavioral strategies was quite broad, it appears from his review that those techniques attempting to increase patient involvement and to encourage an active, ongoing relationship between patient and practitioner are likely to improve patient compliance. Behavioral approaches had the advantage even though educational strategies increased patients' knowledge and improved their skill in taking medication. People, it seems, do not misbehave because they do not know better but because proper behavior, for a variety of reasons, is less appealing.

When Haynes (1979c) later reviewed the literature, he found that educational approaches were even less effective in improving compliance than he had reported 3 years earlier. In his 1979 review, he examined studies that had employed such strategies as programmed instruction, lectures, demonstrations, personal instruction, and personal counseling. Although these educational programs increased patients' knowledge about their disease, none of the studies reported an improvement in either patient compliance or in therapeutic outcome.

In 1987, Haynes, Wang, and da Mota Gomes reviewed the literature on interventions designed to improve adherence and found only two well-designed studies that were able to increase compliance with short-term treatments (1 to 2 weeks in duration). These studies suggested that short-term compliance can be improved to some extent by reducing the prescribed dose to one or two times a day and by giving patients special pill packages and calendars that indicate when and how many pills they should take. Short-term compliance, of course, is easier to achieve than compliance that must continue over a long period.

Later, Haynes and his associates (Macharia et al., 1992) searched the literature for articles on compliance and appointment keeping. They found 23 articles with "scientific merit" that also included an intervention for improving compliance. These studies used a variety of strategies to improve patients' compliance with keeping appointments, including letter and telephone prompts, computer-generated messages to the physician that identified patients who would be visiting the clinic, patient contracts, and educational information. Once again, education was not an effective means of improving adherence, but most of the other interventions were of limited value. For example, contracts improved compliance by about 14%, an increase very typical of the other interventions.

The ineffectiveness of educational and instructional procedures has instigated a growing interest in various behavioral and cognitive strategies for improving patient compliance. These interventions include self-monitoring, home visits, cues and rewards, and peer group discussions. Haynes et al. (1987) found that cues and rewards seem to be the most consistently effective means of improving compliance. Cues include using one's toothbrush or a completed meal as a signal to take one's medication. Rewards might include small sums of money given by the health care provider, or self-reinforcement, such as seeing a movie or treating oneself to a nice meal. Both cues and rewards have been shown to increase the chances that patients will take their prescribed medication.

DiMatteo and DiNicola (1982) recommended four behavioral strategies for improving adherence. First, various *prompts* can be used to remind patients to initiate health-enhancing behaviors. These prompts may be cued by regular events in the patient's life, such as taking medication before each meal, or they may take the form of telephone calls from a clinic to remind the person to keep an appointment or to refill a prescription. A second behavioral strategy, *tailoring the regimen,* involves fitting the treatment to the "habits and rituals, times and places in the individual's daily life" (DiMatteo & DiNicola, 1982, p. 233). Third, these authors suggested a *graduated regimen implementation* that reinforces successive approximations to the desired behavior. Such shaping procedures should be effective with exercise and diet, but of course they are not appropriate to the taking of medications. The final behavioral strategy listed by DiMatteo and DiNicola was a *contingency contract,* an agreement (usually written) between patients and the health care professionals that provides for some kind of reward to patients contingent on their achieving compliance. The ultimate goal of each of these approaches is self-regulation. However, before reaching this goal, patients often need help from others. This outside help, whether from family members or from professionals, ordinarily is given extensively at first and then is gradually withdrawn as patients begin to acquire more control over their health-related behaviors.

Cognitive-behavioral interventions are aimed at improving patients' knowledge of their disease and the consequences of nonadherence to treatment. They also attempt to enhance patients' social support and to increase their self-efficacy for adherence to healthy behaviors. Cognitive-behavioral strategies include training patients to monitor their health-related behaviors, to evaluate those behaviors against a predetermined criterion, and to use positive self-reinforcement for any progress toward meeting the criterion. Several studies have demonstrated the effectiveness of cognitive-behavioral methods in improving patient compliance with a variety of health and medical regimens, including exercise (Atkins, Kaplan, Timms, Reinsch, & Lofback, 1984; Duncan & McAuley, 1993; McAuley, 1993), lithium treatment for bipolar disorders (Cochran, 1984), and weight control for hemodialysis patients (Hegel et al., 1992).

In addition to behavioral and cognitive-behavioral strategies to improve compliance, several novel but simple interventions have shown promising results. Obtaining a *verbal commitment* from mothers increased their adherence to the recommended medical regimen for their children (Kulik & Carlino, 1987). Also, the simple process of a *service fee* for missed appointments was effective in decreasing missed appointments at a college health center (Wesch, Lutzker, Frisch, & Dillon, 1987). *Hypnosis* can be effective in initiating and maintaining dental flossing by college students, increasing the rate from

15% to 67% of students who flossed daily after 8 months (Kelly, McKinty, & Carr, 1988). Hypnosis can also improve compliance in adolescent diabetics who previously showed poor control of their blood glucose (Ratner, Gross, Casas, & Castells, 1990). Finally, an instructional audiotape helped undergraduate women improve their proficiency at breast self-examination (Jones et al., 1993). Although these studies generally used few participants and lacked rigorous controls, they point to potentially promising means of improving patient adherence.

Haynes et al. (1987) proposed several other means of improving adherence to medical recommendations. For all treatment regimens, they suggested that the prescription should be as simple as possible and that patients should receive clearly written instructions on the exact behaviors to follow. For long-term treatments, these authors recommended reminders, rewards, and social support. More specifically, they suggested that health care providers can increase compliance by (1) calling patients who miss an appointment, (2) providing medication that fits easily into a patient's daily schedule, (3) reinforcing the importance of adherence at each visit, (4) tailoring the number of visits to fit the patient's level of compliance, (5) verbally rewarding the patient's efforts to comply, (6) decreasing the frequency of visits as a reward for good adherence, and (7) involving the patient's spouse or other partner.

CHAPTER SUMMARY

Adherence is the extent to which a person's behavior coincides with appropriate medical and health advice. Rates of nonadherence range widely, but in general, about 50% of medical advice goes unheeded.

Several theoretical models attempt to predict and explain compliant and noncompliant behavior. These include the *biomedical model,* which simply looks for demographic and disease characteristics that relate to adherence; the *behavioral model,* which relies on contingency contracts and reinforcement for compliant behaviors; various cognitive learning theories, such as the *self-efficacy model,* which holds that people's beliefs that they can perform certain behaviors strongly predict what behaviors they will enact; the *theory of reasoned action,* which assumes that intentions, attitudes, subjective norms, and motivation predict adherence; and various *health belief models,* which typically include perceived severity of the disease, perceived personal susceptibility, costs/benefits ratio, and perceived barriers to incorporating adherence behaviors into one's lifestyle. Each of these models has some use in predicting and explaining compliance and noncompliance.

Researchers have found little evidence that certain disease and personal characteristics predict compliance. Neither severity of the disease as seen by the physician nor severity of the side effects of the disease are reliable predictors of adherence. Also, no evidence exists that personality traits relate to compliant behavior.

On the other hand, researchers have found some evidence for each of the following predictors of *noncompliance:* (1) long and complicated treatment regimens; (2) lack of social support for adherence; (3) patients' perception of the severity of their illness; (4) patients' cultural beliefs that modern medicine is ineffective; (5) patient's beliefs that their own behavior cannot benefit their health; (6) poor patient-practitioner communication; (7) unfriendly, incompetent, or authoritarian physicians; (8) delays in securing an appointment; and (9) long waiting-room delays.

There are probably as many reasons for noncompliance as there are noncomplying patients, and many of these reasons are difficult to determine with certainty. However, some of these reasons relate to the difficulty of altering lifestyles of long duration. Others result from incomplete practitioner-patient communication, which leaves the patient with erroneous beliefs as to what course of action to follow.

Although many physicians regard nonadherence as a major detriment to people's health, research has failed to find a significant benefit to high levels of compliance. Nevertheless, psychologists have suggested a variety of behavioral strategies to improve compliance, and a combination of these interventions usually increases compliance rates. Effective programs frequently include clearly written instructions, simple prescriptions, follow-up calls for missed appointments, prescriptions tailored to the patient's daily schedule, rewards for compliant behavior, cues to signal the time for taking medication, and involvement of the patient's spouse or support network.

SUGGESTED READINGS

DiMatteo, M. R. (1994). Enhancing patient adherence to medical recommendations. *Journal of the American Medical Association, 271,* 79, 83. In this brief report, DiMatteo reviews the frequency of nonadherence, looks at factors that determine noncompliance, and recommends a cooperative relationship between patient and health care provider.

Hays, R. D., Kravitz, R. L., Mazel, R. M., Sherbourne, C. D., DiMatteo, M. R., Rogers, W. H., & Greenfield, S. (1994). The impact of patient adherence on health outcomes for patients with chronic disease in the Medical Outcomes Study. *Journal of Behavioral Medicine, 17,* 347–360. Does compliance pay off with increased health benefits? This study presents evidence that improved compliance may not result in improved health.

Macharia, W. M., Leon, G., Rowe, B. H., Stephenson, B. J., & Haynes, R. B. (1992). An overview of interventions to improve compliance with appointment keeping for medical services. *Journal of the American Medical Association, 267,* 1813–1817. A comprehensive review of recent research of compliance and appointment keeping, this report suggests methods by which physicians can improve their patients' compliance.

Sherbourne, C. D., Hays, R. D., Ordway, L., DiMatteo, M. R., & Kravitz, R. L. (1992). Antecedents of adherence to medical recommendations: Results from the Medical Outcomes Study. *Journal of Behavioral Medicine, 15,* 447–468. This longitudinal study of patients with three different diseases presents an overview of the various factors that predict compliance and noncompliance.

Identifying Behavioral Factors in Cardiovascular Disease

Jason was determined that he would not undergo coronary bypass surgery, saying, "They're not going to take a vein out of my leg and put it in my heart. No way. I don't care if I die." Jason was not an immediate candidate for cardiac surgery who was refusing treatment but a 15-year-old adolescent whose father had undergone this procedure. The details of the surgery had made a dramatic impression on Jason, and he had become better acquainted with the risk factors for cardiovascular disease than most 15-year-olds.

Despite Jason's determination to avoid cardiovascular disease, he is at increased risk from several sources. Jason's father developed heart disease in his early 40s, and this hereditary factor places Jason at increased risk. His African American ethnic background is another factor that increases his risk, with African Americans experiencing cardiovascular disease and death at higher rates than European Americans (Rogers, 1992; U.S. Bureau of the Census [USBC], 1995).

Although Jason knows that changing certain behaviors would lower his risk for heart disease, he refuses to consider such options. He says that he has no intention of restricting his diet by avoiding high-fat or salty foods. He plans to eat what he wants, and if he has a heart attack, then he has a heart attack. He is, however, strongly opposed to smoking, has felt no urge to experiment with cigarettes, and ridicules those who do. His attitudes about drinking are not as extreme, but he does not drink and feels that he will never be a smoker or a drinker.

Jason is competitive and impatient. His competitive attitude appears in his interactions with his peers and in his motivation for success. He is outgoing and likes to be the center of attention, and his wit allows him to achieve this goal often. However, he sometimes uses his wit to score points at others' expense. His motivation to succeed has not led to outstanding grades, but success in a career (which he has not yet chosen) is very important. Jason believes that success, defined as making a lot of money, is very important. He cannot imagine being happy as an adult without career success and a comfortable life.

Jason's impatience extends to himself as well as to others. His impatience with himself occurs mostly when he cannot meet the high standards he has set for himself. Despite variable academic performance, Jason has a great deal of academic ability, and he judges his own performance critically. He is also critical of others who are less intellectually capable than he and who cannot keep up with his verbal wit. The tendency to be openly critical of others and to use his wit to cut down others restricts his circle of friends to a few who enjoy his intelligence and sense of humor. However, Jason's parents are supportive and encouraging.

This chapter examines the behavioral risks for cardiovascular disease—the most frequent cause of disease in the United States—and looks at Jason's risk from inherent and behavioral factors. But first it describes the cardiovascular system and methods of measuring cardiovascular function.

THE CARDIOVASCULAR SYSTEM

The cardiovascular system pumps blood throughout the body, providing a rapid-transport system for oxygen and nutrients and for the disposal of wastes. During normal functioning, the cardiovascular, respiratory, and digestive systems are integrated: The digestive system produces nutrients and the respiratory system furnishes oxygen, both of which circulate through the blood to various parts of the body. In addition, the endocrine system affects the cardiovascular system by stimulating or depressing the rate of cardiovascular activity. Although the cardiovascular system can be analyzed in isolation, it does not function that way.

This section briefly considers the functioning of the cardiovascular system, concentrating on the physiology underlying cardiovascular disease. The cardiovascular system comprises the heart and the blood vessels. By contracting and relaxing, the heart muscle pumps blood that circulates through the body. The circulation of blood allows the transport of oxygen to body cells and the removal of carbon dioxide and other wastes from cells. The entire circuit takes about 20 seconds when the body is at rest (Davis & Park, 1981), but exertion speeds the process.

The blood's route through the body is pictured in Figure 9.1. Blood travels from the right ventricle of

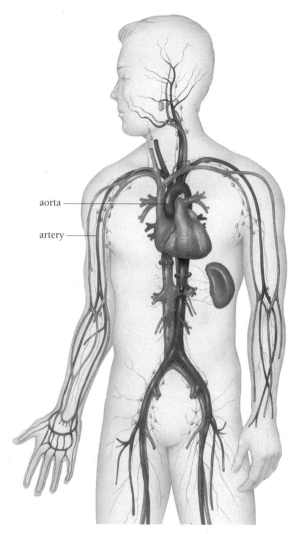

Figure 9.1 *The circulatory system.*
SOURCE: From Ingraham & Ingraham, 1995, p. 671.

the heart to the lungs, where hemoglobin (one of the components of blood) becomes saturated with oxygen. From the lungs, oxygenated blood travels back to the left atrium of the heart, then to the left ventricle, and finally out to the rest of the body. The **arteries** that carry the oxygenated blood branch into vessels of smaller and smaller diameter, called **arterioles**, and finally terminate in tiny **capillaries** that connect arteries and **veins**. Oxygen diffuses out to body cells, and carbon dioxide and other chemical

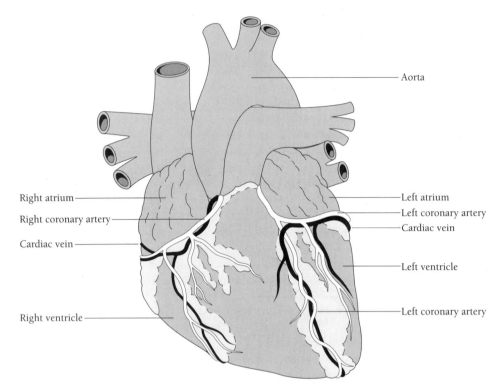

Figure 9.2   Coronary arteries.

wastes pass into the blood so they may be disposed. Blood that has been stripped of its oxygen returns to the heart by way of the system of veins, beginning with the tiny **venules** and ending with the two large veins that empty into the right atrium, the upper right chamber of the heart.

THE CORONARY ARTERIES

The blood supply to the heart muscle, the **myocardium**, is furnished by coronary arteries (see Figure 9.2). The two principal coronary arteries branch off from the aorta, the main artery that carries oxygenated blood from the heart. Left and right coronary arteries divide into smaller branches, providing the blood supply to the myocardium.

With each beat, the heart makes a slight twisting motion, which moves the coronary arteries. The coronary arteries, therefore, receive a great deal of strain as part of their normal function. This movement of the heart has been hypothesized to almost inevitably cause injury to the coronary arteries (Friedman & Rosenman, 1974). This damage can heal in two different ways. The preferable route involves the formation of small amounts of scar tissue and results in no serious problem. The second route involves the formation of **atheromatous plaques**, deposits composed of cholesterol and other lipids (fats), connective tissue, and muscle tissue. The plaques grow and calcify into a hard, bony substance that thickens the arterial walls. The formation of plaques and the resulting occlusion of the arteries is called **atherosclerosis**, shown in Figure 9.3.

A related but different problem is **arteriosclerosis**, or the loss of elasticity of the arteries. The beating of the heart pushes blood through the arteries with great force, and arterial elasticity allows adaptation to this pressure. Loss of elasticity tends to make the cardiovascular system less capable of tolerating increases in cardiac blood volume. Hence, a potential danger exists during strenuous exercise for people with arteriosclerosis.

The formation of arterial plaques (atherosclerosis) and the "hardening" of the arteries (arterioscle-

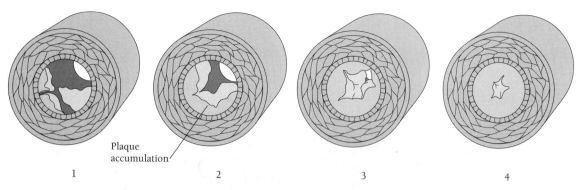

Plaque
accumulation

1   2   3   4

Figure 9.3 *Progressive atherosclerosis.*

rosis) often occur together. Both can affect any artery in the cardiovascular system, but when the coronary arteries are affected, the heart's oxygen supply may be threatened.

CORONARY HEART DISEASE

Coronary heart disease (CHD) arises as a result of atherosclerosis and arteriosclerosis in the coronary arteries. No clearly visible, outward symptoms accompany the buildup of plaques in the coronary arteries; CHD can be developing while a person remains totally unaware of its progress. However, the plaques narrow the arteries and restrict the supply of blood to the myocardium. In addition, blood platelets tend to stick to the plaques, and the blood clots form around the plaques. These blood clots can transform the partially obstructed artery into a completely closed one. Restriction of blood flow is called **ischemia.** If the coronary arteries do not allow enough blood to reach the heart muscle, the heart, like any other organ or tissue deprived of oxygen, will not function properly.

One possible result of restriction of the blood supply to the myocardium is **angina pectoris**, a disorder whose symptoms include a crushing pain in the chest and difficulty in breathing. Angina is usually precipitated by exercise or stress because these conditions increase demand to the heart. With oxygen restriction, the reserve capacity of the cardiovascular system is reduced, and heart disease becomes evident. The uncomfortable symptoms of angina rarely last more than a few minutes, but angina is a sign of obstruction in the coronary arteries.

One approach to the treatment of CHD is surgery and the replacement of the coronary arteries. Bypass surgery replaces the blocked portion of the coronary artery (or arteries) with grafts of healthy veins, usually taken from the patient's leg. The surgeon attaches these grafts so that blood flows through the replacements, bypassing the blocked sections of the coronary arteries (see Figure 9.4). This treatment is generally successful in relieving angina and improving the patient's quality of life.

The number of bypass operations has increased dramatically during the past 25 years, but use of the procedure remains controversial. Bypass surgery is expensive and potentially life threatening, and it may not extend the patient's life significantly (Kolata, 1983). The disease processes that led to blockage of the coronary arteries can also lead to obstruction of the replacement vessels. Therefore, people who have coronary bypass surgery may redevelop CHD, and these patients must change their lifestyle if they are to prevent blockage of the replacement arteries.

Complete blockage of either coronary artery shuts off the blood flow and thus the oxygen supply to the myocardium. Like other tissue, the myocardium cannot survive without oxygen; therefore, coronary blockage results in the death of myocardial tissue, an infarction. **Myocardial infarction** is commonly referred to as a heart attack. During myocardial infarction, the damage may be so extensive as to completely disrupt the heartbeat. In less severe cases, heart contractions may become less effective. The signals for a myocardial infarction include a feeling of weakness or dizziness combined with nausea, cold sweating, difficulty in breathing, and a sensation of

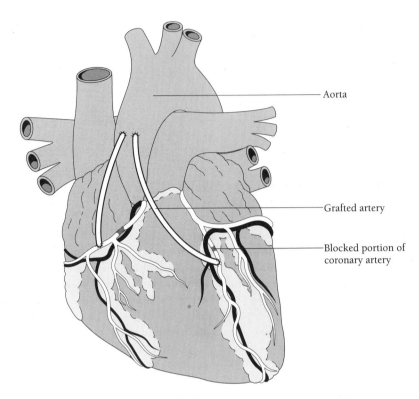

Figure 9.4 Coronary bypass.

crushing or squeezing pain in the chest, arms, shoulders, jaw, or back. Rapid loss of consciousness or death may occur, but the victim sometimes remains quite alert throughout the experience. The severity of symptoms depends on the extent of damage to the heart muscle.

Both angina pectoris and myocardial infarction are typically the result of atherosclerosis, which is most dangerous when it involves the coronary arteries. Continued thickening of the arterial walls restricts the flow of blood, causing angina. If the restriction is severe, heart tissue may die and the heart beat will be disrupted; that is, the person will experience a myocardial infarction.

In those people who survive a myocardial infarction (somewhat more than half do), the damaged portion of the myocardium will not regrow or repair itself. Instead, scar tissue forms at the infarcted area. Scar tissue does not have the elasticity and function of healthy tissue, so a heart attack lessens the capacity of the heart to pump blood efficiently. A myocardial infarction can limit the type and vigor of activi-

ties that a person can safely do, prompting some lifestyle changes. Frequently, these changes result from cardiac patients' uncertainty about which activities are safe and fears about suffering another attack. Such fears have some basis. The coronary artery disease that caused a first attack can cause another, but future infarctions are not a certainty.

The process of cardiac rehabilitation often involves psychologists, who help cardiac patients adjust their lifestyle to minimize risk factors and lessen the chances of future attacks. Preventing heart attack and furnishing cardiac rehabilitation is a major task for the health care system because heart disease is the most frequent cause of death in the United States. This chapter discusses the development and prevention of cardiovascular disease, and Chapter 11 discusses cardiac rehabilitation programs.

STROKE

Atherosclerosis and arteriosclerosis can also affect the arteries that serve the head and neck, thereby restricting the blood supply to the brain. Plaques may become detached from the artery wall, or one of the blood clots that tend to form on plaques may detach and flow through the circulatory system. Any obstruction in the arteries of the brain will restrict or completely stop the flow of blood to the area of the brain served by that portion of the system. A piece of material too small to obstruct an arteriole might completely block a capillary. Oxygen deprivation causes the death of brain tissue within 3 to 5 minutes. This damage to the brain resulting from lack of oxygen is called a **stroke**, the third most frequent cause of death in the United States. But strokes have other causes as well — for example, a blood clot, a bubble of air (air embolism), or infection that impedes blood flow in the brain may also result in a stroke. The arteries serving the brain may be affected by atherosclerosis, which may also impede blood flow to the brain. In addition, the weakening of artery walls associated with arteriosclerosis may lead to an *aneurysm,* a sac formed by the ballooning of a weakened artery wall. Aneurysms may burst, causing a stroke or death.

A stroke damages neurons in the brain, and these neurons have no capacity to replace themselves. Therefore, death of any neuron results in the permanent loss of its function. The brain, however, contains billions of neurons. Rarely do people suffer from strokes that kill *all* neurons controlling a particular function. More commonly, some of the neurons devoted to a particular function are lost, impairing brain function. The remaining healthy neural tissue compensates somewhat, even though no neurons are replaced. For example, one specific area of the brain controls speech production. If this area is completely damaged by a stroke, the victim can no longer speak (but can still comprehend speech). A stroke that damages some of the neurons in this area results in partial loss of fluency and perhaps some difficulty in speaking. The extent of the loss is related to the amount of damage to the area; more extensive damage results in greater impairment. This same principle applies to other types of disabilities caused by stroke. Damage may be so extensive — or in such a critical area — as to bring about immediate death; or damage may be so slight as to go unnoticed.

Degenerative diseases of the cardiovascular system, such as atherosclerosis and arteriosclerosis, are not the only cause of stroke. Blood clots can form around internal wounds in the process of healing and break away to float through the circulatory system. However, the most common cause of stroke is atherosclerosis. Blood clots can form around atheromatous plaques, and a plaque itself may detach from the artery wall, forming a floating hazard in the cardiovascular system that may result in a debilitating or deadly stroke.

BLOOD PRESSURE

When the heart pumps blood, the force must be substantial to power circulation for an entire cycle through the body and back to the heart. In a healthy cardiovascular system, the pressure in the arteries is not a problem because arteries are quite elastic. In a cardiovascular system diseased by atherosclerosis and arteriosclerosis, however, the pressure of the blood in the arteries can produce serious consequences. The narrowing of the arteries that occurs in atherosclerosis and the loss of elasticity that characterizes arteriosclerosis both tend to raise blood pressure and make the cardiovascular system less capable of adapting to the demands of heavy exercise and stress.

Blood pressure measurements are usually expressed by two numbers. The first number represents **systolic pressure**, the pressure generated by the heart's contraction. The second number represents **diastolic pressure**, or the pressure achieved between contractions, reflecting the elasticity of the vessel wall. Both numbers are measured by determining how high in millimeters (mm) a column of mercury (Hg) can be raised in a glass column.

Elevations of blood pressure can occur through several mechanisms. Some elevations in blood pressure are normal and even adaptive. Activation of the sympathetic nervous system, for example, increases heart rate and also causes constriction of the blood vessels, both of which raise blood pressure. The parasympathetic division blocks sympathetic action and returns blood pressure to its baseline rate, so sympathetic activation should not result in permanent increases in blood pressure. Other elevations in blood pressure, however, are neither normal nor adaptive and are symptoms of cardiovascular disorder.

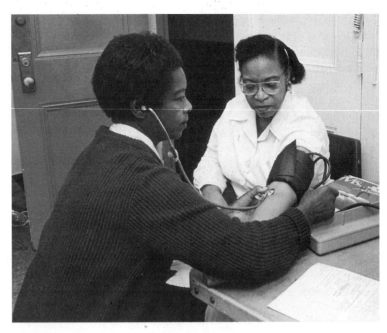

African Americans are more likely to have hypertension than European Americans.

Millions of people in the United States have **hypertension**—that is, abnormally high blood pressure. This "silent" illness is the single best predictor of both heart attack and stroke, the first and third leading causes of death in the United States. Hypertension is of two types—primary or essential hypertension and secondary hypertension. **Essential hypertension,** which accounts for 90% of the hypertension in the United States (Williams & Knight, 1994), refers to elevations of blood pressure that have no identified cause. It is positively related to such factors as age, African American ancestry, weight, sodium intake, tobacco use, and lack of exercise. **Secondary hypertension** is much less common than essential hypertension and stems from other diseases such as arteriosclerosis, kidney disorders, and some disorders of the endocrine system.

Table 9.1 shows the ranges for normal blood pressure, borderline hypertension, and hypertension. Despite beliefs to the contrary, people with hypertension are not able to diagnose their own blood pressure reliably (Baumann & Leventhal, 1985; Meyer, Leventhal, & Gutman, 1985). Therefore, people can have dangerously elevated blood pressure and re-

main completely unaware of their vulnerability to heart disease.

Hypertension tends to progress from elevated systolic blood pressure coupled with normal or slightly elevated diastolic pressure to elevations of both systolic and diastolic blood pressure. Although systolic and diastolic hypertension may occur separately, people—especially older people—with hypertension typically experience elevations of both. Systolic pressure that exceeds 200 mm Hg presents a danger of rupture in the arterial walls (McClintic, 1978). A rupture of the aorta is usually fatal; a rupture of a cerebral artery results in stroke that may be fatal. Diastolic hypertension tends to result in vascular damage that may injure organs served by the affected vessels, most commonly the kidneys, liver, pancreas, brain, and retina.

Because the underlying cause of essential hypertension is unknown, no treatment exists that will remedy its basic cause. Treatment tends to be oriented toward lowering blood pressure through drugs or changes in behavior that can bring about changes in blood pressure. Most treatment for high blood pressure employs drug therapy. Since the 1940s, drugs have been developed that help control blood

Table 9.1 Ranges of blood pressure (expressed in mm of Hg)

	Systolic	Diastolic
Normal	< 140	< 85
Borderline	140–159	85–104
Hypertensive	160 +	105 +

SOURCE: Adapted from the *1984 Report of the Joint National Committee on Detection, Evaluation and Treatment of High Blood Pressure* (p. 8) by the U.S. Department of Health and Human Services (USDHHS), 1984b, Washington, DC: U.S. Government Printing Office.

pressure through three mechanisms: dilating blood vessels, reducing blood fluid volume, and inhibiting the action of the sympathetic nervous system (Davis & Park, 1981). Patients may receive these drugs singly or in combination. All require a physician's prescription, and patients should be periodically monitored while taking them. Because hypertension presents no unpleasant symptoms, many patients are reluctant to continue with a daily medication that may cause unpleasant side effects. (The factors affecting adherence with this and other medical regimens were discussed in Chapter 8.)

Several behaviors relate to both the development and the treatment of hypertension. People with high blood pressure should restrict their sodium intake, which can lower their blood volume and thereby decrease their blood pressure. Obesity is also correlated with hypertension, and many obese people who lose weight lower their blood pressure into the normal range. Regular exercise has also been found effective in controlling hypertension, and exercising is discussed in Chapter 16. Because part of the treatment of hypertension involves behavioral changes, health psychologists have a role to play in changing such behaviors as restricting sodium intake, controlling weight, and maintaining a regular exercise program.

MEASURES OF CARDIOVASCULAR FUNCTION

For 55% of the people with coronary heart disease, a heart attack is the first symptom of a problem (Ellestad, 1986). Therefore, diagnosis of CHD is an urgent issue. Accurate diagnoses depend on reliable measures of the functioning of the cardiovascular system and changes in that functioning.

The most common measurement of cardiovascular function is blood pressure. Blood pressure measurements suggest whether arteries have narrowed or lost elasticity or both. Because high blood pressure has many causes, hypertension does not always signal heart disease. Other techniques can assess cardiovascular function more precisely than the measurement of blood pressure, but none of these other assessments are as simple or as available as blood pressure tests. Although there are no easy methods for the early diagnosis of CHD, several measures besides blood pressure are commonly used to detect potential cardiovascular problems.

MEASUREMENTS OF ELECTRICAL ACTIVITY IN THE HEART

An **electrocardiogram** (ECG) is a measurement of the electrical impulses produced by the heartbeat, and an ECG is capable of revealing abnormalities in the resting heartbeat. People who show an abnormal ECG usually have some type of cardiovascular disorder. However, ECG readings cannot reveal the buildup of plaques in the coronary arteries. Consequently, dangerously advanced CHD may go undetected by an electrocardiogram.

Measurement of the heart's electrical activity taken during exercise is called a **stress test**. This measure is more sensitive and useful than an electrocardiogram in diagnosing heart problems. For example, coronary artery blockage of less than 75% will not be discovered by an ECG, even though such blockage is extensive. A stress test, however, will reveal blockage of around 50%. As Ellestad (1986) pointed out, a 50% blockage in one coronary artery often fails to produce noticeable symptoms, thus stress testing is useful for discovering moderate yet significant levels of coronary artery blockage.

The rationale for the exercise stress test is that a complete assessment of cardiac function cannot be made while a person is at rest (Jones, 1988). In a stress test, measuring electrodes are placed in a standard pattern on the torso, and then the person engages in progressively more strenuous exercise, typically either walking on a treadmill with an increasing slope or riding a stationary bicycle with increasing pedal resistance. As the exercise increases the body's demand for oxygen, the heart increases its action. If coronary arteries are partially blocked, the blood cannot be delivered fast enough to keep up with the increased demand. This restriction results in a pattern of electrical activity with a characteristic waveform that permits trained professionals to make a diagnosis of coronary heart disease.

Stress tests can provide additional diagnostic information about cardiovascular problems. People with angina pectoris may know that restriction of blood flow is the cause of their chest pains, but stress testing can inform them about the severity of the restriction. People with chest pains are sometimes given stress tests to determine whether their pains are a result of ischemia or some other cause. Stress tests are also recommended after myocardial infarction as a way to measure damage to the heart and also after coronary bypass surgery as a way to assess the effectiveness of the procedure (Ellestad, 1986; Jones, 1988). Stress tests are also recommended for previously sedentary people who decide to start an exercise program.

ANGIOGRAPHY

The most accurate method of diagnosis for coronary heart disease is cardiac catheterization and **angiography**. Werner Frossman was the first person to attempt cardiac angiography—on himself in the early 1930s (Tilkian & Daily, 1986). The technique did not develop until the 1940s and 1950s, but it is now a routine diagnostic procedure. Angiography is used for suspected or known coronary artery disease, especially in cases of myocardial infarction in which a stress test has revealed ischemia.

With cardiac angiography, the patient's heart is injected with a dye so that the coronary arteries are visible during X-ray. Injecting the dye involves inserting a catheter into a blood vessel in either the arm or the groin of the patient and then threading it through the circulatory system to the heart. The heart pumps the released dye into the coronary arteries, allowing an X-ray to reveal the extent of the blockage as well as the areas where blood flow is reduced. For a complete diagnostic procedure, three

catheterizations are necessary (Tilkian & Daily, 1986), taking a total time of an hour or more.

Cardiac catheterization and angiography are surgical procedures, but patients are awake and usually only lightly sedated. The procedure is uncomfortable and even painful, and patients are typically anxious about their health as well as the procedure itself. In addition, angiography procedures carry some slight risk of injury or death: The injury rate is around 1%, and the mortality rate is 0.2% (Tilkian & Daily, 1986). Health psychologists can train patients in various techniques to relieve the stress and discomfort involved with this procedure (see Chapter 7).

If angiography reveals substantial blockage of the coronary arteries, surgical intervention—a coronary bypass—may be recommended. Another medical intervention is **angioplasty**. In this procedure, a catheter with an inflatable tip is passed into the obstructed artery and the tip is then inflated. The catheter flattens atherosclerotic deposits, thus improving circulation. Angioplasty was first used successfully in 1977 (Tilkian & Daily, 1986), and at first it was considered appropriate for unblocking only a single coronary artery. However, the procedure now is performed in patients with several blocked arteries. Angioplasty is successful in unblocking obstructed coronary arteries in 90% to 95% of the cases.

Like the coronary bypass operation, angioplasty relieves symptoms of ischemia and improves patients' quality of life; however, approximately 20% to 30% of patients develop renewed blockage of the coronary arteries opened by angioplasty. One advantage of this technique is that it is less invasive than a coronary bypass operation. However, considering the recurrence of blockage, angioplasty does not carry much of a cost advantage (Tilkian & Daily, 1986).

In summary, several techniques measure the functioning of the cardiovascular system. The simplest of these is a blood pressure reading, but this measurement cannot offer a complete diagnosis because it does not reveal the cause for elevations. The electrocardiogram (ECG) can determine cardiovascular abnormalities of a resting heartbeat. However, an exercise stress test is more valid and sensitive because it combines electrical measurement of the heart with the increased demands on the cardiovascular system that exercise produces. This technique can reveal blockage of the coronary arteries if substantial damage has occurred. Angiography, which involves X-raying the heart and coronary arteries, is currently considered the most precise of the diagnostic procedures. However, angiography requires placement of catheters in the heart, an invasive, uncomfortable, stressful procedure. The results of all these diagnostic procedures help health care professionals advise patients about the extent of damage and the possibility of surgery, angioplasty, and lifestyle changes.

LIFESTYLE AND CARDIOVASCULAR HEALTH

Cardiovascular disease (CVD) is the leading cause of death for people in the United States. Included within the category of cardiovascular disease are heart disease, such as myocardial infarction, and disorders of the circulatory system, such as stroke. About one-third of all deaths in the United States are from heart disease and another 7% from stroke. Thus, about 40% of the deaths in this country are attributable to cardiovascular disease (USBC, 1995). During the past 35 years, however, death rates from cardiovascular disease have steadily declined in the United States (see Figure 9.5), and this decrease is due in part to changes in lifestyle.

CHANGES IN LIFESTYLE

Although the people of the United States are not always conscientious about their health, they are becoming more health conscious. For the most part, failure to lead a healthy lifestyle is not because of a lack of knowledge about what constitutes a healthy lifestyle or the lack of availability of health services. Rather, unhealthy lifestyles are frequently the result of psychological factors such as barriers to change or the belief that serious diseases happen only to other people.

Nevertheless, many Americans have abandoned hazards in their lifestyles. Millions have quit smoking, have begun a regular exercise program, monitor

their blood pressure on a regular basis, and have changed their eating habits. Have these lifestyle changes resulted in better cardiovascular health?

CHANGES IN CARDIOVASCULAR DISEASE

Some data suggest that the movement toward better health practices has paid off, at least in terms of reduced mortality from cardiovascular disease. Figure 9.5 shows that the steady decline in CVD mortality rates since the mid-1960s has resulted in a comparable rate for 1993 and 1920.

The United States is only one of many industrialized Western countries that has seen dramatic reductions in cardiovascular deaths and an accompanying change in lifestyle among its population. One study from Finland (Jousilahti, Vartiainen, Toumilehto, Pekkanen, & Puska, 1995), for example, showed nearly a 50% reduction in coronary deaths of 30- to 59-year-old men and women during just the decade from 1972 to 1982. These researchers, who also investigated changes in risk factors, concluded that about one-half of the reduction in deaths was due to a healthier lifestyle, including reductions in total cholesterol, better control of blood pressure, and reductions in cigarette smoking. The authors predicted a decreasing trend of 4% to 5% per year in coronary mortality in this Finnish sample.

In the United States, only about half the people who have heart attacks live long enough to reach the hospital, and emergency medical treatment is a factor in their survival. Those who get to a hospital receive far more aggressive treatment than they would have 30 years ago. However, Guerci and Ross (1989) argued that some of the aggressive emergency treatment for myocardial infarction is unnecessary. Drugs that dissolve blood clots and improvements in emergency cardiac care are the main contributors to the decrease in hospital mortality from heart attack; emergency angiography, angioplasty, and bypass surgery are largely unnecessary. Guerci and Ross concluded that diagnostic angioplasty and preventive bypass surgery might be worthwhile, but a more conservative approach to the treatment of heart attacks would be just as effective and much less expensive.

Is the decline in cardiac mortality a result mostly of changes in emergency coronary care or changes in

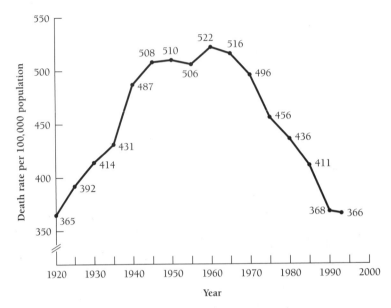

Figure 9.5   Death rates for major cardiovascular disease per 100,000 population, United States, 1920-1993.   SOURCE: Data from *Historical Statistics of the United States: Colonial Times to 1970* (p. 58) by U.S. Bureau of the Census, 1975, Washington, DC: U.S. Government Printing Office; from *Statistical Abstracts of the United States; 1986* (p. 73) by U.S. Bureau of the Census, 1985, Washington, DC: U.S. Government Printing Office; and from *Statistical Abstracts of the United States, 1995* (115th edition). (p. 72) by U.S. Bureau of the Census, 1995, Washington, DC: U.S. Government Printing Office.

lifestyle? No definitive answer is currently possible. Both factors contribute, but as early as 1985, Pell and Fayerweather were able to find evidence that changes in lifestyle may be more critical than improved medical care in reducing deaths from myocardial infarction. Their study found a decline in the rate of *first* acute myocardial infarction among male employees of the DuPont Corporation during the 1950s compared to the 1980s. Not only were fewer men dying of heart attack during the early 1980s than during the late 1950s, but fewer were experiencing nonfatal heart attacks. Sytkowski, Kannel, and D'Agostino (1990) also noted a 19% decrease in the incidence of coronary heart disease in a group of men between 50 and 59 years of age in 1970 compared to a group of similarly aged men in 1950. Among younger men, the decline in sudden death from heart disease has been even greater. Traven, Kuller, Ives, Rutan, and Perper (1995) found a 60% decrease in sudden death from coronary heart disease between 1970 and 1990 in European American men 35 to 44 years old. Traven

et al. concluded that the decline in CHD mortality was due more to changes in lifestyle than to improvements in the treatment of heart disease. Improved medical care may explain some reduction in deaths following myocardial infarction, but it cannot explain the decline in the incidence of first heart attack.

Why have initial myocardial infarctions declined? Some authorities (Pell & Fayerweather, 1985; Sytkowski et al., 1990) have attributed this reduction to the changes in lifestyle that followed publicity given to two reports: the 1964 Surgeon General's report on the close association between cigarette smoking and heart disease and the results from the Framingham Heart Study implicating high serum cholesterol levels in coronary heart disease. The recent decline in cardiovascular mortality is due, at least partially, to reduced incidence of the disease. This reduced incidence stems from behavioral and lifestyle changes that include quitting or not starting to smoke, controlling blood pressure and serum cholesterol levels, making significant changes in diet, and maintaining a regular exercise program.

RISK FACTORS IN CARDIOVASCULAR DISEASE

What causes the dangerous buildup of atheromatous plaques in the arteries? Why do the arteries of some people form scar tissue with no plaque and consequently little damage whereas those of others form occluding plaque or blockage that eventually endangers health and life? Medical research still has no certain answers to these questions, but research has linked several risk factors to cardiovascular disease. A great deal of the information about these risk factors has come from one study, the Framingham Heart Study.

In 1948, epidemiologists began a study of cardiovascular disease that included 5,208 people in the town of Framingham, Massachusetts. The study was a prospective design, thus all participants were free of heart disease at the beginning of the study. The original plan was to follow these people for 20 years to study heart disease and the factors related to its development. The results proved so valuable that the study has continued now for nearly 50 years. With over half the original participants dead, the focus has changed to following the development of cardiovascular disease in the offspring of those original participants (Brown, 1988).

Results from the Framingham Heart Study and other epidemiological studies have brought the concept of *risk factor* into popular usage. By studying a number of variables in a large group of people, epidemiologists can measure relationships between these variables and the subsequent development of a disorder. If people who develop a disorder differ from those who do not on a particular variable, that variable is a risk factor for the development of the disorder. The risk factor approach does not reveal the underlying physiology in the development of the disorder; that is, it does not allow for the identification of a cause. Nor does it allow a precise prediction of who will be affected and who will remain healthy. The risk factor approach simply yields information concerning which conditions are associated with a particular disease or disorder. Chapter 2 covered epidemiology and the risk factor approach.

Risk factors for cardiovascular heart disease include inherent factors such as family history; physiological conditions, such as hypertension; and personal behaviors, such as smoking and diet. Risk factors interact with one another, so a person with several risk factors is generally more vulnerable to CVD than a person with only one.

INHERENT RISK FACTORS

Inherent risk factors result from genetic or physical conditions that cannot be changed through modification of lifestyle. For example, juvenile-onset diabetes is one inherent risk factor for CVD. People who have juvenile-onset diabetes are twice as likely to die of heart disease as those whose sugar metabolism is normal. Age is another inherent risk factor. Older people are more likely to develop heart disease than younger people, and the risk increases with age.

Family history is also an inherent risk factor for CVD. People with a history of cardiovascular disease in their family are more likely to die of heart disease than those with no such history, and Jason is at risk because of his father's history of heart disease at an early age. The inheritance of this predisposition is not the simple action of one pair of genes, but heritability nevertheless seems to be a factor in risk for CVD.

Jason is male, and gender is another inherent risk factor. Men are more likely than women to develop cardiovascular disease prematurely. In fact, men have the same rate of CHD as women who are 15 years older (USBC, 1995). Because of this discrepancy, most early research concentrated almost exclusively on men, but heart disease is also the leading killer of women in the United States. Recent years have seen some trend toward including women in research on cardiovascular disease, but the literature in this area still remains unbalanced.

In addition, a gender discrepancy exists with regard to treatment of men and women with coronary heart disease. Ayanian and Epstein (1991), for example, found differences in the use of diagnostic and therapeutic procedures between women and men hospitalized for heart disease, discovering that women hospitalized for coronary heart disease did not receive the same aggressive treatment as men. Ayanian and Epstein concluded that

> men who are hospitalized for coronary heart disease are more likely than women to undergo major diagnostic and therapeutic procedures. Thus, women may not have equivalent access to these procedures at a time when the incidence of coronary heart disease among women is increasing. (p. 225)

Similarly, Streingart et al. (1991) reported that although female patients were as likely as male patients to have had angina and to have experienced more disability from angina, they were only about half as likely as men to undergo cardiac catheterization or to receive bypass surgery. As Ayanian and Epstein concluded, either men are treated too aggressively or women do not receive sufficiently aggressive treatment for coronary heart disease.

The early exclusion of women from many studies on CHD slowed progress in discovering reasons for the discrepancy in heart disease between women and men. Hormones may be a possible explanation (Williams, 1989), with estrogen offering some protection or testosterone having some damaging effects. Matthews (1989) hypothesized an interaction between behavior and reproductive hormones and opposed as too simplistic the view that estrogen is protective or that testosterone promotes damaging effects.

Ethnic background is another risk for cardiovascular disease mortality, with African Americans at increased risk (Rogers, 1992; USBC, 1995) and Asian Americans and Hispanic Americans at lowered risk (U.S. Department of Health and Human Services [USDHHS], 1994b). Whether this increased risk for African Americans is inherent or related to social, economic, or behavioral factors remains in question. Some evidence indicates that the higher rates of cardiovascular death among African Americans is related to their higher rate of hypertension and that this risk is related to greater cardiac reactivity (Light et al., 1993a; Tischenkel et al., 1989). The tendency to react to stress by increased cardiac function may be a result of inherent factors, but some research (Light et al., 1993a; Treiber et al., 1993) has suggested that African Americans are particularly susceptible to increased blood pressure in reaction to environmental stressors. Of particular interest is the finding that African American college students experience sharply increased cardiac reactivity when presented with racist stimuli (Armstead, Lawler, Gorden, Cross, & Gibbons, 1989). Such differential responding to various types of stressors suggests that ethnic differences in cardiac reactivity may relate to social rather than physiological factors.

Rogers (1992) analyzed the excess of mortality among African Americans, the majority of which is from cardiovascular disease, and found that when sociodemographic and economic factors are controlled, this discrepancy vanishes. Thus, no ethnic differences remain in CVD mortality when age, gender, marital status, family size, socioeconomic status, and family income are controlled. These factors all covary with ethnic background, but they and not some physical correlate of ethnicity may be the underlying reasons for increased mortality among African Americans. The possibility that sociodemographic and economic factors are more important than ethnic background in CVD risk is good news for Jason, who is still at risk from being male but whose family is small and upper-middle class.

Although inherent risk factors cannot be changed, people with these risk factors are not necessarily destined to develop cardiovascular disease. Identifying people with inherent risk factors is important because such high-risk individuals can minimize their overall risk profile through behavioral management and adjustments in lifestyle. For example, even with a family history of heart disease, people can control hypertension, quit smoking, and eat a healthy diet, thus lowering their *combined* risk factors.

PHYSIOLOGICAL CONDITIONS

A second category of risk factors in cardiovascular disease includes the physiological conditions of hypertension and serum cholesterol level.

Hypertension

Hypertension is the single most important risk factor in cardiovascular disease, yet millions of people with high blood pressure are not aware of their vulnerability. Unlike most disorders, hypertension produces no overt symptoms, and dangerously elevated blood pressure levels commonly occur with no signals or symptoms. Most people believe that if their blood pressure is high they will be aware of the elevation (Baumann & Leventhal, 1985; Meyer, Leventhal, & Gutman, 1985). Unfortunately, hypertension ordinarily has no discernible symptoms. At 15, Jason does not monitor his blood pressure, and he takes a rather fatalistic attitude about developing hypertension.

Although the Framingham Heart Study (Dawber, 1980) was not the first to suggest that people with high blood pressure have more cardiovascular problems than those with normal blood pressure, it provided solid evidence of the importance of hypertension. Researchers in the Framingham study divided blood pressure into three categories: normotensive (normal blood pressure), borderline blood pressure, and hypertensive. Regardless of people's age or gender, their risk of cardiovascular disease increased with increases in blood pressure, clearly indicating that high blood pressure is a risk factor.

Another prospective study on heart disease is the Honolulu Heart Program. Like many studies on CHD, the Honolulu study includes only men, but one of its strengths is a sample of participants ethnically and geographically different from those in the Framingham study. Participants in the Honolulu Heart Program were more than 8,000 men of Japanese ancestry between 45 and 68 years of age at the beginning of the study. One report from the Honolulu Heart Program (Reed, MacLean, & Hayash, 1987) found results similar to those from the Framingham study; that is, blood pressure was the best predictor of atherosclerosis.

The relationship between hypertension and weight has long been suspected. The Framingham study confirmed this suspicion with its finding that obesity is the best predictor of hypertension (Dawber, 1980). Reducing weight lowers blood pressure, and lowering blood pressure reduces the risk of mortality. This relationship is true not only for people with hypertension but also for those within the borderline category (Hypertension Detection and Follow-up Program Cooperative Group, 1979).

Also, hypertension seems to be related to anxiety, at least for middle-aged men. As part of the Framingham study, Markovitz, Matthews, Kannel, Cobb, and D'Agostino (1993) hypothesized that height-ened anxiety, heightened anger, and suppressed expression of anger would increase the risk of hypertension. They measured anxiety, anger symptoms, expression of anger, and blood pressure in middle-aged and older men and women. An 18- to 20-year follow-up of those people with normal blood pressure at the beginning of the study revealed that men 45 to 59 who had heightened anxiety were more than twice as likely as middle-age men with lower anxiety levels to develop hypertension. For men 60 or older and for women of any age, none of these factors, including suppression of anger, were associated with later hypertension.

Serum Cholesterol Level

A second physiological condition related to cardiovascular disease is high serum cholesterol level. *Serum* or *blood cholesterol* is the level of cholesterol circulating through the blood stream, and this level is related (but not perfectly related) to *dietary cholesterol,* or the amount of cholesterol in one's food. Cholesterol is waxy, fat-like substance that is essential for human life as a component of cell membranes, insulation for neurons, and an ingredient in the production of certain hormones. The liver manufactures cholesterol, but cholesterol also comes from diet. Dietary cholesterol comes from animal fats and oils but not from vegetables or vegetable products. Although cholesterol is essential, too much may lead to cardiovascular disease.

After a person eats cholesterol, his or her bloodstream transports it as part of the process of digestion. A measurement of the amount of cholesterol carried in the serum (the liquid, cell-free part of the blood) is typically expressed in milligrams (mg) of cholesterol per deciliters (dl) of serum. This measurement is a ratio, but it is generally abbreviated to the cholesterol count. Thus, a cholesterol reading of 210 means 210 mg of cholesterol per deciliter of blood serum. But what does a cholesterol level of 210 mean? Is it good or bad?

Very high levels of cholesterol are dangerous. Physicians have known for several decades that people with a genetic disorder that causes abnormally high levels of cholesterol in the blood, **hypercholesterolemia**, also have an unusually high rate of coronary heart disease, beginning at a very young age. People with CHD also tend to have high serum cholesterol levels. However, until the Framingham Heart Study showed that high cholesterol levels were a risk to the participants, physicians were reluctant to consider high cholesterol levels a danger to the general population (Brown, 1988).

The Framingham study found that men with low levels of serum cholesterol seldom developed coronary heart disease but those with high levels had a substantially elevated risk (Dawber, 1980). For men with intermediate values, the risk was intermediate, suggesting that high levels of cholesterol are not a requirement for CHD. This relationship did not appear in the women in the study, possibly because so few women developed heart disease.

How much cholesterol is too much? In a long-term follow-up of young White men, Klag et al. (1993) found that cholesterol at age 22 predicted incidence of cardiovascular disease, coronary heart disease, and cardiovascular deaths decades later. These researchers divided young men into three groups based on their level of total cholesterol. Men in the top 25% had cholesterol levels of 209 to 315, whereas those in the bottom 25% had total cholesterol levels of 118 to 172. Klag et al. found that men with high cholesterol at age 22 were over 70% more likely to develop cardiovascular disease than men with low cholesterol levels and were twice as likely to develop coronary heart disease and to die of cardiovascular disease.

Earlier, a report for the Multiple Risk Factor Intervention Trial (MRFIT) analyzed data from about 350,000 men and found that men with elevated cholesterol levels also had elevated risks for heart attack and stroke (Stamler, Wentworth, & Neaton, 1986). The relationship between cholesterol level and cardiovascular disease was continuous; that is, the higher the cholesterol level, the greater the risk. As cholesterol levels increased above 245, the risk for CVD increased from three to about four times that of men whose cholesterol level was below 180. Some men with a cholesterol level below 195 also had heart attacks, but at a much lower frequency than those with a higher total cholesterol levels.

Types of Cholesterol. The Framingham study also determined that *total* serum cholesterol may not be the best predictor of cardiovascular disease (Dawber, 1980). A group of researchers involved in this study (Gordon, Castelli, Hjortland, Kannel, & Dawber, 1977) found that not all cholesterol is equally implicated in atherosclerosis. Cholesterol circulates in the blood in several forms of **lipoproteins,** and these lipoproteins can be distinguished by an analysis of their density. The Framingham researchers found that **low-density lipoprotein (LDL)** was positively related to the development of coronary heart disease whereas **high-density lipoprotein (HDL)** was negatively related. Therefore, HDL seems to offer some protection against CVD whereas LDL seems to promote atherosclerosis. A study by Pekkanen et al. (1990) found that low-density lipoprotein was a better predictor of coronary heart disease than was total cholesterol

When too many LDL particles exist in the blood, cholesterol can be deposited in artery walls (Medical Essay, 1993). HDL can retrieve the cholesterol deposited in arteries and transport it to the liver for disposal. However, if there is too much LDL for the HDL to handle, the process of atherosclerosis can begin to clog arteries. Because high LDL levels are positively related to heart disease and high HDL levels are negatively related to heart disease, LDL is sometimes referred to as "bad cholesterol" and HDL as "good cholesterol."

During the past 15 years, much attention has centered on the ratio of total cholesterol to high-density lipoprotein. Total cholesterol is determined by adding HDL, LDL, and 20% of very low-density lipoprotein (VLDL), also called **triglycerides.** A low ratio of total cholesterol to HDL is more desirable than a high ratio. Kenneth Cooper (1988) recommended ratios of less than 4.6 to 1.0 for men and less than 4.0 to 1.0 for women. That is, men should have HDL levels that are at least 22% of total cholesterol; women should have HDL levels that are at least 25% of total cholesterol. Most authorities now believe that a favorable balance of total cholesterol to HDL is more critical than total cholesterol in avoiding cardiovascular disease.

How can people *raise HDL* and thus lower their ratio of total cholesterol to HDL? Presently, two behaviors seem to be related to elevated rates of HDL: moderate alcohol consumption and exercise. We discuss drinking alcohol in Chapter 14 and exercising in Chapter 16. Certain behaviors are also associated with lowering LDL, especially eating. People who eat diets with a high percentage of the calories derived from saturated fats (those from animal sources such as red meats, whole milk, and eggs) tend to have high cholesterol levels; people whose diets include few saturated fats typically have low cholesterol levels and a favorable ratio of total cholesterol to HDL. Research, therefore, suggests that a regular exercise program and moderate consumption of alcohol combined with a diet high in vegetable consumption and low in saturated fats will give people their most favorable ratio of total cholesterol to HDL.

Researchers have also discovered that lipoprotein(a) may be an independent risk for coronary heart disease, at least for White men. (Very few studies have been conducted on women or on African Americans, leaving this risk for them poorly understood.) Lipoprotein(a), or Lp(a), closely resembles low-density lipoprotein, but it has one additional molecule of apoliprotein(a). Schaefer et al. (1994) reported on a prospective, case-control study of men with total cholesterol levels of 265 or higher and LDL levels of 190 or more. A 7- to 10-year follow-up compared Lp(a) levels of men who had developed coronary heart disease (cases) with those of men who had not (controls) and found Lp(a) to be an independent risk factor for coronary heart disease.

Traditional coronary risk factors such as body mass index and cigarette smoking are not correlated with Lp(a) levels (Jenner et al., 1993), suggesting that Lp(a) may be an independent risk factor. However, Lp(a) may not be a risk factor in men with more normal levels of total cholesterol (Ridker, Hennekens, & Stampfer, 1993). Because lipoprotein(a) is quite resistant to dietary change and drug therapy (Schaefer et al., 1994), some physicians (Barnathan, 1993) have argued that even if it is an independent risk factor, it should not be used to screen for CHD because such results would be of little use.

Although total cholesterol levels are not as resistant to change as Lp(a) levels, lowering cholesterol through diet is not easy (Austin, King, Bawol, Hulley, & Friedman, 1987). Elevating cholesterol levels, on the other hand, occurs relatively quickly (Sacks et al., 1981). Many people find it difficult and unpleasant to eliminate enough saturated fat from their diets to substantially lower their serum cholesterol level. Usually, neither drugs nor diet (nor a combination of the two) is capable of changing serum cholesterol more than 20% to 25% (Lipid Research Clinics Program, 1984).

The findings on cholesterol and diet suggest two conclusions. First, cholesterol intake and blood cholesterol are related. Second, the relationship between dietary intake of cholesterol and blood cholesterol relates strongly to habitual diet; that is, eating habits maintained over many years. Lowering blood cholesterol level is possible, but the process is neither quick nor easy.

Cholesterol and the Elderly. Although lowering blood cholesterol may be difficult, it may not be important for people past 70. For years scientists have suspected that high cholesterol levels may not be a risk factor for elderly people, partly because these people are survivors. Recently, evidence has begun to accumulate that supports this hypothesis and even to suggest that high cholesterol may protect older women against heart disease. In 1992, Manolio et al. looked at 22 earlier studies that had investigated the relationship between cholesterol and heart disease in older people. This review showed a slight but statistically significant positive relationship between cholesterol levels above 240 and death from coronary heart disease in both men and women. However, for both genders and especially for women, the risk was much lower after age 65 than before 65.

Since this review, other investigators have reported no association or even an inverse relationship between cholesterol and cardiovascular disease in elderly people. Data from the Framingham study (Kronmal, Cain, Ye, & Omenn, 1993) revealed a significant positive relationship between total cholesterol levels and death from heart disease only up to about age 60. From age 60 to 70, there was no significant relationship, and after age 80 total serum cholesterol levels may actually have a protective effect against death from cardiovascular disease.

In addition, a group of scientists from the Yale University School of Medicine have found that high cholesterol levels should not concern healthy people over the age of 70 (Corti et al., 1995; Krumholz et al., 1994). These studies showed that high total cholesterol did *not* increase all-cause mortality or death from coronary heart disease. Corti et al. found that HDL (the "good" cholesterol) was more strongly

WOULD YOU BELIEVE . . . ?

Cholesterol and Violent Death

Would you believe that lowering your cholesterol level may *increase* your chance of violent death, including suicide? Since the 1980s, evidence has been accumulating that despite the positive relationship between cholesterol levels and incidence of coronary artery disease, there is no positive relationship between serum cholesterol level and all-cause mortality. Curiously, there seems to be a U-shaped relationship between total cholesterol and death from all causes, with both high and low levels of cholesterol associated with higher death rates.

Although the evidence for a relationship between low cholesterol and all-cause mortality has existed for some time, investigators have only recently considered this interesting phenomenon worth researching. The early evidence was mostly embedded in studies designed to investigate some other factor. For example, the 7-year follow-up of the Multiple Risk Factor Intervention Trial (Multiple Risk Factor Intervention Trial Research Group, 1982) found a slight trend for men at risk for heart disease to profit from an intervention to lower cardiac

mortality. When the investigators looked at all-cause mortality, they found no difference between the intervention group and the control group, indicating that death from other causes increased. A later report from the MRFIT study (Iso, Jacobs, Wentworth, Neaton, & Cohen, 1989) indicated more compelling evidence: *The mortality rate for men with total cholesterol below 140 or above 300 was nearly twice as high as the mortality rate of men with cholesterol levels between 180 and 220.*

In 1990, Ingar Holme looked at 19 previous studies (including MRFIT) that had used interventions to lower cholesterol. Results of this review confirmed the effectiveness of reducing total cholesterol on incidence of CHD, but the interventions to lower cholesterol increased total death rates. Later, David Jacobs and his colleagues (Jacobs et al., 1992) held a conference for the National Heart, Lung, and Blood Institute to review and discuss the U-shaped relationship between total cholesterol and all-cause mortality. At that time, the evidence pointed to a strong U-shaped relationship for men but no relationship for women.

These investigators suggested that the excess deaths for people with low cholesterol might be the result of an increase in mortality from lung and some other cancers, digestive and respiratory diseases, and trauma or sudden violent deaths.

The possibility that violent deaths account for the difference was confirmed by two meta-analyses (Cummings & Psaty, 1994; Muldoon, Manuck, & Matthews, 1992), which revealed that men with low levels of cholesterol had significantly higher rates of deaths from violence or suicide. But why should low cholesterol be related to violent death? Researchers looking for the underlying connection have studied psychiatric patients to try to discover a link between low cholesterol and violence. Ross Morgan, Lawrence Palinkas, Elizabeth Barrett-Connor, and Deborah Wingard (1993) studied cholesterol level and depressive symptoms in men 70 and older. They found that depression was about three times higher for men with cholesterol below 160 than for those with higher cholesterol. Marc Hillbrand, Reuben Spitz, and Hilliard Foster (1995) looked at cholesterol

related to heart disease mortality than total cholesterol for those over age 70.

What accounts for the lack of association (or even an inverse relationship in the case of women) between total cholesterol level and incidence of heart disease? One possibility is that cholesterol levels in the elderly may change and thus may not be a reflection of lifelong cholesterol levels. Research (Gordon & Rifkind, 1989; Newschaffer, Bush, & Hale, 1992) indicates that cholesterol levels decrease after age 40. Also, people who have escaped heart disease for their first 70 years may be more resistant to the damaging effects of high cholesterol. Whatever the explanation, it would seem that elderly people can be less concerned than the young and middle-aged about

their total cholesterol or their ratio of total cholesterol to HDL.

BEHAVIORAL FACTORS

A third category of risk factors includes all the behavioral correlates of cardiovascular disease, especially smoking and diet.

Smoking

When the Framingham study began in 1948, little evidence existed to suggest that smoking tobacco would be a risk factor in cardiovascular disease, but the Framingham researchers measured it anyway. During the project, evidence started to mount that

levels of male psychiatric patients who had committed violent crimes and found that the median cholesterol level of these men was 175, considerably lower than the national average. Hillbrand et al. observed a curvilinear relationship between cholesterol levels and frequency of aggression; men with moderately low cholesterol committed the most acts of aggression (but not necessarily the most severe ones) compared to men with either higher or lower levels of cholesterol.

Most of the earlier studies demonstrating a link between lower cholesterol and violent death involved cholesterol-reducing interventions and thus used participants who may have been experiencing the unpleasantness of a low-fat diet or the rigors of a tedious drug program. Could this deprivation have made them irritable and thus aggressive? More recent evidence (Freedman et al., 1995) does not support this hypothesis because it indicates that even a preexisting low level of cholesterol is associated with non-illness mortality — that is, violent death. Although Fowkes et al. (1992), Hillbrand et al. (1995),

and Freedman et al. (1995) found no clear relationship between either aggression or hostility and low cholesterol levels in men, some research with animals by Jay Kaplan and his associates (Kaplan, Manuck, & Shively, 1991; Kaplan et al., 1994) has suggested that monkeys on a low-fat, cholesterol-lowering diet behaved more aggressively than those on a high-fat diet with elevated total cholesterol. In addition, Muldoon, Kaplan, Manuck, and Mann (1992) and Engelberg (1992) have suggested that cholesterol may cause a decrease in brain serotonin activity, which, in turn, may bring about poorer suppression of aggressive behaviors.

The frequently observed relationship between low cholesterol and violent death has led many authorities to rethink the standard recommendation to lower one's cholesterol. Gains from decreased CHD deaths are offset by increased deaths from other causes, including violent deaths. Researchers still have no satisfactory explanation for this intriguing finding, but David Jacobs and his associates (Jacobs, Muldoon, & Rästam, 1995) offered three possible explanations. First, certain diseases

may cause lower cholesterol. This explanation may account for part of the relationship between low cholesterol and all-cause mortality, but it cannot explain the link between low cholesterol and nonillness mortality. Second, some third factor, such as cigarette smoking, age, or socioeconomic status, may relate to both cholesterol and violent death. Although some recent evidence from the Framingham study suggests that smoking may be implicated in excess deaths among people with total cholesterol below 160 (D'Agostino, Belanger, Kannel, & Higgins, 1995), these other factors are unlikely explanations because many of the studies have controlled for their potentially confounding factors. Third, there may be some overarching biological pathway by which serum cholesterol increases rate of violent death. To date, no such biological mechanism has been discovered, so in the meantime, the best advice may be to try to maintain a total cholesterol level that is neither too high nor too low.

cigarette smoking was a risk factor not only for cancer of the respiratory tract but also for cardiovascular illnesses. In a summary report from the Framingham study, Dawber (1980) stated that inhaling cigarette smoke had a proven relationship to cardiovascular disease in men.

Later evidence also linked cigarette smoking to stroke in men of Japanese ancestry living in Hawaii (Abbott, Yin, Reed, & Yano, 1986), but research has not been clear about this relationship in women. The Framingham study did not demonstrate a relationship between smoking and CHD in women (Dawber, 1980), possibly because fewer women in the study smoked and also because fewer women developed cardiovascular disease. In a study on women,

however, Willett, Green and their colleagues (1987) found that smoking increased the risk for CHD. Female smokers' risk for fatal heart attack was 5.5 times greater than for nonsmokers, their risk for nonfatal heart attack was 5.8 times that for nonsmokers, and their risk for angina was also increased. These elevated risks for smokers also apply to the chances of fatal and nonfatal strokes (Colditz et al., 1988). Smoking, therefore, is a risk factor for CVD in women as well as in men. (Smoking and its impact on health are discussed more fully in Chapter 13.)

Diet

Although obesity has long been suspected of being a risk factor for cardiovascular disease, evidence during the past 2 or 3 decades has suggested that diet contributes more to one's chances of developing heart disease than being overweight, which may not even be an independent risk factor for cardiovascular disease. Research during this period has suggested that diet may either increase or decrease one's chances of developing heart disease.

Fats.   Diets high in saturated fat are positively related to heart disease whereas those low in saturated fat protect against heart disease. To reduce the amount of saturated fat in the diet, one can substitute food high in or cooked with oils high in monounsaturated or polyunsaturated fats. Some research has indicated that monounsaturated fats (such as olive oil) and polyunsaturated fats (such as safflower oil) are both good dietary choices.

Other research has indicated that a decrease in overall fat consumption is an even wiser choice. Trevisan et al. (1990) found that the consumption of monounsaturated and polyunsaturated fats was associated with a lower coronary risk than the consumption of butter. In comparing monounsaturated and polyunsaturated fats, however, two studies (Dreon, Vranizan, Krauss, Austin, & Wood, 1990; Mensink & Katan, 1989) showed no advantage in using monounsaturated fats. Other research suggested that substituting dietary protein for fat was more effective in preventing the appearance of new lesions in the coronary arteries (Blankenhorn, Johnson, Mack, Zein, & Vailas, 1990). These studies suggest that people can reduce their risk for cardiovascular disease by substituting diets low in saturated fats for those high in saturated fats.

Vitamins.   Can vitamins reduce the chances of developing heart disease? Some research has suggested that consumption of Vitamin E may protect both women and men against coronary heart disease. Interest in the antioxidant Vitamin E began several years ago when scientists began to notice that oxidized low-density lipoprotein (LDL) may be involved in atherogenesis. Antioxidants seem to protect LDL from oxidation and thus from its potential damaging effects on the cardiovascular system. In addition to Vitamin E, beta carotene, selenium, and riboflavin have been identified as antioxidants. Fruits and vegetables are the main dietary source of these antioxidants, but vitamin supplements are also good sources.

Stampfer et al. (1993) conducted an 8-year follow-up of more than 87,000 female nurses who were between ages 34 and 59 and free of cardiovascular disease (CVD) at the beginning of the study. These investigators divided the group into top and bottom halves of consumers of Vitamin E and found that the women who consumed more Vitamin E were only two-thirds as likely to develop CVD as those who consumed less Vitamin E. Most of the nurses who were high consumers had been taking Vitamin E supplements, and the benefits were not evident until the nurses had been taking supplements for 2 years. This same group of researchers (Rimm et al., 1993) found much the same results with male health professionals. In addition, they found that consumption of Vitamin C was unrelated to coronary heart disease.

A measure of antioxidants in the blood, called serum carotenoids, also seems to protect against coronary disease. Morris, Kritchevsky, and Davis (1994) conducted a 13-year follow-up of men who had high cholesterol levels, but who were free from CHD at the beginning of the study. They found that men with the highest levels of serum carotenoids, compared with those with the lowest levels were less than two-thirds as likely to develop heart disease. These studies suggest that regular consumption of Vitamin E, selenium, beta carotene, and riboflavin probably has some ability to protect against heart disease, especially in smokers.

Fiber.   Fiber is the undigestible part of plants. Human digestive tracts cannot break down this material, so it passes through the digestive tract without being completely digested. Fiber can shorten the time that food stays in the digestive tract and change the metabolism of nutrients.

Does dietary fiber protect against coronary heart disease? During the 1980s, some reputable research and much media controversy centered around the benefits as well as the overselling of fiber, especially fiber from oat bran. Much of the early interest in fiber came from epidemiological studies of diets and disease in countries other than the United States. Connor (1990) reported that physicians working in Africa noticed the lack of cancers of the digestive tract and the low rate of cardiovascular disease among their patients who consumed diets high in fiber, a finding that led some to advocate more fiber in Western diets.

One group of researchers studied the cholesterol-lowering effects of oat bran and found that men who had high cholesterol levels and who ate a large amount (100 grams per day) of oat bran were able to reduce their cholesterol levels by more than 10% (Anderson et al., 1984; Kirby et al., 1981). A later study (Swain, Rouse, Curley, & Sacks, 1990) that varied fiber content of dietary supplements suggested that oat bran has no special ability to reduce cholesterol, but the study did demonstrate that diet can lower cholesterol, even for people whose cholesterol level is within the normal range.

In summary, certain types of polyunsaturated and monounsaturated fats, vitamin E, and dietary fiber seem to have a positive effect in protecting against heart disease. Nevertheless, the effect of specific diets on CVD remains a complex issue. Fortunately, the advice about how to alter behavior to improve or maintain a favorable cholesterol level is rather consistent: Eat a diet low in fat, especially saturated fat from animal sources; eat a diet high in carbohydrates, especially complex carbohydrates from fruits, vegetables, and whole grains; maintain a steady and moderate weight; and exercise regularly. Most of these elements have been shown to increase HDL without raising total cholesterol. This advice is also valid for maintaining a generally healthy lifestyle. As Matarazzo (1984b) once pointed out, the "new" emphasis on behavioral health is not really new. It can be traced back to ancient times and to philosophers and religious thinkers who recommended moderation as a way of life. Science is now discovering the evidence that supports those ancient teachings.

PSYCHOSOCIAL FACTORS

In recent years, researchers have identified a number of psychosocial factors that relate to heart disease. Included among these factors are anxiety level, occupation, attendance at religious services, income, marital status, and education. This section looks briefly at some of this research.

For many years, people have suspected that high levels of anxiety may contribute to coronary death, but only recently has evidence for this belief emerged. Ichiro Kawachi and colleagues (Kawachi, Colditz, et al., 1994; Kawachi, Sparrow, Vokonas, & Weiss, 1994) have reported that men who complained of constant anxiety were three to six times more likely

than less anxious men to die suddenly from heart disease. A prospective study (Kawachi, Colditz, et al., 1994) showed that men who experienced phobic anxiety were three times more likely to suffer sudden death than men who were lower in anxiety. A 32-year case-control follow-up study (Kawachi, Sparrow, et al., 1994) found a similarly elevated risk of sudden death but showed that anxiety was unrelated to the risk for nonfatal myocardial infarction or angina, suggesting that anxiety contributes to the deadliness of the disease.

Psychological and social factors have also been implicated in heart disease for women. In a 20-year prospective study, Eaker, Pinsky, and Castelli (1992) found that some employed women and some homemakers were at increased risk. After controlling for age, systolic blood pressure, ratio of total cholesterol to HDL, diabetes, cigarette smoking, and body mass, they found an increased risk of myocardial infarction or coronary death for employed women and homemakers with little education, heightened tension, and less than one vacation every 6 years. These researchers suggested that stress-related situations caused by feelings of subordination and social isolation may be important psychosocial factors; that is, coronary-prone situations contribute to heart attacks and death from coronary heart disease.

Other factors that relate to heart disease are income level and marital status. Redford Williams and his associates (1992) looked at the survival rates of male and female patients with coronary artery disease and found that those with incomes of $40,000 or more had nearly double the survival rate of those with incomes of $10,000 or less. In addition, unmarried patients who lacked someone in whom they could confide were much more likely to die than were patients who were married, had a confidant, or both. Similarly, Case, Moss, Case, McDermott, and Eberly (1992) found that living alone after having a heart attack was an independent risk for additional heart problems. After 6 months, 16% of heart patients who lived alone had a recurrent cardiac event, but only 9% of patients who lived with others had experienced such an event. Case et al. also found that heart patients with less than 12 years of education had an increased risk for recurrent heart problems.

These studies confirm results from other research on social support and personal control discussed in Chapter 6, which indicated that people who have a wide circle of friends or who feel they can confide in another person and who believe that they have some control over their lives are less likely to die of stress-related diseases. Sudden death from heart disease is related to anxiety and dissatisfaction for both men and women, and people who lack financial or educational resources are probably less able or less likely to seek medical care—conditions that place them at a greater risk for a variety of disorders, including heart disease.

THE TYPE A BEHAVIOR PATTERN

Another behavioral factor that has received a plethora of research attention during the past 20 years is the Type A behavior pattern. At one time, many researchers thought this behavior pattern was an important risk factor for heart disease, but now most believe that the Type A concept is too general and that only one of its components—overt expressions of hostility—contributes to coronary heart disease.

Origin of the Type A Concept

The Type A behavior pattern is a concept originated by Meyer Friedman and Ray Rosenman. Beginning in the 1950s, these two cardiologists worked with a group of researchers to develop the notion that a particular behavior pattern might relate to coronary heart disease. In addition to publishing dozens of technical articles, Friedman and Rosenman have published a popular account of their ideas, *Type A Behavior and Your Heart* (1974). Friedman and Diane Ulmer have written another popular book, *Treating Type A Behavior and Your Heart* (1984), which describes a therapy project designed to alter the Type A behavior pattern. In addition, hundreds of studies by other researchers have tested the concept.

Description of the Type A Behavior Pattern

Friedman and Rosenman (1974) hypothesized that people can be divided into two categories, Type A and Type B, that differ on a number of important behavioral factors. Type As can be characterized as hostile, competitive, concerned with numbers and the acquisition of objects, and possessing an exaggerated sense of time urgency. Friedman and Rosenman originally saw the Type B behavior pattern as

characterized by a lack of time urgency, competitiveness, and hostility, but more recently Kaplan (1992) insisted that Type B is more than the absence of Type A behaviors. Kaplan suggested that the positive qualities of Type B include forgiveness, a sense of humor, healthy humility, high self-esteem, a sense of autonomy and uniqueness, and a balance between achievement and aspirations, demand and realization, and gifts and limitations.

Assessment of the Type A Behavior Pattern

Friedman and Rosenman developed the Structured Interview to assess the Type A behavior pattern. The original Structured Interview was a brief series of questions designed to assess the characteristics associated with the Type A behavior pattern: ambition, competitiveness, time urgency, impatience, and hostility. Psychologist C. David Jenkins put the Structured Interview into a questionnaire format and called it the Jenkins Activity Survey (Jenkins, Rosenman, & Zyzanski, 1965; Jenkins, Zyzanski, & Rosenman, 1979).

Scores on the Structured Interview yield a classification into types, but scores on the Jenkins Activity Survey range from strong Type A to strong Type B, with most scores in between. Its ease of administration has made the Jenkins Activity Survey more widely used in research than the Structured Interview. Despite its widespread use, the Jenkins Activity Survey has had only limited success in predicting coronary heart disease, and Dembroski and Williams (1989) claimed that this limited success was not a failure of the assessment procedure but of the Type A concept.

Type A Behavior and Coronary Heart Disease

Friedman and Rosenman originated the Type A behavior pattern as a result of their observation that most of their coronary patients exhibited these behaviors. An early prospective study, the Western Collaborative Group Study (WCGS), gave initial credibility to the concept of a behavioral risk factor for coronary heart disease (Rosenman et al., 1975). This study found that Type A men were more than twice as likely as Type B men to experience coronary heart disease. This 2 to 1 risk of coronary heart disease seemed to suggest that the Type A concept had some value, and results from the Framingham study tended to support the relationship between Type A behavior and CHD in men and to confirm that a similar relationship exists for women (Haynes, Feinleib, & Kannel, 1980).

However, other research has failed to find strong support for the relationship between the Type A behavior pattern and development of CHD (Ragland & Brand, 1988a, 1988b; Shekelle et al., 1985). The inability of a global Type A behavior pattern to consistently predict heart disease has led investigators to analyze the component behaviors in the Type A pattern to determine whether some one behavior or some constellation of behaviors might yield a more valid predictor. Researchers became increasingly convinced that the global Type A behavior pattern, as defined by extreme ambition, competitiveness, impatience, hostility, and time urgency, is not a risk factor for coronary artery disease (Siegman, Anderson, Herbst, Boyle, & Wilkinson, 1992). Instead, they have focused more and more on one possible toxic component of the Type A behavior pattern—namely, hostility.

HOSTILITY

During the 1980s, Ted Dembroski and his associates (Dembroski & MacDougall, 1985; Dembroski, MacDougall, Costa, & Grandits, 1989; Dembroski, MacDougall, Williams, Haney, & Blumenthal, 1985) suggested that the Type A behavior pattern is too general and that a single component—hostility—is the toxic element that links Type A to coronary artery disease. More specifically, one of these associates, Redford Williams (1989), has presented evidence that one element of hostility—cynical hostility—is especially harmful. Williams contended that people who mistrust others, think the worst of humanity, and interact with others with cynical hostility are harming themselves and their hearts. Furthermore, he suggested that people who use anger as a response to interpersonal problems have an elevated risk for heart disease.

To establish the relationship between hostility and heart disease, researchers must measure hostility, and they have used several instruments, including the Buss-Durkee Hostility Inventory (BDHI), a 75-item, true/false instrument (Buss & Durkee, 1957); the

Cook-Medley Hostility (Ho) Index, a special scale of 50 items from the original Minnesota Multiphasic Personality Inventory (MMPI) (Cook & Medley, 1954); and the Potential for Hostility scale (PoHo), an instrument derived from the Structured Interview. The most frequently used hostility scale in studies of coronary heart disease has been the Cook-Medley (Cook & Medley, 1954), which measures suspiciousness, resentment, frequent anger, and cynical mistrust of others more than it measures the tendency to behave violently (Williams, 1989). This scale offers the advantage of being part of a well-established and widely administered psychological test.

Hostility as a Factor in Coronary Heart Disease

What evidence supports the claim that hostility is the toxic component in the Type A behavior pattern? Using various hostility measures, a number of studies have shown that some form of hostility is associated with coronary heart disease. Hostility increases the risk for CHD (Barefoot, Dahlstrom, & Williams, 1983; Chesney, Hecker, & Black, 1988) and is a better predictor of coronary artery blockage (Williams et al., 1980), heart disease (Dembroski et al., 1989), and all-cause mortality (Barefoot, Williams, Dahlstrom, & Dodge, 1987) than is Type A behavior.

What biological or neurochemical mechanisms can account for the ability of hostile behavior to inflict cardiovascular damage? Chesney et al. (1988) stated that hostility seems to be the strongest correlate of hyperreactivity, the tendency to react or overreact to stressful or emotional situations. Chapter 3 discussed the sequence of physiological responses that occur when a person perceives stress. Among those physical responses are the release of such hormones as epinephrine and cortisol. Chesney et al. suggested that epinephrine probably plays a role in the development of coronary heart disease, and Kuhn (1989) discussed the evidence concerning the secretion of cortisol and the development of CHD. If research in this area continues to indicate that people who are high in hostility have greater cardiovascular reactivity, then the link between a behavioral risk factor and the physical damage underlying cardiovascular heart disease will become more firmly established.

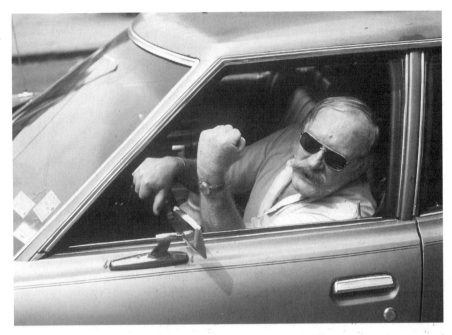

Hostility and expressed anger are risk factors for cardiovascular disease.

Hostility relates to a number of demographic and behavioral factors that are positively related to heart disease. For example, men have higher incidence of premature heart disease than women, older people have higher rates than younger ones, and people in lower socioeconomic levels have more CHD than those in higher levels. Could hostility be a factor in these differences?

Studies have demonstrated that men express more anger and hostility than women and that ethnicity is a factor in anger and hostility. Scherwitz et al. (1991) found that men scored significantly higher on the Cook-Medley Ho scale than women, with African American men scoring higher than African American women and European American men scoring higher than European American women. These researchers noted that differences in hostility could be a factor in the known relationship between gender and heart disease and ethnicity and heart disease. In addition, Colligan and Offord (1988) noted that after people reach age 40, hostility scores go up with age for both men and women. Some Type B men in the original Western Collaborative Group Study changed to Type A after 27 years (Carmelli, Dame, Swan, & Rosenman, 1991), and the Type A

people in that study became even more competitive, exact, and hostile over this same period of time (Carmelli, Dame, & Swan, 1992).

Taken together, these studies suggest that hostility may be related to many of the previously established risk factors for heart disease — namely, being male, having low socioeconomic status and a low level of education, being African American, and aging. This close association of hostility and other risk factors leads to questions about the validity of hostility as a risk for heart disease

Problems for the Hostility Hypothesis

The relationship between hostility and other risk factors for heart disease presents the possibility that hostility is not an independent risk factor for heart disease. That is, any relationship between hostility and heart disease may exist because of the association between hostility and other risk factors rather than because of hostility itself. Additional questions arise from several studies that have failed to show a relationship between hostility and heart disease. In addition, hostility is related to diseases other than heart disease. Although demonstrations that hostility is related to various health problems substantiate the toxic properties of hostility, such evidence does not support its validity as an index of heart disease.

The question of whether hostility is an *independent* risk for heart disease comes from its relationship with ethnicity, age, gender, educational level, and socioeconomic status; hostility also shows close associations with other established risk factors. According to cross-sectional studies, hostility was positively related to stressful life events and negatively associated with social support (Scherwitz et al., 1991); positively related to tobacco and marijuana smoking, alcohol use, and greater caloric intake (Scherwitz et al., 1992); and positively related to higher body-mass index, poorer cholesterol profile, and higher blood pressure (Siegler, Peterson, Barefoot, & Williams., 1992). A 20-year prospective study (Siegler, et al., 1992) substantiated the link between hostility and other risk factors for heart disease, revealing that hostility during young adulthood related to caffeine and alcohol consumption, large body mass, high total cholesterol, high total cholesterol to HDL ratio, smoking, and hypertension during mid-life. Although some of these factors may be the result of hostility, it is difficult to see how others, such as smoking tobacco or drinking caffeine, could be caused by hostility.

Several studies have failed to find a relationship between hostility and heart disease. Using a group of physicians, McCranie, Watkins, Brandsma, and Sisson (1986) failed to find a difference in the incidence of angina pectoris, myocardial infarction (MI), or CHD death over a 25-year follow-up period for those high versus those lower in hostility. Another negative finding was reported by Helmer, Ragland, and Syme (1991), who found no relationship between coronary occlusion and hostility for either men or women, and Hearn, Murray, and Luepker (1989) failed to find a relationship between hostility and either coronary heart disease or all-cause mortality.

Hostile people report more negative life events and have lower levels of social support than do less hostile people (Scherwitz et al., 1991). Why should hostility relate to a variety of health concerns? Houston and Vavak (1991) conducted a study of college students that suggested a possible reason for the frequently reported negative relationship between hostility and good health. They found that highly hostile people, compared with those low in hostility,

experience excessive anger in a variety of situations, feel insecure, and avoid seeking social support. By shunning social support, these students encountered few friends who might encourage them to behave in healthy ways or discourage them from engaging in risky behaviors, such as driving after drinking. Matthews and her colleagues (Matthews, Woodall, Kenyon, & Jacob, 1996) found that family dynamics may play a direct role in the development of hostility and anger in adolescent boys. They observed family interactions involving fathers, mothers, and boys and found that negative behaviors such as criticisms, complaints, and put-downs in family interactions predicted boys' mistrustful, hostile attitudes and their expression of anger 3 years later. Also, Siegel (1984) found that adolescents who outwardly express a great deal of anger have increased risk factors for cardiovascular disease, especially elevated blood pressure. These findings suggest that anger might be a component of hostility that is particularly dangerous.

ANGER

More recently, researchers have narrowed their investigations to specific components of hostility, just as a decade earlier other researchers sought to discover the specific toxic components of the Type A behavior pattern. Are differences in results from studies on hostility and heart disease due to different definitions and different methods of measuring hostility? A study by John Barefoot and his associates (Barefoot, Dodge, Peterson, Dahlstrom, & Williams, 1989) suggested that hostility may be too general and that cynicism and expressed anger may be better predictors of heart disease and death than the global concept of hostility.

Smith (1994) defined anger as an unpleasant *emotion* accompanied by physiological arousal and usually lasting for a relatively short duration. On the other hand, hostility involves a negative *attitude* toward others and may be of long duration. If anger is the toxic element in the Type A behavior pattern, should one avoid becoming angry as protection against heart disease? Research by Aron Siegman and his colleagues (Siegman, Dembroski, & Ringel, 1987) suggested that the mere *experience* of anger probably does not threaten cardiovascular functioning. The *expression* of anger, however, may well be a risk factor for coronary artery disease.

Siegman, Dembroski, and Ringel (1987) found that the *expression* of anger-hostility in angiographic patients was positively related to the severity of their coronary artery disease (CAD). Examples of items that correlated significantly with severity of coronary artery disease were those that involved yelling back when someone yells at you, raising your voice when arguing, and throwing temper tantrums. Siegman et al. also found that the relationship between expression of anger and CAD was independent of traditional risk factors such as cholesterol level and blood pressure (except for patients 65 or older). The significance of this research is that the mere experience of anger did not relate positively to severity of coronary artery disease, but the outward expression of anger did.

Support for the expression of anger as a risk for heart disease came from a study by Mendes de Leon (1992), who found that low socioeconomic White male patients hospitalized for symptoms of heart disease had significantly higher Anger-Out scores than did control patients, who were hospitalized for conditions unrelated to heart disease. As with the study by Siegman et al. (1987), this study showed no difference between the heart patients and the other patients in level of Anger-In. Thus, the expression of anger and not the pervasive feeling of anger seems to lead to coronary heart disease, at least in men.

Anger and Cardiovascular Reactivity

Why should the expression of anger relate to coronary artery disease? Siegman and his colleagues have demonstrated that provoked anger in a laboratory setting increases some measures of cardiovascular reactivity, specifically increases in systolic and diastolic blood pressure. If increased cardiovascular reactivity generally accompanies expressions of anger, perhaps the continual physical or verbal expression of anger over many years may increase one's risk of cardiovascular disease.

In one study of male undergraduates, Siegman, Anderson, Herbst, Boyle, and Wilkinson (1992) measured cardiovascular reactivity in a situation that involved a stressful laboratory situation. Siegman et al. found that participants' heart rate as well as their diastolic and systolic blood pressure increased and that participants generally felt a great deal of anger

after being provoked. However, their *experience* of anger-hostility was unrelated to their level of reactivity. On the other hand, their *expression* of anger-hostility was significantly related to both systolic and diastolic blood pressure but not to heart rate.

These results suggest that men, when provoked, show increased levels of cardiovascular reactivity. However, evidence indicates that women may not experience comparable reactivity when provoked (Siegman, 1993a). In addition, Burns and Katkin (1993) found that provoked men, but not women, showed increased cardiovascular reactivity as they increased their outward expression of anger. Similarly, Smith and his associates (Smith & Brown, 1991; Smith, Sanders, & Alexander, 1990) found gender differences in the cardiovascular reactivity of married couples who were engaged in a potentially hostile confrontation. In the Smith and Brown study, husbands experienced increases in heart rate and systolic blood pressure while attempting to control their wives, but the wives experienced no comparable reactivity while trying to control their husbands. Interestingly, the wives experienced an increase in systolic blood pressure only at the times their husbands were expressing cynical hostility.

In summary, research suggests that provoked anger increases cardiovascular reactivity in cynically hostile men but not in women. If psychophysical factors can cause heart disease, these findings may partially explain the different rates of early CHD for men and women. The findings concerning the risks associated with expressing anger bring up the question, Is it healthier to suppress anger?

Suppressed Anger

Dembroski and his colleagues reported on two studies suggesting that suppressed anger, or Anger-In, was a toxic element in heart disease. Dembroski et al. (1985) found that Potential for Hostility and Anger-In were consistent predictors of severity of coronary artery disease (CAD) for both women and men. Defining suppressed anger (Anger-In) as the "inability or unwillingness in a variety of circumstances to verbally or nonverbally express one's anger, irritation, annoyance and the like against the source of one's frustration" (p. 141), MacDougall, Dembroski, Dimsdale, and Hackett (1985) found a significant relationship between Anger-In scores and CAD for a group of male patients who had received cardiac catheterization. Once again, these researchers found no value in the global Type A behavior pattern as a predictor of coronary artery disease.

Although results from these studies seem to indicate that suppressed anger may be harmful, Dembroski and Costa (1987) argued that for patients in these studies, Anger-In was a *result* of heart disease rather than a contributor to it. Also, Mendes de Leon (1992) contended that the relationship between Anger-In (or the suppression of anger) may result from doctors telling heart patients to avoid situations in which they may be provoked to anger and to keep their angry feelings to themselves. This advice has some validity in light of the findings that an outward expression of anger is predictive of coronary artery disease. But this recommendation should be given to people (especially men) before they develop heart disease. Once people are diagnosed with heart disease, anger, whether expressed or suppressed, seems to exacerbate their condition.

Thus, sufficient research exists to indicate that both the expression and the suppression of anger may be potentially unhealthy. However, expression and suppression of anger do not exhaust all possibilities. Siegman (1993a) suggested that people learn to recognize their anger but to express it calmly and rationally. He presented evidence that when people express anger in a soft, slow voice as opposed to either a loud, rapid voice or nonverbal expressions of anger, they are at a decreased risk of developing hypertension and coronary heart disease.

SUMMARY OF HOSTILITY AND ANGER AS RISK FACTORS

As the Type A behavior pattern was gaining acceptance as a risk factor for cardiovascular disease, some researchers started to question its validity. These questions, in turn, led to investigations of the various components of the Type A behavior pattern, and most of that research demonstrated that hostility was a better predictor of CAD than the global Type A behavior pattern. However, some research has failed to support hostility as an independent risk factor for CAD. One possibility is that hostility itself is multidimensional and that only one of its dimensions—anger—has potentially lethal consequences. Moreover, the mere experience of anger seems to have no detrimental effect on cardiovascular func-

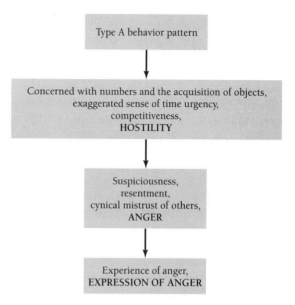

Note: **BOLDFACE** denotes components suggested by research to be the best link to heart disease.

Figure 9.6   *The evolution of expressed anger from the Type A behavior pattern.*

tioning. Rather, the *expression* of anger may be the toxic agent underlying some CAD disease.

Figure 9.6 shows the evolution of the Type A behavior pattern to hostility, to anger, and finally to expressed anger. Although research evidence to date is not unanimous, it does suggest that hostility, defined as the physical and/or verbal expression of anger, may be a behavioral risk factor for the development of cardiovascular disease.

Where does research go next? In the area of hostility and cardiovascular reactivity, Suls and Wan (1993) conducted a meta-analysis of recent studies and found only modest effects for nonprovoked stressors. The most promising area of future research, Suls and Wan predicted, will be provocative interpersonal stressors; that is, researchers should investigate whether people who are consistently provoked to anger by other people are at increased risk for cardiovascular disease. In addition, future researchers must develop more reliable and accurate measures of hostility and anger, and they should use prospective studies that assess both cardiovascular status and hostility/anger periodically throughout the study (Helmers, Posluszny, & Krantz, 1994).

Although the belief that hostility and anger some- how cause heart disease is centuries old (Williams, 1993), psychophysiological research has only re- cently begun to confirm this notion. Still, evidence is lacking that any component of the Type A behav- ior pattern, including hostility and anger, is a strong independent risk for cardiovascular disease in peo- ple generally. Presently, personality factors do not appear to put people (men and women, Black and White, young and old) at the same elevated risk for heart disease as do traditional risk factors, such as cigarette smoking, hypertension, or high cholesterol levels. However, evidence suggests that hostility/ anger interacts with these latter two risks to increase a person's risk for heart disease.

MODIFYING RISK FACTORS FOR CARDIOVASCULAR DISEASE

Psychology's main contribution to cardiovascular health has focused on changing behaviors related to CHD and stroke. Psychologists also participate in cardiac rehabilitation by helping patients change their behaviors so they will lower their risk of hav- ing another heart attack. The role of psychologists in cardiac rehabilitation and other chronic illnesses is discussed in Chapter 11.

Coronary heart disease and stroke are closely as- sociated with several unhealthy behaviors and living habits, presenting the rationale for the involvement of health psychology in modifying risk factors for cardiovascular disease. Most of these behaviors are acquired over many years, and most are somewhat resistant to change. One study (Myers, Coughlin, Webber, Srinivasan, & Berenson, 1995) showed that children at high risk for cardiovascular disease be- cause they had elevated cholesterol levels, were overweight, and had high blood pressure, tended to remain at high risk when they became young adults. Furthermore, nearly all at-risk young adults had been at risk as children, indicating that cardiovascu- lar risk factors begin during childhood and persist into adulthood. Advice to go on a diet or to stop smoking is usually not very effective in altering a person's long-standing behavior. People who enjoy eating eggs and red meats may have quite a bit of trouble giving them up. People who have smoked two or three packs of cigarettes a day for 10 or 15

years may not find it easy to quit. But psychologists have traditionally been concerned with changing be- havior, and many of their techniques can be em- ployed to modify behaviors that place people at risk for developing cardiovascular disease.

Before people will cooperate with programs to change their behavior, they must perceive that these behaviors are risk factors that place them in jeop- ardy. Avis, Smith, and McKinlay (1989) demon- strated that these perceptions can be colored by po- tentially deadly biases. These researchers measured behavioral and biological risk factors for cardio- vascular disease in a random sample of men and women. Among these assessment procedures were questions concerning health-related behaviors and the perception of heart attack risk as well as mea- surements of blood pressure, cholesterol, and weight. The results indicated that these people used the es- tablished risk factors in estimating their overall risk for heart attack, but they also displayed what Neil Weinstein (1984) called optimistic bias; that is, these people tended to believe that someone else would have a heart attack, not them. This tendency to ex- empt oneself from risks, especially behavioral risks, is a strong influence in the development of percep- tion of personal risk, and that perception can affect a person's willingness to change his or her behavior. Both the Avis et al. study and a study by Weinstein (1983) demonstrated that accurate feedback about one's risk status can decrease optimistic bias. A per- son with an accurate perception of risk is more likely to do something about changing the risk fac- tors for coronary heart disease.

The most serious behavioral risk factor in cardio- vascular disease is cigarette smoking, a behavior also implicated in a variety of other disorders, espe- cially lung cancer. For this reason, all of Chapter 13 is devoted to a discussion of tobacco use. Although hypertension and serum cholesterol are not behav- iors and thus cannot be directly modified through psychological interventions, both can be affected in- directly through changes in behavior.

REDUCING HYPERTENSION

Linden (1988) discussed the difficulty of lowering high blood pressure into the normal range because a number of physiological mechanisms act to keep blood pressure at a setpoint. At least eight different feedback systems either raise or lower blood pressure when the body senses that blood pressure is out of the critical zone. Linden proposed that hypertension is perpetuated by the body through the use of these feedback mechanisms, regulating blood pressure to the hypertensive level instead of regulating it into the normal range. Because complex feedback systems act against rather than for the maintenance of appropriate blood pressure, hypertension tends to be difficult to control.

Interventions aimed toward hypertension usually try to control blood pressure through antihypertensive drug therapy. Because hypertension is a disorder that presents few if any symptoms and because medication can cause side effects, patients often fail to comply with the prescribed medical regimen. (Compliance and the role of psychology in improving compliance were discussed in Chapter 8.)

Drugs may be the most common but they are not the only strategy for controlling hypertension. There are also nonpharmacological, behavioral treatments, including stress management (as discussed in Chapter 6.) Other behavioral programs include weight loss, sodium restriction, and limitation of alcohol intake. Langford et al. (1985) demonstrated that changes in behavior could make a difference for people with hypertension. This study examined nearly 500 hypertensive individuals who had been on medication for 5 years and whose blood pressure had been reduced to the normal range with the aid of medication. Participants were taken off their antihypertensive medication and assigned to one of three conditions: a sodium-restricted diet, a weight-loss diet, or a control group. Success with either the weight-loss or the sodium-restricted diet was likely to keep a participant in the normal range without medication. In all, 78% of those who restricted their sodium intake and 72% of those who reduced their weight were successful at maintaining normal blood pressure without medication.

Rose Stamler, Jerry Stamler, and their colleagues have been involved with two long-term trials studying behavioral means to control blood pressure. In one study (R. Stamler et al., 1989), men and women with blood pressure in the high normal range participated in either a control condition or a condition that included attempts to reduce weight (with a low-fat, high-carbohydrate diet), reduce sodium intake, limit alcohol, and increase activity by exercise. The

second study (R. Stamler et al., 1987) also involved diet, but the participants were severely hypertensive. The results of both studies showed that a higher percentage of the participants in the dietary intervention had normal blood pressure without medication when compared to the participants who had not changed their diet.

Relaxation training may also be an effective tool for lowering blood pressure. Davison, Williams, Nezami, Bice, and DeQuattro (1991) found that borderline hypertensive men could reduce their blood pressure to a normal range through relaxation therapy. These findings strongly suggest that hypertension can be modified through behavioral intervention and that continued medication may not be necessary for many hypertensives who are successful in reducing weight, controlling their diet, and learning relaxation techniques.

LOWERING SERUM CHOLESTEROL

Interventions aimed at lowering cholesterol levels can include drugs, dietary changes, or both. Cholesterol-lowering drugs such as *lovastatin* are frequently prescribed for patients with high total cholesterol levels. Lovastatin acts by blocking an enzyme that the liver needs to manufacture cholesterol, and it lowers LDL and raises HDL. Other drugs that lower cholesterol include colestipol, cholestyramine, and gemfibrozil. All have different biological actions that affect cholesterol, but all tend to lower overall cholesterol levels, lower LDL, and raise HDL. All are not equally effective (Lovastatin Study Group III, 1988; Vega & Grundy, 1989), and all the drugs that lower cholesterol are prescription medications that cost money and have side effects. These factors make drug treatment less attractive and less cost-effective than other interventions. Experts (Kinosian & Eisenberg, 1988; Wilson, Christiansen, Anderson, & Kannel, 1989) have concluded that dietary modification is a more appropriate approach to lowering cholesterol levels for the majority of the population. Can people learn to adjust their eating habits sufficiently to affect serum cholesterol levels?

To determine the effects that dietary counseling has on high levels of cholesterol, Bloemburg, Kromhout, Goddjin, Jansen, and Obermann-de Boer (1991) conducted an experimental study on hypercholesterolemic men. Participants were randomly assigned either to an experimental group, which received individualized dietary advice aimed at lowering total cholesterol, or to a control group, which was seen only for cholesterol testing. The goal of the experiment was to lower total cholesterol by 38 points without lowering HDL, and although the experimental group did lower their cholesterol levels, the intervention did not achieve the target levels of cholesterol.

Educational messages aimed at an entire city may have some value in reducing both cholesterol and high blood pressure. As part of the Stanford Five-City Project, Winkleby, Flora, and Kraemer (1994) conducted a 6-year educational program aimed at people in the two treatment cities. Their purpose was to provide future researchers with information on which subgroups can most profit from community-wide CVD interventions. In general, they found that an educational intervention program, which made use of television, radio, and the print media, was generally effective in motivating people to change their behavior. Older people with high blood pressure and high cholesterol levels made the most lifestyle changes, and less educated Hispanic women with high smoking rates and low levels of CVD knowledge made the fewest changes.

Does lowering cholesterol result in decreased deaths from coronary heart disease? Although reductions in total cholesterol do not produce comparable reductions in all-cause mortality (refer back to Would You Believe . . .?), they do bring about decreases in deaths from heart disease in men. Holme (1990) reviewed earlier studies that had included interventions designed to lower cholesterol. At that time, many of these studies had reported a 1 to 2 ratio between cholesterol reduction and reductions in coronary heart disease incidence; that is, for every 1% reduction in cholesterol, a 2% drop in incidence of CHD occurred. However, Holme's analysis revealed an even greater reduction in coronary disease, provided people are able to reduce their total cholesterol by at least 8% to 9%. A later review by Jacobs et al. (1992) confirmed the benefits of cholesterol lowering for men but failed to show similar decreases in coronary heart disease deaths for women. Little research has concentrated on women, and many cholesterol-lowering trials have excluded female participants, resulting in scant and sometimes inconsistent findings. Walsh and Grady (1995) reviewed nine available studies and concluded that healthy women showed no benefit from cholesterol lowering, but another study (Verschuren & Kromhout, 1995) showed a strong relationship between cholesterol level and CHD mortality. These discrepancies may be resolved through additions to the sparse research.

Jacobs et al. (1992) also found that reductions in cholesterol levels were associated with decreased coronary heart disease deaths for men, but this analysis, similar to the Holme report, showed that such reductions resulted in an increased number of deaths from other causes. The recommendations for cholesterol lowering, therefore, are complex. For men, lowering total cholesterol by at least 8% to 9% will probably result in a 15% to 20% reduction in CHD, but unless total cholesterol is over 240, the reduction of heart disease may be offset by mortality from other causes. For women, lowering cholesterol will not produce the same benefits or risks as for men, but women with existing coronary artery disease may benefit.

MODIFYING THE TYPE A BEHAVIOR PATTERN

If the Type A behavior pattern or some component of it is a risk for CHD, modifications should decrease the risk. The most comprehensive program to assess the possibility that changes in Type A behavior might decrease coronary disease was conducted by Meyer Friedman and his colleagues in San Francisco (Friedman & Ulmer, 1984). They assigned people who had suffered a heart attack to either standard cardiac rehabilitation by a cardiologist or to an experimental group that received the standard cardiac rehabilitation advice and care plus participating in group therapy oriented toward changing their Type A behaviors. Friedman and his colleagues (Friedman et al., 1984; Friedman & Ulmer, 1984) reported that by the end of the third year, participants who had received therapy not only changed their behavior but they also had a reduced recurrence of heart attacks. Patients who received behavior-change therapy decreased their risk for heart attack recurrence by half, suggesting that the Type A behavior pattern can be changed and that change decreases the likelihood of a second heart attack.

Although preventing recurrent heart attacks is important, a more desirable type of prevention is to avoid a first heart attack. Friedman and Ulmer (1984) suggested that modern industrial society rewards competitiveness, hostility, time urgency, and concern with material possessions, making people with the Type A behavior pattern uninterested in change. Nevertheless, findings from the Montreal Type A Intervention Project indicated that Type A individuals can change their behavior before they have a heart attack (Roskies et al., 1986).

Earlier, we discussed research strongly suggestive that hostility and its anger component are the toxic elements in the Type A behavior pattern. If this is so, then a reduction in hostility and anger should prove therapeutic. Redford Williams (1989) has suggested that becoming more trusting is the antidote to cynical hostility. He outlined a 12-step program through which people can decrease their cynicism and hostility and thus lower their risk of heart disease. The steps constitute a type of cognitive therapy in which people become aware of their attitudes, stop cynical thoughts, reason with themselves, and practice trust and relaxation.

Anger, too, can be dealt with in a therapeutic manner, and clinical health psychologists have recommended a variety of strategies for coping with anger. The goal of intervention strategies is not to eliminate anger but to cope with it. Deffenbacher (1994) agreed with Siegman (1993a, 1993b) that neither the suppression of anger nor its violent expression can be recommended. Instead, he listed several techniques for managing anger that research has shown to be effective. One such strategy is relaxation training, which we discussed in Chapter 6. Another approach involves learning new social and communication skills. Perpetually angry people can learn to negotiate with others, to be more assertive, and to become aware of cues given by others that typically provoke angry responses. In addition, people can remove themselves from provocative situations before they become angry, or they can do something else. In interpersonal encounters, people can call "time out," count backward from 10, or use self-talk as a reminder that the situation won't last forever. Humor is another potentially effective means

of coping with anger, but one must be careful with its use. Sarcastic or hostile humor can incite additional anger, but silliness or mock exaggerations often defuse potentially volatile situations.

Also, Deffenbacher and Stark (1992) presented evidence that cognitive and relaxation coping skills are effective means of dealing with anger. They used a combination of progressive relaxation, deep breathing exercises, tension-reducing training, relaxing to the slow repetition of the word "relax," and relaxation imagery, in which the person imagines a peaceful scene. People who learned these skills experienced significant reductions in anger compared with people in a no-treatment control group. Moreover, the relaxation group maintained its ability to cope with anger after 1 year.

In summary, angry people can be taught to recognize their anger and to express it verbally in a soft, slow voice or to cope with it by a variety of other strategies designed to prevent the anger from turning to rage or fury. Because anger has some association with heart disease, people at risk for cardiovascular disease who also have problems with anger control can reduce that risk through these various coping and relaxation strategies.

CHAPTER SUMMARY

Cardiovascular disease, which includes coronary artery disease (CAD) and stroke, is the leading cause of death in the United States and most European countries. However, deaths from cardiovascular disease have been steadily declining in the United States, partly because of better medical procedures but also because of healthier lifestyles adopted by many Americans.

Cardiovascular disease can result from atherosclerosis, a thickening of the arterial walls. Although the exact causes of atherosclerosis are not yet fully understood, an accumulating body of evidence points to certain risk factors. The Framingham Heart Study, a prospective study of cardiovascular disease that has gathered data for nearly 50 years, has shown that these factors include such inherent risks as family history of heart disease and physiological conditions such as hypertension and high serum cholesterol levels. In addition, behavioral conditions such as smoking and imprudent eating relate to heart disease, as do certain psychosocial factors and the hostility/anger component of the Type A behavior pattern.

Some of the risk factors can be changed through psychological interventions. Hypertension is subject to some modification, and behavioral interventions have been moderately successful in lowering high blood pressure. Diets that are low in fatty foods help maintain healthy cholesterol levels, but once elevated, total cholesterol levels are resistant to change through behavioral means. However, research suggests that long-term changes in diet can lower total cholesterol as much as 7% to 10%, perhaps without reducing HDL. Hostility and expressed anger—the toxic components of the Type A behavior pattern—can also be modified through behavioral interventions.

SUGGESTED READINGS

Cooper, K. H. (1994). *Dr. Kenneth H. Cooper's antioxidant revolution.* Nashville, TN: Nelson. In this very readable book, Kenneth Cooper, one of the early promoters of aerobic exercise for a healthy heart, discusses the value of antioxidants, including vitamin E.

Rosenman, R. H. (1993). Relationships of the Type A behavior pattern with coronary heart disease. In L. Goldberger & S. Breznitz (Eds.), *Handbook of stress: Theoretical and clinical aspects* (2nd ed., pp. 449–476). New York: Free Press. A co-founder of the Type A behavior pattern concept, Rosenman reviews research linking this concept to coronary artery disease and also discusses the role of hostility and anger in CAD.

Siegman, A. W. (1994). From Type A to hostility to anger: Reflections on the history of coronary-prone behavior. In A. W. Siegman & T. W. Smith (Eds.), *Anger, hostility, and the heart* (pp. 1–21). Hillsdale, NJ: Erlbaum. One of the leading advocates of the notion that anger is the toxic component of the Type A behavior pattern discusses the evolution of Type A to hostility to anger.

Williams, R. B., Jr. (1993). Hostility and the heart. In D. Goleman & J. Gurin (Eds.), *Mind/body medicine: How to use your mind for better health* (pp. 65–83). Yonkers, NY: Consumer Reports Books. Redford Williams traces the development of the Type A behavior pattern to hostility, making an argument that hostility is the critical component in the Type A behavior pattern and suggesting how to reduce this and other psychosocial risks.

10 Identifying Behavioral Factors in Cancer

Victoria was a 16-year-old high school junior when she was diagnosed with **non-Hodgkin's lymphoma**, cancer of the lymphatic system. She had noticed a lump on her head and knew of no reason for it. Her mother took Victoria to her pediatrician, who referred her to several specialists. A dermatologist was one of the specialists, and he took a biopsy and diagnosed lymphoma.

The dermatologist did not explain his reasoning or the procedures. Even when he told Victoria and her mother that the lump was lymphoma, he didn't really explain what it was or what she should expect. He did, however, refer her to an **oncologist**, a physician who specializes in the treatment of cancer. The oncologist conducted further tests and confirmed the diagnosis.

Victoria's parents were not pleased with her medical care and took her to a large research hospital that specializes in children's cancer. The hospital physicians repeated some of the testing and rapidly confirmed the diagnosis of lymphoma. The treatment she received there was different — the staff was always completely honest and ready to explain any facet of the diagnosis and treatment. They were also prepared to deal with her reaction to her diagnosis, the first of which was anger. She was angry with everyone for a while.

Her doctors' understanding helped her assimilate her diagnosis and accept the treatment, which consisted of a 3-month regimen of intensive chemotherapy followed by 6 months of less intensive treatment. Her experience during the 3 months of intensive chemotherapy was terrible. She lost 30 pounds, she experienced muscle atrophy and coordination problems, and her hair fell out. But the treatment worked: The tumor started to shrink from the first treatment.

Victoria's life was disrupted by her illness as well as by the treatment. In addition to the difficulties of traveling to the hospital to receive treatment and coping with its side effects, she was faced with changes in her life due to her illness. Her friends treated her differently, becoming awkward around her and not knowing what to say. Victoria knew that they had never been faced with a life-threatening illness in someone their own age. "I didn't think it could happen to anyone I know," she said. She had been dating a young man for about 3 months when she was diagnosed, and she thought that her illness would end their relationship. She told him that if he couldn't handle it, she would understand. He said that he thought he could, and he did.

Victoria could not attend school during her treatment but received home schooling and graduated from high school with her class. She remembers that keeping up with the school work was not difficult but being alone was. Rather than going to school and being with her friends, she had to study at home by herself. She believes that the experience has changed her, making her less sociable and less outgoing.

Victoria's lymphoma went into remission and has remained so. Although her diagnosis and treatment were difficult and painful, she said that she always thought, "It could have been worse." She never believed she was going to die and never tried to live each day as though it was her last. She did, however, lose her feeling of invincibility.

In this chapter, we examine cancer, the second most frequent cause of death in the United States and many other industrialized countries. We look at the demographics and risk factors for cancer and then discuss behavioral changes that can help to alter risk factors. First, however, we define cancer and describe its biology.

WHAT IS CANCER?

The first medical document to describe cancer was the *Ebers Papyrus,* written around 1500 B.C. That document did not give a detailed description of cancer, only a description of the swellings that accompany some tumors. Hippocrates gave the disorder the name *cancer,* and the Greek physician, Galen, first used the word *tumor.* These ancient physicians did not know much about cancer, however, because they did not have microscopes or use dissection, two procedures that greatly facilitated an understanding of cancer (Braun, 1977).

The 19th century was a time of rapid growth of biological knowledge, and that knowledge furthered the understanding of cancer. The great physiologist, Johannes Muller, discovered that tumors, like other tissues, consisted of cells and were not formless collections of material. However, their growth seemed unrestrained by the mechanisms that control other body cells.

The finding that tumors consist of cells did not shed light on what causes their growth. During the 19th century, the leading theory of cancer was that a parasite or infectious agent caused the disorder, but researchers could find no such agent. Because of this failure, a mutation theory arose holding that cancer originates because of a change in the cell, a mutation. The cell continues to grow and reproduce in its mutated form, and the result is a tumor.

Research during the late 19th and early 20th centuries found that a large number of agents—chemical, physical, and biological—cause cancers (Braun, 1977). Interestingly, each of these different agents can cause identical tumors. For example, a chemical such as benzene and a physical agent such as X-rays can precipitate the same tumor at the same site. Cancers can even develop in laboratory cell cultures, apparently spontaneously. This diversity of origin complicates the search for the cause of cancer because cancer does not have a single cause.

Nor are cancers unique to humans. All animals get cancers, as do plants. Indeed, any cell that is capable of division can be transformed into a cancer cell (Braun, 1977). In addition to the diverse causes of cancer, many different types exist. However, different cancers share certain characteristics, the most common of which is the presence of **neoplastic** tissue cells. Neoplastic cells are characterized by new and nearly unlimited growth that robs the host of nutrients and that yields no compensatory beneficial effects. All true cancers share this characteristic of neoplastic growth.

Neoplastic cells may be **benign** or **malignant,** although this distinction is not always easy to determine (Levy, 1985). Both types consist of altered cells that reproduce true to their altered type. Benign and malignant neoplasms have some differences: Benign growths tend to remain localized whereas malignant tumors tend to spread and establish secondary colonies. The tendency for benign tumors to remain localized usually makes them less threatening than malignant tumors, but not all benign tumors are harmless. Malignant tumors are much more dangerous because they invade and destroy surrounding tissue and may also move or **metastasize** through blood or lymph and thus spread to other sites in the body.

The most dangerous characteristic of tumor cells is their autonomy—that is, their ability to grow without regard to the needs of other body cells and without being subject to the restraints of growth that govern other cells. This unrestrained tumor growth makes cancer capable of overwhelming its host, damaging other organs or physiological processes, or using nutrients necessary for body functions. The tumor takes priority, becoming like a parasite on its host (Braun, 1977).

Malignant growths can be divided into two main groups—**carcinomas** and **sarcomas.** Carcinomas are cancers of the epithelial tissue, cells that line the outer and inner surfaces of the body such as skin, stomach lining, and mucous membranes. Sarcomas are cancers that arise from cells in connective tissue such as bone, muscles, cartilage, and lymph. These two main groups have many types, most of which are named for the cell type from which they originate. For example, the pigment of the skin is called melanin, so carcinoma of these pigmented skin cells is called melanoma. Cancers of the muscles are called myosarcomas. In addition to the two main groups, other types of cancers appear, the most common of which originate from blood cells and are known as leukemias. These three types of cancers—carcinomas, sarcomas, and leukemias—account for over 95% of malignancies (Braun, 1977). Victoria's cancer, lymphoma, was one of the rarer types of cancer.

Carcinomas and sarcomas are not equal in occurrence. Humans have about five times more connective tissue than epithelial tissue, but carcinomas account for about 85% of all cancers in adults (Braun, 1977), and sarcomas account for only 2%. The rate of sarcoma development stays constant regardless of a person's age, but the rate of carcinoma increases markedly with age. The reason for the increased frequency of carcinoma has to do with its exposure to substances that promote cancer. Environmental carcinogens would be much more likely to come into contact with the epithelial tissue that covers the body (inside and out) than the connective tissue inside the body.

Braun (1977) estimated that 70% of cancer is due to exposure to some environmental agent, but inheritance also plays a role in the development of neoplasms. Although cancer itself is not inherited, there can be a genetic predisposition to the disease (Moolgavkar, 1983). Our primary concern however, is with those behaviors and lifestyles that have been identified as risk factors in the development of cancer.

MORTALITY RATES FROM CANCER

Although some people may believe that cancer rates are skyrocketing, such is not the case. True, overall mortality rates from cancer have gradually increased during the 20th century. As Figure 10.1 shows, the total death rates from cancer in the United States has risen from 64 per 100,000 people to 206 per 100,000 from 1900 to 1993. Several factors have

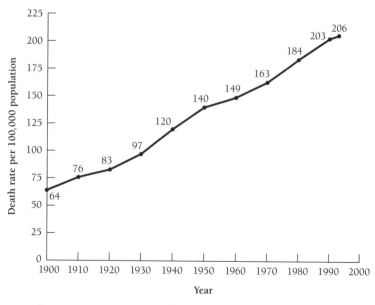

Figure 10.1   Death rates from cancer per 100,000 population, United States, 1900–1993.
SOURCE: Data from *Historical Statistics of the United States: Colonial Times to 1990, Part 1* (p. 68) by U.S. Bureau of the Census, 1975, Washington, DC: U.S. Government Printing Office; *Statistical Abstracts of the United States, 1995* (115th ed., p. 92) by U.S. Bureau of the Census, 1995. Washington, DC: U.S. Government Printing Office.

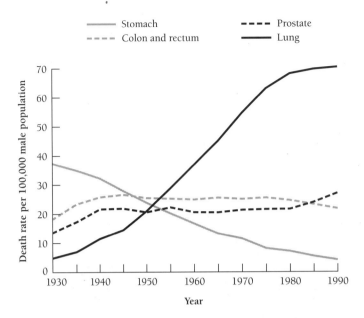

Figure 10.2 **Age-adjusted cancer death rates for selected sites, men, United States, 1930–1990.**
SOURCE: *National Cancer Program 1983–1984 Director's Report and Annual Plan, FY 1986–1990* by National Institutes of Health, 1985, Washington, DC: U.S. Government Printing Office; *Fact Book* by National Institutes of Health, 1993 (p. 47), U.S. Department of Health and Human Services, Washington, DC: U.S. Government Printing Office.

contributed to the continuing increase in cancer mortality rates. First, some small portion of the reported gain is due to improved methods of diagnosis and does not represent a real increase in cancer rates. Second, lung cancer death rate for women has risen sharply since about 1965, and for men that increase began as early as 1950. Third, cancers from acquired immune deficiency syndrome (AIDS), especially Kaposi's sarcoma and non-Hodgkin's lymphoma, have greatly increased in recent years. Fourth, the control or elimination of other diseases, especially cardiovascular disease, means that people are living long enough to develop and die from cancer (Doll, 1991). A fifth possible source of the increase in cancer mortality during the 20th century is an increase in environmental carcinogens, such as pesticides (Leiss & Savitz, 1995). Environmental causes, however, account for only a small fraction of cancer deaths compared with lifestyle and individual behavior (Doll & Peto, 1981)

With the exception of lung cancer, the mortality rates for cancer have stabilized during the past 30 years. When cancer mortality rates for selected body sites are examined, an interesting picture emerges. For men, the four leading sites are lung, prostate, colon and rectum, and pancreas, with lung cancer

deaths far exceeding the sum of the other three leading sites (USDHHS, 1993b). For young males below the age of 25, leukemia is the leading cause of cancer deaths (USDHHS, 1993b). Figure 10.2 shows that from 1930 to 1990, deaths from lung cancer for men have increased about tenfold, with a marked increase since 1950. However, the death rate from stomach cancer has steadily declined. Since 1950, death rates from cancers of the colon and rectum and the prostate have both leveled off.

For women, the four cancer sites leading to the largest number of deaths are lung, breast, colon and rectum, and pancreas, but for girls under the age of 16, the primary cause of cancer deaths is leukemia. Stomach cancer death rates for women, like those for men, have shown a consistent decline during the past 65 years. Unfortunately, the death rate from lung cancer among women has shown a sharp rise since about 1965. In 1985, for the first time, women's deaths from lung cancer exceeded those from breast cancer, and that trend has continued (USDHHS, 1993b). Whereas lung cancer death rates for men are beginning to level off, those for women continue to rise rapidly but still remain lower for women than for men. Figure 10.3 reveals that breast cancer has shown a consistent rate since 1930 and that mortal-

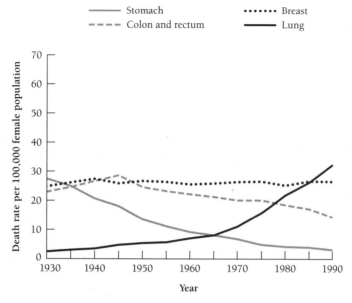

Legend: Stomach ——— Breast •••••• Colon and rectum ———— Lung ———

Figure 10.3 *Age-adjusted cancer death rates for selected sites, women, United States, 1930–1990.*
SOURCE: *National Cancer Program 1983–1984 Director's Report and Annual Plan, FY 1986–1990* by National Institutes of Health, 1985, Washington, DC: U.S. Government Printing Office; *Fact Book* by National Institutes of Health, 1993 (p. 47), U.S. Department of Health and Human Services, Washington, DC: U.S. Government Printing Office.

ity from cancer of the colon and rectum has declined steadily since 1945. From these data we see that except for lung cancer, mortality rates from cancer for both men and women have shown little, if any, increase during the past 60 years. The one disturbing trend, of course, is the increased mortality from lung cancer. For men, this increase was rapid and steady until about 1980. Since then, the data show a gradual leveling off of lung cancer deaths among men. For women, the sharp upturn in lung cancer did not begin until the mid-1960s.

In summary, death rates from cancer have shown an almost straight-line rise since 1940 (see Figure 10.1), but most of the recent increases have been due to more accurate means of diagnosing cancer; a decline in cardiovascular death rates, which means that people now live long enough to die of cancer; the rapid rise of AIDS-related cancer deaths; and mostly to a sharp increase in lung cancer, which is closely tied to cigarette smoking. Most cancer deaths are related to individual behaviors and lifestyles and are therefore avoidable. Despite the continuing rise in cancer mortality, many cancer researchers see some good news about cancer trends, including a 2-decade decline in cancer deaths for both men and women under the age of 55 (see box—Would You Believe . . . ?)

RISK FACTORS FOR CANCER

Although genetic and environmental factors account for some cancers, the leading risk factors for cancer are behavioral. Whelan (1978) and Doll and Peto (1981) have estimated that about two-thirds of all cancer deaths in the United States are caused by either smoking cigarettes or eating unwisely. Cigarettes and diet are not the only known behavioral risk factors; alcohol, exposure to ultraviolet light, sexual behavior, and stress are also associated with cancer. In addition, certain environmental factors, such as asbestos and pesticides, have been linked to cancer.

SMOKING

Of all the factors that have contributed to the rise of cancer deaths in the United States, the primary one has been cigarette smoking. Currently, about 400,000 people a year die prematurely of smoking-related causes; more than one third of these deaths are from smoking-related cancers (USDHHS, 1995). Although the vast majority of these deaths are due to lung cancer, smoking is also implicated in deaths for several other cancer sites, including the lip, oral

WOULD YOU BELIEVE . . . ?

Good News About Cancer

Would you believe that we have more good news than bad news regarding death rates from cancer? Although cancer mortality rates have gradually increased since 1900 (see Figure 10.1), many cancer experts are quite optimistic. How is it possible to be optimistic when death trends are moving upward and media reports tell of the myriad genetic, environmental, and behavioral factors that cause cancer?

Let's look first at some of the media reports. On February 9, 1994, the Lake Charles (Louisiana) *American Press* carried a story on cancer rates under the headline, "Study: Nonsmoking Cancer Rates Increase." The lead paragraph stated, "White men born during the middle of the baby boom are three times as likely to get cancer unrelated to smoking as their grandfathers were" (p. 32). On the same day, an article appeared in the Houston Chronicle under the byline of David Brown of the *Washington Post*. The *Chronicle's* headline read, "Baby Boomers Have Greater Cancer Risk, Researchers Report," and the lead paragraph stated that "a white man of the baby boomer generation has about twice the risk of developing cancer as his grandfather, and a white woman of the same age has about a 50 percent greater risk than her grandmother" (Brown, 1994, p. 2A).

Both newspaper stories were based on the same research, an article in the *Journal of the American Medical Association* by Devra Lee Davis, Gregg Dinse, and David Hoel (1994) that reported on decreasing deaths from cardiovascular disease and increasing cancer mortality among Whites in the United States. The article was subtitled "Good News and Bad News." Both the good news and the bad news referred to current cancer rates.

The bad news is that the all-age mortality rates for cancer are increasing; Americans over 20 have a higher *incidence* of cancer compared with those born from 1888 to 1897; and women now have a five times greater incidence of smoking-related cancer than women born during the later years of the 19th century. The good news is that cancer *death rates* are going down for both men and women below the age of 55 (see Figure 10.4 and Figure 10.5) and that smoking-related cancer for men in nearly all age groups has leveled off.

The Davis et al. study included a 10% sample of the U. S. population across nine regions of the country, but it was limited to European Americans. This study found that from 1973 through 1987, death from cardiovascular disease decreased 42% for people under 55 and 33% for people 55 to 84. On the other hand, death rates for cancer decreased 17% for people under 55, but they increased 12% for people 55 to 84.

Davis et al. found that although a larger proportion of the older population died of cancer in 1987 than in 1973, the all-cause death rate for the elderly was down, meaning that cancer accounted for a larger *proportion* of deaths in 1987 than it did in 1973. Although fewer people died, relatively more people died of cancer.

Although Davis et al. stated that not all increases in cancer were linked to the aging of the population and smoking patterns, other cancer researchers believe that the declining mortality rate from cardiovascular and other diseases accounts for much of the increase in cancer deaths among the elderly. In an editorial in the same issue of the *Journal of the American Medical Association,* Anthony B. Miller (1994) pointed out that as CVD deaths go down, other causes will inevitably rise. In other words, people who in the past might have died of cancer during old age instead died of heart disease or stroke before they reached that age.

One of the world's foremost cancer researchers, Sir Richard Doll (1991), also attributed the increase in cancer deaths to the control or elimination of other diseases, especially heart disease. Doll suggested that the mass media tend to perpetuate a pessimistic view of science's progress against cancer. In recent years, scientists have identified most of the causes of cancer and have determined that most of the identified causes are avoidable. Nevertheless, the media suggest that "our success in discovering avoidable causes . . . is outweighed by the spread of new hazards" (Doll, 1991, p. 675). Although Doll recognized some new hazards, such as Kaposi's sarcoma and non-Hodgkin's lymphoma that are associated with AIDS, he suggested that new hazards are not a cause for pessimism. He also argued that better treatment and changes in lifestyle have brought about a decrease in cancer mortality for both men and women below the age of 65.

Although media reports frequently focus on the negative trends in cancer mortality, ample evidence exists that the good news on cancer death rates outweighs the bad news.

cavity, pharynx, esophagus, pancreas, larynx, trachea, urinary bladder, and kidney (CDC, 1993). In addition, Siegel (1993b) reviewed recently published research and concluded that smoking is a causal factor in leukemia.

What Is the Risk?

Epidemiologists generally agree that cigarette smoking is a strong risk factor for cancer in humans, but they disagree as to the strength of that risk. A study in Czechoslovakia (Kubik, 1984) reported that the

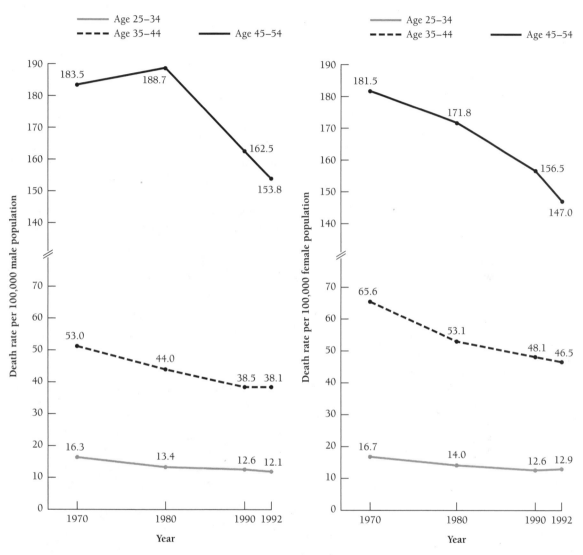

Figure 10.4 Cancer death rates by age, men, United States, 1970 to 1992. SOURCE: Data from *Statistical Abstracts of the United States, 1995* (p. 98) by U.S. Bureau of the Census, 1995, Washington, DC: U.S. Government Printing Office.

Figure 10.5 Cancer death rates by age, women, United States, 1970 to 1992. SOURCE: Data from *Statistical Abstracts of the United States, 1995* (p. 98) by U.S. Bureau of the Census, 1995, Washington, DC: U.S. Government Printing Office.

incidence of lung cancer in men 40 to 64 years of age who had been heavy smokers was 50 times greater than it was in nonsmokers, indicating that smokers in this group were 50 times as likely as nonsmokers to develop lung cancer. Another study

of Seventh-Day Adventists in California (Fraser, Beeson, & Phillips, 1991) also found a relative risk of over 50.0 for smokers. The high risk in these two studies is not typical of other studies, which usually find the relative risk of lung cancer for smokers to be about 8.0 to 9.0. For example, Lubin, Richter, and Blot (1984) found that lung cancer was nine times higher among smokers than among nonsmokers, and a study by Schoenberg, Wilcox, Mason, Bill, and Stemhagen (1989) found that female smokers' relative risk for all types of cancer was about 8.5.

More recently, Risch et al. (1993) found that female smokers were at a somewhat greater risk than male smokers for developing lung cancer. In this case-control study, women who ever smoked were 9.2 times more likely to have lung cancer than women who never smoked. Men who ever smoked were only 8.3 times more likely to develop lung cancer than men who never smoked. Risch et al. suggested two reasons women may be at a greater risk than men for lung cancer. First, women find it harder to quit smoking, but the researchers could find only weak support for this hypothesis. A more tenable hypothesis is that women, for still unknown reasons, are more susceptible to lung cancer at a given level of cigarette smoking.

The nearly tenfold risk that cigarette smokers have of dying of lung cancer is the strongest link between any behavior and a major cause of death. In Chapter 2 we saw that a relative risk of 1.3 can suggest causality and that a relative risk of 2.0 or greater is considered strong. Thus, cigarette smokers' relative risk in the vicinity of 9.0 for lung cancer clearly establishes smoking as a primary contributor to death from lung cancer—the leading cancer-related death for both men and women. This link is so well established that epidemiologists now have moved beyond conducting research in this area and, instead, are more concerned with the risk to passive smokers—that is, people exposed to the smoke of others. (See Chapter 13 for a review of this research.)

Cigarette smoking may also contribute to breast cancer. Although an earlier study (Smith, Sowers, & Burns, 1984) found no evidence for a relationship between smoking and either breast cancer or ovarian cancer, a later prospective study by Calle, Miracle-McMahill, Thun, and Heath (1994) found a small but statistically significant relative risk for dying of breast cancer among women who smoked. After following a large number of healthy women for 6 years, these researchers found that women who smoked, compared with those who never smoked, had a relative risk of 1.26 for dying of breast cancer. Moreover, they discovered a dose-response relationship. Women who smoked 40 or more cigarettes daily had a relative risk of 1.74, whereas, those who smoked 10 to 19 cigarettes a day had a relative risk of only 1.19. Also, the number of years of smoking history was directly related to risk of breast cancer. Finally, women who began smoking before the age of 16 had about a 60% greater risk of dying from breast cancer than those who began at age 20 or later; women who began between 17 and 19 had a 40% greater risk compared to those who started after their 20th birthday. Because of the dose-response relationship in terms of number of cigarettes smoked daily, number of years smoked, and age of initiation, this study presents powerful evidence that smoking at least slightly increases women's chances of dying of breast cancer.

Approaching the contribution of cigarette smoking to cancer from a little different perspective, Po-Huang, Nomura, and Stemmermann (1992) conducted a 22-year prospective study of about 8,000 Japanese American men living in Hawaii. At the end of that period, 1,389 men had developed cancer. Po-Huang et al. estimated that nearly 30% of all cancers could be attributed to smoking. More specifically, they reported that cigarette smoking was the source of 85% of lung cancers, 46% of oral-bladder cancers, and 16% of all other cancers.

These studies leave no doubt that cigarette smoking is a primary factor in the incidence of cancer, especially lung cancer. Research reports vary somewhat with regard to the level of risk of lung and other cancers for cigarette smokers, but such fluctuations are partially explained by the fact that cancers are multidetermined. Besides smoking, such factors as polluted air, socioeconomic level, occupation, nationality, and building material in one's house have all been linked to lung cancer. Each of these has an additive or possibly an interactive effect with smoking (Millar, 1983; Radford & Renard, 1984), so studies of different populations may yield quite different risk factor rates. In addition, the number of cigarettes consumed (Doll & Hill, 1956; Kubik, 1984; Risch et al., 1993) is directly related to risk factor rates for lung cancer, and this dose-response relationship is perhaps the clearest evidence implicating cigarette smoking in lung cancer.

What Is the Perceived Risk?

Despite their heightened vulnerability to cancer, many smokers do not perceive that their behavior puts them at risk. They show what Weinstein (1984) referred to as an *optimistic bias* concerning their chances of dying from cigarette-related causes. In one study of high school students, Reppucci, Revenson, Aber, and Reppucci (1991) found that both smokers and nonsmokers recognized a significant relationship between smoking and lung cancer. However, the smokers judged their chances of developing lung cancer as average despite evidence suggesting that they have nearly a tenfold chance compared with nonsmokers of dying of this disease. A study of low socioeconomic status smokers and former smokers in Australia (Chapman, Wong, & Smith, 1993) found much the same results. In this study, 45% of current smokers endorsed the statement that there is no strong evidence that smoking causes cancer whereas only 24% of the ex-smokers agreed with this statement. Also, 42% of smokers versus only 19% of former smokers believed that lung cancer is caused by something other than smoking. In addition, Brownson et al. (1992) found that both current and former smokers were less likely to believe that cigarette smoking caused lung cancer, and current smokers were less likely than ex-smokers to endorse this belief.

These findings are similar to those of Jemmott, Croyle, and Ditto (1988), who investigated the self-delusional beliefs of both college students and physicians and found that both groups underestimated the life-threatening potential of any illness or condition that directly affects them. Also, van Assema, Pieterse, Kok, Eriksen, and de Vries (1993) found that adults in the Netherlands held beliefs and attitudes that justified their cancer-related risk behaviors. These researchers compared smokers with non-smokers, heavy drinkers with light and non-drinkers, high fat consumers with low fat consumers, and people exposed to artificial tanning light with people not exposed to artificial tanning light. As expected, they found that people who engaged in cancer-related risk behaviors had more positive attitudes toward those risks. For example, smokers were more likely than nonsmokers to say that smoking tastes good, smells good, is sociable, or is good for one's nerves; heavy drinkers believed that alcohol produces relaxation, allows them to interact better with others, and helps them work out problems; high fat consumers were more likely than low fat consumers to believe that fatty food tastes good and is gratifying; and users of sun lamps were more likely than nonusers to believe that artificial light made them look more beautiful and healthy.

People in these studies had some difficulty acknowledging that their risky behaviors actually placed them at risk. Other people seem to lack knowledge about risk factors for cancer sufficient to enable them to change risky behaviors. Pérez-Stable, Sabogal, Otero-Sabogal, Hiatt, and McPhee (1992) surveyed Latinos and Anglos in the San Francisco/Oakland area to learn the extent of their knowledge about cancer and found many erroneous beliefs in both groups. More than half the Latinos and one-third of the Anglos believed that cancer could be caused by sugar substitutes or by bruises from being hit; nearly one-third of the Latinos and more than 10% of the Anglos thought that eating pork could cause cancer; and about half the Latinos and one-fourth of the Anglos believed that having cancer was a death sentence. Although a significant number of both groups held unsubstantiated beliefs about which behaviors can cause cancer, 26% of the Latinos and 19% of the Anglos said there is little one can do to prevent cancer. Also, a substantial number of both groups held unlikely notions about the symptoms of cancer. For example, 39% of the Latinos and 25% of the Anglos said that dizziness was a symptom of cancer. Finally, 35% of the Latinos and 23% of the Anglos said that they would rather not know if they had incurable cancer. Because this Bay area sample is quite representative of the U.S. population (except being somewhat underrepresentative at the extremes of income and age), the findings probably reveal a reasonably accurate portrait of the country's beliefs concerning cancer, beliefs that are not accurate.

Is Smoking Ever Safe?

Is smoking ever safe? Are filter tip cigarettes, pipes, and cigars safer than nonfiltertip cigarettes? Prior to 1960, fewer than half the cigarettes consumed in the United States were filtertips. Given a 25- to 35-year lag between the onset of smoking and the development of lung cancer, comprehensive studies on this issue were not available until the mid-1980s. One study (Lubin, Blot, et al., 1984) of nearly 8,000 lung cancer patients in several countries of Western Europe revealed that lifelong nonfilter cigarette smokers were nearly twice as likely to develop lung cancer as were lifelong filter smokers, thus indicating some safety benefit of filtertips in comparison with nonfilter cigarettes. This finding does not, of course, mean that filtered cigarettes are safe. The problem of filters versus nonfilters is compounded by the fact that the "tar" and nicotine content of nonfilter cigarettes has declined over the years so that some of them yield fewer potential carcinogens than some filter cigarettes. Furthermore, Wynder, Goodman, and Hoffmann (1984) reported that filtertip smokers puff more often, deeper, and longer than do nonfilter smokers. The overall benefit of filter cigarettes is yet to be determined and an accurate evaluation from epidemiological studies may be impossible. Figures 10.2 and 10.3 show a continued rise in mortality from lung cancer 20 to 30 years after filters became the more popular form of cigarettes. Any subsequent decline in lung cancer mortality may be due not only to fewer people smoking but also to cleaner auto exhaust systems and reduced occupational hazards, both of which have a *synergistic* effect when combined with cigarette smoke. In other words, these environmental hazards join with cigarette smoking to produce more than an *additive* effect. Their combined effects *multiply* to produce greater susceptibility than would result merely by adding the individual risk factors.

Another question concerns the use of cigars and pipes and their relative risk for cancer. Lubin, Richter, et al. (1984) compared the smoking habits of lung cancer patients with those of nonsmoking controls. The relative risk for cigarette-only smokers was 9.0, meaning that cigarette smokers were nine times more likely than nonsmokers to die from lung cancer. In comparison, the risks for cigar-only and pipe-only smokers were 2.9, and 2.5, respectively. Interestingly, when cigars or pipes were combined with cigarettes, the relative risk for lung cancer increased dramatically. Cigars and cigarettes combined yielded a 6.9 risk whereas pipes and cigarettes raised the relative risk to 8.1, or nearly as high as cigarettes alone. On the other hand, these researchers found no risk for either cigar or pipe

smokers who had never inhaled. However, cigars, pipes, snuff, and chewing tobacco have been found to be related to cancer of the mouth, pharynx, and esophagus (Mahboubi, 1977), and use of snuff and chewing tobacco has been associated with pancreatic cancer (Heuch, Kvale, Jacobsen, & Bjelke, 1983).

In summary, the leading behavioral risk for lung cancer deaths is cigarette smoking. Although not all cigarette smokers die of lung cancer, and although some nonsmokers develop this disease, clear evidence exists that smokers have an increased chance of developing some form of cancer, particularly lung cancer. The more cigarettes per day they smoke and the more years they continue this practice, the more they are at risk. If a person must smoke, cigars and pipes are safer, especially if one does not inhale.

DIET

Another risk factor for cancer is an unhealthy diet. Simone (1983) estimated that nutritional factors account for 60% of all cancer in women and 40% of all cancer in men. Poor dietary practices are associated with cancers of the breast, stomach, uterus, endometrium, rectum, colon, kidneys, small intestine, pancreas, liver, ovary, bladder, prostate, mouth, pharynx, thyroid, and esophagus.

Foods That May Cause Cancer

Unwise eating includes selecting foods high in carcinogens, either as a natural component or as a food additive. "Natural" foods—those without added chemicals or preservatives—are not necessarily safer than those containing preservatives, and some may be less so. Also, the lack of preservatives can result in high levels of bacteria and fungi. Spoiled food is a risk factor in stomach cancer, and the sharp decline in this cancer (see Figures 10.2 and 10.3) is due in part to increased refrigeration during the last 65 years and to lower consumption of salt-cured foods, smoked foods, and foods stored at room temperature.

Dietary fat contributes to high cholesterol—an established risk for cardiovascular disease, but is such a diet also a risk for cancer? A number of studies have investigated this question, especially as it relates to breast cancer. In general, the evidence for a direct relationship between fat consumption and breast cancer is somewhat complex.

Studies with Seventh-Day Adventists (Mills, Annegers, & Phillips, 1988), postmenopausal women in New York state (Graham et al., 1992), and female nurses (Willett et al., 1987a; Willett et al., 1992) found no relationship between fat consumption and elevated risk of breast cancer. These groups of women may not be typical of all women in the United States because even those in the upper 20% of fat intake may be eating only slightly more fat than those in the bottom group. For this reason Paolo Toniolo and his associates (Toniolo, Riboli, Protta, Charrel, & Coppa, 1989) investigated the link between dietary fat and breast cancer among Italian women who have a much greater variation in fat intake than U.S. nurses. These researchers also looked at the source of dietary fat in a case-control study that compared breast cancer patients with healthy women. Toniolo et al. found little difference between breast cancer patients and healthy woman in consumption of carbohydrates and vegetable fats. However, the cancer patients had a slightly higher consumption of protein and nonvegetable fats.

When the researchers looked more closely at this difference, they found that the breast cancer patients' slightly elevated consumption of fat was due almost entirely to their very high consumption of milk, high-fat cheese, and butter. Women who consumed half their calories as fat had breast cancer rates that were three times higher than average. In addition, both saturated fats and animal protein were implicated in increased breast cancer rates. This study also found that women at a below normal risk for breast cancer consumed less than 30% of their calories as fat, less than 10% as saturated fat, and less than 6% as animal protein.

Dietary fat also seems to be related to the growth and spread of cancer. Verreault et al. (1988) studied dietary habits of Canadian women with newly diagnosed breast cancer and found a direct relationship between consumption of fat in the year previous to diagnosis and severity of the disease. They also found that the relationship varied with the type of fat consumed and the age of the patient. High intake of saturated fat was directly related to cancer severity in older women but not in younger patients. One puzzling finding emerged from this study: Both high

and low consumption of polyunsaturated fat were directly related to severity of breast cancer. In summary, much more research is needed before we can draw firm conclusions concerning the relationship between various kinds of fat consumption and incidence and severity of breast cancer.

Diet may also be related to lung cancer. As part of the Western Electric study, Shekelle, Rossof, and Stamler (1991) followed a large group of men for 24 years and found that increases in dietary cholesterol were directly related to their chances of developing lung cancer. Men who consumed high levels of cholesterol had nearly twice the rate of lung cancer as men who were low consumers of cholesterol, and men who consumed an intermediate level had an intermediate risk. However, the increased risk seemed to be limited to dietary cholesterol from eggs. These authors concluded that cholesterol itself probably does not contribute to lung cancer, but something in eggs does.

Foods That May Protect Against Cancer

If certain eating practices increase the risk for cancer, do other dietary measures protect against this disease? Which foods should people consume to reduce the risk for cancer? In recent years, many health promoters have talked enthusiastically about the protective value of vitamin A, vitamin C, and selenium. What evidence is there to support these claims?

Deficiencies in vitamin A result in deterioration of the stomach's protective lining, and this situation has prompted several investigators to look for a possible association between cancer and low intake of vitamin A and **beta-carotene**, a form of vitamin A found in plentiful supply in vegetables such as carrots and sweet potatoes. The work of many of these early investigators was reviewed by Peto, Doll, Buckley, and Spron (1981, p. 207), who concluded that there is a "slightly lower than average incidence of cancer among people with an above average intake of beta-carotene." The studies reviewed typically revealed relative risk factors in the range of 1.5 to 2.0, indicating that people with low beta-carotene intake, compared with those with high intake, were about 1.5 to 2 times more likely to develop various types of cancers. Because this inverse relationship between beta-carotene and cancer incidence could

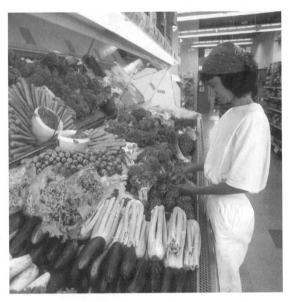

A diet high in fruits and vegetables offers protection against both cancer and cardiovascular disease.

be due to some other factor, the authors were reluctant to conclude that beta-carotene is truly protective. Since this review, other studies (Byers, Graham, Haughey, Marshall, & Swanson, 1987; Hinds, Kolonel, Hankin, & Lee, 1984; Hunter et al., 1993; Stehr et al., 1985) have tended to support the hypothesis that moderate amounts of vitamin A and beta-carotene probably provide some protection against lung and stomach cancer.

Vitamin C (ascorbic acid) has been suggested by some health promoters (Cameron, Pauling, & Leibowitz, 1979; Pauling, 1980) as an effective protector against cancer. Ascorbic acid acts as a nitrite scavenger, thus inhibiting the formation of **nitrosamine** carcinogens. For this reason, vitamin C does appear to have some *potential* to protect against cancer. However, the evidence in support of this hypothesis is not overwhelming. Epidemiological studies with humans have yielded only weak evidence that vitamin C provides effective protection against cancer (Newberne & Suphakarn, 1983). More recently, Hunter et al. (1993) in their study of the 89,000 nurses found no protective value of either vitamin C or vitamin E for breast cancer.

Selenium is an important trace element found in grain products and in meat from grain-fed animals. It enters the food chain through the soil, but not all

soils throughout the world contain equal amounts of selenium. In excess, selenium is toxic, but in moderate amounts, it may provide some protection against cancer. Newberne and Suphakarn (1983) reviewed studies that found some association between deficiencies in selenium and incidence of cancer in animals. In addition, some researchers have found evidence that people residing in areas low in dietary selenium are at increased risk of developing cancer. For example, a study (Salonen, Alfthan, Huttunen, & Puska, 1984) of middle-aged residents from two counties in Finland (where daily selenium intake is less than half of that contained in the average U.S. diet) found that people with low selenium concentrations had excessive rates of cancer. These findings suggest that moderate levels of selenium provide some protection against cancer, but most U.S. diets probably satisfy these requirements.

Although evidence has revealed some protective value against cancer for certain nutrients such as vitamin A and selenium, more research must be conducted to determine the precise relationship between various nutrients and specific cancer sites in humans. Indeed, Graham (1983) warned that some nutrients, such as vitamin C, may inhibit cancer at one site but promote tumor formation at another site. Nevertheless, evidence suggests that some of the same unwise eating practices associated with coronary heart disease (see Chapter 9) are also implicated in the development of cancer. Diets high in animal fat have been found to be related to both diseases whereas high-fiber diets (fruits, vegetables, and whole grain cereals) can be recommended as a possible protection against both.

Evidence that high-fiber diets provide protection against cancer is limited mostly to colon and rectum cancers. Rosen, Nystrom, and Wall (1988) found that high-fiber diets from grain cereals protected both men and women from colorectal cancer. These researchers found high negative correlations (-.75 for men and -.67 for women) between cereal consumption and incidence of colorectal cancer. A study conducted with Mormons in Utah (Slattery et al., 1988) found that some fiber is better than others. More specifically, fiber from fruits and vegetables seemed to offer more protection against colon cancer than fiber from cereals and other grains. In this second study, colon cancer patients were compared to randomly selected controls on food consumption. The researchers found a significantly decreased risk for colon cancer in men who ate diets high in fruit and for women who ate diets high in vegetables, but neither men nor women received any apparent protection from eating grains.

Other studies have found that fruits and vegetables offer little protection against colon cancer. For example, Steinmetz, Kushi, Bostick, Folsom, and Potter (1994) used a prospective design to study 42,000 Iowa women 55 to 69 years old. They found that women who consumed lots of fruits and vegetables and those who ate high-fiber diets had a somewhat reduced chance of colon cancer. However, except for garlic, no specific fruit or vegetable protected against colon cancer. Vegetables that offered no protection included those high in vitamin C, fruit and vegetable juices, carrots, broccoli, cabbage, and potatoes. The lack of associations in this study may have been due to the narrow range of fruit and vegetable consumption of these women.

Although the role of fruits and vegetables in protecting against colon cancer is still uncertain, some evidence seems to suggest that fruit consumption can be a weapon against lung cancer. In the study of Seventh-Day Adventists mentioned earlier, Fraser et al. (1991) found a strong inverse relationship between fruit consumption and lung cancer. Compared with people who ate fruit fewer than three times a week, those who ate fruit three to seven times a week were less than one-third as likely to develop lung cancer, and Seventh-Day Adventists who consumed fruit two or more times daily were only about one-fourth as likely to get lung cancer. These participants led a generally healthy lifestyle—half did not eat meat, only 4% smoked—and very few developed lung cancer over the 6-year follow-up. A healthy diet may protect against cancer, but more research is needed before specific recommendations concerning fruit consumption can be proposed.

ALCOHOL

For cancers of all sites, alcohol is not as strong a risk factor as either smoking or imprudent diet. Scherr et al. (1992) found no relationship between alcohol consumption and cancer mortality among three populations of older people.

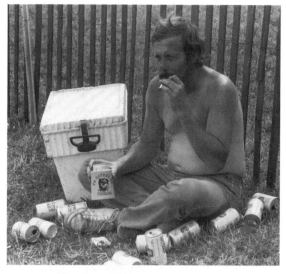

Risks from smoking, drinking, and sun exposure can have a synergistic effect, multiplying the chances of developing cancer.

Alcohol has been implicated in cancers of the tongue, tonsils, esophagus, pancreas, and liver. Pancreatic cancer has a special affinity to alcohol consumption. A prospective study in Norway (Heuch et al., 1983) found that alcohol consumption showed a stronger risk than any other factor for pancreatic cancer. Frequent users of alcohol were more than five times as likely to develop cancer of the pancreas than were nondrinkers.

Some evidence also exists tying alcohol consumption to liver cancer. The liver has primary responsibility for detoxifying alcohol. Therefore, persistent and excessive drinking often leads to **cirrhosis** of the liver, a degenerative disease that curtails the organ's performance of its job. Cancer is more likely to occur in cirrhotic livers than in healthy ones (Leevy, Gellene, & Ning, 1964). However, because liver cancer is quite rare and because alcohol abusers are likely to die of a variety of other causes first (Monson & Lyon, 1975), alcohol-related liver cancer is responsible for relatively few deaths in the United States (USDHHS, 1993b).

During the 1980s, a controversy arose over a possible link between alcohol consumption and breast cancer. Two studies (Schatzkin et al., 1987; Willett et al., 1987b) reported that women who drank alcohol had about a 50% increased chance of developing breast cancer. The findings applied to all levels of drinking, with women who drank more heavily being at increased risk. In addition, the risk was greatest for premenopausal women who were thin.

These studies, however, had some methodological shortcomings (see Feinstein, 1988), and later studies challenged their findings. A study by the American Health Foundation (Harris & Wynder, 1988) compared women with breast cancer with female hospital patients who were free of breast cancer. After adjusting for age at first pregnancy, the researchers found no evidence that alcohol contributed to the development of breast cancer. The authors did not entirely rule out a weak association between alcohol and breast cancer in certain groups—such as thinner women—but found no compelling evidence that alcohol contributed to the development of this malignancy. Two later studies (Chu, Lee, Wingo, & Webster, 1988; Rosenberg, Palmer, Miller, Clarke, & Shapiro, 1990) supported these findings, concluding that alcohol consumption does not significantly increase the risk of breast cancer. These results present a complex picture of the relationship between alcohol and breast cancer. Although drinking may increase the risk of breast cancer in some women, it is not a large risk for women as a group.

Alcohol also has a synergistic effect with smoking, so people who both smoke and drink heavily have relative risk for certain cancers exceeding that of the two independent risk factors added together. For example, Flanders and Rothman (1982) reanalyzed earlier studies and found a synergistic effect of alcohol and tobacco on cancer of the larynx. They concluded that exposure to both substances increased the risk for laryngeal cancer by about 50% more than would be expected if the effect were merely additive. These data suggest that people who both drink excessively and smoke heavily could substantially reduce their chances of developing laryngeal cancer by giving up one or the other unhealthy practice. Quitting both, of course, would reduce the risk still more.

Alcohol and tobacco do not have this same strong synergistic effect on all cancer sites. Herity (1984), for example, reported that alcohol and tobacco have largely independent effects on oral and lung cancers, with only some slight interaction. This finding does not mean that alcohol consumption is unrelated to cancers of the mouth and lungs, but only that its synergistic effects with cigarette smoking are minimal.

PHYSICAL ACTIVITY

Can exercise cause cancer, or does it have a protective effect? Evidence is beginning to suggest that both alternatives may be possible, although much more research is needed before scientists can give a definite answer. Several studies have reported on the relationship between physical activity and breast cancer, but those reports have yielded somewhat inconsistent results. For example, Dorgan et al. (1994) found a moderate risk of breast cancer for physically active women in the Framingham Heart Study. However, this study included only a small number of women who exercised frequently and who also developed breast cancer. Furthermore, these results contradict several other studies. An early study by Paffenbarger, Hyde, and Wing (1987) found no associaiton between breast cancer and physical activity whereas other studies (Bernstein et al, 1994; Frisch et al., 1985; Vena, Graham, Zielezny, Brasure, & Swanson, 1987) reported that physical activity *decreases* the risk for breast cancer.

As for colon cancer, physical activity seems to offer some protection to both men and women. Slattery, Schumacher, Smith, West, and Abd-Elghany (1990) found that regular exercise offered both women and men some protection against colon cancer and concluded that physical activity may buffer some of the harmful effects of a high-fat, high-protein diet.

Evidence for a relationship between physical activity and prostate cancer is mixed, with some studies showing a positive association and others a negative relationship. In a case-control study, Le Mardchand, Kolonel, and Yoshizawa (1991) compared men with prostate cancer with a group of controls and found that older men who had spent most of their lives in sedentary or low-activity jobs had lower rates of prostate cancer than men who had worked on more active jobs. For younger men, however, no relationship emerged between work at physically active jobs and incidence of prostate cancer. One weakness of this study was the lack of assessment of leisure-time activity, which may affect overall activity levels. In contrast, Lee, Paffenbarger, and Hsieh (1992) measured all types of activity and found that physically active men had a much reduced rate of prostate cancer compared with men who exercised infrequently or not at all. These researchers followed nearly 18,000 Harvard alumni for more than 20 years but found only one case of prostate cancer among highly active men and more than 400 cases in less active men. The authors hypothesized that physical activity may protect against prostate cancer because it affects testosterone, a hormone that seems to increase the risk of prostate cancer. Lee et al. hypothesized that exercise moderates the production of testosterone, a potential risk for prostate cancer. The potential risks and benefits of physical activity for cancer are discussed more fully in Chapter 16.

ULTRAVIOLET LIGHT

Exposure to ultraviolet light, particularly from the sun, has long been recognized as a cause of skin cancer (Levy, 1985). Both cumulative exposure and occasional severe sunburn seem to relate to subsequent risk of skin cancer. Since the mid-1970s, the incidence of skin cancer has risen dramatically, but because this form of cancer has a low mortality rate, it has only slightly affected total cancer mortality statistics. Not all skin cancers, however, are innocuous. One form, malignant melanoma, can be deadly. Malignant melanoma is especially prevalent among light-skinned people exposed to the sun. Precise figures are unavailable, but Doll and Peto (1981) estimated that sun exposure accounts for 1% to 2% of all cancer deaths.

Although skin cancer is associated with a behavioral risk (voluntary exposure to the sun over a long period of time), it also has a strong genetic component. Light-skinned, fair-haired, blue-eyed individuals, compared with dark-skinned people, are 45 times more likely to develop skin cancer (Allison & Wong, 1967), and light-skinned people are a higher risk the nearer they live to the equator. Chrombie (1979) found that in Britain and North America, melanoma incidence increased with decreasing geographical latitude. In contrast, on the European continent, incidence was higher among people living *farther* from the equator. One possible reason for

this apparent paradox is that in Europe, skin pigmentation is distributed geographically, so that light-skinned Scandinavians reside in the north and dark-skinned Mediterraneans live in the south. Chrombie concluded that differences in skin color overwhelm the opposing effects of increasing ultraviolet light in southern climates.

What are the implications of these findings for fair-skinned North Americans? The message is clear. Fair-skinned people who have outdoor occupations should avoid prolonged and frequent exposure to the sun by taking protective measures, including using sunscreen lotions and wearing protective clothing while exposed to the sun.

A great deal of sun exposure occurs in people who want a tan, and sometimes those people not only expose themselves to the sun but also frequent tanning salons. Tanning salons are not a safe addition or alternative to sun exposure. For light-skinned people there may be no such thing as a safe tan. The American Cancer Society's slogan, "Fry now, pay later," is an ominous warning, but justified given the evidence that risk of skin cancer increases for people who receive too much exposure to the sun.

SEXUAL BEHAVIOR

Some sexual behaviors also contribute to cancer deaths, especially cancers resulting from acquired immune deficiency syndrome (AIDS). Two common forms of AIDS-related cancers are Kaposi's sarcoma and non-Hodgkin's lymphoma. Kaposi's sarcoma is a malignancy characterized by soft, dark blue or purple nodules on the skin, often with large lesions. The lesions can be so small as to look like a rash but can grow to be large and disfiguring. They can not only cover the skin but can also spread to the lung, spleen, bladder, lymph nodes, mouth, and adrenal glands. Until the 1980s, this type of cancer was quite rare and was limited mostly to elderly men of a Mediterranean or Jewish background. However, AIDS-related Kaposi's sarcoma occurs in every age group and in both men and women. But not all people with AIDS are equally susceptible to this disease; gay men with AIDS are 10 times more likely to develop Kaposi's sarcoma than people with AIDS due to intravenous drug use or hemophilia (Silverberg,

1991). For reasons scientists do not yet understand, Kaposi's sarcoma is now decreasing in all AIDS patients (Doll, 1991; Silverberg, 1991). Among Danish AIDS patients, this cancer declined from 31% before 1985 to only 13% in 1990 (Lundgren, Melbye, Pedersen, Rosenberg, & Gerstoft, 1995) . However, the proportion of AIDS patients who died of Kaposi's sarcoma has remained about the same because, for some reason, patients who were more recently diagnosed with Kaposi's sarcoma had more advanced HIV infection.

Non-Hodgkin's lymphoma is characterized by rapidly growing tumors that are spread through the circulatory or lymphatic systems. Most people with non-Hodgkin's lymphoma, like Victoria, do *not* have AIDS, but a positive human immunodeficiency virus (HIV) test combined with aggressive non-Hodgkin's lymphoma is sufficient to establish an AIDS diagnosis. Like Kaposi's sarcoma, non-Hodgkin's lymphoma can occur in AIDS patients of all ages and both genders, but unlike Kaposi's sarcoma, its incidence is rising. The greatest risk for AIDS-related cancers continues to be unprotected sex with an HIV-positive partner.

Other sexual practices put both women and men at risk for cancer. For women, early age at first intercourse and a large number of sex partners are both strongly suspected in the development of cancer of the cervix, vagina, and ovary. However, some of the danger is offset by physiological changes in women's bodies resulting from pregnancy and childbirth that seem to protect against breast, ovarian, and endometrial cancers. These cancers are less common in women who have had children early in life compared with those who have had children later in life or who have no children. That is, a strong inverse relationship exists between development of breast cancer and age of first childbearing (Levy, 1985). Having a first child later in the childbearing years does not confer the same protection as it does during early years.

The presence of invasive cervical cancer has become a basis for diagnosing AIDS (CDC, 1992), but the majority of cases of cervical cancer are unrelated to HIV infection. Cancer of the cervix accounts for approximately 2.5% of all cancer deaths among women in the United States (Stern, 1991), but some women are at greater risk than others. Its incidence is disproportionately higher among women in low socioeconomic groups, those who have had many sex partners, those whose first sexual intercourse experience occurred early in life, and those who have had early pregnancies. Cervical cancer is related not only to the sexual behavior of women but also to the sex practices of their male partners. When men have multiple sex partners, specifically with prostitutes and also at an early age, their female sex partners are at an increased risk of cervical cancer. Poor sexual hygiene is also implicated in this disease, and evidence suggests that the use of barrier forms of contraception, including diaphragms and condoms, will lower the risk for cervical cancer (Levy, 1985).

Men's sexual behavior can also put them at risk for cancer. Studies by Daling et al. (1982, 1987) and by Peters and Mack (1983) found that men who engage in receptive anal intercourse were at increased risk. Indeed, men who have many sexual partners or who are the receptive partner in anal intercourse are 33 times more likely to get anal cancer than men who avoid this sexual behavior or who have fewer partners.

EMOTIONAL FACTORS

Cigarette smoking, improper diet, excessive use of alcohol, exposure to the sun, and certain sexual behaviors are leading behavioral risk factors for cancer. In addition, emotional factors such as stress, depression, and suppression of emotion have been investigated as possible precursors to cancer. What are the results of these investigations?

Stressful Life Events

Do stressful life events lead to cancer? A definitive answer to this question requires *prospective studies* that begin with people free of cancer and follow them for several years. *Retrospective studies* that begin with cancer patients and then measure their levels of stress several years earlier are less conclusive because having cancer may prompt people to recall and exaggerate earlier stressful events. Greer and Morris (1978) criticized retrospective studies for relying too heavily on the imperfect memories of cancer patients, people admittedly under stress at the time of recall and whose recollections, therefore, could be biased. Also, difficulty often arises in determining the exact time of the onset of cancer, so that cause and effect are clouded. Prospective studies measure such stressful events as loss of job, divorce, and death of a family member *before* a diagnosis of cancer.

Personality factors, such as denial of unpleasant experiences and inability to express anger, may relate to development of cancer. Cooper and Faragher (1993) conducted a quasi-prospective study of women who attended a breast-screening clinic. The study was quasi-prospective in the sense that none of the women had been diagnosed with breast cancer prior to filling out a questionnaire that asked about personality patterns, previous stressful events, and coping strategies. However, these women had breast conditions sufficient for them to seek a diagnosis. After filling out the questionnaire and receiving a diagnosis, they were placed into one of three groups: breast cancer, cyst, and benign condition. The benign group and a fourth group of women who came to the clinic for a general medical check-up served as control groups.

Cooper and Faragher found that personality, life events, and coping styles all play a part in determining the consequences of stress on the development of breast cancer. Factors that *positively* related to cancer were bereavement and other loss-related events and denying the existence of problems, including loss-related events. Factors *negatively* associated with breast cancer were the ability to express anger and living a busy lifestyle. Perhaps the most interesting finding—and one that surprised the author—was that regular exposure to stressful situations *lessened* a woman's chances for breast cancer, whereas experiencing a single major life event increased the risk. Cooper and Faragher speculated that women who are regularly exposed to large amounts of stress are more likely to direct their anger outward and to maintain a busy lifestyle, both of which relate to lower rates of breast cancer.

In summary, although some retrospective evidence suggests a relationship between some stressful life events and subsequent development of cancer, no clear prospective evidence is available to demonstrate that stressful life events are strong predictors of cancer. Cooper and Faragher's study suggested that the inability to externalize emotions relates positively to breast cancer. What other evidence exists that suppression of emotion increases one's chances of cancer?

Suppression of Emotion

The inability to express emotion is a stronger predictor of cancer than recollections of stressful life events (Cox & Mackay, 1982). To avoid the problems of biased memory encountered in the stressful life events approach, Greer and Morris (1978) conducted a prospective study to investigate the effects of emotional suppression and stressful life events on the later development of cancer. They began with a group of women admitted to a hospital for **biopsy** of a lump in the breast. After removal of the sample of tissue and its microscopic examination, about 40% of these women showed a malignancy and the rest had benign tumors. Before the women knew the results of the tests, all were in a stressful situation. Patients were divided into (1) those who suppressed emotion, (2) those who were extreme in their expression of feelings, and (3) those who were apparently normal in their emotional response. A 5-year follow-up revealed that the suppression or denial of anger was significantly related to increased chances of a later diagnosis of breast cancer. On the other hand, such factors as extraversion, depression, sexual inhibition, and stressful life events were not significantly related to a diagnosis of breast cancer. Thus, with levels of stress held constant, suppression of anger seems to be a better predictor of breast cancer than earlier life events.

Dattore, Shontz, and Coyne (1980) avoided problems with the accuracy of recalling life events in a study in which male patients at a Veterans Administration hospital had previously filled out the Minnesota Multiphasic Personality Inventory (MMPI). At the time of testing, all men were free of any diagnosed medical or psychiatric symptoms. Ten years later, these researchers used medical records to divide the participants into a cancer group and a noncancer group. When they examined earlier MMPI scores, they found that the cancer group was more likely than any other participants to have suppressed emotion during a period of years prior to the onset of cancer. Again, these results suggest that people's attitude, including their suppression of emotion, may relate to their subsequent development of cancer.

Later, we examine the effects of emotional suppression on survival of cancer patients. First, however, we look at the relationship between depression and cancer.

Depression

Several studies have examined the relationship between clinical depression and the subsequent development of cancer. The study cited earlier (Dattore et al., 1980) showed that cancer patients not only were more likely to suppress emotion but also to score high on the depression scale of the MMPI years before they developed cancer. An even earlier study (Whitlock & Siskind, 1979) had found that a greater number of previously depressed men had died of cancer of all sites than would be expected from actuarial data. For women, the researchers found no significant relationship.

A larger follow-up study (Shekelle et al., 1981) randomly selected more than 2,000 men ages 40 to 55 from a health study designed primarily to investigate causes of coronary heart disease. These investigators analyzed the data for any possible relationship between depression, as measured by the MMPI Depression scale, and mortality from cancer 17 years later. For men initially assessed as depressed, the risk for death by cancer of several sites was twice as great as it was for nondepressed participants. A follow-up report on this study (Persky, Kempthrone-Rawson, & Shekelle, 1987) showed that depression was a risk factor for dying of cancer but not for developing it. That is, this investigation found an increased rate of cancer *deaths* for men who were significantly depressed 20 years earlier but not a higher *incidence* of cancer. Persky et al. concluded that depression may promote established cancers, but it probably does not initiate them.

However, a later study by Zonderman, Costa, and McCrae (1989) showed no significant relationship between depression and either cancer morbidity or mortality. These investigators followed participants in the National Health and Nutrition Examination Survey for 10 and 15 years and found no difference in cancer incidence or cancer deaths between cheerful people and depressed people. An earlier investigation (Kaplan & Reynolds, 1988) had reported essentially the same results. This study, which was part of the Alameda County study, found an association between depression and deaths from *noncancer* causes, but no relationship between levels of depression at baseline and either cancer incidence or cancer mortality 17 years later. These findings held true for lung, breast, prostate, and colon cancers as well as cancer of all sites.

Differences among these studies may be due to different methods of assessing depression. Studies that reported an association between depression and subsequent development of cancer generally have used the MMPI to define depression whereas studies that have indicated no such relationship relied on other measures of depression. Therefore, the Depression scale of the MMPI, but not other measures of depression, seems to predict cancer incidence and mortality.

PERSONALITY FACTORS

Do personality traits predict cancer? Are some people more susceptible than others to the development of cancer? In this chapter we have reviewed evidence that certain behaviors and lifestyles are related to cancer, but we have not addressed the question of the cancer-prone personality. Since the days of the Greek physician Galen (A.D. 131–201), people have theorized about the relationship between personality types and certain diseases, including cancer.

Interaction of Personality with Other Factors

British psychologist Hans Eysenck is one of several researchers who have speculated on the complex interaction among genetic factors, stress, behavior, and personality in the development of cancer. Eysenck (1984, 1991c) argued that cancer has many causes and that establishing a causative link between a single factor and the development of cancer would be nearly impossible. To prove causation, Eysenck contended, evidence must show that an agent is both *necessary* and *sufficient* to cause the disease. For example, because not all heavy smokers die of lung cancer, smoking is not a sufficient cause; and because some nonsmokers die of lung cancer, smoking is not necessary. Although most epidemiologists do not confine causation to such a narrow definition (see Chapter 2 on criteria for establishing causation), Eysenck's point about multiple causation is well taken. Instead of postulating a single causal agent in lung cancer, Eysenck theorized a complex model where stress, smoking, personality, and heredity are all co-factors in the development of cancer.

The first co-factor, *stress,* may relate directly to cancer. Some evidence (Horne & Picard, 1979) links stressful life events to cancer, but the relationship is neither overwhelming nor clear-cut. A second co-factor, *smoking,* may directly correlate with lung cancer, and evidence of this relationship is massive. In addition, smoking may relate to stress, which in turn may be associated with cancer. A third co-factor, *personality,* relates to cancer, and some evidence (e.g., Cooper & Faragher, 1993) indicates that suppression of anger is positively related to cancer.

Finally, *heredity* may influence cancer through several pathways. First, genetics may relate directly to cancer, and we reviewed studies (Colditz et al., 1993; Slattery & Kerber, 1993) that have demonstrated the impact of family history on cancer. Second, genetic factors may influence behavioral factors, such as smoking, that may relate directly or indirectly to cancer. Also, genetics influence personality, which as we have seen, may relate directly or indirectly to cancer.

The Cancer-Prone Personality

During the 1980s, Eysenck, along with Yugoslav physician and psychologist Ronald Grossarth-Maticek and others (Eysenck, 1988; Grossarth-Maticek, Eysenck, Vetter, & Frentzel-Beyme, 1986), developed a model for the cancer-prone personality. Using questionnaires and personal interviews, Eysenck and Grossarth-Maticek were able to place about 90% of their sample into one of four distinct personality groups or types. Type I included people for whom close interpersonal relations are important and who have a helpless and hopeless reaction to stress. These people also have a rational, nonemotional reaction to life events and do not easily express strong feelings such as anger or fear. These characteristics have been associated with the cancer-prone personality.

People classified as Type II are easily frustrated by others and by things that happen to them. They tend to blame others for their distress and unhappiness and typically react to frustration with anger, aggression, and emotional arousal. Type III people shift back and forth between Type I and Type II be-

haviors and have no consistent reaction to life events. Type IV individuals are the most psychologically healthy, having a strong sense of autonomy and a basic feeling of personal well-being.

Eysenck (1988) reported on results from a study in Yugoslavia for which participants were recruited by selecting the oldest person in every second household in one town. This method resulted in a pool of relatively old people, mostly from 59 to 65 years of age. Ten years later, deaths from cancer and heart disease were compared across the four personality types. More than 45% of the deaths among Type I people were due to cancer whereas only 5% of deaths among Type II people resulted from cancer. This finding alone suggested a strong link between a helpless, hopeless, nonemotional reaction to powerful events and the development of cancer. When the researchers looked at the deaths from cardiovascular disease (CVD), they found that about 30% of deaths among Type II individuals were due to cardiovascular disease, but fewer than 10% of the deaths among Type I people resulted from CVD. Thus, Type I individuals with a helpless, hopeless attitude seem to be prone to cancer mortality whereas Type II people who react with strong emotion to life events are more likely to die from heart disease.

Type III personalities—those who shift back and forth between Type I and Type II reactions—were not vulnerable to either cancer and heart disease. After 10 years, only 5% of them had died from cancer and 10% from cardiovascular disease. Among Type IV personalities, only about 5% had died of cancer and heart disease combined. Thus, cancer deaths were high only among Type I individuals—those people with a nonemotional, helpless, and hopeless reaction to life.

Grossarth-Maticek et al. (1986) replicated this study in Heidelberg, Germany, using somewhat younger participants. Once again, cancer was overwhelmingly the leading cause of deaths among Type I people whereas heart disease was the leading cause of deaths for Type II personalities. After 10 years, nearly 18% of Type I participants had died of cancer, but only 2% had died of cardiovascular disease. For Type II people, about 5% died from cancer and 15% from heart disease and stroke. Grossarth-Maticek and his associates examined a second group in Heidelberg that was similar to the first in age, sex, and smoking habits but differed in being under severe stress. Because stress plays a role in both cancer and heart disease, death rates in the stressed group far exceeded those of the normal, nonstressed group. The pattern of death, however, was even more pronounced in the stressed group than it was in the normal group. Almost 40% of deaths among Type I individuals were due to cancer but only 7% to heart disease. For Type II participants, only 1% of deaths resulted from cancer compared with 28% from cardiovascular disease.

Other researchers (Van der Ploeg & Vetter, 1993; Vetter, 1993), have criticized the research of Grossarth-Maticek and his colleagues (1986) as well as others for its methodological weaknesses. In answer to these criticisms, Eysenck (1993) reanalyzed the Heidelberg data by combining the normal and the stressed groups and extending the follow-up another 4.5 years. He found much the same results as Grossarth-Maticek—Type I individuals were much more likely to die of cancer than of heart disease whereas very few Type II participants succumbed to cancer.

Grossarth-Maticek and Eysenck were not the first to discover a link between personality traits and cancer. Other investigators have supported the notion that a hopeless, helpless feeling and a nonemotional reaction to stressful life events are related to subsequent development of cancer. Simonton and Simonton (1975) discussed the influence of feelings of helplessness and hopelessness on subsequent development of cancer. They have also developed psychotherapeutic strategies designed to change personality traits among cancer patients. These strategies include getting patients to change their hopeless feelings into optimistic beliefs, visualize being cancer free, learn relaxation techniques, and become convinced that they have some control over their illness. Also, Greer and Morris (1975) found that people who repress feelings, especially hostility, tend to develop cancer more than those who openly express their emotions. Shaffer, Graves, Swank, and Pearson (1987) reported on a 30-year follow-up of nearly 1,000 Johns Hopkins medical school students who had answered questions on a series of psychological tests and questionnaires. As a result, the researchers were able to assign students to one of six groups. Thirty years later, only 1% of physicians in the group characterized by "acting out" behaviors and

by overt expression of emotion had developed cancer. However, physicians who suppressed their emotions and who were characterized as loners were 16 times more likely to have developed cancer than physicians in the acting-out group.

Results from these studies point to the possibility that certain personality types are more vulnerable than others to cancer. However, just as further research led to refinement of the Type A behavior pattern as a factor in heart disease (see Chapter 9), additional research is needed to sift out the precise personality characteristics that tend to correlate with cancer.

FACTORS BEYOND PERSONAL CONTROL

Most, but not all, cancer risk factors result from personal behaviors and lifestyles, and these factors are subject to modification. Other factors, however, are largely beyond personal control, including family history, age, and environmental exposure to potential carcinogens.

Breast cancer has long been suspected to relate to family history, and research has confirmed this link. In one recent investigation, Colditz et al. (1993) followed 118,000 women in the Nurses' Health Study for more than 12 years to see whether family history might predict incidence of breast cancer. Using women whose mothers had no history of breast cancer as the comparison group, Colditz et al. found that women whose mothers were diagnosed with breast cancer before age 40 were more than twice as likely to have breast cancer, and those whose mothers were diagnosed with breast cancer after age 70 were one and a half times more likely to develop this cancer. Having one sister with breast cancer more than doubles a woman's chance of developing this same disease, and having both a sister and a mother with breast cancer increases a woman's risk by about two and a half times. Slattery and Kerber (1993) found similar results with a sample of Mormon women in Utah. In this study, women with the strongest family history of cancer had three times the risk of breast cancer compared with those with the lowest risk. The risk was greatest if one's mother or sister had breast cancer, less if the relative was an aunt or grandmother, and still less if she was a cousin or great-grandmother. Slattery and Kerber estimated that about 17% to 19% of all breast cancer is attributable to family history.

As we discussed earlier (see box—Would You Believe. . .?), cancer death rates are coming down for people under 55. Age, however, is a direct and powerful risk factor for cancer death; that is, the older people become, the greater their chances of developing and dying of cancer. Figure 10.6 shows a steep incline in cancer mortality by age for both men and women, but especially for men. Of course, age is also an increasing risk for many illnesses, including cardiovascular disease. Indeed, cancer mortality does not increase as rapidly with age as does cardiovascular mortality. Yet, advancing age remains a strong, largely uncontrollable risk factor for cancer.

Other risks largely beyond personal control include such environmental carcinogens as exposure to radiation, asbestos, pesticides and other chemicals, and living near a nuclear facility. Besides asbestos, Shaw (1981) mentioned arsenic, benzene, chromium, nickel, vinyl chloride, and various petroleum products as being suspected in a number of cancers. About 4% of all cancer deaths have been attributed to exposure to carcinogens in the workplace and another 3% to exposure to ultraviolet light and X-rays (Doll & Peto, 1981).

Children often are unknowingly exposed to pesticides and other carcinogens that could possibly place them at risk for cancer. Leiss and Savitz (1995) studied children under age 15 in the Denver area who had been diagnosed with cancer and compared them to children with no such diagnosis. They interviewed parents about the use of home pesticides such as extermination agents that contained chlordane heptachlor, Diazinon, and chlopyrifos; yard treatment that contained 2,4-D and carbaryl; and pest strips that contained dichlorvos. In general, Leiss and Savitz found no significant relationship between exposure to any of these chemicals and total number of cancers. However, they found some slight tendency for the chemicals used by exterminators to relate to brain tumors and lymphomas; for those used in yard treatment to be associated with soft tissue sarcomas; and for exposure to pest strips to predict leukemias. Obviously, these results produce no clear conclusions, and much more study is necessary to discover the precise relationship between home pesticides and childhood cancers.

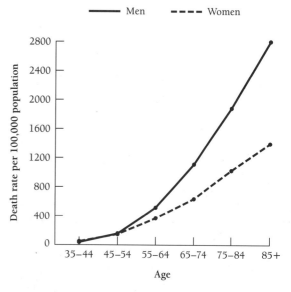

Figure 10.6. *Cancer death rates by age and gender, per 100,000 of U.S population, 1992.* SOURCE: Data from *Statistical Abstracts of the United States, 1995* (p. 98) by U.S. Bureau of the Census, 1995, Washington, DC: U.S. Government Printing Office.

Does living near a nuclear plant increase the chances of dying of cancer? Jablon, Hrubec, and Boise (1991) investigated this question by comparing cancer mortality rates of people living in U.S. counties where nuclear facilities were located with the rates of people living in counties without such facilities. This large-scale study included more than 40 million people and covered the years 1950 to 1984; the researchers found no increased cancer mortality for people living near nuclear electrical generating plants.

This finding, along with results of other studies on possible environmental carcinogens, suggests that very few cancers are caused by factors beyond one's personal control. Smoking and diet remain the two primary contributors to cancer mortality.

PSYCHOSOCIAL FACTORS AND SURVIVAL OF CANCER PATIENTS

Once people develop cancer, can they improve their chances of survival through nonmedical means? More precisely, do psychosocial factors such as social support, a "fighting spirit," or marital status play a role in the survival of cancer patients? Are nonmedical interventions successful in prolonging the lives of cancer patients? Can psychotherapy be an effective tool in changing behaviors associated with the cancer-prone personality?

Despite some negative findings, a growing body of research indicates that psychosocial factors are important in cancer survival. Early studies (Derogatis, Abeloff, & Melisaratos, 1979; Pettingale, Morris, Greer, & Haybittle, 1985) found that patients who fight angrily against the diagnosis of cancer tend to live longer than those who calmly accept their fate. Interestingly, those cancer patients who were poorly adjusted to their illness outlived those who were more psychologically adjusted and more accepting of their cancer diagnosis. Specifically, the long-term survivors had higher levels of anxiety, depression, and guilt as well as stronger feelings of alienation. Patients who did not survive the first year were less hostile, better adjusted to their illness, and showed less anger and fewer feelings of discontentment.

Failure to find any advantage for psychosocial factors has come from several studies (Cassileth, Lusk, Miller, Brown, & Miller, 1985; Jamison, Burish, & Wallston, 1987; Richardson, Zarnegar, Bisno, & Levine, 1990). These studies found no advantage for adjustment to diagnosis or any other personal factor but rather that the stage of cancer predicted survival. None of these studies, however, included specific assessments of the factor of social support. Such social support can come from at least two sources — marital status and supportive psychotherapy.

Married people seem to be able to survive cancer better than unmarried persons. Goodwin, Hunt, Key, and Samet (1987) identified three components in the increased survival time of married people. First, married patients were more likely to be diagnosed earlier than unmarried persons; second, they were more likely to receive early treatment. For reasons that Goodwin et al. were unable to identify, even after controlling for these two factors, married persons still had better survival rates. A later study (Reynolds & Kaplan, 1990) clarified this point, finding that women with social support were less likely to die of cancer of all sites than were socially isolated women, and men with few social connections had shorter cancer survival rates. Spiegel

(1993) discussed the importance of the quality of the marital relationships, saying that people who are unhappily married have health disadvantages but that good marriages are a valuable source of social support. Adequate social support, like marriage, seems to lower one's risk of dying of cancer or to prolong the life of people who have cancer.

In addition to a fighting spirit and marital status, certain types of psychotherapy may relate to survival time of cancer patients. Recall that Hans Eysenck and Ronald Grossarth-Maticek have identified a personality syndrome (called Type I) that seems to be linked to cancer. Moreover, they have reported research indicating that behavior therapy techniques can be used to teach Type I cancer patients to express their emotions more readily and consequently increase their survival time (Eysenck, 1987, 1988, 1991a, 1991b; Grossarth-Maticek & Eysenck, 1989; Grossarth-Maticek, Vetter, Frentzel-Beyme, & Heller, 1988). In one study, Grossarth-Maticek and Eysenck (1989) allowed 100 women with advanced breast cancer to select or reject chemotherapy. Half chose this standard medical treatment and the other half rejected it. Each of these groups was then divided on the basis of age, social background, extent of cancer, and medical treatment into an experimental group that received behavior therapy and a control group that received no psychotherapy. This procedure yielded four subgroups of 25 women each. Survival time for terminal breast cancer patients who received neither chemotherapy nor behavior therapy was 11 months; for those receiving chemotherapy only, survival time was 14 months; for those receiving psychotherapy only, survival time was 15 months; and for those receiving both chemotherapy and behavior therapy, survival time was 22.4 months. Astonishingly, women who received only behavior therapy—consisting of relaxation training, desensitization, and creative motivation—lived one month longer than those who received only chemotherapy. With such small numbers, this difference would not be statistically significant, yet the finding that behavior therapy might be as effective as chemotherapy suggests a crucial role for psychologists in treating cancer patients, at least for those who are classified as Type I.

David Spiegel and his colleagues (Spiegel, 1992, 1993; Spiegel, Kraemer, Bloom, & Gottheil, 1989)

have also found that therapy is important in cancer survival. Spiegel et al. randomly assigned women with metastatic breast cancer to either regular treatment or regular treatment plus participation in a support group. The support groups consisted of weekly 90-minute meetings in which the women were free to express fears and other negative emotions. Spiegel (1993) reported that he had expected the groups to benefit the women emotionally, but he had not expected the experience to lengthen their lives. However, the women who participated in the group therapy lived an average of 18 months longer than comparable women who received only medical treatment.

The studies reporting significantly extended lives for cancer patients dramatically demonstrate the value of such interventions. As Spiegel (1993, pp. 331–332) commented:

> The added survival time was longer than any medication or other known medical treatment could be expected to provide for women with breast cancer so far advanced. Something about the intense social support the women experienced in the sessions appeared to influence the way their bodies coped with the illness. Living better also seemed to mean living longer.

MODIFYING RISK FACTORS FOR CANCER

Psychologists have been involved in treating emotional problems that result from a diagnosis of cancer, and these treatment interventions appear in Chapter 11. Here, we discuss the role of psychologists in preventing cancer by changing those risky behaviors that relate to the development of malignancies. Most cancer deaths can be attributed to risk factors that have strong behavioral components, and the two leading risk factors for cancer — smoking and imprudent diet — are also important risk factors for cardiovascular disease. Therefore, changing certain behaviors will likely lower one's risk of developing both diseases.

Quitting smoking and starting to eat wisely are two habits that most strongly relate to lowered risk for various types of cancers. Smoking is doubly condemned, once as a risk factor for cardiovascular disease and again for its relationship to cancers of the

lung, stomach, and oral cavity. (Health psychology's role in quitting smoking is discussed in Chapter 13.) A diet high in saturated fat is also a doubly dangerous habit because it is implicated not only in cardiovascular disease but also in cancers of the kidneys, bladder, digestive tract, reproductive system, breast, and liver. Conversely, a vegetarian diet, or one with an abundant supply of fruits, vegetables, and grains, is associated with low incidence of many types of cancer. (Eating and dieting are discussed in Chapter 14.)

Excessive drinking is a risk factor for cancer and should be avoided, especially in combination with smoking. Other behaviors to avoid are getting too much sunlight and frequent exposure to X-rays. Certain emotional states, such as chronic depression and an abundance of stressful life events may also lead to the onset of cancer. Various psychological therapies can help reduce depression and thus decrease a person's risk for cancer. Stressful life events cannot be avoided, but treatments that help people cope in an active and effective manner with stress include relaxation training, biofeedback, and cognitive-behavioral therapy. As discussed in Chapter 6, such treatments often mediate the harmful effects of these events.

Another risk factor for cancer is the feeling of hopelessness and helplessness, especially when combined with a nonemotional reaction to powerful life events. Psychologists can use their therapeutic skills to teach people to express emotion openly and to assume more control over their lives. This hopeless/helpless stance also relates to survival of cancer patients and, once again, behaviors that express these feelings are amenable to modification through behavior therapy. A diagnosis of cancer is no longer considered a death sentence. Improved medical treatments have reduced death rates from most cancers. But in addition to advanced medical procedures, certain psychological interventions can play a role in both preventing and treating cancer.

CHAPTER SUMMARY

Cancer is the second leading cause of death in the United States. With the exception of lung cancer, however, cancer mortality rates have remained relatively stable over the past 35 years and are actually going down for people under 55. Approximately two-thirds of cancer deaths in the United States are associated with lifestyle and personal behavior, with cigarette smoking and imprudent eating being the two leading psychosocial risk factors. In addition, research has related alcohol, ultraviolet light, sexual behavior, emotional reactions, and personality characteristics to cancer.

Cigarette smoking is the leading risk factor for lung cancer. Although cigarette consumption in the United States has decreased during the last 30 years, lung cancer rates have continued to increase, especially for women. Cancers of the mouth, pharynx, and esophagus have also been associated with cigars, pipes, snuff, and chewing tobacco as well as cigarette smoking.

Poor dietary habits, especially high-fat diets, are related to cancers of the digestive and excretory systems, breast, and uterus. Women who consume half their calories in fat have an elevated chance of developing breast cancer, but the relationship between specific diets and various cancers is quite complex. Currently, no convincing evidence exists that proper diet is a cure for cancer, but several studies suggest a preventive effect for certain nutrients, such as beta-carotene and selenium.

Alcohol is probably only a weak risk factor for cancer. Nevertheless, it has a synergistic effect with cigarette smoking; when the two are combined the total relative risk is much greater than the two factors added together. Lack of physical activity and exposure to ultraviolet light are additional risk factors for cancer. Also, certain sexual behaviors relate to cervical and anal cancers as well as cancers associated with AIDS—Kaposi's sarcoma and non-Hodgkin's lymphoma.

Some emotional experiences, including stressful life events, predict certain cancers, but the evidence for this link is somewhat inconsistent. Depression and the suppression of emotion, especially anger and hostility, may be related to the incidence of cancer, but a causal link has not yet been established. A pattern of personality traits, including a hopeless, helpless attitude and a rational, nonemotional reaction to life events also relates to cancer.

Psychosocial factors can predict length of survival time for people with cancer. Poor adjustment and a nonacceptance of the cancer diagnosis are *positive* traits for cancer patients and tend to prolong their lives. For several reasons, cancer patients who are married tend to live longer than those who are not. Supportive therapy that allows the expression of negative emotions increases survival time and demonstrates the power of psychosocial factors in cancer survival.

Psychologists can help people modify risk factors for cancer through techniques oriented toward quitting smoking and changing eating habits. In addition, some evidence exists that behavior therapy and some other therapies can be effective in changing personality characteristics of people who are prone to cancer.

SUGGESTED READINGS

Dollinger, M., Rosenbaum, E. H., & Cable, G. (1991). *Everyone's guide to cancer therapy.* Kansas City: Somerville. For anyone with cancer or who has a loved one or family member with cancer, this very readable book contains answers to commonly asked questions.

Eysenck, H. J. (1988, December). Health's character. *Psychology Today, 22,* 28–35. Hans Eysenck discusses the work of Ronald Grossarth-Maticek, who found Type I personality characteristics to be highly related to the development of cancer. Eysenck also discusses the effectiveness of behavior therapy intervention in prolonging survival time of terminal cancer patients.

Ott, P. J., & Levy, S. M. (1994). Cancer in women. In V. J. Adesso, D. M. Reddy, & R. Fleming (Eds.), *Psychological perspectives on women's health* (pp. 83–98). Washington, DC: Taylor & Francis. Peggy Ott and Sandra Levy discuss psychological aspects of cancer in women, with emphasis on breast and gynecological cancers. Pertinent topics include prevention, psychological adjustment to cancer, and psychological factors in survival rates.

Living with Chronic Illness

Brenda was concerned about her mother, Sylvia, who seemed to be more and more forgetful. At first, Brenda attributed the lapses in Sylvia's memory to her age. She was 81 and entitled to be forgetful at times, but the times were becoming progressively more frequent and disturbing. One day when she was visiting her mother, Brenda noticed that the electric stove in the kitchen was still turned on to the highest setting. She turned it off without saying anything to Sylvia. Later that afternoon, Brenda asked her mother what she had fixed for dinner and was quite surprised when Sylvia replied that she had forgotten to eat. Could it be that Sylvia had turned on the stove and then forgotten to cook anything? The question bothered Brenda.

Several months later when Brenda was visiting her mother, Sylvia suddenly became angry and accused her daughter of throwing away her reading glasses. "You threw out my glasses," Sylvia shouted. "You don't want me to read the newspaper. What are you trying to do to me?" Brenda tried to assure her mother that she had not thrown out her glasses and that she wasn't trying to do anything to her, but Sylvia remained unconvinced.

As time passed, Sylvia's failing memory became even more disconcerting to Brenda. Sylvia often forgot to eat, to bathe, to comb her hair, or to feed her cat. Moreover, she repeatedly confused the names of her children, lost interest in reading and watching television, failed to understand directions, and had difficulty making herself understood.

Sylvia was aware of her loss of memory and would become angry at herself when she could not think of names for simple objects like the chair, the table, or the radio. Her memory for past events seemed to be largely unaffected. She frequently showed old photo albums to Brenda and told stories about the people in the pictures. However, she had little memory for what happened the day before or even the minute before. One day when Brenda was preparing to leave, she said to Sylvia, "I'm going home now, Mother. Do you understand?" Sylvia replied that she did, but when Brenda started for the door, Sylvia asked, "Where are you going?"

Brenda had two brothers and an older sister, but they lived in other cities, and the closest was more than 200 miles away. Brenda knew that she would be the one primarily responsible for her mother. She wondered whether her mother might have Alzheimer's disease, so she sought the opinion of Sylvia's physician. The doctor was unable to confirm a diagnosis and pointed out that no absolute diagnosis of Alzheimer's is possible while the patient is still living. Only by eliminating other possible causes of Sylvia's dementia, the doctor told Brenda, could he determine that Sylvia was likely to have Alzheimer's disease.

This chapter looks at the consequences of living with chronic illnesses, such as Alzheimer's disease, cancer, cardiovascular disease, diabetes, and AIDS, but other chronic illnesses share many elements with these. The physiology of the diseases varies, but the emotional and physical adjustments, the disruption of family dynamics, the need for continued medical care, and the necessity for self-mangement also apply to such chronic diseases as asthma, arthritis, kidney disease, head injury, and spinal cord injury.

THE IMPACT OF CHRONIC ILLNESS

Long-lasting, chronic illnesses are now far more common in the United States than short-term, acute diseases. At any point in time, half the U.S. population is affected by chronic illness, and virtually everyone will eventually develop some type of chronic illness (Taylor & Aspinwall, 1993). Most of these conditions are not severe or life-threatening, but the number of people affected presents a major problem for the medical profession and for health psychology because such conditions affect not only the person with the illness but friends and family members as well. As Chapter 1 explained, the patterns of death and illness in the United States have changed during the past 100 years. Whereas acute illnesses such as pneumonia and influenza were once among the leading causes of death, today such chronic illness as heart disease and cancer have become the leading causes of death. Acute illnesses do not last long; people are either cured relatively quickly or die rapidly. Chronic illnesses, on the other hand, are lingering and if fatal, they cause death only after a lengthy period of illness. During this period symptoms are not necessarily constant. People with chronic illnesses may feel relatively well at times and very sick at other times, but they are never completely healthy.

According to Howard Leventhal and his colleagues (Leventhal, Meyer, & Nerenz, 1980; Leventhal, Nerenz, & Steele, 1984; Meyer, Leventhal, & Gutman, 1985), people tend to conceptualize illnesses as acute rather than chronic. These researchers have found that people with a chronic illness (namely, hypertension) thought about this disorder as though it were an acute illness, believing that they would not be in treatment for the rest of their lives and that they would eventually recover. These beliefs would be correct about an acute illness, but they represent a distorted view of a chronic illness like hypertension. The research of Leventhal and his colleagues suggests that people have trouble understanding that chronic illnesses will continue indefinitely; instead, they tend to apply their knowledge of acute illness to any disorder they develop.

Arluke (1988) also discussed the difficulty that people have in conceptualizing chronic illness, but his emphasis was on society rather than the individual. He pointed out that our view of illness and the role that sick people assume—the sick role—is oriented toward acute illness. With acute illness, the sick person has the privilege of relief from normal responsibilities and the duty to try to get well. With chronic illness, this role is often inappropriate because the person may not need or wish to have relief from normal responsibilities, and although the person may be able to improve, ordinarily he or she cannot get well.

Serious chronic illness presents a crisis in people's lives that frequently goes beyond adjusting to the illness itself. For instance, chronic illness may change the way patients see themselves, produce financial hardships, and severely affect relationships with family members and friends.

Recognizing how pervasive a chronic illness is to a person's life, Moos and Schaefer (1984) analyzed physical illness in terms of crisis theory. *Crisis theory*—based on the ideas of Erich Lindemann, Erik Erikson, and others—deals with the impact of disruptions on established patterns of personal and social functioning. This theory holds that individuals need to operate in a state of equilibrium. When that state is disrupted for any reason, including illness, people rely on previously successful ways of responding in an effort to restore balance. A crisis exists when events are so unusual or major that habitual patterns of coping are inadequate. People then experience heightened feelings of anxiety, fear, and stress. Because people cannot tolerate a crisis state for very long, they will adopt new ways of responding. Some of these new patterns of coping may lead to healthy adaptation, but others result in unhealthy adjustment and psychological deterioration. The crisis itself is neither healthy nor pathological. Rather, it is a turning point in a person's life, resulting in either a healthy adjustment to the precipitating event or a psychologically unhealthy adaptation. Crisis theory suggests that chronic illness would not inevitably bring about psychological distress. A person might react to the illness in either a positive or a negative manner.

IMPACT ON THE PATIENT

In one way or another, all patients must cope with their illness. They must deal with the symptoms of the illness and manage the stress of treatment procedures. These tasks are not easy. As Chapter 7 explained, all people who enter into the health care system must cope not only with their illness but also the stresses of receiving treatment. Because of the time course of chronic illnesses, patients with these conditions are faced with problems beyond those that patients with an acute illness must manage.

Several studies have explored the impact of chronic illness on the lives of patients. Anita Stewart and her colleagues (1989) evaluated the functioning of a large group of patients with a variety of chronic illnesses. These researchers found that patients with chronic illnesses showed worse social and physical functioning, poorer mental health, and greater pain than patients without chronic illnesses, demonstrating that chronic illness produces a variety of problems. Hypertension had the least whereas gastrointestinal disorders and heart disease had the highest impact. Patients with more than one chronic condition showed greater decrements in functioning than patients with only one chronic illness. Devins et al. (1990) investigated the degree of intrusiveness for chronic illnesses, finding that the degree of intrusiveness correlated with the time required for treatment of the condition, the symptoms, the amount of fatigue, and the degree to which the illness interfered with daily activities. These two studies show

that chronic illnesses differ in their impact, not in terms of severity but in how much they disrupt patients' lives. Even serious illnesses that have few symptoms and allow patients to function at near normal levels do not produce the adjustment problems caused by less serious but more intrusive illnesses.

A major impact of chronic illness involves the changes that occur in how people think of themselves; that is, the diagnosis of a chronic illness changes self-perception. Fife (1994) studied cancer patients to investigate how they understood and integrated the meaning of their illness into their lives and how their diagnosis changed their perceptions of themselves. She found that understanding the meaning of their illness on a personal level was an important part of their coping. Many of the cancer patients in the study had been forced to reevaluate their lives, relationships, and body image as a result of their illness and treatment. Some had found positive as well as negative aspects in the experience. None of them, however, had remained as they were before their diagnosis, and none imagined that their lives would ever be the same.

People with chronic illnesses tend to adopt a number of coping strategies to deal with their illness. Christine Dunkel-Schetter and her colleagues (1992) identified several of these strategies, including attempts to focus on the positive aspect of one's illness. Although these researchers studied cancer patients, they found coping strategies similar to those of people with other chronic illnesses. In addition to focusing on the positive, the patients who experienced the least emotional distress tended to seek social support and to try to distance themselves emotionally from their illness. Those who experienced more emotional distress tended to cope by using strategies of cognitive or behavioral avoidance, such as wishing that the situation would go away or avoiding the situation by misusing drugs, alcohol, or food. In summary, people with chronic illnesses—like other stressed people—use a variety of coping strategies, but some strategies are more effective than others.

Like patients with acute illnesses, those with chronic diseases must develop and maintain relationships with health care providers (Moos & Schaefer, 1984), but the nature of these relationships is not the same for patients with chronic illnesses as it is for patients with acute illnesses. People with a chronic illness may have a somewhat hopeless attitude toward their condition, and this despair is often reflected in their relationship with their physician. Conversely, people with an acute illness usually believe that modern medicine can quickly cure their disorder, and this hopeful attitude often results in an optimistic feeling toward their health care provider.

Gallagher (1988) noted that the basis for medical authority comes from the respect that patients have for their health care providers. Patients with acute illnesses are not likely to challenge this authority, but those with chronic illnesses frequently question their doctor's knowledge and competence, perhaps because they have the unrealistic belief that physicians should be able to cure them. These challenges may come through alternative sources of knowledge that patients acquire through personal experience with the illness or through personal contact with other patients. Patients may also challenge a treatment regimen that they believe is not helping them. Either of these challenges can result in failure to follow the prescribed regimen, and noncompliance is a substantial problem in the treatment of chronic illness. Health care providers are frequently frustrated by patients who fail to adhere to their prescribed regimens and therefore may find that treating patients with chronic illness is less satisfying than treating other patients. These feelings may alter their relationships with chronically ill patients and negatively affect treatment.

Gallagher also noted that medical authorities often fail patients with chronic illnesses by concentrating on the physical aspects of the illness while neglecting to provide practical advice on how to cope with it. For example, people who have experienced a heart attack often participate in a program of rehabilitation that includes dietary changes. The medical advice includes lowering the amount of fat in their diet and restricting sodium intake. The advice might even include a list of the foods to avoid and the foods to eat, but this advice would not include information on how to order such a meal in a restaurant or how to cook such a meal. Nor do physicians necessarily feel competent in giving such advice (Mittelmark, Luepker, Grimm, Kottke, & Blackburn, 1988).

Such deficits have led to the creation of support groups for patients with chronic illnesses as well as the growing involvement of health psychology in providing interventions aimed at coping with chronic illnesses. These services supplement traditional health care and help chronically ill patients to maintain compliance with the prescribed regimen and sustain a working relationship with health care providers. Unfortunately, these interventions tend to appeal to White, middle-class women, a group well served by traditional mental health services (Taylor & Aspinwall, 1993).

Another problem that people with physical illnesses must solve is the management of emotion and negative feelings (Moos & Schaefer, 1984). The management of negative emotion is an even more serious task for those with chronic illness than for the acutely ill because their illness will last longer and have a more uncertain course. According to Moos and Schaefer, the uncertainty of chronic illness results in a state of provisional equilibrium, a tenuous condition that may be shattered at any moment by changes in the illness. This uncertainty is an additional emotional burden and one that medicine has traditionally neglected. Health care professionals often expect some negative emotional reactions and fail to label these reactions as problems to be diagnosed. People with adverse emotional effects experience a decreased quality of life and may be less likely to adhere to treatment regimens (Taylor & Aspinwall, 1993). Diagnosing emotional problems can be difficult in those with chronic illness because the physical manifestations of the illness or treatment may be similar to the symptoms of depression.

Again, health psychologists have created interventions for many chronic illnesses that emphasize the management of emotions. Support groups have also addressed this need by providing emotional support to patients or family members who must confront an illness with little chance of a cure. Meyer and Mark (1995) performed a meta-analysis on studies dealing with the effectiveness of psychosocial interventions with cancer patients to determine whether these interventions are effective in helping patients. They included studies that used a variety of behavioral, informational, and educational methods. This meta-analysis revealed that all these types of interventions showed beneficial effects for emotional and functional adjustment measures as well as measures of treatment-related and disease-related symptoms.

Moos and Schaefer also discussed the need for sick people to be able to maintain a sense of competence and mastery. This task, however, is not easy. As Chapter 7 discussed, interactions with the health care system tend to deprive people of not only their sense of competence and mastery but also their rights and privileges; that is, health care tends to result in the "nonperson" treatment for sick people. Gallagher (1988) pointed out that people with chronic illnesses are sometimes expeced to manage their own condition and sometimes urged to rely on care from medical professionals. Thus, these patients have to take responsibility for and control of their treatment sometimes and completely relinquish control of their condition at other times. Such a situation is especially difficult and may lead to repeated feelings of loss of control.

Fife (1994) mentioned the loss of personal control and threats to self-esteem as two of the changes that patients with chronic illnesses must face. The patients in her study described a feeling of increased vulnerability related to putting themselves in the hands of health care professionals. In addition, many of the participants in the study mentioned changes in the way others thought of them and how they considered their own worth. Their illness had restricted their feelings of competence and their planning for a future.

Sustaining personal relationships was the final task of coping with physical illness mentioned by Moos and Schaefer (1984). Social support is an important factor in maintaining health (Berkman & Syme, 1979; Wiley & Camacho, 1980), and the family is the major source of social support for many people. When people become ill, their behavior often changes, and the relationships and the expectations of their friends and family members undergo significant shifts. These changes are partly due to their role as sick people. However, people who are chronically ill do not fit the sick role as well as those who are acutely ill. Therefore, chronic illness

can have a great impact on the family of the chronically ill.

IMPACT ON THE FAMILY

Illness is a crisis not only for people who are ill but also for the families of sick people. As Sylvia's illness progressed, she became unable to live alone. She sometimes wandered about her neighborhood in the middle of the night, forgot to eat, set fires in her house to burn old letters, and behaved in other dangerous ways that made living alone an impossibility. Brenda realized that her mother needed constant care and vigilance, so she and her husband, Bob, decided to move Sylvia into their home. Sylvia resented this notion, claiming that nothing was wrong with her and that Brenda was trying to steal her money. With much rancor and bitterness all around, the move was made. Although Sylvia had previously spent a great deal of time in her daughter's house, this move confused and disoriented her. She couldn't find her personal belongings and had trouble understanding how to move from one room to another. She became increasingly angry at Brenda, her primary caregiver, and complained to Bob that "that woman (meaning Brenda) is mean to me." Paradoxically, her fury was directed almost exclusively at Brenda, the person who spent so much time and effort caring for her. Brenda was unable to continue her law practice and care for her mother, so she gave up her practice to be with Sylvia 24 hours a day. Bob tried to relieve his wife whenever possible, but he too was a lawyer, and his income was important, so he worked longer hours than he did before Brenda gave up her job. During the 3 years that Sylvia lived with Brenda and Bob, Brenda felt stressed and confined. Often she wondered who was the real victim of her mother's disease.

In adults like Sylvia, chronic illness may cause a redefinition of identity (Fife, 1994; Moos, 1984) and a change in relationships with others. Chronic illness in children also changes the lives not only of the patients but of the entire family, as parents and siblings try to maintain a family life while coping with therapy for the sick child.

The relationship between married partners often undergoes changes when one develops a chronic illness. Palmer, Canzona, and Wai (1984) analyzed coping responses in married couples when one partner underwent kidney dialysis for renal failure. They found that this illness changed the role of the married couple and that those couples with flexible roles adapted better than those couples with fixed, inflexible roles. For example, one woman was so accustomed to being the submissive partner in her marriage that she failed to summon medical assistance when her dominant husband became unconscious as a result of a failure in the dialysis procedure. Her inaction contributed to his death.

The couples studied by Palmer et al. experienced strain in their relationships due to lack of understanding and lack of support. These problems tended to grow out of a discrepancy between the patients' view of their problems and the partners' view of the patients' problems. Interestingly, the treatment itself was not a major problem in the relationship, but these marital relationships suffered as a result of the treatment. Many couples became closer but not more satisfied, because the closeness was a result of dependency and came at the price of sacrificing one partner for the other's needs. Research by Helgeson (1993) confirmed the changes in couples' relationship as a result of chronic illness. Although couples initially experienced changes in their relationships, partners reported that their relationship had returned to what it was before the illness. However, their beliefs in a return to "normal" did not correspond to objective reports, suggesting that couples make changes in the ways that they relate to each other but that they may be unaware of the extent of those changes.

Chronically ill parents can also experience changes that produce problems in their relationships with their children, and these changes are most pronounced for children with a terminally ill parent (Christ et al., 1993). As part of the sick role, a parent may lose the authority to discipline a child, or a sick parent may be protected from children's misbehavior because of the illness. Children may avoid consulting a sick parent so as not to burden the parent additionally, resulting in decreased closeness. Children may be even less comfortable than adults with sick people and may change their behavior toward their sick parent as a result. Children may fear or experience changes in family life and

their role in the family may change as a result of a parent's illness. Young children may even feel guilt for their parent's illness because they do not understand that their misbehavior played no role in the development of the illness. Many of the children in the Christ et al. study exhibited this or other misunderstanding of their parent's illness, and many children expressed fears that their other parent would also get sick.

Changes in family relationships that occur as a result of sickness can greatly affect spouses, children, and other family members. Sick people adopt new behaviors because their physical symptoms frequently impose adjustments and because their interpersonal relationships are changing. For adults, these changes are the result of a redefinition of identity, but for children who are sick, illness can be an important factor in their identity formation.

Although the rates of illness for children have fallen dramatically in the 20th century, a significant number of children still experience chronic illnesses (Newachek & Taylor, 1992). The majority of these illnesses are relatively minor, such as respiratory allergies; some of the chronic illnesses that affect children, such as cancer, asthma, rheumatoid arthritis, and diabetes, limit mobility and activity. For the 11% of children with more severe chronic conditions, about half reported that they were affected about half the time and another one-fifth said the condition bothered them most or all of the time. The bothersome aspects of their illnesses included time they must spend in bed and lost school days as well as restrictions on activities and mobility. For some children, these restrictions are very difficult, leading to isolation, depression, and distress whereas other children cope more effectively (Brunnquell & Hall, 1984). Children who tend to be physically active and who have formed friendships based on activity find restrictions difficult. Health care providers and parents can help these children make adjustments by offering alternative or modified activities.

Families of sick children tend to be emotionally and physically fatigued (Garrison & McQuiston, 1989; Moos, 1984). Furthermore, a child's chronic illness can lead to marital problems and sibling jealousy. Moos pointed out that the dependence of sick children can easily lead to overdependence, and sick children can learn to manipulate the family by becoming angry or depressed when they do not get their way.

Sick children change family dynamics, but they do not change family roles. A child who is ill requires a great deal of emotional support, most of which is supplied by mothers. Moos mentioned that mothers can be so drained by the demands of a sick child that they have little emotional energy left for their husband, a situation that may cause the husband to feel angry and abandoned. Fathers of sick children may experience a great deal of conflict over their feelings of anger and abandonment. This conflict is often linked to their concern for the health of the sick child, the financial demands of the entire family, and their own difficulty in expressing emotions.

Moos recommended that families try to find some positive aspect of their child's illness. One example of this would be to look for ways that the crisis might bring the family closer together and make family members feel less reluctant to express their feelings. Moos also suggested that families should find ways to express their negative emotions, such as anger and frustration over their situation. Families with sick children should also set aside time for themselves and not spend all their energy caring for the sick child. As a result of their own unmet emotional needs, many parents have joined support groups for families of children with chronic illnesses. These support groups can help families manage their emotions as well as receive information about their child's condition.

Chronic illness tends to disrupt normal family functioning and place added stress on the patient. Although some common elements are found in all chronic diseases, special problems exist for people living with cardiovascular disease, cancer, diabetes, AIDS, and Alzheimer's disease.

FOLLOWING A CARDIAC REHABILITATION PROGRAM

Charlie had been retired less than 2 years when he began to experience signs of coronary heart disease. During his years working at a chemical plant, he had had a number of different jobs. For almost 15

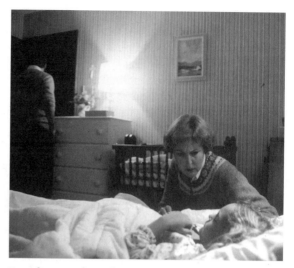

Providing care for a chronically ill child can create emotional and financial stress and alter family dynamics.

years his jobs included a lot of physical activity, but his job in industrial relations was both stressful and sedentary. During this time, he developed hypertension and started taking medication. Also, he first began to have trouble with his weight and to feel more quickly out of breath when he changed from an active job to a sedentary one. After his retirement, his exercise was limited to fishing and hunting, and he continued to smoke and enjoy eating. One day he felt a deep, severe pain in his chest, shoulders, and arms. He immediately interpreted this pain as a heart attack, called for help, and was taken to a hospital.

An angiogram revealed that Charlie had 100%, 99%, and 95% blockage of three coronary arteries. The physicians who treated him decided that he was not a good candidate for angioplasty and that he should have coronary bypass surgery. Charlie thought, "Let's get this thing over with so I can start recuperating," and the arrangements were made for triple bypass surgery.

In the intensive coronary care unit (ICCU), Charlie developed a respiratory complication that prolonged the normally painful and stressful stay in ICCU. Charlie started to wonder if he would survive, and at one point, he became convinced that the hospital staff was going to leave and abandon the care of all the patients in ICCU. Charlie decided to leave when the shift changed rather than stay in the hospital, and, in his attempt to leave the hospital, he disconnected the intravenous lines and electrode leads to the monitoring machinery. He stayed only because he was restrained.

Despite the complications and the bypass surgery, Charlie recovered from his heart attack and cardiac surgery with no serious damage to his heart. As part of his rehabilitation program, he was advised to quit smoking, lose weight, and begin regular exercise. Charlie quit smoking immediately but found losing weight difficult. At first he lost some weight but then regained it. Charlie's exercise program consisted of walking a quarter of a mile for one week and then increasing the distance by one quarter mile per week until he could walk two miles in 30 minutes. Charlie now finds the distance no problem but has difficulty walking at that pace. However, he feels better when he sticks to his exercise schedule, so he tries to exercise at least every other day.

In addition to changing his lifestyle, Charlie takes several medications for his heart and blood pressure. Once a year he undergoes a complete medical examination that includes an exercise stress test. Although he experienced depression that lasted for over a year after his cardiac surgery, Charlie says that he feels fine now, 3 years after his heart attack. His wife and family are pleased at his recovery, but they want him to be even more concerned about losing weight and sticking to his regimen for rehabilitation.

Charlie's cardiac rehabilitation program included lifestyle changes as well as medication. Cardiac rehabilitation programs can encompass a number of conditions and include a variety of activities. People with hypertension may not only take medication to lower blood pressure but also participate in programs to lower the risk factors for cardiovascular disease. People with angina pectoris and those with blockage of the coronary arteries are candidates for lifestyle changes and possibly for coronary bypass surgery as well. People who have experienced a heart attack participate in cardiac rehabilitation programs to restore their physical, social, and economic usefulness. Approaches to altering risk factors for cardiovascular disease include interventions to lower blood pressure and serum cholesterol as well as to change the hostility components of Type A behavior. This chapter concentrates on the rehabilitation programs that assist people who have undergone cardiac surgery or have experienced a heart attack.

Are rehabilitation programs effective in increasing the life expectancy of those who have experienced a heart attack? An evaluation of cardiac rehabilitation programs (Oldridge, Guyatt, Fischer, & Rimm, 1988) showed a significant difference between those who participated in a program of cardiac rehabilitation and those who did not. Although people who participated in the programs had lower death rates from cardiovascular disease, their rate of nonfatal heart attacks was the same as that of patients who had not participated in cardiac rehabilitation. These results are somewhat puzzling, but they suggest some value of programs for cardiac rehabilitation.

Most programs of cardiac rehabilitation are similar to the one that Charlie has followed. They include adherence to a regimen of medication, smoking cessation, a gradual increase in exercise, and dietary changes to lower fat intake. The exercise components vary according to the extent of damage to the heart and may include attendance at exercise classes supervised by health care personnel who can provide emergency care for cardiac complications. Health psychologists have formulated and implemented programs that supplement the standard cardiac rehabilitation programs. In addition to researching the problems with implementing lifestyle change programs, health psychologists have researched and designed interventions for the adjustment problems of heart disease patients and their families.

LIFESTYLE CHANGES

Programs for cardiac rehabilitation emphasize lifestyle changes and, in that respect, are similar to the programs designed to prevent cardiovascular disease. However, cardiac rehabilitation patients have already experienced dramatic signs of the disease and thus may be more highly motivated to change their behavior than people trying to prevent the disease. Their behavior, then, may differ from those at risk for heart disease, and so we can consider research in the context of cardiac rehabilitation.

One approach that has been successful with people who have experienced heart disease is a program originated by Dean Ornish and his colleagues (Ornish et al., 1990). This program tested the possibility of reversing coronary artery damage by introducing substantial changes in lifestyle. Although similar to the interventions that attempt to alter risk factors, this program was more comprehensive and imposed more stringent modifications. Diet, an important part of the program, was much more restricted in its allowance of fat than most cardiac rehabilitation or cholesterol-lowering diets. The American Heart Association's guidelines recommend that no more than 30% of calories come from fat. In the Ornish program, participants were allowed only 10% of calories from fat, necessitating a vegetarian diet with no added fats from oils, eggs, butter, or nuts. Ornish (1995) contends that a diet in which 30% of calories come from fat is not sufficient to *reverse* coronary artery disease (CAD), although such a diet may be sufficient to *prevent* the development of CAD. In addition to the dietary restrictions, participants received stress management training and were encouraged to stop smoking, moderate their alcohol intake, and start exercising. A control group in this study followed a typical program intended to lower risk factors for people with coronary heart disease, including eating a low fat-diet, quitting smoking, and increasing physical activity.

After 1 year of the program, Ornish and his colleagues (1990) found that 82% of their patients in the treatment group showed a regression of plaques in the coronary arteries, a truly difficult achievement. Compared with the control group, patients in the treatment group had significantly less blockage of their coronary arteries, and those who most faithfully followed the program showed the most dramatic changes. This study demonstrated that a change in the coronary arteries can occur without the use of drugs that alter cholesterol levels and without coronary bypass surgery.

Programs that attempt to lower risk factors for cardiovascular disease share many goals with the programs that assist in cardiac rehabilitation. Both types of programs emphasize increases in physical activity, decreased smoking, lowered dietary fat, and moderation of alcohol intake. However, the psychological impact of heart surgery or heart attack differs from the impact of simply being at risk for heart disease. Cardiac patients have reported a variety of psychological reactions after developing heart disease.

PSYCHOLOGICAL REACTIONS AFTER HEART DISEASE

Patients recovering from heart disease, as well as their spouses, often experience a variety of psychological reactions that include depression, anxiety, anger, fear, guilt, and interpersonal conflict. In addition, some patients suffer serious psychiatric disturbances, such as delusions and paranoia.

Depression is the most common and persistent problem for survivors of a heart attack. Holahan, Moos, Holahan, and Brennan (1995) found that cardiac patients reported more serious depression after 1 year than did healthy people. Women with cardiac problems were especially vulnerable to depression, but both women and men benefited from social support and active coping efforts. Holahan et al. suggested that cardiac rehabilitation programs could benefit from addressing issues of social support and coping strategies. In addition, Frasure-Smith, Lespérance, and Talajic (1995) found that depressed survivors of heart attack were more likely than nondepressed survivors to suffer additional cardiac problems during the year following their heart attack. Frasure-Smith et al. also found that the association between depression, anxiety, and a history of major depression with recurrent cardiac events was as great as the risk associated with having had a previous heart attack.

When married men suffer a heart attack, their wives tend to be the most affected family members, and the marital relationship is changed in many ways. Michela (1987) discussed how the mutually dependent relationship that characterizes marriage can change immediately after the husband's discharge from the hospital. Patients recovering from a heart attack have physical limitations, and their regimen for rehabilitation makes demands on the time of wives and other family members. Michela studied couples in which the husbands were recovering from a heart attack and found that both husbands and wives experienced depression. Furthermore, the feelings of depression were highly correlated with feelings of helplessness. Both husbands and wives experienced feelings of anger, but the husbands' feelings of anger decreased over time more than their wives' anger did.

Michela found that the dynamics and activities of the couples changed as well. Wives did more for their husbands after the heart attack, but the husbands who had a heart attack did less for their wives and less for themselves. Both husbands and wives expressed more affection, and about 25% reported increased marital satisfaction. For most of the couples, satisfaction with their marriage remained unchanged after the husband's heart attack despite the negative feelings and changes in the nature of their relationship.

The emotional support provided by spouses can be important in recovery from heart disease, and married people tend to receive more emotional support than their unmarried counterparts (Kulik & Mahler, 1993). This emotional support is related to emotional adjustment, quality of life, and compliance with lifestyle changes such as exercise and smoking cessation. Kulik and Mahler's study found that receiving emotional support and not marriage itself was the important factor. Surprisingly, they found that emotional support was not related to subsequent cardiac health.

The belief that sexual activity increases the chances of subsequent heart attack can affect both husbands and wives. This belief, however, is a myth—a myth that probably has its basis in the elevation of heart rate during sex, especially during orgasm. Heart rate does not rise to a dangerous level during sex, so sexual activity poses little threat to those who have experienced a heart attack. Despite these reassurances, the couples in Michela's study were more comfortable with a gradual return to sexual activity.

Many people attach special significance to the heart, and therefore cardiac surgery can be a psychologically meaningful and fearful experience. The risk of death from heart surgery is a real fear, but Goldman and Kimball (1985) discussed the tendency of cardiac patients to perceive the risk of death as 50–50, even when their surgeon had repeatedly presented risk figures that were more accurate and more optimistic. Charlie's feelings were not consistent with Goldman and Kimball's results; he never felt that he was in danger of dying from the surgery, and he felt eager to proceed with his recovery. Scheier et al. (1989) found that such optimism is beneficial in recovery from cardiac bypass surgery, but Fitzgerald, Tennen, Afflect, and Pransky (1993) suggested the beneficial element in recovery from heart surgery is the feeling of control that accompanies optimism.

Some survivors feel guilty because they have survived when others have not. Between 15% and 50% of the people who have undergone cardiac surgery experience very serious psychological disturbances during the days after their surgery (Goldman & Kimball, 1985). These reactions often include delusions and paranoia that are comparable in magnitude to psychotic reactions. The origin of such severe psychological problems following cardiac surgery is not understood, but the incidence of such problems relates to the length of time patients spend on the heart pump during their surgery. However, these symptoms rarely last longer than 2 or 3 days. Charlie's delusion that the hospital staff would abandon him and the other ICCU patients is typical of the type of disturbance common among cardiac surgery patients, but his disturbance lasted only a few hours rather than a few days.

Although most patients report improvements attributable to their cardiac surgery (Goldman & Kimball, 1985), not all do. Psychological problems cause difficulties in those who do not report improvement. Charlie is one of the majority of patients who feel benefited by surgery. His depression decreased after a year, and he now feels neither physical nor psychological problems due to his heart disease and surgery.

In summary, both heart attack and cardiac surgery can cause psychological problems for patients and their families. Depression is the most common and persistent psychological problem for those who have undergone cardiac surgery. Not only do patients experience depression, but the wives of men who have had heart attacks also feel depressed. Fear and anxiety are also frequent emotions and both can introduce a source of conflict into families that changes the nature of marital relationships. Some patients experience symptoms of severe psychological problems within several days after surgery, but these symptoms persist for only a few days.

PSYCHOLOGICAL INTERVENTIONS IN CARDIAC REHABILITATION

Psychological interventions with cardiac patients usually begin while patients are still in the hospital. Although many cardiac patients see no need for psychological assistance and may even be upset if someone else requests psychological attention for them, psychological counseling can ameliorate the experience of hospitalization, counteract some of the anxiety of being monitored while in intensive care, and increase the patient's confidence in the hospital's equipment and personnel. Families, too, need to understand the ramifications of the patient's heart disease, and most cardiac care programs include information to refute the common misconceptions about recovery from heart disease.

Thompson and Meddis (1990a, 1990b) implemented and evaluated a program of in-hospital counseling for heart attack survivors and spouses. Their intervention consisted of four 30-minute counseling sessions that took place while the patients were still in the hospital. The patients reported significantly less depression and anxiety, and these differences persisted in a 6-month follow-up. The spouses of the heart attack victims also participated in the counseling, and these spouses too reported less anxiety, both immediately and after 6 months. This program demonstrates that a simple psychological intervention can be effective in dealing with anxiety and depression, the most common psychological problems of cardiac patients and their families.

Another research project (Fontana, Kerns, Rosenberg, & Colonese, 1989) evaluated the effect of social support on recovery after hospitalization for heart disease. These researchers found social support lessens the experience of both stress and distress and that social support was more important in the first 6 months after hospitalization than in the next 6 months. These results suggest the value of both psychological interventions for the patients and support groups for the families. Families that understand car-

diac rehabilitation can help the patients by improving the critical factor of social support.

In summary, cardiac rehabilitation programs attempt to help heart patients increase their level of physical, social, and psychological functioning. These programs typically include regimens for lifestyle changes as well as interventions aimed at reducing the harmful psychological effects of coronary heart disease on patients and their families. In addition to the pain and distress associated with hospitalization, heart attack and cardiac surgery cause anxiety and depression that may become a permanent part of the lives of heart patients and their families. Interventions that offer counseling for patients and families while the patients are still hospitalized have been effective in decreasing anxiety and depression. Other research has demonstrated that social support is important to patients recovering from heart disease, and interventions targeting families can help provide such support to those patients.

COPING WITH CANCER

In Chapter 10, we met Victoria, who had been treated for non-Hodgkin's lymphoma when she was 16 years old. Her diagnosis and treatment had been very stressful, not only for Victoria but for her parents and three siblings. After her initial inpatient treatment, she took part in 3 months of intensive and then 6 months of less intensive chemotherapy. The hospital in which she received treatment was over 500 miles from her home, and transportation to the hospital was one of those sources of stress for her family. The nausea that she experienced as one of the side effects of the chemotherapy prohibited flying, so her parents drove her to her appointments and then brought her home. This arrangement was time-consuming, requiring the entire family to concentrate on Victoria and her treatment, often to the neglect of other family members' needs.

Victoria could not attend school, where she had been a popular and outgoing student, but she took part in a home schooling program so that she continued to earn high school credits. Rather than going to school, she had to stay home and study. Being isolated from her friends and alone at home all day was one of the more stressful aspects of the 6 months of less intensive therapy. Victoria believes that the experience changed her into a more introspective and less outgoing person.

Her friends also had trouble in knowing how to treat her. Having a peer with a potentially fatal illness was something beyond their experience, and the awkwardness they felt resulted in their avoiding her. Victoria thought her boyfriend would also be alienated by her illness, but he was not, and their relationship continued throughout her treatment and afterward.

Victoria's family experienced all the aspects of a family in crisis, but they coped with the crisis and supported Victoria and her treatment. This support was important to Victoria, who had always been close to her family and felt distant from her friends during her treatment. As the experts (Moos, 1984) recommend, Victoria and her family managed to find some positive aspects to her illness, and the family maintained their closeness throughout her treatment.

According to the American Cancer Society, more than 1 million people in the United States were diagnosed with cancer in 1995. Most of those people experienced feelings similar to those of Victoria, who was not only fearful and anxious but also angry. Indeed, the diagnosis of cancer nearly always has a significant psychological impact on the patient. Helping people cope with their emotional reactions to this diagnosis and preparing them for the negative side effects of some cancer treatments are important jobs for psychology-oriented health care providers.

PSYCHOLOGICAL IMPACT OF CANCER

Although some cancer patients suffer from psychosocial problems as a result of their illness, serious distress and depression are not universal. The percentage of patients suffering from psychological problems depends on how these problems are defined. Most cancer patients experience some depression after receiving a diagnosis of cancer, but when clinical depression is used as a criterion, the prevalence among cancer patients may not be any greater than it is among other hospitalized patients. For example, Derogatis et al. (1983) found that only about 6% of their cancer patients were clinically depressed. Bieliauskas (1984) reviewed earlier studies and concluded that "while some cancer patients are significantly depressed, the widespread notion that cancer patients are generally depressed is not supported by the evidence" (p. 38).

When other psychosocial problems are considered along with depression, the role of emotional disturbances in cancer increases. Derogatis et al. (1983) found that 47% of their patients suffered from some sort of psychiatric disorder, with chronic mild distress and anxiety accounting for most of these problems. Telch and Telch (1985) reviewed earlier studies and concluded that "cancer has a major psychological impact on the lives of patients" (p. 326). They cited one study that reported 39% of mastectomy patients in need of psychiatric treatment for anxiety, depression, and sexual problems. In contrast, only 12% of benign breast disease patients manifested these disorders. Other studies reviewed by Telch and Telch reported somewhat lower percentages (18% to 25%) of cancer patients with psychosocial problems. These data suggest that the majority of cancer patients do not suffer serious psychological problems.

Problems Associated with Cancer Treatments

Currently, nearly all medical treatments for cancer have negative side effects that may add stress to the lives of cancer patients. These therapies include surgery, radiation, chemotherapy, hormonal treatment, and immunotherapy. The first three are the most common and also the most stressful.

Andersen (1989) reported that cancer patients undergoing surgery, compared with other surgery patients, have overall higher levels of distress and slower rates of emotional recovery. The high distress of cancer surgery patients correlates with a greater rejection of these patients by their physicians. In one study Andersen reviewed, attending physicians on a cancer unit offered less emotional support and were less likely to address the needs of their patients than were physicians on other surgical units. Physicians may be less supportive because cancer patients are more distressed, or cancer patients may be more distressed because their physicians are less supportive. For whatever reason, cancer surgery patients are likely to experience more rejection, stronger fears, and less emotional support than other surgery patients.

Andersen reported that most patients who receive radiation therapy anticipate their treatment with fear and anxiety, fearing such side effects as loss of hair, burns, nausea, vomiting, fatigue, and sterility. Most of these conditions do occur, so patients' fears are not unreasonable. However, patients are seldom adequately prepared for their radiation treatments, and thus their fears and anxieties may exaggerate the severity of these side effects. Andersen's review indicated that the emotional side effects of radiation treatment lessen after the physical side effects diminish, usually by 12 months after treatment.

Chemotherapy is also frequently accompanied by unpleasant side effects that precipitate stressful reactions in cancer patients. Burish, Meyerowitz, Carey, and Morrow (1987) reported that at least half those cancer patients treated with chemotherapy experience nausea, fatigue, depression, weight change, hair loss, sleep problems, and loss of appetite. Sexual problems are also common, regardless of the cancer site. Burish et al. reported that 70% of women interviewed 3 years after chemotherapy had decreased or no sexual interest, and 85% of men in treatment for Hodgkin's disease had lost their sexual drive.

Victoria described her chemotherapy treatments as "terrible." Some of the procedures were painful, and the side effects made Victoria feel helpless and out of control. During the course of her chemotherapy treatments, Victoria experienced nausea and vomiting. She lost her appetite and all interest in eating, so she lost 30 pounds. Her hair fell out, and she experienced a significant loss of coordination and decreased ability to concentrate. Years later, she believes that she has not regained her former concentration ability. Many cancer patients have similar unpleasant experiences during chemotherapy.

Not only do many patients become nauseated by chemotherapy, but some experience anticipatory nausea; that is, they become conditioned to nausea by certain sights and smells that precede the treatment. Andersen (1989) mentioned several psychological interventions that have demonstrated some success in controlling anticipatory reactions, includ-

ing hypnosis, progressive muscle relaxation with guided imagery, systematic desensitization, diversion of attention, and biofeedback.

Stress in Former Cancer Patients

More than half of all cancer patients survive at least 5 years (National Center for Health Statistics, 1995) and many show no physical signs of the illness during that time (Burish et al. 1987). However, many of these people continue to manifest psychological reactions to cancer. Burish et al. indicated that cancer patients in remission often suffer from stress and other psychological problems for years before they are able to resume a normal lifestyle. The longer the remission, the more likely it is that the patients will be able to experience a quality of life comparable to their lives before cancer. However, many former cancer patients remain anxious about recurrence and carefully monitor every physical symptom for signs of cancer. Victoria was especially frightened about a relapse during the two years after she was pronounced to be in remission. As the years have passed, her fears have decreased, but she is still anxious about the possibility of recurrence.

Paradoxically, some patients become accommodated to their treatment and find returning to normal functioning to be quite difficult. Burish et al. suggested that some patients become distressed after they leave the protective environment of the hospital and cited one study in which radiation patients reported higher levels of anger and depression as the end of their treatment approached. Similarly, parents of leukemia patients became more anxious at the time that their children's chemotherapy was over. Burish et al. (1987, p. 162) concluded that "leaving treatment meant a loss of security and decreased social support. Possibly, treatment also provided a sense of increased control by giving patients an active means of trying to control the cancer."

In addition to these temporary stresses, former cancer patients sometimes experience a number of more permanent problems. Burish et al. suggested that some former patients retain a feeling of vulnerability, a pervasive dread that their disease will return. They cited one study that found former cancer patients with no signs of the disease had more general health worries and lower feelings of self-control than did a group of controls. These authors cited other studies that reported former cancer patients to have recurring fears and anxieties, such as frightening implications of everyday aches and pains, concern that they may pass the disease genetically to their children, and worries about their ability to have children. Whether or not these fears are justified, an important point remains: Many cancer patients never completely recover from the distress of having had that disease.

Few follow-up studies have investigated the effects of cancer beyond 5 years after treatment. However, Byrne and her colleagues (1989) investigated the long-term impact of cancer by studying the patterns of marriage and divorce in adults who had survived cancer between 5 and 15 years earlier when they were children or adolescents. These investigators found that the former cancer patients were less likely to be married than the controls and that those who married had slightly shorter marriages. However, their analysis revealed that those individuals who had survived cancers of the central nervous system accounted for most of the difference. The marriage patterns among former cancer patients who had tumors in other sites were similar to those of people who had not developed cancer during childhood or adolescence. This study measured only one aspect of adjustment after childhood cancer, but this aspect is an important index of normal adjustment. The results indicate that cancer did not prevent most of these people from marrying and that their marriages were comparable in length to those of people who had no history of cancer.

PSYCHOLOGICAL TREATMENT FOR CANCER PATIENTS

We have seen that the diagnosis of cancer is frequently experienced as a major crisis and that it often leads to anger, depression, anxiety, and other emotional reactions. Each of these feelings is likely to have harmful effects, not only on the patient's psychological health but also on relationships with family members and the medical staff. For this reason, individual or group psychotherapy or a combination can be important in cancer treatment programs.

Psychologists are sometimes involved in helping cancer patients learn relaxation training for reduc-

ing pain, insomnia, and nausea; self-instruction, for helping patients learn to talk to themselves in a constructive rather than a negativistic manner; and problem-solving skills, for enhancing patients' sense of personal control (Telch & Telch, 1985). Many of these coping strategies are directed at reducing the deleterious effects of such medical interventions as chemotherapy, surgery, and radiation. Telch and Telch reviewed several studies on the effectiveness of these coping strategies and found some evidence of the efficacy of various behavioral techniques, including deep muscle relaxation to alleviate post-chemotherapy nausea. However, they found little support for programs aimed at increasing personal control through problem-solving skills.

Some researchers (Dunkel-Schetter & Wortman, 1982; Wellisch, 1981) have emphasized the advantages of social support groups as part of the treatment for cancer patients. Discussions about fears, anxieties, and uncertainties faced by all cancer patients may be easier in a group of people with similar problems. Dunkel-Schetter and Wortman suggested that cancer patients may feel they do not wish to burden friends and families with the additional emotional difficulties that would arise from an open discussion of their illness. As a result, friends and family members may withdraw emotionally and physically, leaving cancer patients with less social support at a time when their need for support has increased.

Support groups for cancer patients are generally aimed at increasing social support and reducing emotional distress. Studies on several such groups have indicated their effectiveness in helping cancer patients manage their emotional reactions. In addition, several studies have found that patients who participate in such groups lived longer than those who received only medical care.

David Spiegel and his colleagues (Spiegel, 1992, 1993; Spiegel & Bloom, 1983; Spiegel, Bloom, & Yalom, 1981; Spiegel, Kraemer, Bloom, & Gottheil, 1989) have studied the beneficial effects of support groups to emotional adjustment and survival in breast cancer patients. The support groups met twice weekly for 1 year. One group included a supportive environment in which the women were free to express negative emotions, and the other included a similar support group plus hypnosis. After

12 months, patients in both support groups were less tense, depressed, fatigued, and phobic than the untreated participants. In addition, patients in the hypnosis support group experienced significantly lower levels of pain than those who received either support group therapy alone or no treatment. The support group experience was also associated with extended survival, with the women in support groups living an average of 18 months longer than those who received only medical treatment.

Fawzy I. Fawzy and his colleagues (1993) studied the effects of a psychiatric group intervention for patients who had undergone surgery for malignant melanoma. Similar to Spiegel's breast cancer patients, the melanoma patients who participated in the group showed improved coping ability. They also experienced fewer recurrences of their cancer compared to a group that had received only medical care. Six years after their initial treatment, only 3 of the 34 patients in the therapy group had died, compared to 10 of the 34 patients in the comparison group. Therefore, psychosocial interventions may show double benefits of helping cancer patients cope with their illness and increasing survival time.

The special problems of helping young cancer patients cope has been discussed by Wellisch (1981). First, young children with cancer are typically removed from the secure environment of home and family, their source of both physical and social support. Parents often have added emotional and financial burdens, which may have a negative impact on their relationship with the child. In addition, Wellisch observed that many chronically ill children believe they are to blame for their condition, reasoning that they have done something bad to cause their own cancer. Wellisch recommended that children with cancer should return to a normal routine as soon as possible, including resumption of schoolwork.

Adolescent cancer patients have some of the same needs as younger children, but they have additional problems concerning newly formed sex roles and autonomy. The uncertainties about the future that affect all cancer patients make vocational choice and possible marriage and family life special issues for adolescents with cancer. In addition to an uncertain future, adolescent cancer patients are even more strongly affected than adults by the physical changes that often accompany cancer treatment (Wellisch, 1981). The loss of a limb, scars from surgery, or hair loss from chemotherapy can be a frightening experience, a threat to self-esteem, an assault to self-confidence, and an impediment to peer acceptance.

Victoria had no surgery and thus no scars, but her hair fell out, and her peers treated her differently; these occurrences were distressing. Her parents arranged for home schooling in the attempt to keep her occupied and to allow her to continue her education. This strategy was wise because it allowed Victoria to graduate with her high school class and to be prepared to go to college. She never believed that she was going to die, so she was anxious to engage in activities that would allow her to continue her life and be as normal as she could during her treatment.

Patients frequently feel socially obligated to appear cheerful and optimistic (Lazarus, 1984b). Because cancer patients face many uncertainties about their treatment and prognosis, they may feel especially burdened to express an optimism they may not feel (Dunkel-Schetter & Wortman, 1982). The dishonesty of appearing optimistic and striving for a cheerful acceptance of cancer may be more harmful than beneficial. One study (Derogatis, Abeloff, & Melisaratos, 1979) found that women with metastatic breast cancer who freely expressed negative emotions outlived women who appeared to be better adjusted to their illness. Therefore, an honest expression of negative feelings may be both emotionally and physiologically healthy for cancer patients. However, pessimism, hopelessness, and depression are negative feelings that are not healthy. As Norman Cousins (1983) emphasized, a sense of hope—a fighting spirit—can be beneficial in recovering from all diseases.

ADJUSTING TO DIABETES

Dawn was diagnosed with **diabetes mellitus** when she was 4 years old. She has no clear memories of life without diabetes, and no facet of her life has been unaffected by the disease. She remembers being ostracized by other children during elementary school because they were afraid that playing with her would make them sick, too. She hid her condition during junior high and high school, but her attempts to fit in led her to neglect her diabetes regimen.

Diabetes mellitus is a chronic illness of unknown origin with no cure. Speculations concerning the origin include heredity, viral infection, autoimmune disease, and stress (Wertlieb, Jacobson, & Hauser, 1990). The disorder is caused by problems in the secretion of the hormone **insulin**, and deficiencies of insulin lead to difficulties in the metabolism of sugar. The two types of diabetes mellitus are insulin-dependent diabetes mellitus (IDDM), also known as juvenile-onset diabetes or Type I diabetes. The other type is variously known as noninsulin dependent diabetes mellitus (NIDDM), adult-onset diabetes, or Type II diabetes. This second type appears during adulthood, typically when a person is past the age of 30. Type II diabetics are most often overweight, female, and poor (Blevins, 1979). The characteristics of both types of diabetes are shown in Table 11.1. Both require lifestyle changes in order for the patient to adjust to the disease and to minimize health complications. Diabetes is one of the chronic disorders that requires daily monitoring and relatively strict compliance to both medical and lifestyle regimens.

THE PHYSIOLOGY OF DIABETES

Before examining the psychological issues in the management of diabetes, let's look more closely at the physiology of the disorder. The **pancreas**, located below the stomach, is both a ducted and a ductless gland. (The secretions distributed by its ducts are involved with digestion and food metabolism and thus it is considered part of the digestive system.) The **islet cells** of the pancreas constitute an endocrine gland. They produce several hormones, two of which, glucagon and insulin, are critically important in metabolism. **Glucagon** stimulates the release of glucose and therefore acts to elevate blood sugar levels. The action of insulin is the opposite. Insulin decreases the level of glucose in the blood by causing tissue cell membranes to open so glucose can enter the cells more freely. Disorders of the islet cells produce difficulties in sugar metabolism. Diabetes mellitus is a disorder caused by insulin deficiency. If the islet cells do not produce adequate insulin, sugar cannot be moved from the blood to the cells for use. Excessive sugar accumulates in the blood and also appears in abnormally high levels in the urine. If unregulated or poorly regulated, diabetes may cause coma and death.

The administration of insulin can control the most severe symptoms of insulin deficiency but it does not cure the disorder. Nor do insulin injections mimic the normal production of insulin by the islet cells. Lack of insulin prevents the blood sugar level from being regulated by the body's control mechanisms. This inability to regulate blood sugar often causes diabetics to have other health problems. Elevated levels of blood sugar seem to be involved in the development of (1) damage to the blood vessels, leaving diabetics prone to cardiovascular disease (diabetics are twice as likely as other people to have hypertension and to develop heart disease); (2) damage to the retina, leaving diabetics at risk for blindness (diabetics are 17 times as likely to go blind as nondiabetics); and (3) kidney diseases, leaving diabetics prone to renal failure. In addition, diabetics, compared with nondiabetics, have more than

Table 11.1 Characteristics of insulin-dependent and noninsulin-dependent diabetes mellitus

Insulin-dependent	Noninsulin-dependent
Onset occurs before age 15	Onset occurs after age 30
Patients are underweight	Patients are overweight
Patients experience frequent thirst and urination	Patients experience frequent thirst and urination
Affects equal numbers of men and women	Affects more women
Has no socioeconomic correlates	Affects more poor than middle-class people
Requires insulin injections	Requires no insulin injections
Carries risk of kidney damage	Carries risk of cardiovascular damage

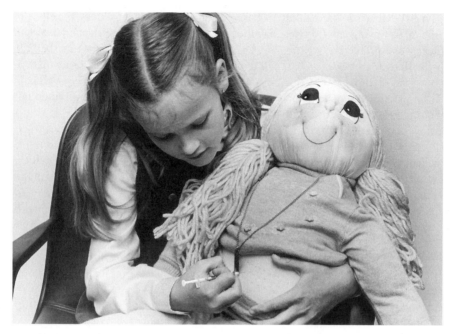

Learning to inject insulin is one of the skills that children with Type I diabetics must master.

double the risk of cancer of the pancreas (Everhart & Wright, 1995). Dawn experienced damage to her retinas at age 17, and the laser surgery left her vision permanently impaired. She is not blind, which her doctors feared she would be, but she has no night vision, and she can focus only if given time. These visual impairments prevent her from qualifying for a driver's license.

THE IMPACT OF DIABETES

The diagnosis of any chronic disease produces an impact on patients for two reasons: first, the emotional reaction to having a lifelong incurable disease, and second, the adjustments to lifestyle required by the disease. For the juvenile-onset variety of diabetes, both children and their parents must come to terms with the child's loss of health (Kovacs et al., 1990) and the management of the disorder, which includes careful restrictions in diet, insulin injections, and recommendations for regular exercise. Dietary restrictions include careful scheduling of meals and snacks as well as adherence to a set of allowed and disallowed foods. Juvenile-onset diabetes typically requires daily injections of insulin, and in-

jections can be a source of fear and stress. Regular medical visits are also required; these may frighten the children and create scheduling difficulties for the parents.

Dawn did a poor job of taking care of herself when she was a teenager. She learned to give herself insulin injections when she was 6 years old, and her compliance with this aspect of her care has always been good. Eating was a problem. She never developed a taste for sweets, so avoiding them was not difficult, but she was always a finicky eater, and did not like to eat three meals a day. She found skipping meals easy and saw it as a good strategy for losing weight. However, one diet put her in the hospital because of a very low blood sugar level.

Noninsulin-dependent (Type II) diabetes often does not require insulin injections, but this type of diabetes does require lifestyle changes and oral medication. Because the majority of people with Type II diabetes are overweight, a frequent component of treatment is weight loss. Type II diabetics must deal with dietary restrictions and attend to their schedule of oral medication. Diabetes often affects sexual functioning in both men and women, and diabetic women who become pregnant often have problem pregnancies. Type II diabetes is more likely to cause circulatory problems, leaving adult-onset diabetics prone to cardiovascular problems.

Some diabetics deny the seriousness of their condition and ignore the need to restrict diet and take medication. Others become aggressive and they either direct their aggression outward and refuse to comply with their treatment regimen or they turn their aggression inward and become depressed. Finally, many diabetics become dependent and rely on others to take care of them and therefore take no active part in their own care. All these reactions can interfere with the management of blood sugar levels and lead to serious health complications, including death.

Kovacs et al. (1990) studied the psychological functioning of the mothers of insulin-dependent children for 6 years after the diagnosis and found that mothers initially reacted to the diagnosis of Type I diabetes with anxiety, fear, guilt, and depression. Kovacs et al. found that mothers' initial reaction was not related to either the medical aspects of their children's illness or the children's levels of anxiety and depression. The mothers generally found coping easier the longer their children had the disease, and the mothers' distress was related to how difficult they found the management of their children's diabetes. This study demonstrated some effects of chronic illness on the family and highlights the complexity of the adjustment to chronic illness by the affected individual and the family.

Dawn was able to deny the seriousness of her condition until she experienced kidney failure at age 22. She was put on kidney dialysis, and eventually received a kidney transplant. In the hospital, she became aware of the dangers of her condition in a way that she had never been before. Not only did she understand that she might die, but the possibility of nerve damage and amputation of a limb made her more vigilant about self-care. Now, she monitors her blood sugar at least three times a day, eats regularly, and gives herself appropriate insulin injections.

HEALTH PSYCHOLOGY'S INVOLVEMENT WITH DIABETES

Health psychologists are involved in both researching and treating diabetes. Research efforts have concentrated on the ways that diabetics understand and conceptualize their illness, the effect of stress on glucose metabolism, the dynamics of families with diabetic children, and the factors that influence compliance with medical regimens by diabetic patients. The treatment efforts of health psychologists have been oriented toward improving compliance with medical regimens so diabetics can control their blood glucose levels and minimize health complications.

Stress has been hypothesized to play two roles in diabetes: as a possible cause of diabetes and as a factor in the regulation of blood sugar in diabetics (Wertlieb et al., 1990). The role of stress as a cause of diabetes is only one possibility, but several research groups have demonstrated effects for stress on blood glucose. Gonder-Frederick, Carter, Cox, and Clarke (1990) found that an active stressor (solving math problems) had more effect on the blood glucose level of diabetics than did a passive stressor (viewing a gory movie). Not all the diabetics they studied showed blood glucose changes in response to stress, but more than half of them did. More recently, Goldston, Kovacs, Obrosky, and Iyengar (1995) conducted a longitudinal study that looked at the role of stress in metabolic control for school-age children with insulin-dependent diabetes. They found that the extent to which stressful negative events disrupted the children's life was a strong predictor of metabolic control, but *number* of negative stressful life events made little or no contribution to blood glucose regulation. Dawn sees stressful negative events as major problems in her management of her condition. She has trouble staying on her regimen when she is having trouble with her boyfriend. These researchers speculated that even positive life events, such as an outstanding personal achievement, can affect metabolic control.

Another line of research concerns diabetic patients' understanding of their illness and how their understanding affects their behavior. Gonder-Frederick, Cox, Bobbitt, and Pennebaker (1986) studied the accuracy of diabetic patients' beliefs about their symptoms. These researchers pointed out that both the patients and health care workers assume that the patients recognize the symptoms of high and low blood glucose levels. Thus the perception of symptoms is important in the management of diabetes. They found that diabetics use their symptoms as a guide to action, but the accuracy of patients' beliefs varied widely. All patients had some inaccurate beliefs. For example, 58% of the diabetics had inaccurate beliefs about high and 42% had inaccurate beliefs about low blood glucose levels. These patients were more likely to have *beliefs* that suggested problems than they were to have problems; that is, their reports of symptoms were false alarms. Patients also overlooked symptoms that indicated problems, but the tendency toward false alarms was the more frequent type of error. Gonder-Frederick and her colleagues also found that the women in the study were more vigilant in both correctly and incorrectly perceiving symptoms, whereas the men were more likely to miss symptoms. These researchers suggested that diabetics should be taught how to perceive symptoms accurately.

Compliance of young diabetics with their treatment regimen is quite poor, and studies (Glasgow et al. 1989; Johnson, Freund, Silverstein, Hansen, & Malone, 1990; Johnson, Tomer, Cunningham, & Henretta, 1990; Orme & Binik, 1989) have shown that several factors underlie compliance. Compliance in one area does not predict compliance in any other. For this reason, the attempts of health psychologists to improve adherence to treatment regimens for diabetes have met with only partial success. One innovative approach has been to study the effectiveness of self-monitoring of blood glucose levels. This type of measurement allows diabetics to adjust insulin and diet to achieve better control of their glucose levels. However, several studies (Wysocki, 1989; Wysocki, Green, & Huxtable, 1989) have indicated that this technique is not as effective as it could be because patients do not use this information to alter treatment. Even when they have measured their blood glucose, patients tended to rely on estimates of their needs rather than on the measurement's assessment of their needs. Even worse, patients tended to estimate the measurements as more normal than they actually were, which minimized their perception of need for treatment. These cognitive distortions again highlight the importance of cognitive factors in managing chronic illness.

More promising results have come from a study (Ratner, Gross, Casas, & Castells, 1990) that demonstrated the effect of hypnosis on compliance with a diabetic treatment regimen. The only change in management strategy was the use of hypnosis. The participants were adolescents, a group that is especially bad at complying with diabetic treatment regimens. The adolescents who had been hypnotized showed blood glucose and hemoglobin values consistent with compliance. Although hypnosis diverges from the traditional management strategy for diabetes, this study suggests that the technique may be helpful in enhancing compliance even with adolescent diabetics.

The role of health psychology in diabetes management is likely to expand because some research indicates that behavioral components can add to the effectiveness of educational programs for diabetic patients. Goodall and Halford (1991) contended that education alone is not adequate in helping diabetics follow their regimen. They concluded that situational factors such as stress and social pressure to eat the wrong foods affect adherence, and they suggested that a behavioral skills training component might be a valuable addition to diabetes management training. Toobert and Glasgow (1991) confirmed the role of problem-solving skills in improving diabetics' adherence to diet, exercise, and blood glucose testing. Therefore, behavior-oriented management programs can teach diabetics skills that help them to maintain a healthier lifestyle.

In summary, diabetes mellitus is a chronic disease that results from failure of the islet cells of the pancreas to manufacture sufficient insulin, affecting blood glucose levels and producing effects in many organ systems. The disease can become apparent in either childhood or adulthood, but the juvenile-onset variety is typically more serious, and the patients require insulin injections to survive. Diabetics must maintain a strict regimen of diet, exercise, and insulin supplements to avoid the serious cardiovascular, neurological, and renal complications of the disorder.

As with other chronic diseases, a diagnosis of diabetes mellitus produces distress for both patients and their families. Health psychologists have studied the factors involved with adjustment to the disorder and those that affect compliance with the necessary lifestyle changes. Adolescent diabetics are especially likely to be poor at adherence, but the technique of self-monitoring blood glucose level has not been effective in enhancing adherence. Skills and problem-solving training programs have shown more success in helping diabetics manage their disorder.

DEALING WITH HIV AND AIDS

Glenn Burke had always wanted to play baseball, and he had enough skill to become a major league player. From 1976 to 1979, he was a gifted outfielder for the Los Angles Dodgers and Oakland Athletics and played for the Dodgers in the 1977 World Series. Burke's promising career was never fulfilled—not because he lacked ability but because players, managers, and general managers suspected that he was gay, and they made his life as a ballplayer miserable. Burke *was* gay, but he did not acknowledge his sexual orientation openly until 2 years after he left baseball. He was also an African American, and the combination of being gay and African American probably cut short his baseball career. Prejudice in organized baseball in the late 1970s was so strong that the Dodgers offered to pay Burke for an expensive honeymoon—if only he would get married. After he was traded to the Oakland Athletics, Billy Martin, the controversial manager of the Athletics (as well as several other teams) told Burke, "I don't want no faggot on my team," and the team promptly refused to sign Burke to an extended contract.

After his baseball career came to a premature end, Burke continued to have difficulties. He spent some time in San Quentin prison and more time as a homeless person on the streets of San Francisco. Eventually he contracted AIDS, but he fought hard against the disease and survived many months longer than doctors had predicted. After developing AIDS-related illnesses and losing nearly 100 pounds from his once-powerful athletic frame, he died in May 1995 at the age of 42. Unlike many gay men who develop AIDS, Burke reconciled with his family and was cared for by his sister during his final months.

AIDS is a disorder in which the immune system loses its effectiveness, leaving the body defenseless against bacterial, viral, fungal, parasitic, cancerous, and other opportunistic diseases. Immune deficiency itself is not fatal, but without the immune system, the body cannot protect itself against the many organisms that can invade it and cause damage. (For a more complete discussion of the immune system and its function, see Chapter 4). The danger from AIDS comes from the opportunistic infections that start when the immune system no longer functions

effectively. The result of AIDS is similar to the immune deficiency in children who have been born without immune system organs and are susceptible to a variety of infections. AIDS is the result of exposure to a contagious virus, the **human immunodeficiency virus (HIV)**. Presently, two variants of the human immunodeficiency virus have been discovered; HIV-1, which causes most AIDS cases in the United States, and HIV-2, which is responsible for most AIDS cases in Africa, although some HIV-2 cases have appeared in the United States. The progression from HIV infection to AIDS is not inevitable, and, indeed, a few HIV-infected people, such as former Los Angeles Laker basketball star Magic Johnson, have remained free of AIDS symptoms for many years.

INCIDENCE OF HIV/AIDS

AIDS appears to be a relatively new disease, with the first cases reported in the United States in 1981. However, some scientists (Corbitt, Bailey, & Williams, 1990; Froland et al., 1988) now believe that the disease dates at least to the 1950s. In fact, Lawrence Altman (1995) has suggested that isolated cases of AIDS in humans may be thousands of years old and that only relatively recently has the mobility of the population allowed the disease to spread from its apparent origins in Africa to the rest of the world.

During the 1980s, both the number of new cases and the number of deaths from AIDS increased rapidly until HIV infection is now one of the leading causes of death in the United States (CDC, 1994a) and the leading cause of death for all people 25 to 44 years of age (1995b).

In 1992, the Centers for Disease Control and Prevention (CDC, 1992) revised its definition of HIV infection so that incidence figures from 1993 and subsequent years are not directly comparable to earlier figures. This new and expanded definition includes adolescents and adults who are infected with HIV and whose CD4+ T-lymphocyte cell count (formerly called helper T-lymphocytes) has fallen to 200 per cubic millimeter, about one-fifth that of a healthy person, or whose CD4+ T-lymphocyte cell count is less than 14% of total lymphocytes (CDC, 1992). This definition added three clinical conditions to the AIDS classification: pulmonary tuberculosis, recurrent pneumonia, and invasive cervical

WOULD YOU BELIEVE . . . ?

Recovery from HIV Infection

Would you believe that it may be possible to recover from HIV infection? Although many people who have been infected with HIV take several years to develop any symptoms of illness, HIV experts generally hold that, once infected, it is impossible to eliminate the virus from one's body.

In 1995, however, Yvonne Bryson and her colleagues at UCLA reported on a child who had been infected with HIV at birth but who now appears to be free from infection. The identity of this child is being kept secret to protect his privacy, but Bryson et al. reported that his mother was HIV positive when she was 4 months pregnant with him. The child was tested 19, 33, and 51 days after he was born, and all three tests were positive for HIV. Nevertheless, when he was tested again at one year of age, the results were negative, and annual retesting has continued to show no HIV infection.

Some HIV researchers (McClure et al., 1995) have disputed the Bryson et al. report, claiming that the original samples were contaminated

and that the child was not initially infected. Bryson et al. claimed that the sequencing of the viral DNA was essentially the same in the samples, which would rule out contamination. In addition, they contended that the strain of HIV was similar for child and mother, which indicates that he was infected during birth. They concede that the child may have dormant HIV in lymph nodes or in his brain, but he shows no signs of HIV infection, including negative blood tests.

The child whom Bryson et al. studied is not an isolated case. Some similar cases (McDowell & Mondi, 1995) were less convincing, but later research (Newell et al., 1996) has presented evidence from seven children, all of whom were infected but seem to have shed HIV infection. Researchers from the Institute of Child Health in London estimated that about 2.7% of children infected with HIV from their mothers may be able to tolerate the virus or get rid of it.

If these children were infected with HIV and now are not, then their

condition is puzzling in two ways. First, HIV infection has been considered to be invariably permanent. Once infected, there is no known mechanism through which HIV can be eliminated from the body. The people who become HIV infected may not have symptoms of any illness for years, but the infection remains. Second, the immaturity and lack of efficiency of infants' immune systems typically leads to greater vulnerability for newborns. Instead, these children's immune systems have accomplished a task on which thousands of adult immune systems have failed.

The HIV experts do not understand either how recovery from HIV can take place or how infants' immune systems could accomplish such a task. If these few children have managed to rid themselves of HIV, then they offer hope in several ways. First, HIV infection may not be permanent. Second, when researchers understand how HIV can be shed, they may use this knowledge to develop a vaccine or even a cure for HIV.

---

cancer. The CDC also revised its classification for HIV in children less than 13 years of age, but this new definition, which was separate from that of adolescents and adults, did not add appreciably to the number of children with HIV (CDC, 1994f). By 1994 nearly all the new cases of HIV infection in children were due to perinatal transmission—that is, transmission of HIV from mother to infant during the birth process (CDC, 1994f).

The 1993 definition brought both uniformity and simplicity to the diagnosis of AIDS, but it also distorted the data on yearly incidence of the disease. Its immediate effect was to more than double the number of AIDS cases reported in 1993 over that reported in 1992 (see Figure 11.1). However, the 1993 figure can also be misleading because it brought into

the classification a large backlog of people who, in previous years, would not have been classified as having AIDS. Subsequent to 1993, the incidence figures should decline yet remain higher than those of the early 1990s, and Figure 11.1 shows this pattern. What would be the 1993 incidence of AIDS if the earlier definition were used? The Centers for Disease Control and Prevention (CDC, 1995b) estimated that the 1993 rate would be about 3% higher than the 1992 count and that the 1994 count would be at the lowest level since 1989. With the expanded definition, however, incidence of AIDS will remain at a rate higher than 1992 until this disease is brought under better control.

Better control has already begun. Figure 11.1 indicates that from 1990 to 1992 the *rate of increase* for

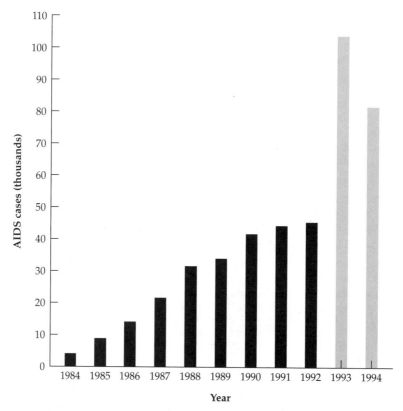

Figure 11.1 **Incidence of AIDS cases by year, United States, 1984 to 1994.** SOURCE: Data from *Statistical Abstracts of the United States, 1994* (114th ed.) by U.S. Bureau of the Census, 1994, p. 139, Washington, DC: U.S. Government Printing Office; and *Morbidity and Mortality Weekly Report, 44,* Update: Acquired immunodeficiency syndrome—United States, 1994, p. 65, Centers for Disease Control and Prevention, 1995, USDHHS, Washington, DC: U.S. Government Printing Office. NOTE: Data for 1993 and 1994 are based on the expanded definition of AIDS and are not comparable to earlier data.

new cases declined. Most of this decline (that is, a slower growth) was a result of gay and bisexual men taking more precautions to avoid AIDS (CDC, 1994g; Ekstrand et al., 1994). HIV infection, of course, is not an equal opportunity disease; men are much more likely than women to develop the disease, and African Americans and Hispanic Americans are considerably more vulnerable than European Americans. In 1994, 82% of new AIDS cases were men, 18% were women. Despite making up only 12% of the United States population, African Americans accounted for 39% of new AIDS cases; Hispanic Americans, who make up about 10% of the U.S. population, accounted for 19% of AIDS cases (CDC, 1995b).

The 1990s have brought about an evolution in the demographics of HIV infection. The Centers for

Disease Control and Prevention (1994g) reported that from 1992 to 1993 the proportion of AIDS-related opportunistic illnesses in gay and bisexual men *decreased* 1% whereas the proportion of injection drug users with these diseases increased 8% and the proportion of heterosexuals increased 23%. This slight decline in the rates for gay men and the 1993 definition, which included invasive cervical cancer, combined to increase women's proportion of AIDS cases. In 1992, women accounted for about 14% of AIDS cases, but this proportion jumped to 18% in 1994. African American and Hispanic American women represented 77% of all women with AIDS in 1994, which means that the combined number of European American, Asian/Pacific Islander, and Native American women accounted for only 23% of the cases among women and only about 4% of the total AIDS cases in 1994 (CDC, 1995c).

Although women have accounted for an increasingly higher percentage of AIDS cases, the proportion of male to female *deaths* remained fairly constant from 1987 to 1992 (see Figure 11.2). During those years, about 89% deaths from HIV infection were men and about 11% were women. However, because the incidence of cases has risen faster for women than for men (largely because of the revised definition of HIV infection), in subsequent years women will account for an increasingly higher percentage of deaths from AIDS. AIDS is currently the fourth leading cause of death for women ages 25 to 44 (CDC, 1995c) and the leading cause of death for women of this age in several U.S. cities (Selik, Chu, & Buehler, 1993).

Figure 11.2 shows that the number of deaths from HIV infection declined sharply in 1994 despite the gradual increase in incidence of the disease. This continued increase in the total number of cases and the recent decrease in deaths indicates that patients are now surviving longer. Why are HIV-infected individuals now living longer? Drugs such as azidothymidine (AZT) and interleukin-2 probably account for some of the increase in survival time (Lenderking et al., 1994; Kovacs et al., 1995), but early detection and aggressive lifestyle changes may be more important contributors. Folkman (1993) cited several strategies adopted by HIV patients that may prolong their lives. First, these patients often give up unhealthy habits (such as smoking, drinking alcohol, and taking drugs) while adopting healthy ones (eating a better diet and getting more rest). Second, HIV patients become more vigilant about their health and monitor their symptoms. Third, they exercise more control over their treatment, which may include healing therapies such as visualization, meditation, megavitamins, and yoga. Even though people now are living longer with the disease, there is still no cure for AIDS.

SYMPTOMS OF HIV AND AIDS

HIV progresses over a decade or more through four stages, but people vary greatly in the length of time at each stage. During the first stage of HIV infection, symptoms are not easily distinguishable from those of other illnesses. Within a week or so of infection,

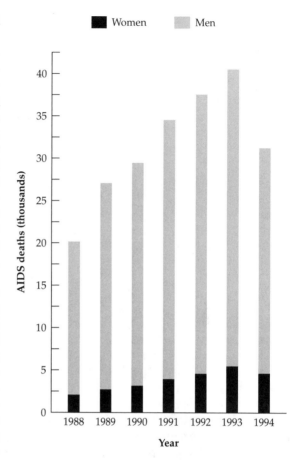

Figure 11.2   Incidence of AIDS cases, by gender, United States, 1988 to 1994.   SOURCE: Data from *Statistical Abstracts of the United States, 1995* (115th ed.), p. 97, by U.S. Bureau of the Census, 1995, Washington, DC: U.S. Government Printing Office.

people frequently experience fever, sore throat, skin rash, headache, and other mild symptoms (McCutchan, 1990). This relatively short first period of from 1 to 8 weeks is typically followed by a latent period that may last as long as 10 years during which patients are asymptomatic or experience only minimal symptoms. During the third stage, patients typically have a cluster of symptoms that formerly was known as AIDS-related complex (ARC). This cluster includes swollen lymph nodes, fever, fatigue, night sweats, loss of appetite, loss of weight, persistent diarrhea, white spots in the mouth, and painful skin rash. During the final stage, the patients' CD4+ T-lymphocyte cell count drops to 200 or less per cubic millimeter of blood (healthy people have a CD4+

count of 1,000). As their immune system begins to lose its defensive capacities, patients become susceptible to various opportunistic infections involving the lungs, gastrointestinal tract, nervous system, liver, bones, and brain. Symptoms include greater weight loss, general fatigue, fever, shortness of breath, dry cough, purplish bumps on the skin, and AIDS-related dementia. At this point, HIV has become full-blown AIDS, from which no person has ever recovered.

The diseases associated with HIV and AIDS are caused by a variety of agents, including viruses, bacteria, fungi, and parasites. The supply of CD4+ T-lymphocytes is depleted, so the immune system no longer has a mechanism for fighting infections within cells. The AIDS virus damages or kills the part of the immune system that fights viral infections, leaving no way for the body to fight HIV. But HIV does not destroy the antibodies that the immune system has already manufactured, so the immune system response that occurs through antibodies circulating in the blood remains intact. Therefore, being HIV positive does not often cause a person, for example, to develop infections with the bacterium that causes strep throat or the virus that causes influenza. Most HIV-infected people have antibodies to fight against these common agents. Instead, HIV results in infection from otherwise rare organisms, which leads to such diseases as *Pneumocystis carinii* pneumonia and Kaposi's sarcoma, the two leading causes of death among AIDS patients.

During the first 7 years of the AIDS epidemic, *Pneumocystis carinii* pneumonia occurred in 80% of AIDS patients (Saah et al., 1995), but for some reason, incidence of both *Pneumocystis carinii* pneumonia and Kaposi's sarcoma began to decline during the late 1980s and early 1990s (Doll, 1991; Silverberg, 1991). Moreover, the *proportion* of AIDS patients dying from these two illnesses will probably continue to drop with the 1993 definition of AIDS that added invasive cervical cancer, pulmonary tuberculosis, and recurrent pneumonia to the list of AIDS-related opportunistic diseases.

THE TRANSMISSION OF HIV

Although HIV is an infectious organism with a high fatality rate, the virus is not easily transmitted from person to person. The main routes of infection are from person to person during sex, from mother to child during pregnancy or birth, and from direct contact with blood or blood products (Glasner & Kaslow, 1990). Concentrations of HIV are especially high in the semen and blood of infected people. Therefore, contact with infected semen or blood is a risk. Other body fluids do not contain such a high concentration of HIV, making contact with saliva, urine, or tears much less of a risk. No evidence exists that any sort of casual contact spreads the infection. Eating with the same utensils or plates or drinking from the same cup as someone who is infected does not transmit HIV, nor does touching or even kissing someone who is infected. Insect bites do not spread the virus, and even being bitten by someone who is infected will not infect the person who is bitten.

People most at risk for HIV infection are gay men and intravenous (IV) drug users, a fact that is hardly news to people in those two high-risk groups. Yet many gay men (especially young ones) and many injection drug users (both women and men) engage in behaviors that put them at risk for HIV infection. What are these high-risk behaviors?

Male-Male Sexual Contact

Although the rate of HIV infection among gay and bisexual men has declined slightly in recent years (CDC, 1994g), male-male sexual contact still accounts for the largest number of HIV infections in the United States. Among gay and bisexual men, unprotected anal intercourse is an especially risky behavior, particularly for the receptive partner. Because the delicate lining of the rectum is often damaged during anal intercourse, the receptive person is at high risk if his partner is infected with HIV. The damaged rectum makes an excellent route for the virus to enter the body, and semen of infected men has a high concentration of HIV. Therefore, unprotected anal intercourse is one of the high-risk behaviors for a receptive partner. Unprotected oral sex with an infected partner is also a risky practice because HIV can enter the body through any tiny cut or other lesion in the mouth.

Although most older gay men now use condoms routinely, many younger ones engage in unsafe sexual practices, especially after using alcohol or other drugs. Stall, McKusick, Wiley, Coates, and Ostrow (1986) were among the first to report that alcohol may contribute to unsafe sexual practices among gay men. Since that time, several additional studies have also shown a link between risky sexual behaviors and use of drugs. For example, Penkower et al. (1991) looked at several potential factors related to receptive anal intercourse and found that heavy drinking, heavy drug use, and being 35 or younger were each significantly related to this unsafe practice. These same three variables also predicted number of sexual partners, willingness to have anonymous sex, and failure to use condoms. In another study, Lemp et al. (1994) surveyed young gay and bisexual men in the San Francisco/Berkeley area and found that most of them reported some form of intoxication during unprotected anal intercourse. Moreover, most of these 17- to 22-year-old men had begun unprotected anal intercourse and drug injection use after 1988, by which time information on risky sexual behaviors was widespread in the Bay area. Results of these and other studies suggest at least two possibilities. First, risk-taking individuals may engage in a variety of dangerous behaviors, including use of intoxicants and unprotected sex; second, the use of intoxicants may cloud people's decision-making ability with regard to potentially dangerous sexual practices.

Injection Drug Use

Another high-risk behavior is the sharing of unsterilized needles by injection drug users, a practice that allows the direct transmission of blood from one person to another. Injection drug use is the second most frequent source of HIV infection among men in the United States and the most frequent source for women. The Centers for Disease Control and Prevention (1994g) reported that the proportion of AIDS-related opportunistic illnesses attributable to injection drug users increased 8% from 1992 to 1993.

Use of injection drugs persists in spite of people's knowledge that this practice puts them at risk for HIV infection. Loxley and Hawks (1994) examined the persistence of risky drug injection use and risky sexual behaviors in a sample of current or recent drug users. They found no difference in knowledge about HIV/AIDS between people who engaged in

very risky drug injection and sexual behaviors and those who practiced relatively safe drug and sexual behaviors. In their sample, very risky drug injection practices and very risky sexual behaviors both seemed to have been related more to the specific situation than to lack of knowledge of their consequence. For example, being intoxicated or not having immediate access to sterile drug equipment were better predictors of risky behaviors than knowledge of the causes of HIV infection. Also, Sibthorpe and Lear (1994) found that about one-fifth of current injection drug users had quit using drugs for at least 1 year but then restarted. Of 180 participants who had quit, only 1 cited concern about HIV as a reason for quitting. These results suggest that relapse is a problem in drug cessation and that knowledge of the possible consequences of a risky behavior is not generally sufficient to change that behavior.

Currently, about half of AIDS cases for women are due to exposure to injection drug use, and African American women with AIDS are considerably more likely than White women with AIDS to have contracted the disease through intravenous drug use. Astemborski, Vlahov, Warren, Solomon, and Nelson (1994) studied women who were injection drug users and found that the greater the number of male sex partners these women had, the higher was their prevalence of HIV infection. Astemborski et al. also found that trading sex for drugs or money was independently related to HIV infection. For those women who had not traded sex for drugs or money during the past 10 years, about one in four injection drug users tested positive for HIV; but for those who had exchanged sex for drugs or money with more than 50 partners, nearly half were HIV positive. Women who trade sex for injection drugs are at high risk for HIV infection from two sources—unsafe sex with a partner who injects drugs and use of contaminated needles. However, Freeman, Rodriguez, and French (1994) found that the greater of the two risks is from sex with drug-using partners. Thus, heterosexual contact, independent of injection drug use, is a source of HIV infection.

Heterosexual Contact

Heterosexual contact is the leading source of HIV in Africa (Eckholm & Tierney, 1990) and the fastest growing source in the United States (CDC, 1994g).

For women, heterosexual activity is still second to IV needle sharing as a leading source of HIV infection, but it is a more rapidly increasing mode of transmission (CDC, 1995c).

Ickovics and Rodin (1992) reviewed studies on the biological and psychosocial factors relevant to women with HIV or AIDS and found that male-female sexual contact accounted for one-third of the cases of women with AIDS. By far the most frequent form of this contact was sex with an injection drug user, which accounted for about 60% of the cases due to sexual contact. Ickovics and Rodin found that having sex with a bisexual man accounted for only about 6% of AIDS cases among adult and adolescent women. These results agree with those of Freeman et al. (1994), who found that women who traded sex for drugs were at greater risk of HIV from sexual contact with drug-injecting partners than from the use of unsterile drug equipment.

Some evidence suggests that those women with the most dangerous practices are the least likely to be tested for the virus. In a national sample of heterosexual women currently in a relationship with IV drug-using male partners (Tortu, Beardsley, Deren, & Davis, 1994), women with only one sex partner were about twice as likely to have HIV testing as women with multiple partners who exchanged sex for drugs or money. Not surprisingly, drug and alcohol use was highest among women who had multiple sex partners and who also traded sex for drugs or money. In another study, Edlin et al. (1994) surveyed young men and women in the inner city of three large metropolitan areas and found that 30% of the women who traded sex for drugs or money were HIV positive compared with 9% of those who did not exchange sex for drugs or money. Results of these two studies indicate a strong association between HIV infection in women and their practice of trading sex for drugs or money.

Women seem to be more vulnerable than men to HIV through heterosexual contact. Research suggests that although men are susceptible to HIV through sexual contact with women, they are relatively safe if they take reasonable precautions. Padian, Shiboski, and Jewell (1991) recruited 379 couples from several HIV counseling and testing sites in California. Of this number, only one man was a possibility for having received HIV infection through sexual contact with his female partner. However, Padian et al. reported that this couple had had numerous unprotected sexual contacts, including several times when they noted vaginal and penile bleeding during sexual intercourse. In addition, they had had intercourse immediately after the women had had sex with another man who was at a high risk for HIV. The results of this study show that it is difficult but not impossible for exclusively heterosexual men to receive the human immunodeficiency virus from sexual contact with women. Other studies have found that although both men and women are vulnerable to HIV infection if they engage in unprotected heterosexual contact, their chances of becoming infected are somewhat low. For example, Fullilove et al. (1992) studied the prevalence of HIV in a representative sample of unmarried 20- to 44-year-old men and women living in San Francisco. Of nearly 880 men tested, 66 were HIV positive, but of those, only 4 had neither engaged in male-male sexual activity nor injected drugs. Thus, fewer than .05% of heterosexual men who do not inject drugs tested positive for HIV. Of 890 women tested, only 1 who did not inject drugs tested positive. Again, though HIV infection is rarely transmitted from one partner to another during heterosexual intercourse, unprotected heterosexual intercourse is not completely safe.

Heterosexual men and women who regularly use condoms, of course, are safer than those who do not. De Vincenzi (1994) conducted a prospective study of HIV-negative men and women whose only risk of HIV was a stable heterosexual relationship with an infected partner. Over a 20-month follow-up, none of the HIV-negative partners who used condoms consistently for vaginal and anal intercourse tested positive for HIV despite 15,000 episodes of intercourse. However, for those couples who used condoms inconsistently, 10% became HIV positive. Similarly, Avins et al. (1994) studied heterosexual men and women in alcohol treatment programs and found that inconsistent use of condoms as well as having heterosexual contact with multiple partners placed people at a relatively high risk for HIV infection.

Evidence suggests that unsafe heterosexual behaviors are related to noninjection drugs, such as crack, alcohol, and marijuana. Edlin et al. (1994)

found that inner-city young men who were regular crack smokers were about three times more likely than those who did not use crack to be HIV positive. In addition, Hingson, Strunin, Berlin, and Heeren (1990) found that adolescents who drank heavily or who used marijuana were much less likely to use condoms than adolescents who were not heavy drinkers or marijuana users, and Lowry et al. (1994) found that high school students who used marijuana, cocaine, and other illicit drugs were more likely than students with no history of substance abuse to have had sex with four or more partners and not to have used a condom at last sexual intercourse. These studies once again indicate an association between use of drugs and dangerous sexual practices, although cause and effect has not been determined.

Other Modes of Transmission

Other means of HIV transmission include exposure to infected blood through transfusions and during the birth process. During the early history of the AIDS epidemic, some people, especially hemophiliacs, were exposed to HIV through receiving blood transfusions. However, since 1986, all donated blood has been routinely tested for HIV, and blood transfusion is no longer a risk. Donating blood, of course, has never carried a risk for infection with HIV.

However, children born to HIV-positive women are still at risk. The Centers for Disease Control and Prevention (1995c) estimated that 7,000 infants are born to HIV-infected women in the United States each year. Of that number, 1,000 to 2,000 are themselves infected with HIV, so that presently HIV infection is the seventh leading cause of death in children 1 to 4 years of age (CDC, 1994f).

Children infected with HIV perinatally—that is, during the birth process—suffer a variety of developmental disabilities including intellectual and academic impairment, psychomotor dysfunctions, and emotional and behavioral difficulties (Levenson & Mellins, 1992). In addition, many of these children are born to mothers who ingested drugs during pregnancy and are thus put at further risk for developmental difficulties. The drug zidovudine (ZDV) has been used with very limited success to reduce perinatal transmission of HIV (CDC, 1994e), but it has been used somewhat more successfully after

birth to enhance children's cognitive abilities and improve their social and emotional behaviors (Wolters, Brouwers, Moss, & Pizzo, 1994).

PROTECTIVE MEASURES

Except for infants born to HIV-infected mothers, most people have some control in protecting themselves from the human immunodeficiency virus. Fortunately, HIV is not easily transmitted from person to person, making casual contact with infected persons a low risk. People can protect themselves against infection with HIV by changing those behaviors that are high risks for acquiring the infection—namely, having unprotected sexual contact or sharing needles with an infected person. The majority of people in the United States, Canada, and Europe who are infected have become so in one of these two ways. Limiting the number of sex partners, using condoms, and avoiding shared needles are three behaviors that will protect the largest number of people the United States and Canada from HIV infection.

However, other protective measures may be applicable for some people. Health care workers who participate in surgery, emergency care, or other procedures that bring them into contact with blood should be careful to prevent infected blood from entering their body through an open wound. For example, many dentists and dental hygienists now wear protective gloves, and health care workers are taught to adhere to a set of standard protective measures.

The tendency to base judgment on appearances can be dangerous when it comes to HIV infection. Because HIV infection typically has a long asymptomatic incubation period, people can be contagious and still appear healthy. Choosing sex partners based on the appearance of health can be very risky. Even with the widespread concern about AIDS and infection with HIV, many people continue to engage in high-risk behaviors. As we have seen, alcohol and other noninjection drugs are often linked to unsafe sexual practices. In addition to research cited earlier, two studies have shown that some people at risk often appear oblivious of any personal threat from the disease. Biglan et al. (1990) questioned adolescents about their high-risk sexual behaviors. They found that adolescents who engaged in one type of high-risk sexual behavior were also likely to engage in other high-risk behaviors. For example, adolescents who had sex with multiple partners whom they they do not know very well were also not likely to use condoms. Moreover, these high-risk sexual behaviors were related to other health-risk behaviors such as smoking and drinking. In the other study, Kelly et al. (1990) found that 37% of the patrons of gay bars reported engaging in unprotected anal intercourse and having somewhat naive beliefs about the potential danger of AIDS. Those who avoided this high-risk behavior were more likely to attribute safety to their own behavior (as opposed to luck, chance, or fate), be more knowledgeable about high-risk practices, have fewer sex partners, be older, consider safety an accepted norm in their social contacts, and be more realistic about their own risk.

Many people who engage in high-risk behaviors do so as part of a pattern of taking risks. Thus, psychological programs constructed to change high-risk sexual behaviors must consider the optimistic bias, naive beliefs, or disregard for safety among people who are at greatest risk.

PSYCHOLOGISTS' ROLE IN THE AIDS EPIDEMIC

Psychologists play many roles in the AIDS epidemic — counseling people about being tested for HIV, changing high-risk behaviors, helping patients deal with deteriorating mental abilities, conducting bereavement therapy for dying patients and for friends of deceased patients, and investigating the behavioral manifestations of AIDS.

People with high-risk behaviors may have difficulty deciding whether to be tested for HIV, and psychologists can provide both information and support for these people. A significant minority of gay and bisexual men, injection drug users, and a larger proportion of heterosexual men and women with multiple partners and inconsistent use of condoms have never been tested for HIV. People in this last group may be unaware of their risk and deny a need to be tested. Because HIV infection has a long incubation period, at-risk heterosexual men and women may contaminate others for years before they learn they have HIV.

Folkman (1993) reviewed several studies of gay and bisexual men and found that between 18% and

41% of these men at risk for HIV either had never been tested or did not know the results of their test. Folkman pointed out that the decision to be tested has both benefits and costs. The benefit, of course, is that people can find out their serostatus as soon as possible. Such knowledge can eliminate uncertainty and reduce anxiety, even if the results are positive. A positive HIV test can lead to early treatment, which can prolong a person's life. Another potentially positive benefit of early testing is the reduction or elimination of behaviors that place others at risk. Folkman's review found that gay and bisexual men reduced risky sexual behaviors and most informed their primary partner. Some, however, continued unprotected anal intercourse, a small minority failed to tell their primary sex partner, and somewhat more HIV-positive men neglected to inform nonprimary partners.

What are the costs of receiving an HIV-positive test result? Does such information increase anxiety, depression, anger, and psychological distress? Folkman also reviewed research on this question and found some interesting results. Several studies indicated that HIV-positive gay men manifested more psychological distress than a nonclinical population. However, Folkman (1993, p. 667) also cited evidence suggesting that gay men have "a high lifetime prevalence of major psychiatric disorders, including increased generalized anxiety disorder and major depression" and that most of these men had psychiatric problems prior to learning of their HIV-positive status. Folkman (p. 668) further explained that "wrestling with the meaning of one's sexual orientation in terms of identity, affiliations, and life goals and disclosing sexual orientation to others will have significant psychosocial effects." In addition, Folkman cited evidence that receiving a positive HIV test result may not increase general anxiety and depression and may even lead to improved interpersonal relations. She also reported that patients who used active coping skills rather than avoidant coping tended to have less severe psychological distress. Avoidant coping includes a denial of reality and a clinging to illusory hope.

Studies reviewed by Folkman included only gay or bisexual men with HIV infection, but Fleishman and Fogel (1994) studied a more representative sample of HIV-infected men and women. In this

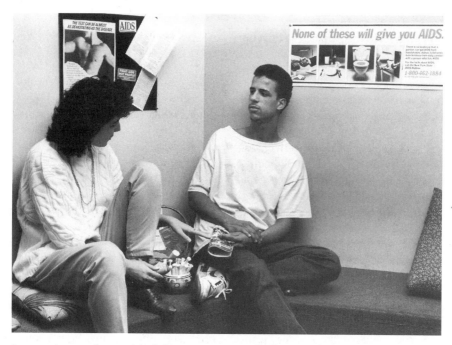

Interventions to change risky behaviors are currently the most effective way to decrease the transmission of HIV.

large national sample, more than 40% of persons with AIDS were diagnosed with clinical depression, a percentage considerably higher than that reported in other studies. Fleishman and Fogel found that HIV patients with a history of drug use were the most likely to engage in avoidant coping, the least likely to use positive coping, and the least likely to seek social support. These nonproductive coping mechanisms frequently characterize people with a history of drug use and may not be a reaction to an HIV diagnosis (Khantzian, 1980). The findings suggest that people with positive HIV test results have somewhat more psychological distress than people who are not at risk for HIV, but some of that distress may have existed prior to the knowledge that the person is HIV infected.

In summary, acquired immune deficiency syndrome (AIDS) is the result of depletion of the immune system due to infection with the human immunodeficiency virus (HIV). When the immune system fails to defend the body, a number of diseases may develop, including bacterial, viral, fungal, and parasitic infections that are uncommon in those who have functioning immune systems.

HIV progresses into AIDS through four stages, but throughout most of the time, an HIV-positive person has few or no symptoms and may unknowingly infect others with the virus. For this reason, frequent blood tests for people in high-risk categories are essential to control the spread of AIDS. The modes of transmission of HIV are behavioral, with receptive anal intercourse and the sharing of needles for intravenous drug injection the two behaviors that have spread the infection to the most people in the United States. However, unprotected heterosexual contact with an infected partner accounts for an ever-increasing proportion of people with HIV.

Psychologists have used a variety of interventions to help patients reduce high-risk behaviors, to cope with their illness, and to manage their symptoms. In addition, psychologists have been involved in the study of the effects of HIV on the central nervous system and have provided counseling services for those seeking to be tested and for those whose tests reveal infection. These programs not only encourage protective behaviors but also emphasize the role of positive health in combating AIDS.

LIVING WITH ALZHEIMER'S DISEASE

Alzheimer's disease, a degenerative disease of the brain, is a major source of impairment among older people, affecting as many as four million patients in the United States (Davis et al., 1992). Medical researchers identified the brain abnormalities that underlie Alzheimer's disease in the late 19th century. In 1907, a German physician, Alois Alzheimer, reported on the relationship between autopsy findings of neurological abnormalities and psychiatric symptoms before death. Shortly after his report, other researchers began to call the disorder Alzheimer's disease.

Although Alzheimer's patients show behavioral symptoms of cognitive impairment and memory loss, the disease can be diagnosed definitively only through autopsy. A microscopic examination of the brain of those with Alzheimer's disease reveals "plaques" and tangles of nerve fibers in the cerebral cortex and hippocampus. These tangles of nerve fibers are the physical basis for Alzheimer's disease.

The underlying mechanisms in the development of the disease are not yet completely understood, but research has identified two different forms of the disease; one that occurs before age 60 and the other that occurs after age 70. The early-onset type is quite rare, representing less than 1% of all Alzheimer's patients (Mayeux & Schupf, 1995). Early-onset Alzheimer's seems to be due to a genetic defect, and at least three different genes have been implicated on chromosomes 1, 14, and 21 (Marx, 1992; Mayeux & Schupf, 1995; Travis, 1995).

The late-onset type seems to be related to apolipoprotein E, a protein involved in cholesterol metabolism (Goedert, Strittmatter, & Roses, 1994; Mayeux & Schupf, 1995). One form of apolipoprotein, the E4 form, is a risk factor for development of the tangles of neurons that are characteristic of Alzheimer's disease. Other forms of apolipoprotein, the E2 and E3 forms, may offer some protection against the development of Alzheimer's disease (Cotton, 1994). This research on the physiology underlying Alzheimer's disease offers the promise of identifying the causes of this disease and suggests the possibility of treatment for those at risk and perhaps even for those with the disease.

The incidence of Alzheimer's disease rises sharply with advanced age (Evans et al., 1989; Hebert et al., 1995; Paykel et al. 1994). Evans et al. (1989) found that more than 10% of all people over age 65 showed symptoms that indicated a probable diagnosis of Alzheimer's disease. These people showed symptoms of serious cognitive, language, and memory deficits. Evans et al. also found a strong association between age and Alzheimer's disease, with only 3% of the people between ages 65 and 74 demonstrating symptoms of the disease; 18.7% of the people between ages 75 and 84 manifesting symptoms; and 47.2% of their sample over age 85 showing symptoms of Alzheimer's disease. The increase does not continue, however, and people who have not developed symptoms of Alzheimer's disease by their mid-80s are less likely to do so than people in their 70s (Ritchie & Kildea, 1995). The high number of people over 85 years old who have existing symptoms of probable Alzheimer's disease casts a pall over the otherwise encouraging figures on increasing life span. They indicate that as the population ages, this disease and its management will become an increasingly pressing social and medical problem.

Because the symptoms of Alzheimer's include a number of behavior problems that are also symptoms of psychiatric disorders, the disease can be difficult to diagnose. These symptoms include memory loss, language problems, agitation and irritability, sleep disorders, suspiciousness and paranoia, incontinence, and sexual disorders (Rabins, 1989). These behavioral symptoms can be the source of much distress to the patients as well as to their caregivers. Reifler and Larson (1989) discussed the association between Alzheimer's disease and old age and also the association between Alzheimer's disease and psychiatric symptoms. The most common psychiatric problem among Alzheimer's patients is depression. Rabins (1989) estimated that between 15% and 40% of Alzheimer's patients exhibit symptoms of depression, and depression is especially common among people in the early phases of the disease. Those people who retain much awareness of their problems find their deterioration distressing and respond with a feeling of helplessness and depression.

The memory loss that characterizes Alzheimer's disease may first appear in the form of small, ordinary failures of memory, but the memory loss progresses to the point that Alzheimer's patients fail to recognize family members and forget how to perform even routine self-care (Rabins, 1989). In the early phases of the disease, patients are usually aware of their memory failures, making this symptom even more distressing. This chapter opened with the case of Sylvia, who was typical of many Alzheimer's patients in that she became angry with herself for not being able to recall people's names and for forgetting words in the middle of a sentence. She knew that she should be able to say the right name or word, a situation that sparked frustration and fury.

Sylvia's language problems highlight a related cognitive deficit. The inability to utter the intended word is quite common among Alzheimer's patients. Sometimes patients substitute other words for the one they intended, but the substitutes are not always good matches, posing communication problems. This language disability can lead to frustration and, if patients withdraw from attempts to communicate, can promote isolation.

Patients with Alzheimer's disease often exhibit symptoms of agitation, irritability, and even violence. Sylvia was no exception. A gentle, even passive woman during the first 80 years of her life, she frequently became aggressive and threatening as her disease progressed. She accused Brenda of mistreating her and on one occasion cut up all her old photos of Brenda. In some cases, Sylvia's explosive agitation was related to her memory failure. Sometimes she would have an explosive outburst while getting dressed because she had forgotten how to complete the task and had become confused and frustrated. At other times she would become angry because her daily routine had been disrupted and she was uncertain about how she should behave.

The common symptoms of paranoia and suspiciousness may also relate to cognitive impairments. Rabins (1989) noted that Alzheimer's patients may forget where they have put belongings, and because they cannot find their possessions, accuse others of taking them. However, suspicious and accusatory behaviors are not limited to misplaced belongings. Like many Alzheimer's patients, Sylvia concentrated her suspicions and accusations on her primary caregiver, leading Brenda to become resentful and emotionally distressed.

Although difficulties in staying asleep are common among older adults, Alzheimer's patients have even more severe problems than their peers. As a result, these patients tend to wander at all times of the day and night (Rabins, 1989). This behavior can disturb those who sleep in the same house and provide opportunities for the patients to injure themselves. After Brenda and Bob moved Sylvia into their house, this problem became so serious that they were required to retain a "sitter" who watched Sylvia at night. The sitter was instructed to gently lead Sylvia back to her bedroom whenever she roamed around at night.

Incontinence and sexual disorders are acutely distressing problems to both the patients and their caregivers. Incontinence is very common in patients with advanced cases of Alzheimer's disease. In the year before she died, Sylvia lost all control over her bowel movements. Even more distressing to Brenda, she seemed also to have lost her awareness of normal excretory functions and showed no appreciation for her daughter's extra work in cleaning her. Also distressing to Brenda was her mother's inappropriate sexual behavior, a common disorder among Alzheimer's patients. Sylvia would sometimes masturbate in public and use obscene language, behaviors that were totally uncharacteristic of her earlier life. A pattern of behavioral symptoms, such as Sylvia's, is strong indication of Alzheimer's disease and the only means of diagnosis before autopsy.

HELPING THE PATIENT

Presently, no cure for Alzheimer's disease exists; the most effective treatment for the disease would be one that prevented or reversed the degeneration of neurons in the brain. Reifler and Larson (1989) maintained that incurability and untreatability are two different things and that Alzheimer's patients are the victims of this confusion. They contended that the physical symptoms and other accompanying disorders of Alzheimer's disease can be treated but not cured. Other researchers, however, are less optimistic, maintaining that few treatments have demonstrated significant benefits for patients with Alzheimer's disease (Cohler, Groves, Borden, & Lazarus, 1989; Davis et al., 1995).

In 1984, the Secretary's Task Force on Alzheimer's Disease reviewed a number of drug treatments for the disease and found little evidence that any are effective in reversing the cognitive deficits or lost learning ability or memory that accompany it. Since that time some authorities have speculated that the drug tacrine (a cholinesterase inhibitor) may be an effective treatment. Davis et al. (1992) conducted a double-blind, placebo-controlled study of tacrine and found that the tacrine group performed slightly better than the control group on an Alzheimer's disease assessment scale. However, this difference was not clinically meaningful and appeared only because test scores of the control (nontreatment) group worsened. In addition to drugs aimed at slowing or reversing cognitive decline of Alzheimer's patients, physicians sometimes prescribe the same drugs that they recommend for psychiatric patients with depression, paranoia, sleep disorders, and agitation. Such drugs provide a type of secondary treatment for Alzheimer's patients because they are helpful in managing patients whose behavior is a problem for their caregivers.

In addition to drugs, several researchers have advocated behavioral approaches in treating Alzheimer's patients. Rabins (1989) advocated a behavioral approach designed to modify the environment of Alzheimer's patients so they can adjust better to their lives. He suggested an analysis of the antecedents of the patient's problem behaviors. By identifying the events that precede problem behaviors, family members can eliminate or reduce those events and thus perhaps decrease the patient's undesirable behaviors. Rabins listed a number of ways to change these antecedents, including changes in the environment and in the patient's behaviors. For example, he suggested that patients with awareness of their memory loss could learn to write notes as a way of keeping track of the important things in their lives. For those who get lost in their own homes, Rabins recommended labeling the doors.

Hall (1994) described a somewhat different tactic for dealing with patients with Alzheimer's disease and other dementias. Called the Progressively Lowered Stress Threshold model, this approach divides symptoms into cognitive or intellectual problems, affective or personality changes, losses in the ability to plan, and lowering of stress thresholds that cause episodes of dysfunctional behavior. This model holds that dysfunctional episodes are caused by stresses such as fatigue, changes in environment or routine, inappropriate levels of stimulation, performance demands that exceed capability, and physical stressors. Hall maintained that this model provides an assessment of behavior problems and allows for interventions to minimize dysfunctional episodes by helping caregivers to structure the environment, establish a routine for the patients, minimize fatigue, and identify pain. For example, Hall cited an example of patients who yelled throughout the day, 60% of whom were found to have fractures that had not been identified, causing them considerable pain. This behavioral management program offers a way to approach the care of patients with Alzheimer's disease so as to allow them prolonged periods of functioning while providing their caretakers with a way to approach the demands of caring for a person with diminishing capabilities.

Although none of these therapies will cure Alzheimer's, most will help control undesirable behaviors and alleviate some of the distressing symptoms of the disease. In the early phases of Alzheimer's disease, both patients and their families are distressed by its symptoms, but as the patients worsen and lose awareness, the stress of Alzheimer's becomes more severe for the family.

HELPING THE FAMILY

As with other chronic illnesses, Alzheimer's disease affects not only patients but also their families. For Alzheimer's disease, however, the symptoms of the illness are particularly distressing to the families (Cohler et al., 1989; Mohide, 1993). The memory impairments are disturbing because patients may fail to recognize their spouses and children. Cognitive impairments lead to changes in personality, and the one affected no longer seems like the same person. The suspiciousness that Alzheimer's patients frequently manifest can lead to accusations that hurt family members, and Alzheimer's patients who are violent upset normal family functioning. Families tend to find dangerous or embarrassing behaviors especially distressing (Barrett, Ford, Stewart, & Haley, 1994). In addition to this emotional burden, the

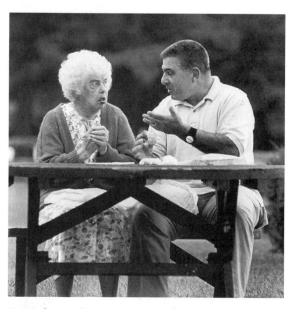

Caring for an Alzheimer's patient can produce high levels of stress, making caregivers vulnerable to illness.

problems of taking care of an Alzheimer's patient greatly disrupt family routine.

For instance, arguments between Brenda and Bob increased during the time Sylvia lived with them. Brenda neglected her own appearance, became absorbed in her caregiving duties, and lost interest in sexual relations with Bob. Before Sylvia's illness, Brenda and Bob shared interests in the law, movies, books, and traveling. Although she could have arranged to do so, during the 3 years her mother lived with them, Brenda never took a vacation or even went to a movie.

In the United States, the caregiver role is occupied mostly by women (Cohler et al., 1989; Pearlin, Turner, & Semple, 1989), and an unmarried woman has the greatest likelihood of becoming the primary caretaker for Alzheimer's patients (Modesti & Tryon, 1994). The National Long-term Care Survey (Stone, Cafferata, & Sangl, 1987) showed that family caregivers are usually the patients' wives or daughters. For Alzheimer's patients with spouses who are able to provide care, the caregiving falls to the spouse, and men as well as women fill this role. These spouses may not be able to provide the necessary care with ease because the spouses are elderly

and may be in poor health themselves. Therefore, adult children often become involved in caregiving, sometimes by assisting one parent to provide care for the other. Daughters and daughters-in-law are called on to help more often than sons or sons-in-law, whose assistance is typically in the form of helping their wives or sisters (Cohler et al., 1989). The gender inequity also exists in the assistance that adult children provide to parents who are caregivers, with men receiving more assistance in caring for their wives than women receive in caring for their husbands.

Not only must people who care for Alzheimer's patients have the time and energy for this task, but they must also take care of their other obligations as well. Often the demands of caring for an Alzheimer's patient conflict with job or career, and family members are usually not free to leave jobs because caregiving is an economic as well as an emotional strain. Many families exhaust their financial and emotional resources to provide care for an Alzheimer's patient (Pearlin et al., 1989).

In some ways, Brenda was more fortunate than the typical caregiver. Bob's income was sufficient, and Brenda suspended her career to care for her mother. Brenda could have continued with her career and hired a full-time nurse, but she felt that she should be the one to provide care. According to Cohler et al. (1989), Brenda's feelings are typical of caregivers for Alzheimer's patients.

Alzheimer's caregivers frequently experience feelings of loss for the relationship that they once shared with the patient. This sense of loss may be similar to bereavement, only the person is still alive (Perlin et al., 1989). During her times alone, Brenda found herself reminiscing more and more about her childhood and the pleasant times she enjoyed with her mother. She knew that Sylvia would never regain the loving personality that marked her earlier life. The woman Brenda once knew no longer lived in her mother's body, and she grieved over her loss.

Caregivers experiencing the stress and strain of their role exhibit a number of symptoms of their own distress, including fatigue, frustration, helplessness, grief, embarrassment, guilt, and depression (Mace & Rabins, 1981). Anger seems to be the most common negative emotion, and Gallagher, Wrabetz,

Lovett, Del Maestro, and Rose (1989) found that 67% of Alzheimer's caregivers reported feelings of anger. These researchers found that somatic symptoms, such as sleep problems and low energy, were less common than negative emotions but that 30% of the caregivers in their study reported some somatic symptoms. These caregivers did not make greater use of medical services than people of similar ages who were not providing care to Alzheimer's patients, but they did average nearly three times as many stress symptoms. Between 20% and 50% of caregivers experience symptoms of depression (Gallagher et al., 1989; Modesti & Tryon, 1994). The study by Gallagher et al. found that 25% of their participants met the criteria for clinical depression and another 20% experienced nonclinical depression. These studies suggest that depression and negative emotions appear frequently in those who provide care for Alzheimer's patients.

Janice Kiecolt-Glaser and her colleagues (Kiecolt-Glaser et al., 1991; Kiecolt-Glaser & Glaser, 1989; Kiecolt-Glaser, Glaser, et al., 1987) have explored the effect of caring for Alzheimer's patients on immune functioning. As part of their studies in psychoneuroimmunology, these researchers have conceptualized Alzheimer's caregiving as a chronic stressor, one that can lower immune functioning and leave the caregiver vulnerable to illness. Kiecolt-Glaser, Glaser, et al. (1987) compared caregivers of Alzheimer's patients with a matched control group and found that the caregivers were more distressed, exhibited a poorer immune response, and developed more infectious illnesses. They also found that the level of impairment of the Alzheimer's patient was related to the level of distress in the caregiver; the more impaired patients had more distressed caregivers. These results indicate that the chronic stress of providing care for Alzheimer's patients lowers immune system functioning and increases vulnerability to infectious illness.

A further report (Kiecolt-Glaser, Dyer, & Shuttleworth, 1988) from this ongoing study indicated that the type of support caregivers receive from *their* friends and family can affect their immune systems. Caregivers who received positive support had better immune functioning than those who received little support or negative support, such as criticism of how they provided care. The people who received negative support from friends and family showed the poorest immune functioning of anyone in the study. This finding emphasizes the importance of support and the need for assistance in coping for caregivers of Alzheimer's patients.

Gallagher et al. (1989) recommended cognitive-behavioral therapies to manage the negative emotions that accompany caregiving, pointing out that this type of therapy has been successful in dealing with these emotions when they arise in other situations. They also suggested that people who care for Alzheimer's patients may benefit from participation in support groups. Many support groups exist to provide social support and information about caring for Alzheimer's patients. Participation in a group that encourages an open, honest sharing of feelings, including negative feelings, can provide support that families may not be able to give. This additional support may be needed because of the strain imposed on the family and friends of the patient, people who would otherwise be the main sources of support. Support groups can also be sources of information about caring for the patients and about community resources that provide respite care.

In summary, Alzheimer's disease is a progressive, degenerative disease of the brain that affects cognitive functioning, especially memory. The cause of the disease is not known, but increasing age is a risk factor. As many as 47% of people over age 85 exhibit symptoms. The other symptoms of Alzheimer's disease include language problems, agitation and irritability, paranoia and suspiciousness, sleep disorders, depression, incontinence, and sexual problems. These symptoms are also indicative of some psychiatric disorders and make Alzheimer's disease distressing to both patients and caretakers.

No effective medical treatment exists for the disease, although researchers are active in seeking drug treatments that may halt or reverse the cognitive deficits. The available treatments consist of pharmacological methods, behavior modification, cognitive therapy, and alterations of the patient's environment to manage the symptoms. Treatment may also be desirable for those who provide care to Alzheimer's patients because a high percentage of these caregivers experience stress and stress-related problems, depression being the most common. Individual therapy or increased social support from an Alzheimer's support group can help the caregivers and families of Alzheimer's patients cope with the stress of providing care.

CHAPTER SUMMARY

Chronic illnesses affect not only the afflicted person but friends and family members as well. Unlike infectious diseases that last for a relatively short time, chronic illnesses like heart disease, cancer, diabetes, AIDS, and Alzheimer's disease may persist for years.

Long-term chronic illnesses frequently bring about a crisis in people's lives, change the way patients see themselves, produce financial hardship, and disrupt family dynamics. Chronically ill patients have physiological, social, and emotional needs that are different from those of healthy people, and finding ways to satisfy these needs is part of the coping process. The social and emotional needs may be neglected while health care professionals attend to the patient's physical needs. Health psychologists and support groups have been involved in providing for the emotional problems associated with chronic illness.

Although coronary heart disease is the leading cause of death in the United States, an increasing number of people survive a heart attack. These people and those who undergo cardiac surgery typically engage in a cardiac rehabilitation regimen that consists of medication, smoking cessation, regular exercise, and a recommendations for a low-fat, low-salt diet. One such program that lowered dietary fat to 10% of consumed calories succeeded in reducing coronary artery plaques in a significant number of patients. In addition to these standard regimens, some programs attempt to alter the Type A behavior pattern and thus successfully reduce the chances of a recurring heart attack. Many cardiac patients suffer prolonged anxiety, sleep disturbance, and concern about a second heart attack. Also, spouses frequently experience depression and sexual anxieties. For this reason, psychological interventions in cardiac rehabilitation often include counseling with spouses.

The diagnosis of cancer may sound like a death sentence to some, but an increasing number survive this illness. Pain is a frequent problem with cancer patients, with about two-thirds suffering from severe pain. Cancer patients frequently suffer depression, marital stress, and other emotional and psychological disorders as well, but these experiences are not inevitable, and some evidence suggests that they are only slightly elevated in cancer patients.

The standard medical treatments for cancer—surgery, chemotherapy, and radiation—all have negative side effects that often produce added stress. These side effects include changes in body image, loss of hair, nausea, fatigue, and sterility. Psychological interventions, including relaxation, individual psychotherapy, and support groups can help patients cope with the unpleasant side effects of cancer.

Diabetes, both insulin-dependent and noninsulin-dependent, requires changes in lifestyle, including constant monitoring and compliance with the treatment regimen. People with juvenile-onset (Type I) diabetes must receive insulin injections, usually daily. In addition, they must adhere to the treatment regimen prescribed for adult-onset (Type II) diabetes, namely dietary restrictions, careful scheduling of meals, avoidance of certain foods, regular medical visits, and routine exercise. When these requirements are followed, most diabetics live relatively normal lives, with few additional psychological problems. Health psychologists, using cognitive-behavioral techniques, can help diabetics adhere to treatment regimens.

AIDS is the result of depletion of the immune system due to infection with the human immunodeficiency virus (HIV). Its main sources of transmission are receptive anal intercourse and unsterile drug needles, but it has also been transmitted through vaginal intercourse and from mother to fetus. Psychologists are involved with AIDS through counseling those infected with HIV and encouraging behaviors that protect against AIDS.

Alzheimer's disease is perhaps more stressful for family members than any of the other chronic illnesses. It affects mostly the elderly, although some middle-aged people have developed Alzheimer's. The disease cannot be diagnosed with certainty without autopsy, so it can be confused with other dementia illnesses. Symptoms of Alzheimer's include memory loss, language problems, agitation and irritability, sleep disorders, suspiciousness, wandering, incontinence, and loss of ability to perform routine care. Alzheimer's disease, like AIDS, is presently incurable, so no medical treatment will reverse the course of the illness. Psychological interventions with Alzheimer's disease usually include support groups for family members and individual counseling for the primary caregiver, who frequently experiences more stress than the patient.

SUGGESTED READINGS

Cousins, N. (1983). *The healing heart: Antidote to panic and helplessness.* New York: Norton. Norman Cousins describes his heart attack and his recovery in this readable, personal book about living with heart disease. Cousins's approach was unorthodox, but his advice led to an optimistic view of the process of recovery and coping.

Fife, B. L. (1994). The conceptualization of meaning in illness. *Social Science in Medicine, 38,* 309–316. Betsy Fife examines patients' search for meaning in their illness. She studied cancer patients, asking them about the social circumstances of their illness and how they came to understand it and their lives. Although she studied cancer patients, the responses could apply to those with any chronic illness.

Heston, L. L., & White, J. A. (1991). *The vanishing mind: A practical guide to Alzheimer's disease and other dementias.* New York: Freeman. This practical book provides valuable information for family members and other caregivers who deal with Alzheimer's disease and other dementias.

Holland, J. C., & Lewis, S. (1993). Emotions and cancer: Who do we really know? In D. Goleman & J. Gurin (Eds.), *Mind/body medicine: How to use your mind for* *better health* (pp. 85–109). Yonkers, NY: Consumer Reports Books. In addition to examining the evidence on emotions and cancer in a nontechnical format, Holland and Lewis review various adjunctive therapies for cancer, including psychotherapy, imagery, and support groups. They also give advice for coping with cancer and for helping someone with cancer deal with the emotional and physical problems of the disease.

Shilts, R. (1987). *And the band played on.* New York: St. Martin's Press. This book chronologically tells the story of the AIDS epidemic, the epidemiology research, and the medical and governmental reactions. Shilts's approach is as interesting and involving as a novel, but it also provides factual information (as well as personal opinion) about AIDS.

Taylor, S. E., & Aspinwall, L. G. (1993). Coping with chronic illness. In L. Goldberger & S. Breznitz (Eds.), *Handbook of stress: Theoretical and clinical aspects* (2nd ed., pp. 511–531). New York: Free Press. Shelly Taylor and Lisa Aspinwall summarize the research on coping with chronic illness, including the stresses that accompany chronic illness, the variety of coping strategies that people use to deal with such illnesses, and interventions to help people cope more effectively.

3

Behavioral Health

12

Staying Healthy

In Chapter 1 we met Dwayne and Robyn, two college students with different conceptions of health. Dwayne gives little thought to his health and has a variety of unhealthy behaviors whereas Robyn is very health conscious and leads a generally healthy lifestyle. The differences in their conceptions of health extend to their views of control of health, with Robyn believing that she can control her future health by her present behaviors and Dwayne believing that his health is largely beyond his control.

These attitudes also extend to their safety-related attitudes and behaviors. Dwayne believes that accidents are inevitable and unavoidable, so he does little to protect his safety. This attitude does not mean that Dwayne is not concerned with his safety, but he thinks that he can do little to prevent unintentional injury. For example, he rarely wears his seatbelt, arguing that people wearing and not wearing seatbelts are about equally likely to be injured in an auto crash. Robyn's views are quite different. She also believes that some accidents are unavoidable, but she sees most unintentional injury as the result of failing to think through the consequences of risky behavior.

Despite the differences in their views on safety, neither Dwayne nor Robyn takes many safety risks. Dwayne's failure to wear his seatbelt is a risk, but he is otherwise a careful driver; he obeys other traffic laws, rarely drives over the speed limit, and does not combine drinking with driving. Although Dwayne does not believe that his behavior is risky, he pays very little attention to his safety, an attitude that is consistent with his belief in the inevitability of accidents.

Consistent with her health-consciousness, Robyn always wears seatbelts, whether she is driving or is a passenger. In addition, she owns a car with an airbag, and the airbag played a role in her decision to purchase her current automobile. Robyn, however, has driven after she has been drinking. She has never actually been drunk when driving, but when she was a teenager, she drove after drinking and rode with someone who had been drinking on several occasions. It has been several years since she has done either, and now she considers her earlier behavior to have been foolish.

Although Dwayne and Robyn have different attitudes toward health and safety, each fails to be completely consistent in following a risky or safe lifestyle. Dwayne's disregard for his health and Robyn's concern with hers, however, reflect significant differences. Research indicates that healthy habits tend to be related, just as unhealthy behaviors also tend to go together. Hawkins (1992) studied the relationship between health-enhancing behaviors and health-risking behaviors of 10th to 12th graders and found that high school students who engaged in such unhealthy behaviors as smoking, carrying a weapon, and driving while drinking were less likely to use seatbelts, eat a healthy diet, get adequate sleep, or have healthy dental habits. Moreover, adopting a healthy lifestyle seems to begin early. A survey (Donovan,

Jessor, & Costa, 1993) of a large group of middle school children and a large group of high school students found a high degree of interrelationship among health-enhancing behaviors for both groups. For middle school students (7th and 8th graders), using seatbelts, eating a healthy diet, exercising regularly, and avoiding being too sedentary all correlated with each other.

PREVENTING INJURIES

Unintentional injuries, suicides, and violent deaths from homicides are 3 of the 10 leading causes of death in the United States, and they account for three of every four deaths among young people age 15 to 24 (USBC, 1995). More specifically, among young adults in this age group, unintentional injuries account for 40% of their deaths; homicides, 22%; and suicide, 13%. In addition to the large number of fatal injuries from these three causes, an even larger number of people suffer nonfatal injuries every year. Because injuries are a leading killer of young people, they are responsible for more lost years of life than any other source, and nonfatal injuries are responsible for increased health care costs and lost work and school days. Clearly, violent death and injury are major health problems in the United States, and health psychologists are beginning to be involved in strategies to reduce their number (Spielberger & Frank, 1992; Williams & Lund, 1992).

UNINTENTIONAL INJURIES

Unintentional injuries are the the fourth leading cause of deaths in the United States, accounting for 4% of the total. For young people 5 to 24, however, they account for 72% of all deaths (USBC, 1995). Just as older people could reduce their risk of heart disease, cancer, and chronic obstructive pulmonary disease by changing their behavior, young people could decrease their risk of unintentional injuries by altering their behavior. Most deaths among high school students are the result of behaviors that contribute either to unintentional or intentional injuries.

Among those behaviors that result in unintentional injuries are failure to use seatbelts, disdain of bicycle and motorcycle helmets, and riding with a driver who has been drinking. Kann et al. (1995) reported that nearly 20% of students in grades 9 to 12 rarely or never used seatbelts while riding in a car or truck driven by someone else and that male students were less likely than female students to use seatbelts. Of students who had ridden a motorcycle during the past year, 40% rarely or never wore a motorcycle helmet. Kann et al. also found that nearly 93% of those who had ridden a bicycle rarely or never used a helmet. During the month preceding the survey, more than one-third of students had ridden with a driver who had been drinking alcohol. Kann et al. found some gender and ethnic differences in frequency of behaviors that contributed to unintentional injuries, but there were more similarities than differences among the various groups. Table 12.1 shows that high school boys are less likely to use seatbelts than high school girls, but that the two are quite similar with regard to other dangerous behaviors. Also, African American students engaged in each of these risky behaviors somewhat more frequently than European American youth, especially in their reluctance to wear seatbelts or use motorcycle helmets. However, differences in seatbelt use by European Americans and African Americans tend to disappear when one takes belief in destiny into consideration (Colon, 1992), with African Americans holding stronger beliefs in the role of destiny in traffic crashes. Table 12.1 shows that different ethnic groups are quite similar in risk taking behaviors. For example, a very high percentage of high school students in all these ethnic groups rarely or never wore a bicycle helmet.

This survey revealed that young people, regardless of gender or ethnicity, are willing to engage in a variety of risky behaviors. Because high school students and other young people frequently have more than their share of motor vehicle and other unintentional injuries, many injury-prevention programs target this age group.

Motor Vehicle Injuries

Automobile crashes continue to contribute to more fatal and nonfatal injuries than any other single factor, even though deaths from motor vehicle accidents in the United States have dropped steadily during the past 25 years (USBC, 1995). Despite more severe penalties for drunken driving, a high

Table 12.1 Percentage of high school students who participated in behaviors that contribute to unintentional injuries, by gender and ethnicity—United States, Youth Risk Behavior Survey, 1993

Ethnic group	Rarely or never used seatbelts	Rarely or never used motorcycle helmets	Rarely or never used bicycle helmets	Rode with a driver who had been drinking alcohol
White	17.3%	37.2%	91.9%	34.1%
Female	11.5	36.3	93.1	33.5
Male	22.6	37.4	90.8	34.7
Black	30.3	48.4	97.1	39.3
Female	26.2	52.3	96.4	37.3
Male	34.5	46.9	97.6	41.3
Hispanic	19.6	59.8	94.6	42.3
Female	17.2	52.3	94.2	39.7
Male	21.9	58.3	94.9	42.3
Total	19.1	40.0	92.8	36.3
Female	14.3	39.0	93.6	34.5
Male	23.8	40.4	92.2	36.3

SOURCE: by L. Kann, C. W. Warren, W. A. Harris, J. L. Collins, K. A. Douglas, M. E. Collins, B. I. Williams, J. G. Ross, & L. J. Kolbe. "Youth Risk Behavior Surveillance—United States, 1993," 1995 *Morbidity and Mortality Weekly Report, 44*, No. SS-1.

percentage of fatal car crashes involve a driver who was legally intoxicated. Honkanen (1993) suggested that alcohol's major contribution to motor vehicle injuries as well as other unintentional injuries comes from two sources: greater risk-taking behavior and impaired psychomotor functioning.

A nationwide survey (Williams & Wells, 1993) indicated that 40% of fatally injured drivers had a positive blood alcohol concentration (BAC) of at least 0.10, and more than 20% had a BAC of 0.20 or higher. The survey also showed that alcohol-related fatal motor vehicle crashes were most frequent among young men who were not wearing seatbelts. Also, fatalities were closely associated with late-night driving, fixed-object crashes, rollovers, and crashes on curves. Among men 21 to 40 years of age, 60% of motor vehicle fatalities involved drivers who were legally intoxicated at the time of the accident.

Besides alcohol, another major contributor to motor vehicle injuries is failure to wear seatbelts. Studies in the late 1980s consistently demonstrated the effectiveness of seatbelts in saving lives. Seatbelt use cuts the probability that a person will die in a motor vehicle accident by 30% to 50% (Wagenaar, Maybee, & Sullivan, 1988), and seatbelts are effective in preventing fatal injuries irrespective of the occupant's age, size of vehicle, travel speed, type of

road, type of crash, time of year, or geographical area (Evans, 1987).

Seatbelts also reduce nonfatal injuries to both drivers and front seat passengers. Data on nearly 900 front seat passenger car occupants (Conn, Chorba, Peterson, Rhodes, & Annest, 1993) showed that about half of them were not wearing a seatbelt at the time of a crash. Those not wearing seatbelts tended to be younger and to have been drinking at the time of the accident. Looking at all passenger cars, front seat occupants not wearing seatbelts were more than four times as likely to have suffered serious injury as front seat occupants who were wearing seatbelts. For small cars, the difference was much less, but for large cars the chances of a serious injury were 10 times greater for front seat occupants who were not wearing a seatbelt. Thus, Dwayne is incorrect in his belief that wearing a seatbelt makes little difference in the outcome of an auto crash. The evidence is clear that the use of seatbelts lowers one's chance of serious injury in almost all types of motor vehicle crashes.

Other Unintentional Injuries

The total number of unintentional fatal injuries is divided almost equally between motor vehicle accidents and all other unintentional fatal injuries. Since

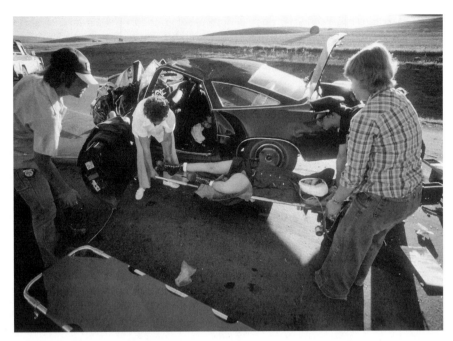

Automobile crashes continue to be the leading cause of both fatal and nonfatal injuries in the United States.

1970, both have declined by more than 40% (USBC, 1995), and death from occupational injuries alone dropped by 37% during the decade from 1980 to 1989 (Stout, Jenkins, & Pizatella, 1996). After motor vehicle fatalities, the most frequent causes of unintentional fatal injuries are falls, drowning, fires, and poisoning (USBC,1995). Alcohol has been a contributor to each of these as well as to bicycle injuries.

For adolescents and adults, alcohol is involved in nearly as high a percentage of bicycle-associated fatal injuries as it is in automobile fatalities. Almost one-third of fatally injured bicyclists 15 years old or older tested positive for alcohol, and nearly one-fourth were legally intoxicated (Li & Baker, 1994). Again, men were more likely than women to test positively for blood alcohol. More than half the legally intoxicated bicyclists killed were between 25 and 34, and even among fatally injured bicyclists 15 to 19 and not yet old enough to purchase alcohol legally, nearly one in seven had a positive BAC. A case-control study in Finland (Olkkonen & Honkanen, 1990), where bicycling is an important mode of transportation, showed that intoxicated bicyclists had more than a tenfold risk of an accidental injury compared with bicyclists who had not been drinking. The study also revealed that bicycle injuries were more likely to result from falling than from collisions. In other words, drunk bicycle riders seem to need neither another vehicle nor a fixed object (other than the road) to injure themselves.

Besides alcohol, failure to use bicycle helmets is an important contributor to unintentional injuries. More than 600,000 bicyclists a year are injured badly enough to require medical attention, more than 1,300 die of various injuries while riding a bicycle, and nearly 90% of those who received fatal head injuries could have survived if they had been wearing protective helmets (Sacks, Holingreen, Smith, & Sosin, 1991). Nearly 90% of the fatalities resulted from collisions with motor vehicles, most of the victims were males, and about half were children or adolescents. If only half the bicyclists had complied with helmet use, more than 1,000 lives would have been saved between 1984 and 1988.

In addition to alcohol and failure to wear protective helmets, smoking is a frequent source of injuries, with more than 1,400 people dying each year and nearly 3,800 receiving nonfatal injuries due to

WOULD YOU BELIEVE . . . ?

Smokers and Accidents

Would you believe that smokers have far more accidents than non-smokers—even though many of the accidents have nothing to do with fires? Interestingly, research shows that smokers have significantly more nonfire-related accidental injuries than nonsmokers. Among the nonthermal injuries are those related to motor vehicle crashes, occupational accidents, and suicide. Jeffery Sacks and David Nelson (1994) reviewed the literature and found that smokers, compared with nonsmokers, have a 50% increased risk of motor vehicle crashes and are more than twice as likely to be injured on the job. In addition, smokers have a much greater chance of committing suicide than nonsmokers.

Sacks and Nelson discussed several reasons for the increased risk of nonfire-related injuries among smokers. First, some evidence suggests that carbon monoxide or nicotine from cigarettes may be associated with reduced night vision as well as increased errors in driving judgment, either of which could result in accidental injury.

Second, the relationship between smoking and nonthermal injuries is complicated by smoking's association with a number of other factors, any one of which may relate to increased accidental injuries. These confounding factors include increased alcohol and drug consumption, lower educational and socioeconomic status, decreased levels of social support, and reduced use of seatbelts and other safety devices.

A third explanation for smokers' elevated risk of injuries is their increased chances of smoking-related illnesses, such as cardiovascular disease and cancer. Sudden heart ailments can precipitate a motor vehicle accident, and both cardiovascular disease and cancer may contribute to depression and thus to suicide. In addition, Sacks and Nelson cited evidence that medication for these two diseases can increase the risk of accidental injury.

Fourth, and perhaps the most important reason, is that smokers are more likely to become distracted by the act of lighting a cigarette or by dropped embers. Also, smoke may obscure one's vision, cause eye irritations, eye blinking, and coughing—all of which may increase one's risk of injury. This explanation probably accounts for much of smokers' increased risk of auto accidents and some of their elevated risk for occupational accidents. *However, smokers who work on jobs where smoking is prohibited still have more occupational injuries than nonsmokers!* Thus, if you smoke but work at a job that does not permit smoking, you nevertheless have a greater chance of being injured than if you did not smoke.

---

smoking-related fires and burns. Smoking is the leading cause of fire-related deaths and the second leading cause of fire-related injuries. Moreover, 11% of those who die in smoking-related fires are children (Miller, 1993). Smoking-related injuries, however, are not limited to fires and burns (see box, Would You Believe . . . ?)

In conclusion, a number of behavioral factors, such as alcohol consumption, nonuse of safety devices, and cigarette smoking contribute to a variety of fatal and nonfatal accidental injuries. Next, we look at strategies for preventing these unintentional injuries.

STRATEGIES FOR REDUCING UNINTENTIONAL INJURIES

During the past 2 decades, psychologists have been playing an increasingly important role in developing and implementing strategies for reducing unintentional injuries. Prior to 1970, psychologists, like nearly everyone else, referred to unintentional injuries as *accidents,* a term with connotations of chance, fate, or inevitability (Loimer & Guarnieri, 1996; Williams & Lund, 1992). During the 1970s and 1980s, physician William Haddon, Jr. (Haddon, 1970, 1972, 1980; Haddon & Baker, 1987), began to change the way psychologists and many others looked at unintentional injuries. Rather than viewing them simply as a consequence of unavoidable human error (as Dwayne still does), health psychologists now see unintentional injuries as resulting from a complex of conditions, including individual behaviors, dangerous environmental conditions, and lack of tough legislation and enforcement. Health psychologists are beginning to become concerned with each of these three areas (Rosenberg & Fenley, 1992; Spielberger & Frank, 1992).

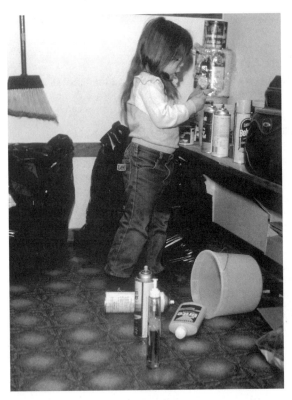

Homes include a number of safety hazards for young children.

Changing the Individual's Behavior

Changing an individual's behavior is one component of a comprehensive program to reduce unintentional injuries. Most of the emphasis on reducing unintentional injuries through changes in the individual's behavior has centered on home safety, motor vehicle safety, and bicycle safety. In all three areas, however, individually oriented interventions have been, at best, only moderately successful.

Strategies to Prevent Home Injuries. Lizette Peterson and her colleagues (Peterson, Gillies, Cook, Schick, & Little, 1994; Peterson & Schick, 1993) have been concerned with injuries to children, including injuries resulting from child abuse (Peterson & Brown, 1994). Using a behavior analysis approach suggested by Skinner (1953), Peterson and Schick examined minor unintentional injuries experienced by 8-year-old children with respect to their antecedents, the event itself, and the consequences of the event. Using this analysis as a guide,

the experimenters developed categories of rules for injury prevention. Their analysis revealed that most of the preventable injuries could have been avoided if children had followed these nonrestrictive rules, that is, rules that permitted children their normal range of activities. This strategy holds some promise of reducing unintentional injuries in the home, provided parents are willing and able to implement such a program.

Injuries from falls in the home are a serious threat to the health of many older persons, but strategies to change individual behavior have not been a very effective means of reducing these unintentional injuries. These strategies have included use of relaxation therapy, reflective safety tape, assertiveness training, exercise, and safety information (Steinmetz & Hobson, 1994). One recent study (El-Failzy & Reinsch, 1994) compared an experimental group of older adults who received an educational intervention with a control group that did not receive such information. Both groups had received a home safety assessment that included ways of making the home safer. Although the participants in the educational intervention group gained information regarding the benefits of the proposed changes, they did no better than people in the control group in implementing safety precautions. Similarly, a study of more than 3,000 older members of the Kaiser Permanente health maintenance organization found that a program emphasizing home safety, exercise, and risky behaviors reduced the number of falls by only 7% (Hornbrook et al., 1994). Moreover, this study reported that participants' chances of avoiding falls serious enough to require medical treatment were not significantly improved by the intervention. Results from these studies suggest that interventions aimed at changing behavior of individuals are not, by themselves, sufficient to reduce unintentional injuries.

Strategies to Prevent Motor Vehicle Injuries. Much of the decline in motor vehicle deaths is due to safer cars and roads, but socially oriented programs and a variety of interventions aimed at changing the behavior of individuals have also contributed to this decline (Robertson, 1996). One individually oriented strategy for reducing alcohol-related traffic injuries is the designated driver approach, whereby

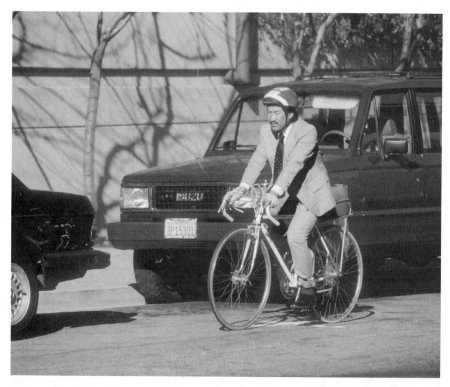

Wearing bicycle helmets could reduce fatal head injuries by 90%, but a majority of bicyclists fail to take this precaution.

one person is supposed to abstain from alcohol and be responsible for driving and the overall safety of others in the party. Although this concept has been part of the social norm for a number of years, controversy still exists as to its effectiveness in reducing traffic-related injuries. Some research suggests that participation in a designated driver program does not affect enjoyment of the social occasion for either the passengers or the driver (Shore, Gregory, & Tatlock, 1991). Other research (Glascoff, Knight, & Jenkins, 1994) indicates that many designated drivers do not remain abstinent and that alcohol consumption by passengers increased when they had a designated driver. DeJong and Wallack (1992) have argued that the promotion of designated driver programs by the media, bars, restaurants, the alcohol industry, and different public service groups has deflected attention away from problems that have caused the vast majority of traffic deaths—namely, alcohol-impaired drivers. DeJong and Wallack further contended that the focus should be on increas-

ing public awareness of the consequences of drunk driving and on the social, environmental, and economic factors that influence alcohol consumption. Although they suggested that powerful economic interests are behind the designated driver concept and that these programs may encourage some underaged adolescents to binge drink, DeJong and Wallack argued that these programs can be one of several strategies for reducing the number of alcohol-impaired drivers. Other strategies might include strictly enforcing laws against the sale of alcohol to minors, increasing taxes on alcoholic beverages, and setting up sobriety checkpoints. (We discuss some of these approaches in the section on changing laws.)

Strategies to Prevent Bicycle-Related Injuries.
Fatal and nonfatal bicycle injuries continue as important health problems in the United States. If all bicyclists would wear helmets, fatal head injuries could be cut by nearly 90% (Sacks et al., 1991).

Unfortunately, however, only about 7% of high school students regularly wear a helmet while riding a bicycle (Kann et al., 1995). This situation suggests that strategies to prevent bicycle-related injuries have not been as successful as those that have greatly reduced motor vehicle injuries.

One intervention to reduce bicycle injuries has been counseling or advising by a physician. This strategy, however, has been only marginally successful, perhaps because medical schools have traditionally placed little or no emphasis on training physicians to counsel patients regarding preventive medicine (Chi-Lum, 1995). Also, physicians are less likely to stress injury prevention than illness prevention (Moser, McCance, & Smith, 1991). Moreover, some research (Price, Desmond, & Losh, 1991) suggests that patients did not want their doctors to discuss such injury prevention topics as seatbelt use, although they did desire counseling about home safety issues.

Physician counseling with children on the importance of wearing bicycle helmets does not seem to increase use of helmets, even though a very high percentage of pediatricians report that they discuss bicycle helmet use with their patients. A survey of over 1,200 pediatricians (Ruch-Ross & O'Connor, 1993) found that only 30% of them always wore a helmet while bike riding, and 40% never wore a helmet. In addition, only one third of those with children under 18 reported that their children always wore a helmet. Physicians have not been effective in promoting helmet wearing among children (Cushman, James, & Waclawik, 1991). A 2- to 3-week follow-up on a group of children whose families received physician counseling and take-home pamphlets and a control group whose families received neither revealed that only 7.2% of the intervention group had purchased helmets compared with 7.0% of the control group. These modest gains for both groups were probably due to increased media exposure and a campaign offering a $5.00 discount on the purchase of bicycle helmets.

How can physicians get children to wear bicycle helmets? Carol Runyon and Desmond Runyon (1991) offered several suggestions. First, they acknowledged that educational programs do not work. Second, they suggested that an effective campaign must focus on changing children's beliefs regarding the magnitude of the risk for serious head injury and the effectiveness of helmets in preventing those injuries. Next, they proposed that interventions must also address the "nerd" factor—that is, reduce children's beliefs that bicycle helmets are "nerdy" looking. In addition, they called for increased availability of low-cost helmets that look attractive to children. To be effective, Runyon and Runyon contended, campaigns should be repeated in different contexts, using a variety of media.

Some research findings support these suggestions. For example, one study (Frank, Bouman, Cain, & Watts, 1992) indicated that changes in beliefs regarding the seriousness of injuries can lead to changes in safety-oriented behaviors, and another (Sacks et al., 1991) reported that bicycle helmets, if worn by all cyclists, could save 500 lives and prevent 1,500 head injuries a year. In addition, Stevenson and Lennie (1992) found that poor helmet design and being derided by one's peer group (the "nerd factor") were barriers to bicycle helmet use. This finding supports the theory of reasoned action and the theory of planned behavior (see Chapter 7), both of which suggest that behavior follows intentions, and intentions are, in part, shaped by subjective norms. Thus, if children believe that their peers regard bicycle helmets as fashionable (the social norm), they will more likely wear one. As for cost, Cushman et al. (1991) found that an affordable price for bicycle helmets contributed more to the purchase of helmets than did physician counseling. Thus, theory and research have combined to provide possible effective strategies for increasing helmet use. However, the problem of implementing these tactics on a individual basis remains a huge hurdle to the regular use of bicycle helmets. As with other unintentional injury topics, changing the environment or enacting and enforcing legislation may be more efficient means of reducing fatal and nonfatal injuries.

Changing the Environment

A second strategy for reducing unintentional injuries is to make changes in the environment. Such an approach includes building safer cars and roads, manufacturing better bicycle and motorcycle helmets, and making the home and workplace safer. Although some of the changes may require new legislation, others have been and can be made without changing laws. For example, people's demand for safer cars was an incentive for automobile manufacturers to build cars with seatbelts and airbags long before legislation mandated passive restraints. Similar environmental changes can be effective means of reducing unintentional injuries.

One example of modifying the environment was reported by Paul, Sanson-Fisher, Redman, and Carter (1994), who trained volunteers to go into the homes of people with young children and check for unsafe conditions. More than three of every four homes had multiple safety hazards, but after residents became aware of these hazards, they made significant reductions in the number of dangerous environmental conditions. A more comprehensive approach (Davidson et al., 1994) targeted changing a major part of 5- to 16-year-old children's environment. This program, conducted in Harlem and called the Safe Kids/Healthy Neighborhoods Injury Prevention Program, included such environmental interventions as (1) renovating playgrounds; (2) involving children and adolescents in safe, supervised activities, such as dance, art, sports, and carpentry; (3) conducting injury and violence prevention classes; and (4) providing bicycle helmets and other safety equipment. In a comparison of injuries during and after the years of the intervention with injuries during preceding years, the targeted age group showed a decline of 44%, indicating that a comprehensive program to alter specific environmental conditions can successfully reduce the rate of injury.

However, when people must make a major effort or a substantial financial commitment toward a safer environment, multifaceted community interventions are less successful. A comprehensive injury prevention program in an African American community in Philadelphia (Schwarz, Grisso, Miles, Holmes, & Sutton, 1993) consisted of (1) making simple modifications in the home such as providing smoke detectors, water thermometers, night lights, poison prevention supplies, and emergency telephone numbers; (2) inspecting the home to inform residents of hazards and ways to eliminate or reduce them; and (3) educating residents about specific injury prevention practices. After 12 months, residents in the intervention homes had more knowledge of injury prevention and had more safety supplies available than did residents in the control homes. However, the investigators found no difference between the intervention group and the control group in home hazards that required a major effort to correct. These results agree with those of other studies (Hsu & Williams, 1991), which suggest that lack of money and lack of control over one's environment lead to an inability to comply with many injury-prevention strategies that call for changes in one's environment.

Changing the Law

In general, legal interventions that require safety, such as airbags and automatic seatbelts, have been more effective than either educational programs or environmental manipulations (Zador & Ciccone, 1993). However, legislation aimed at punishing unsafe behaviors, such as driving too fast or driving while intoxicated, are not very effective unless the punishment is quite severe. There is little evidence that laws increasing the penalties for getting caught driving while intoxicated or speeding had any measurable effect on motor vehicle fatalities. On the other hand, laws that increase the certainty of punishment, that mandate seatbelt use, or that increase liquor and beer taxes have been effective modes of reducing drunk driving fatalities (Evans, Neville, & Graham, 1991).

Laws mandating the use of bicycle helmets have also been effective in preventing head injuries. The frequency of helmet use among children in grades 4, 7, and 9 changed in connection with the passage of laws (Dannenberg, Gielen, Beilenson, Wilson, & Joffe, 1993). One Maryland county passed a mandatory helmet law and coupled it with an educational safety campaign. A second county received only the educational intervention, and a third county received very little educational information. Helmet use rose from 11% to 37% in the first county after the law was passed, from 8% to 13% in the county that received an extensive educational intervention, and from 7% to 11% in the third county. Differences in helmet use between the second and third counties were not significant, indicating again that educational campaigns are not effective. Although the law was more effective than education alone, the majority of children in the first county still did not routinely wear helmets. Those who did were more likely to have friends who wore helmets, to believe that the law was good, and to use car seatbelts. Interestingly, having a previous injury or having a friend who was injured while riding a bicycle did not contribute to a child's use of a helmet. This study suggests that laws can increase injury-prevention behaviors, but that many people will continue to engage in unsafe behaviors. Presently, a combination of interventions aimed at the individual, the environment, and the law, combined with severe penalties for noncompliance, offers the most promise in preventing unintentional injuries.

PREVENTING SUICIDE

Suicide is the eighth leading cause of death in the United States and the third leading cause for young adults 15 to 24 (USBC, 1995). Kann et al. (1995) found that almost one-fourth of high school students had seriously considered suicide during the past year, nearly 9% had actually attempted suicide during the preceding 12 months, and almost 3% had sought medical attention as the result of a suicide attempt.

Different factors relate to suicide in people of different ages, and effective suicide prevention strategies focus on those contributing factors. Compared with younger people, elderly people who killed themselves used more lethal methods, suggesting that they were more committed to a successful attempt (Lester, 1994). Suicide for younger people was more likely to be a response to an unhappy interpersonal relationship. These findings suggest that suicide prevention programs should be tailored to specific age groups. For the elderly, psychiatric treatment for depression and restricting access to lethal methods of suicide is appropriate. For younger adults, crisis counseling and educational programs may be better choices.

Alcohol relates to suicide and suicide attempts in people of nearly every age. One study (Eckardt et al., 1981) found that alcohol was involved in as many as 30% of all suicide attempts. This finding does not mean that alcohol caused many attempts; some people may decide to kill themselves while sober and then use alcohol as an anesthetic. However, an inability to control alcohol consumption is related to a person's chances of attempting suicide.

For example, Gomberg (1989) found that 40% of alcoholic women have attempted suicide whereas fewer than 9% of nonalcoholic women have attempted to take their own lives. Moreover, Eckardt et al. reported that problem drinkers are from 2 to 15 times more likely to succeed at committing suicide than light or nondrinkers. This association does not mean that use of alcohol is responsible for suicides; the relationship could be due to general feelings of despair and hopelessness that lead some people to both abuse alcohol and to attempt suicide.

Suicides occur in all age groups from preadolescence to old age, but the people most often targeted for intervention are adolescents, young adults, and the elderly. Many high schools have suicide-prevention programs, including mental health teams for counseling at-risk students and their surviving peers, written formal suicide policies, and programs for training teachers and counselors to identify and work with threats of suicide (Malley, Kush, & Bogo, 1994). Other school-based interventions include classes to increase the likelihood that students who come into contact with a suicidal classmate will act responsibly. Kalafat and Elias (1994) compared a group of 10th-grade students who had participated in such classes with a group of controls. Students who had taken part in the intervention classes gained more knowledge about suicidal peers and had more favorable attitudes toward helping troubled schoolmates than did the controls.

An intervention that is available to all age groups is the telephone hot line service that allows suicidal people to call suicide prevention centers and talk to trained volunteers. However, a meta-analysis of studies over a 70-year period indicated that traditional hot line services had little or no effect on the rate of suicide for people who call (Dew, Bromet, Brent, & Greenhouse, 1987).

A more effective telephone-based approach was developed in Italy and oriented toward the elderly. It differed from the traditional hot line in that trained workers contacted elderly people at risk for suicide (De Leo, Carollo, & Dello Bueno, 1995). This two-faceted service, called Tele-Help/Tele-Check, provided elderly people with a portable alarm system so they could call any time of the day or night if they needed help (Tele-Help). The second aspect of this service (Tele-Check) consisted of trained staff members making contact with elderly clients twice a week to monitor their medical and psychological condition and to offer emotional support. De Leo et al. examined the effectiveness of Tele-Help/Tele-Check among a large group of elderly people living at home, most of whom lived alone. Although Tele-Help/Tele-Check is not solely a suicide prevention program, De Leo et al. reported that it was effective in reducing suicides. During a 4-year period, only one person in the intervention community had committed suicide compared with an expected rate of more than seven. This study suggests that when older people receive emotional and social support, they feel less despair and alienation and have more reasons to live.

In summary, strategies to prevent suicide must focus on factors that relate to suicidal behaviors in various age groups. For adolescents, those factors are often interpersonal and may involve estrangement from family members and unhappy romantic relationships. For elderly people, isolation and depression are more prominent risk factors. Programs directed toward identifying and alleviating such factors as depression, alienation, and despair probably offer some promise for reducing suicide rates.

PREVENTING VIOLENCE

Homicide is the 9th leading cause of death in the United States and the second leading cause for young people 15 to 24 (USBC, 1995). In addition, violent, intentional deaths are the fifth leading cause of mortality in children 1 to 4 years of age and the fourth leading cause for children 5 to 14 (National Center for Health Statistics, 1995). Although violence affects the entire society, young people are more likely to be both perpetrators and victims of violence.

Youth and Violence

In a study of a nationally representative sample of 9th to 12th graders, Kann et al. (1995) found that high school students engaged in a number of behaviors that placed either themselves or others in danger. Nearly one-fourth of these students had carried a gun, knife, or club during the 30 days preceding

the survey; almost 42% had been in a physical fight during the previous 12 months, and 4% had to seek medical help for injuries sustained in a fight. In this study, similarities among ethnic groups generally outweighed differences. For example, 11% of European American, 15% of African American, and 13% of Hispanic American high school students had carried a weapon to school during the 30 days preceding the survey.

However, high school is not the time aggressive and violent behaviors begin. Elementary and middle school children frequently carry weapons, often in self-defense, but the outcome can still be lethal. Webster, Gainer, and Champion (1993) reported that nearly half of inner-city 7th- and 8th-grade boys carried knives and one-fourth carried guns. Among 7th- and 8th-grade girls, 37% carried a knife. Moreover, these junior high school students carried guns more for aggressive purposes than for defensive reasons. Similarly, Cotten et al. (1994) reported that carrying a weapon tended to give middle school students more security and confidence, attitudes that foster rather than diminish aggressive behaviors.

Young African American men are much more likely to die from homicide than any other segment of United States society, including young European American men and African Americans in other age groups. For example, the death rate from homicide by firearms is more than 10 times higher among male African Americans ages 10 to 34 than it is for male European Americans of the same age (USBC, 1995). For all age groups, African Americans are nearly eight times more likely to be victims of murder than European Americans. In other words, although African Americans make up only 12% of the total population of the United States, almost half the murder victims in this country are African Americans. Figure 12.1 contrasts the homicide rates by ethnicity and gender of the victim from 1980 to 1992. (Note that the overall murder rate in recent years has not escalated, despite the belief of many people that it has.)

Although young African American men are far more likely than any other group to become victims of violence and murder, studies that focus on age, ethnicity, and gender may overlook the basic causes of homicide. In an article titled "Violence in

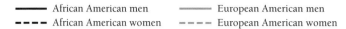

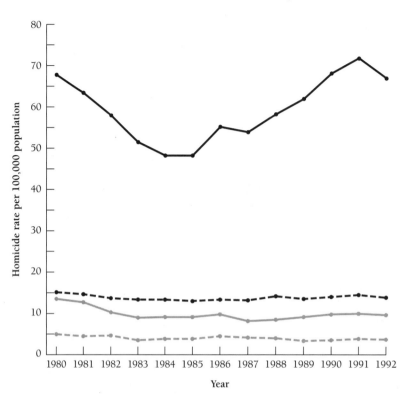

Figure 12.1   Homicide rates in the United States by ethnicity and gender of victim, 1980 to 1992 (rates per 100,000 of specified population).   SOURCE: Data from *Statistical Abstracts of the United States, 1995* (115th ed.). By U.S. Bureau of the Census, 1995, p. 202. Washington, DC: U.S. Government Printing Office.

American Cities: Young Black Males Is the Answer, but What Was the Question?" Michael Greenberg and Dona Schneider (1994) obtained mortality data in three New Jersey cities and discovered that violent death rates for all ethnic groups were elevated in poor, overcrowded urban areas. Under such conditions, moreover, women as well as men and middle-aged and elderly populations as well as young people all have high rates of death from homicide. Greenberg and Schneider argued that the underlying causes of high rates of violence are economic and political and are largely independent of age, gender, or ethnicity.

Domestic Violence

Another group of victims of violence consists of those who have been injured by a member of their own family or by a former family member. Ann Car-

den (1994, p. 541) contended that "violent crimes occur more frequently within families than among strangers." By any estimation, domestic violence is a major health problem in the United States; it includes physical and sexual abuse of children, spouses, and the elderly. Van Hasselt, Morrison, Bellack, and Hersen (1988) calculated the annual number of violent crimes perpetrated against family members and concluded that between 1.4 and 1.9 million children are physically abused, between 80,000 and 250,000 children are sexually abused, 500,000 elderly people are abused, one in seven women who have ever been married are raped by their husbands, and 1.8 million spouses are abused. Because of the reluctance to report family violence, these figures are probably underestimates. Indeed, a more recent study of a national sample of households (Sorenson, Upchurch, & Shen, 1996) found that nearly 3 million married couples had some form of physical violence in their marriage during the past year. This study also found that younger people with low levels of education and income were most likely to be involved in domestic violence.

One reason for the continuation of domestic violence is that many people find such behavior acceptable, at least under some circumstances. A survey of American couples (Straus, Gelles, & Steinmetz, 1980) found that 25% of wives and over 30% of husbands considered violence an acceptable way to resolve some disputes. Both women and men behave violently toward each other, but women are more likely to be verbally violent, whereas men are more likely to be physically violent (Thompson & Walker, 1989). This tendency and men's generally larger size and superior strength result in the greater likelihood that women will sustain injury.

Carden's review found that more than 6 million people 12 years old and older are victims of violent crimes every year and that 39% of these adolescents and adults are intentionally injured by a family member, an ex-family member, or a close relative. According to Carden, "a woman is more likely to be physically assaulted, raped, or murdered by a current or former male partner than by any other assailant" (p. 544).

Strategies to Prevent Violence

Although violence has received much publicity in recent years, prevention programs remain largely ineffective. The effectiveness of programs to reduce violence against children seems to be limited mostly to getting children to report violence and to stop blaming themselves for the violent acts of their parents (Finkelhor, Asdigian, & Dziuba-Leatherman, 1995). Carden (1994) suggested that interventions to reduce the incidence of domestic violence must be multi-dimensional and based on research of their underlying causes. Neither sociopolitical nor psychological approaches are sufficient by themselves, Carden stated, but when they are combined with community involvement and professional counseling for the abuser, some progress is possible.

Researchers who have examined all types of violence (Guerra, 1994; Walker, Goodwin, & Warren, 1992) generally agree that psychological interventions alone will not be successful in halting domestic violence, and that any effective program must be based on an understanding of the root causes, which include poverty, overcrowded housing, the ready availability of weapons, acceptance of interpersonal violence, and myriad other social problems.

BENEFITING FROM HEALTH CAMPAIGNS

We have seen that injury prevention programs that focus on the individual's behavior are not generally effective. Moreover, such prevention efforts are not always economically feasible. For these reasons health psychologists sometimes direct injury and disease prevention programs toward groups of people.

This section examines some of the programs that have attempted to change the behavior of groups so as to lower the risk factors for disease. These programs can be divided into (1) those that provide information through various media and are designed to educate a targeted group of people about health-related conditions and ways by which they can change to a healthier lifestyle, (2) those that focus on one particular workplace and are intended to improve employee health, and (3) those that involve an entire community and attempt to change health-related behaviors of people in that community.

INFORMATION CAMPAIGNS

Health information campaigns that use mass media to change health-related behaviors are capable of reaching regions as large as an entire nation. Such campaigns may focus on a single disorder or promote a comprehensive prevention program. Traditional methods of educational and informational programs assume that, when people are provided with information about the dangers of their behavior, they will make appropriate changes.

Unfortunately, information alone is usually not a very effective means of changing well-entrenched behaviors. Passive procedures such as listening to lectures, reading, and viewing films have a generally dismal record of getting people to change health habits. Similarly, programs that threaten people with disease, disability, or death also have not proven to be a useful method of changing health-related behaviors. Many studies attest to the general ineffectiveness of traditional educational methods. A brief review of some of these studies suggests the types of procedures to avoid.

Green (1984) found that health education programs designed to impart information were ineffective as a means of changing behavior. Indeed, some health education programs may be counterproductive and actually *increase* the behaviors they seek to decrease. Evidence exists that driver education programs may increase motor vehicle crashes, and drug education programs can increase drug use. Robertson (1984) reviewed a number of studies on driver education and concluded that these programs actually contribute to an increased frequency of motor vehicle crashes, because driver education programs allow teenagers to begin driving at an earlier age. The crash rates are higher for younger drivers compared with those of other age groups, making younger drivers more likely to be involved in accidents and thus more dangerous.

Similarly, Stuart (1974) compared the incidence of alcohol, marijuana, and LSD use in a group of teenagers who had participated in a drug education program in their school with the incidence in another group who had not been exposed to the drug education course. He found that students in the drug education course were more likely to use all these drugs and were more likely to sell marijuana and LSD.

In another, mostly ineffective prevention program, Biglan et al. (1987) found that a behavior modification intervention in which teachers trained students how to refuse offers to smoke produced lower rates of smoking for students who were current smokers; however, this strategy may have increased smoking rates among boys who were not already smokers. These researchers also found that the antismoking messages delivered by parents had no effect on smoking rates and that commonsense approaches are not necessarily effective. Biglan et al. (1987) summarized the pitfalls of untested educational efforts when they said that "we cannot simply assume that well-intentioned programs will necessarily be beneficial" (p. 625).

Stephen Ramirez (1995) has used his experiences in health promotion with underserved populations to offer five specific suggestions for more effective health education programs. First, Ramirez recommended that such programs should be comprehensive rather than categorical—that is, they should address the whole person's needs rather than a specific unhealthy behavior. Second, the program should be integrated into institutions and communities rather than offered in a single setting. Third, Ramirez contended that health promotions be multifaceted and tailored to the needs of specific groups. Fourth, he proposed an innovative combination of community, business, law enforcement, religious, education, and media groups, which could offer opportunities and activities that more traditional health education programs cannot. Fifth, Ramirez called for agencies to offer follow-up and support mechanisms that help individuals and groups maintain healthy behaviors.

Many of Ramirez's suggestions are exemplified by The Passport To Health program (Wellness Management, 1995), an intervention that involves students, teachers, and parents in learning about health in a school-based program aimed at fourth to sixth graders. Two sessions per month during the school year cover a wide variety of health-related topics, such as nutrition, drug awareness, bicycle helmet safety, first aid, community involvement, and hospital tours. Pretest-posttest evaluations have shown that 35% of the students in the program made positive lifestyle behavior changes. Although this program did not use a control group, results of the posttest suggest that Passport To Health can be an effective intervention for young people who are at risk for unhealthy behaviors.

Fear Appeals

Information campaigns based on fear can be effective if they do not arouse too much fear. Moderate levels of fear can motivate people to initiate health-related behavior, whereas campaigns that arouse either no fear or too much fear are generally ineffective.

In a classic study, Janis and Feshbach (1953) examined three levels of threat in connection with a program designed to persuade students to use better dental hygiene. The high-fear approach used explicit, unpleasant photographs of the consequences of neglecting dental hygiene. The materials used in the medium- and mild-threat conditions were correspondingly less frightening. Janis and Feshbach found that the high-fear appeal was least effective in prompting positive dental health attitudes, whereas the mild-fear approach was the most successful.

In two later studies, Job (1988) and Self and Rogers (1990) explored the use of fear in health promotion. Job's report concluded that fear-provoking messages detailing the unpleasant consequences of a behavior are unlikely to promote change. Self and Rogers found that without reassuring people about their ability to cope, attempts to frighten them had a negative effect on health behaviors. Job contended that fear can be useful under certain circumstances: (1) People are fearful *before* they receive the health communication; (2) the fear-arousing event appears imminent; (3) specific guidelines are provided on what behaviors one should perform to reduce the fear; (4) people begin with a low level of fear that can realistically be reduced by performing a desirable health-related behavior; and (5) a strong possibility exists that reducing fear will serve as a negative reinforcer. Careful campaigns can include these elements, but Job concluded that positive reinforcement is probably more effective than the use of fear.

If fear is ineffective, what elements should be included in positive health campaigns? Rimer and Glassman (1984) investigated the factors underlying effective persuasive health messages. They found that comprehension of the message was not enough; that is, people who understood the message still failed to act on it. Being able to recognize and recall the information is unrelated to performance of the recommended behavior. Rimer and Glassman concluded that comprehension is a necessary but not sufficient step in translating a persuasive message to behavior change.

Mass Media Campaigns

Mass media health campaigns that do not rely on fear can be an effective means of influencing people to change their health-related behaviors. Messages about health and health behaviors come to us in a variety of the mass media, including the morning, noon, afternoon, and evening news as well as other television programs. Radio messages frequently parallel the ones on television, with both special reports and shows devoted solely to health. Also, newspapers carry health news as feature stories and publish regular columns that answer health questions.

In addition, dozens of magazines explore health-related topics as well as the behaviors that relate to the development and maintenance of health.

Advertisers in all these media use the public's interest in health to sell a variety of products, and paradoxically, some of these products, such as high-fat snack and fast foods, may contribute to health risks, As Richard Winett (1995) pointed out, health psychologists should have campaigns sufficiently strong to compete with commercial interests that tempt people to behave unwisely.

Do media messages work to change health behaviors, or does their number only confuse people with seemingly contradictory information? Because of the abundance of mass media health campaigns, difficulties arise in assessing their effectiveness. Many government-sponsored public service messages appear nationwide, thus precluding any possibility for comparison with a group that has not seen the message. Without such a comparison or control group, evaluation is very difficult. In any case, many public service campaigns do not include formal assessments of effectiveness.

Media campaigns based solely on informing people of the consequences of unwise health behaviors are typically not very effective. Simply learning that one's habits are risky is usually not sufficient because many people believe they will be exempt from the negative consequences of their behavior, a tendency that Neil Weinstein (1980) called optimistic bias. In 1995, Weinstein and Klein found that optimistic bias was resistant to change—people tended to preserve the beliefs that they were less likely than others to suffer from their risky behaviors, despite various types of information they received. This study demonstrated that media campaigns must be carefully designed to include more than information if they are to be effective in prompting changes in behavior.

Maccoby and Alexander (1980) assessed the effectiveness of a media campaign that was part of a communitywide heart health promotion. These researchers organized a media-only campaign in one area and a media plus individual attention campaign in another community. In comparing these two communities, Maccoby and Alexander found that during the first year of the program, the media-only group lagged behind the group receiving the more comprehensive intervention. The group that received the media-only program improved only slightly in their health knowledge, decreased their cholesterol intake, and cut down on smoking. The number of people in this group who quit smoking was not significantly different from what it would have been without any intervention. During the second year, however, the media-only group made greater gains, almost catching up with the community that had received the more comprehensive intervention. Maccoby and Alexander concluded that a health campaign using only media could be effective in changing some health behaviors.

In a slightly different design and using smoking prevention as the targeted behavior, Brian Flynn and his associates (Flynn et al., 1992, 1994) compared the effectiveness of a school intervention program with a school intervention plus a communitywide mass media campaign. Fourth- to sixth-grade students in two communities received only the school-based intervention whereas those in two matched communities received both the school-based program and a variety of television and radio spots that promoted an attractive lifestyle rather than attempting to sell a specific message. The media campaign was designed to counter the effects of cigarette (and beer) commercials that promote glamorous and easy-going lifestyles and only incidentally mention a brand name. Flynn and his associates exposed the students to one of the two interventions for 4 years and then followed them for another 2 years. At the end of the follow-up period, both groups, as expected, increased their cigarette consumption, but students exposed to both the mass media campaign and the school-based intervention had a much lower rate of weekly smoking than those who had received only the school-based intervention. These results support those of Maccoby and Alexander (1980) and others in suggesting that multifaceted programs are generally more effective than single interventions.

Media campaigns have also been effective in getting people to stop smoking. Cummings, Sciandra, and Markello (1987) evaluated the impact of a series of newspaper articles designed to encourage people in a particular geographic area to stop smoking. Of those smokers who saw the articles, 13% were en-

couraged to try to quit and 4% succeeded. The rate of quitting is not nearly so high as it would be with more personal interventions (see Chapter 13), but in the area served by the newspaper, 4% equaled 9,600 people. This impressive total indicates that a sufficiently intensive campaign can make a significant impact on some health-related behaviors.

Several researchers have developed novel uses of media in health promotion. Davis (1988) reported on a program that encouraged television stations to report on health issues by distributing a prepackaged video news release to the stations. This video called attention to the new warnings about smokeless tobacco. A total of 22% of the stations aired the video within 6 days of receiving it, and a similar percentage indicated that they had held the video for future use. Thus nearly half the TV stations agreed to show the prepackaged news release. Another media campaign distributed a 13-segment antismoking video program to people with home videocassette players (Marston & Bettencourt, 1988). Only about half the people who received the programs watched all 13 segments, but of those who did, 40% quit smoking for at least 3 months and 30% were still not smoking after 12 months. The cost of the videos (about $60) makes this program more expensive than most other mass media campaigns but less expensive than most smoking clinics.

Another creative use of television involves local-access cable television programs to deliver health information. Katz (1985) discussed one such program that had concentrated on arthritis. This cable television program attracted a fairly high number of viewers, most of whom had arthritis. Katz argued that local-access cable television is a low-cost method for providing health programming.

Mass media campaigns are capable of reaching millions of people, but two issues remain: the misunderstanding of health messages and advertising that includes biased information. With regard to the first issue, Yeaton, Smith, and Rogers (1990) evaluated the ability of college students to comprehend the health information contained in press reports. They chose reports from newspapers and magazines and presented them to college students. Their results revealed that the overall rate of misunderstanding approached 40%, with most rates falling between a third and a half. These rates of misunderstanding suggest that even college students frequently misunderstand health-related information disseminated by media campaigns.

The second problem involves advertising claims. As Freimuth, Hammond, and Stein (1988) put it, health advertising is a case of prevention for profit. Advertisements frequently claim that certain products will make people healthier or help them lower particular risk factors. Some of this advertising conveys accurate information, but much health advertising distorts scientific findings to make the product appear more attractive or effective than it actually is. Freimuth et al. cited a campaign that included the National Cancer Institute's cancer prevention message in the advertising for Kellogg's All-Bran cereal. The campaign was controversial because of its health claims but effective in terms of profits. To be effective in terms of improved health behaviors, advertising must be accurate and should avoid exaggerated claims.

Although some advertising presents accurate information about health, all of it is ultimately aimed at selling products. Many of these products do not promote a healthy lifestyle, and some can even be dangerous. Story and Faulkner (1990) analyzed prime-time television to determine the content of programming and commercials concerning one aspect of health—food. They found that food references occurred about five times per 30 minutes of viewing and that 60% of food references in both sources were for low-nutrition beverages and sweets. Some differences existed between the foods discussed in programs (coffee and soft drinks were the most commonly mentioned) and those discussed in commercials (fast-food restaurants and cereals were the most commonly advertised). This analysis demonstrates that although some mass media coverage is oriented toward health promotion, the majority is directed toward selling products and has little regard for health considerations.

Health advertising can parallel other types of marketing (Lefebvre & Flora, 1988; Winett, 1995). This sophisticated application of marketing techniques to health promotion is called social marketing and involves analyzing the audience; analyzing the type of media that would be most effective for the message; considering the mixture of products, places, and types of promotions to include in the campaign; and tracking the effectiveness of the campaign. Social marketing has many advantages over the traditional information campaigns, which usually consist of public service announcements using ineffective fear appeals. The mass media offer the potential to send health messages to large segments of the population, and several studies have indicated that some types of mass media campaigns can be effective in imparting information and even in prompting people to alter their behavior.

However, programs that include some amount of personal contact along with media campaigns are generally more persuasive than media-only campaigns. According to a study of medical services utilization (Worksite Wellness Works, 1995b), people who had access to a 24-hour telephone-based nurse advice line and self-care reference books used fewer medical services than people with the standard insurance coverage. For each $1 invested in this program, the sponsoring insurance group saved $4.75 for the people who had telephone access to a nurse. In addition, those with access to the nurse's advice by telephone were less likely to use medical services than those with only the self-care information. Therefore, the telephone component of this program appears to have added savings.

One type of health promotion campaign that has become increasingly common is the workplace wellness program. Both workplace wellness programs and communitywide health campaigns aim to reach large groups of people. The workplace programs do not typically contain media presentations, but the communitywide health campaigns are usually a combination of media appeals and group or individual interactions.

WORKPLACE WELLNESS PROGRAMS

Workplace wellness programs are run by companies with the goal of attaining and maintaining employee health. These programs seek to make the workplace healthier by making changes in the work environment and in employees' health behaviors. Kizer (1987) noted that workplace wellness programs are part of the wellness movement, a philosophy that prevention is better and cheaper than cure. Kizer explained that two additional factors have influenced the growing trend toward company involvement in employee health: insurance costs and the desire of executives to be healthier.

The cost of insurance has grown dramatically in recent years because the cost of health care has increased. These health care costs have been passed along to employers who pay their employees' insurance premiums. Thus, companies benefit financially by having healthier employees, and employers have become increasingly interested in controlling their costs. Restricting health care payments or raising the amount paid by employees are two strategies to decrease employers' health care costs, but these measures have been unpopular with employees and ineffective in containing health care costs (Kizer, 1987). An alternative strategy is to have healthier employees who use fewer health services.

The second factor in the development of workplace wellness programs was the healthier lifestyles of some company executives. According to Kizer, many middle-aged executives became interested in a healthier lifestyle to reduce their risk for heart disease. The changes in diet, weight, smoking, and exercise that lower the risk for heart attack can also lead to improved health and energy. Many of these executives simply wanted to share their newfound healthy lifestyle with employees, but they also appreciated the increased productivity and positive attitude of a healthier workforce. Pelletier (1984) pointed out that an enthusiastic chief executive officer is often the impetus for a company's workplace wellness program.

The strategy of promoting health awareness and healthy behaviors among employees has become much more common in the United States, although the United States has lagged behind the Scandinavian countries, Germany, Japan, and Canada in supporting worksite wellness programs (Pelletier, 1984). The number of U.S. companies that support workplace wellness has grown rapidly in recent years. Fielding and Piserchia (1989), reporting on the first National Survey of Worksite Health Promotion Activities, said that 65% of the surveyed companies had one or more areas of health promotion activity, and more than half of those had been added within the 5 years before the survey. Davenport

(1995), reporting on a 1992 survey, said that 80% of companies employing more than 50 people had wellness programs.

Nathan (1984b) discussed the advantages and disadvantages of health promotion in the workplace, pointing out that workplace prevention efforts benefit from a captive audience. In addition, programs in the workplace are typically convenient for employees, with many programs scheduled before and after work and even during lunchtime. Some companies allow employees to participate in health programs during work time. One problem with workplace programs is directly related to the advantage of having a captive audience: Employees may not feel free to decline participation, even if the program is ostensibly voluntary. Workers sometimes feel uneasy about attending programs that include treatment for drug or alcohol abuse. Employees may also feel pressured to participate in their company's programs to lose weight, stop smoking, and exercise more. Nathan recommended that participation records be kept separate from other employment records to ensure privacy, and Kizer (1987) argued that all employee participation should be voluntary.

Components of Worksite Wellness Programs

According to Kizer, a workplace health program is within the reach of any company, regardless of its size or the amount of money available for the program. A no-smoking policy alone does not cost the company anything and pleases more employees than it displeases. As smoking has become increasingly unpopular and employees have begun to complain about co-workers' smoking, many companies have banned smoking (Laabs, 1994). In 1991, 32% of companies prohibited smoking. By 1993, the number had grown to 56%, and 96% of companies hoped to be smoke free by the year 2002. This wish is consistent with the growing number of state and city ordinances that limit smoking in many types of buildings.

Smoking is often a major focus of worker wellness programs due to its association with a number of diseases and thus with greater absenteeism and increased health care costs. Smokers experience 31% higher health claims costs than nonsmokers (Anderson, Brink, & Courtney, 1995). Therefore, programs that decrease smoking have greater economic benefits to companies than other types of wellness programs.

Companies that prohibit smoking often offer their employees assistance in quitting and cooperate with their employees to construct a no-smoking policy. Research has indicated that such policies tend to gain better acceptance than policies unilaterally formulated by companies without employee consultation (Laabs, 1994). In their enthusiasm to control employees' smoking, companies may succeed in getting employees to enroll in smoking cessation programs but not to quit permanently.

Kizer (1987) also mentioned the policy of discouraging (but not prohibiting) alcohol use at company social functions. He proposed that nonalcoholic drinks be made available and that no employee be pressured into drinking. However, an analysis of medical costs (Anderson et al., 1995) showed that drinkers had lower medical costs than those who did not drink, indicating that cutting down on alcohol consumption for nonproblem drinkers should not be a high priority for companies trying to save on medical costs.

Other low-cost programs include changing the foods in vending machines and company dining facilities to more nutritious options and then posting the calorie count of these foods. This strategy could save money in medical costs because unhealthy diet is associated with higher medical costs for workers (Anderson et al., 1995).

Many of the workplace health programs have started with an exercise component (Davenport, 1995; Kizer, 1987) and then have expanded to offer a variety of health-promoting activities. Some large companies have created and implemented comprehensive wellness programs such as the Johnson & Johnson Company's Live for Life program (Nathan, 1984a), the Control Data Corporation's Staywell program (Naditch, 1984), Quaker Oats's Live Well, Be Well (Davenport, 1995), and the Coca-Cola Company's HealthWorks fitness program (Worksite Wellness Works, 1995a). Most of these programs include components oriented toward smoking cessation, weight control, management of blood pressure, stress management, regular exercise, and health knowledge, often integrated into a health risk assessment for each employee and a plan to reduce employees' risk into the low category.

Table 12.2 Frequency of workplace health promotion activities

Type of Activity	Percentage of Companies Offering Activity
Smoking Cessation	35.6%
Risk Assessment	29.5
Back Problem Prevention and Care	28.5
Stress Management	26.6
Exercise/Fitness	22.1
Off-the-Job Accident Prevention	19.8
Nutrition Education	16.8
Blood Pressure Control and Treatment	16.1
Weight Control	14.7

SOURCE: Adapted from "Frequency of Worksite Health Promotion Activities" by J. E. Fielding and P. V. Piserchia, 1989, *American Journal of Public Health, 79,* p. 16.

Most workplace programs are less comprehensive, but many include at least some of these components. Fielding and Piserchia (1989) found that smoking cessation programs were the most frequent type offered by companies, with 36% of the companies surveyed offering them. Table 12.2 shows the health promotion activities offered by these companies. The average number of components was 3.2, and the majority of companies paid the entire cost of the program rather than sharing the cost with employees.

Creating a Wellness Program

A variety of workplace health programs now exist, along with different philosophies and recommendations for implementing them. Kizer (1987) and Feldman (1984) were early advocates of such programs and made recommendations about how to set up health promotion programs in companies. The number of programs and their duration has allowed research on their effectiveness and in reviewing worksite health promotion programs, Russell Glasgow and his colleagues (Glasgow, McCaul, & Fisher, 1993) concluded that several elements make them more effective. Their conclusions tend to be consistent with the recommendations from Kizer and Feldman. Companies that want to start health promotion programs need to consider several factors in creating an effective one.

Employee involvement should start at the planning stage to maximize employee participation. Well-meaning programs that no one attends are not helpful. Employee involvement can include determinations of what types of programs employees want and recommendations for tailoring the programs to fit their lives. Kizer pointed out the value of an internal analysis of employee health to determine employees' needs and to help in setting the goals for the program. He estimated that in many companies 20% of employees will be healthy, 60% will be nearly healthy, and 20% will be at high risk because of their lifestyle.

Early research (Zavela, Davis, Cottrell, & Smith, 1988) indicated that employees who were healthy, near healthy, and unhealthy all participated in workplace health promotions in nearly equal numbers, but the Glasgow et al. review showed that healthy workers, women, and executives are more likely to participate. Therefore, programs should attempt to find ways to reach less healthy, male, and blue-collar workers. Activities to increase employees' awareness of the program and of their own personal risk can address this problem. In addition, Glasgow et al. recommended that workers receive incentives for designing and participating in programs that increase accessibility and convenience.

Glasgow et al. emphasized the involvement of management, and other research (Sloan & Gruman, 1988) confirmed the importance of this factor. The perceived support of supervisors was a significant factor in employee participation. In addition, Sloan and Gruman found that perceived risks of illness motivated people to participate in order to reduce those risks. This finding suggests that boosting employees' awareness of personal risk can be an effective strategy in increasing their participation.

Although programs with multiple components are more expensive than simpler programs, the multiple components offer the advantage of being attractive to a wider variety of employees. Glasgow et al. suggested that a variety of intervention options is a desirable strategy for companies to include in their health promotion program. Not only do such programs attract more participants, but they also have the potential to be more effective in helping employees manage a variety of health risks.

Effectiveness of Workplace Health Promotions

Workplace health promotion programs can be effective in increasing worker health and productivity and in decreasing employer health care costs. In Johnson & Johnson's Live for Life program, for example, the average cost increase for inpatient treatment of participants was only 57% of that for nonparticipants (Bly, Jones, & Richardson, 1986). Live for Life participants also had a lower rate of hospital admissions and fewer days in the hospital, but no differences emerged in the number of outpatient services or other health care costs. The program was therefore somewhat effective in decreasing expensive hospital care, but it did not affect outpatient health care expenses. Davenport (1995) presented more optimistic estimates of savings, citing savings of over $400 per year for each employee who participated in a risk management program. Davenport contended that employers save $3 for every $1 that they invest in workplace wellness programs.

The estimates of greater savings for more elaborate programs are consistent with descriptions of various types of workplace programs by Gebhardt and Crump (1990), who identified three levels of fitness and wellness programs that have demonstrated some success in reducing the cost of coronary heart disease (CHD) to employers. Level I programs consist of information designed to make workers more aware of risk factors for heart disease; Level II programs attempt to modify lifestyles; and Level III programs create a fitness environment designed to help workers maintain healthy lifestyles. Gebhardt and Crump reported that Level III programs are generally more cost effective than the simpler ones. The cost of the programs is more than offset by reductions in absenteeism, work-related injuries, and employee turnover. These programs are effective even though only 15% to 30% of white-collar workers and 3% to 5% of blue-collar workers choose to participate.

Several workplace health promotions have incorporated money or other types of prizes as incentives. Windsor, Lowe, and Bartlett (1988) investigated the effect of a multicomponent smoking cessation program versus the effect of a cash incentive on success in quitting smoking. They found that the employees who took part in the multicomponent program were most successful; but that the cash incentive had no effect on quitting. Cummings, Hellmann, and Emont (1988) also reported on a smoking cessation program that used a contest as part of the program. Rather than using support groups, this program placed participants in a noncompetitive partnership. Only 14% of the smokers participated, but a third of them were abstinent 3 months later. Jason, Jayaraj, Blitz, Michaels, and Klett (1990) evaluated a workplace smoking cessation program with several components, including support groups, incentives, and competition. They found that the combination of components increased participation among smokers to over 80%. Six months later, 42% of those participants were no longer smoking. This last program, which was the most successful, included one element that the less successful programs did not: competition.

Cohen, Stunkard, and Felix (1987) compared three workplace weight-loss programs and also found that competition was an effective element. Team competition was most effective whereas some elements of individual competition were counterproductive, especially with women. The most effective use of competition was team competition against a natural business competitor. For example, a smoking cessation competition between two banks in the same community would be a good use of the competition element. Such a competition would make use of the support that each bank's employees could offer fellow employees, and that support could be mobilized against a business that was already a competitor.

Workers' health habits can be tied to rebate programs that apply to their health care coverage (Anderson et al., 1995; Davenport, 1995). In such programs, workers who reduce their risk or stay in a low-risk category receive monetary rewards, which they apply to cover the costs of their cafeteria health care plan, allowing employees to choose from an array of benefits. The incentive programs allow for employees to pay for health care for themselves and their family through the rebates their employers give for low health care expenditures due to a healthy lifestyle and low risks. In general, these reward systems work better than punishment systems in which people who have high-risk profiles must pay for their risky behaviors.

In summary, workplace wellness programs have become increasingly common in the United States. They encompass a wide variety of components, the most common of which is smoking cessation, but most companies with programs offer several components. To be successful, programs must include the components that employees are interested in, the programs must be voluntary, and the health information collected during the program must be kept confidential. Group and company support, convenience, and competition help make workplace health promotion campaigns more effective. A workplace health promotion program can be implemented at little cost, and the savings come about through lowered hospital use, decreased absenteeism, and a more energetic workforce.

COMMUNITY CAMPAIGNS

If an entire company with thousands of employees can participate in a multicomponent health campaign, can an entire community become more healthy through changes in lifestyle? Communitywide health campaigns have tested that question with interventions aimed at changing risk factors in an entire community. In 1721, Cotton Mather originated what might be considered the first community health campaign in the United States. Through the use of pamphlets and oratory, he sought to persuade the citizens of Boston to accept smallpox inoculations (Faden, 1987). Until quite recently, most community health campaigns were similar to Mather's — organized and administered by private citizens who had a strong belief in the benefits of the measures they advocated. Currently, communitywide capaigns are usually government efforts that include massive funding for design, implementation, and evaluation.

These communitywide campaigns also differ from traditional public health measures, which include such sanitation programs as purification of water and safe treatment of sewage. Historically, public health campaigns have attempted to improve health by making the *environment* less hazardous whereas community health campaigns seek to change *individual* behavior.

Weiss (1984) discussed the rationale and advantages of community health promotion programs, pointing out that such programs combine educational efforts oriented toward lifestyle change with community organization and social support. Community programs can motivate changes that are difficult for individuals to accomplish, such as changing the types of foods available at restaurants and supermarkets, creating exercise facilities in public parks, and restricting smoking in public places.

Community interventions also have the potential to reach people in moderate-risk categories whereas many other types of interventions concentrate on those at high risk. As Altman (1995) pointed out, the majority of cases of most chronic diseases occur to those in the moderate-risk range, and communitywide interventions are an effective way of reaching those people. In addition, many chronic illnesses share some risk factors, and programs that target behaviors such as a high-fat diet, smoking, and a sedentary lifestyle can lower the risk for several disorders, decreasing their occurrence.

The first major communitywide program for the prevention of cardiovascular disease started in 1972 in North Karelia, a mostly rural county in eastern Finland with 180,000 inhabitants (Puska, 1984). This county had a very high rate of cardiovascular disease as a result of the high-risk behaviors of its inhabitants. The Finnish government organized a program aimed at (1) reducing smoking, serum cholesterol levels, and blood pressure through mass health communication; (2) organizing individual and group services; (3) training local health personnel; and (4) bringing about changes in the environment. The program avoided fear appeals and emphasized practical ways to accomplish behavior changes.

The initial evaluation, which occurred 5 years into the project, compared the residents of North Karelia to those of another county in eastern Finland. Five years is not long enough to show reductions in cardiovascular morbidity and mortality, but it is sufficient time to demonstrate changes in CVD

risk factors such as cigarette smoking, serum cholesterol, and systolic and diastolic blood pressure. The 5-year follow-up showed that health-related behaviors of North Karelia residents changed in the desired direction. Middle-aged men experienced a 17.4% decrease and women an 11.5% decrease in cardiovascular risks compared to the reference county. A 10-year evaluation showed maintenance or further decreases in these target factors, with the result that men in North Karelia experienced a 22% decrease in cardiovascular mortality whereas the men in the comparison county experienced only a 12% decrease (Puska, 1984). Furthermore, the rate of disability payments for cardiovascular disease changed, and 5 years into the program North Karelia had a 10% lower rate of payment for cardiovascular disabilities than the comparison region. This savings more than paid for the entire community intervention program.

In 1981, the U.S. Department of Health and Human Services sponsored a health campaign called Health Style (Davis & Iverson, 1984). The Office of Health Information and Health Promotion implemented this program in nine test communities throughout the nation. The campaign was primarily an educational awareness program through the public media, and it included a wide range of health-related behaviors. Its goals were to increase awareness, lead people to assess their lifestyles, prompt information seeking, and boost community activities oriented to health. As an awareness campaign, Health Style was fairly successful, but the program did little to change behavior.

Groups of researchers have carried out several communitywide intervention programs in the United States including the Stanford Five-City Project (Farquhar et al., 1984; Fortmann, Taylor, Flora, & Jatulis, 1993; Fortmann, Taylor, Flora, & Winkleby, 1993; Taylor et al., 1991; Winkleby, Flora, & Kraemer, 1994), the Pawtucket Heart Health Project (Lasater et al., 1984), the Minnesota Heart Health Program (Blackburn et al., 1984; Lando et al., 1995), and the Community Intervention Trial for Smoking Cessation (COMMIT Research Group, 1995a, 1995b).

Most community interventions have tried to reduce risks for cardiovascular disease. For example, in the Stanford Five-City Project, two communities received educational interventions to change behaviors related to coronary heart disease risk. These interventions took the form of television and radio programs and announcements, booklets given to residents, weekly newspaper columns, changes in school curricula, and cookbooks and booklets with low-fat recipes and information about quitting smoking, as well as talks, seminars, and workshops. Three cities served as controls: two with residents who participated in the same measurements as the treatment cities but received none of the educational materials, and one city in which the research team collected only information about mortality and morbidity without questioning individuals.

The goal of the Stanford Five-City Project has been to stimulate and maintain lifestyle changes that result in a communitywide reduction of cardiovascular disease. Several reports from the research team at 5- and 6-year follow-ups have shown small but in some cases, significant decreases for the two treatment cities. Farquhar et al. (1990) reported on a 5-year follow-up that showed a significant decrease in cholesterol levels, resting pulse rate, and blood pressure in the treatment compared to the control cities. The smoking rate decreased in both treatment and control cities (Fortmann, Taylor, Flora, & Jatulis, 1993), but the decrease was greater in the cities that received the educational intervention.

The educational intervention was less successful in changing people's eating habits as reflected in their weight (Taylor et al., 1991). Although the people in the treatment cities gained less weight during the 6-year follow-up, both men and women in all age groups gained rather than lost weight. The study also showed small but favorable changes in cholesterol levels (Fortmann, Taylor, Flora, & Winkleby, 1993). Although nutritional knowledge increased over the duration of the study and intake of saturated fat decreased, only men lowered their serum cholesterol levels, and those changes did not represent significant differences between treatment and control cities.

The treatment cities showed greater decreases in overall mortality rates and risk factor scores for coronary heart disease (Farquhar et al., 1990). However, the project demonstrated that many people have changed their health habits, even without the

community intervention and that the interventions tended to produce greater changes during the initial years of the program than during the later years.

The North Karelia Project, the Stanford Five-City Project, the Pawtucket Heart Health Project, and the Minnesota Heart Health Program all have attempted to decrease the risk for cardiovascular disease by altering risk factors in the study population. Each program has included unique elements, but all have made use of community resources, involved the media, and collected data to evaluate their effectiveness. Several of the programs have shown short-term positive changes but have failed to show significant long-term benefits.

The Community Intervention Trial for Smoking Cessation (COMMIT) is one of the few examples of a community intervention with goals not limited to risk factors for cardiovascular disease (COMMIT Research Group, 1995a, 1995b). The COMMIT group targeted smoking in an attempt to reduce the risk for lung disease. They located 22 communities, which they divided into intervention and control sites. The research focused on heavy smokers and attempted to increase quit rates through public education, community events, health care providers, and workplace programs. Despite these efforts, both the intervention group and the comparison group showed similar quit rates, with 3% of heavy smokers quitting in both groups of communities. This 3%, however, represents about 3,000 heavy smokers who quit. In contrast, the campaign was successful for light-to-moderate smokers who were significantly more likely to quit in the intervention communities than in the comparison communities.

Worden, Flynn, Merrill, Waller, and Haugh (1989) reported on a more promising communitywide campaign targeted at attempts to curtail alcohol-impaired driving. Drink calculators were dispensed at bars and liquor stores, and bartenders and television announcements demonstrated their use. One community received all the materials, another saw only the television announcements, and a third acted as a control. After 6 months of the intervention, the researchers surveyed nighttime drivers for their blood alcohol content. They found that the community that received the full intervention had 5.3% fewer drivers with blood alcohol levels over 0.05 grams per deciliter than the control community. The community that received only the television announcements had 1% fewer drivers with the target blood alcohol level than did the control community. The researchers also found that heavy drinkers and young drivers were more likely to use the drink calculators. Even though the differences were small, effectiveness with these high-risk groups seems promising.

Another communitywide campaign was aimed at increasing the use of social support networks. According to the Alameda County study, social support is a significant factor in health (Camacho & Wiley, 1983). One group of researchers (Hersey, Klibanoff, Lam, & Taylor, 1984) formulated the Friends Can Be Good Medicine campaign, an intervention that consisted of both media and community activities. The media materials included television and radio public service announcements, brochures, a workbook, bumper stickers, posters, and billboards. The local activities included talk show appearances, a short film shown in local theaters, and a series of workshops. The research team compared evaluations made before the intervention to those made a year later. The results indicated that this campaign affected people's knowledge, attitudes, and behavioral intentions. In addition, behaviors that enhanced social support increased as people learned to trade favors with a friend and to share personal feelings with friends and family. This campaign also demonstrated particular effectiveness with a high-risk group—people who had experienced the death of someone close to them within the past year. The community gains persisted at the 1-year follow-up.

Communitywide campaigns have demonstrated that health interventions can be successful. Community residents' attitudes and behavioral intentions have changed in response to information obtained through media, and several communitywide campaigns have demonstrated behavior changes and even lower disease rates. The magnitude of changes in behavior and health risks has been small, leading to the question, Are they worth the effort? Is communitywide involvement necessary to bring about lower risk, or would an approach oriented toward only those who are at risk be more efficient?

The strategy of identifying and treating only people at high risk was the approach taken by the Multiple Risk Factor Intervention Trial (MRFIT) study (see Chapter 9). This study identified men at high risk for cardiovascular disease and compared them with another group that received standard medical care. The intervention behaviors were similar to those targeted by the North Karelia program and other cardiovascular community studies. However, programs like MRFIT provide treatment to individuals rather than to entire communities. Which approach is more effective?

Communitybased interventions for cardiovascular disease have greater potential benefits than interventions with high-risk individuals (Kottke, Puska, Salonen, Tuomilehto, & Nissinen, 1985). Interventions with individuals at high risk for CVD typically deal with people in the top 10% of a risk category, and the goals usually include lowering cholesterol by 20% and lowering diastolic blood pressure to 90 millimeters of mercury. Kottke et al. maintained that achieving these goals would decrease deaths due to CVD by 28%. However, few such interventions achieve these goals. On the average, they decrease cholesterol levels by only about 10% and lower diastolic blood pressure to about 95. If an entire population achieved these modest goals (and projects like the one in North Karelia demonstrate that these goals are possible), the decrease in deaths due to cardiovascular disease might be as high as 50%. Kottke et al. also maintained that populationwide interventions were the only way to achieve a reduction in death rate of that magnitude.

If population approaches to lowering risk factors for the major causes of death are the best approach, what are the impediments to their implementation? One problem, of course, is the magnitude of the required intervention. Reaching practically every member of a society is an enormous task. The studies on communitywide campaigns have revealed some of the elements that might make such projects feasible. Varied media components, involvement of community organizations, reliance on existing social networks, and mobilization of the community's health care services have been successful components all of the communitywide campaigns.

A second problem is the length of time that such programs require. Susser (1995) argued that the benefits of public health campaigns must occur over a period of years for significant effects to appear. In addition, because of the trend toward healthier habits for the population in general, obtaining significant differences between intervention and control communities is difficult.

A third problem is expense; both the complexity and length of such programs require a considerable commitment of time and money. Many community-wide programs have assessed their cost effectiveness, with generally positive results. Disease is often more expensive than prevention, and the North Karelia study demonstrated cost savings after only 5 years (Puska, 1984).

Wikler (1987) discussed a different sort of problem with government-sponsored health programs, including media and community health campaigns. His concerns were with the ethics of interventions that affect everyone in a community. Such programs differ in their ethical implications from all other types of research. In both experimental and descriptive research, human participants must have the right to decline participation, to withdraw from the study at any point, and to be informed of the consequences of their participation. Researchers do not make these principles known to the residents in a community in which a health campaign takes place. Residents may listen to the media messages, read the brochures, and attend the community activities or not, but those residents will still be exposed to the campaign.

Wikler also explored the possibility that the emphasis on individual behavior might undermine other types of public health measures oriented toward making the environment safer. If people are held responsible for their individual health, Wikler fears they will also be blamed for their individual illnesses. He argued that this attitude might influence such things as insurance rates, with higher premiums or loss of employment for those who fail to comply with health advice and even the withholding of health care for the noncomplying people who become ill. These provocative possibilities are issues to consider before beginning nationwide health campaigns.

Communitywide health campaigns have demonstrated that health changes can come about through such interventions. These programs are expensive, and they pose difficult ethical questions. However, communitywide health campaigns can be cost effective, and lowered mortality poses no ethical problem. Critics of such programs argue that we cannot afford them, either financially or ethically. Advocates argue that we cannot afford to continue without them, financially or ethically.

ADOPTING A HEALTHY LIFESTYLE

Injury prevention programs and various health campaigns have both demonstrated some effectiveness in encouraging people to change to a safer or more healthy lifestyle. Research (Cornelius, 1991; Donovan et al., 1993; Hawkins, 1992) has consistently shown that health-related behaviors tend to be related to each other and also to risky behaviors. In other words, some people have adopted a generally healthy lifestyle whereas others engage in a variety of unhealthy behaviors.

How can health psychologists help people give up unhealthy patterns of behavior and adopt more healthy lifestyles? Presently, the answer lies in cooperation with health psychologists working as members of prevention teams consisting of biomedical experts, social workers, educators, epidemiologists, and other representatives from the biological, social, and behavioral sciences. Using a team approach, prevention scientists can use a variety of strategies to enhance people's health.

Consistent with evidence presented earlier in this chapter, Steven Schinke (1994) recommended that prevention efforts adopt a team approach and use multifaceted programs. These programs should be based on sound theoretical models, such as the theory of reasoned action (Ajzen & Fishbein, 1980), the stages of change theory (Prochaska & DiClemente, 1983), or other models that we discussed in Chapters 7 and 8. The theory of reasoned action, for example, suggests that one determinant of people's intention to behave is their subjective norm—that is, their perception of the social pressures put on them to behave in a particular manner. Using this concept, programs designed to prevent young people from smoking should emphasize the observation that most people do not smoke and that the most popular students are even less likely to smoke than other students.

The stages of change theory also has implications for prevention science. During the precontemplation stage, mass media campaigns can arouse interest in the possibility of change; during the contemplation stage, individualized intervention will probably be more effective than mass media programs that target everyone; during the action stage when people are making an effort to change, intervention strategies should reinforce newly acquired healthy behaviors; and during the maintenance stage, programs should be directed at preventing a relapse to earlier, unhealthy behaviors.

Schinke recommended that prevention programs, in addition to being based on a sound theoretical model, should be selective in their choice of target populations. Interventions aimed at an entire population, including those who are not at risk, are usually more expensive and less effective than those that carefully select a group of people most at risk. For example, programs to prevent people from abusing drugs should be targeted toward those most likely to begin drug abuse. Designers of these programs should look at biopsychosocial factors that relate to drug use and aim their interventions at people who are most vulnerable. Schinke also noted that prevention programs must be sensitive to cultural differences among the targeted populations. In some cultures, for example, carrying a weapon is the norm whereas in other cultures almost no one carries a gun or knife as a weapon. Finally, Schinke contended that program evaluation must be an integral part of prevention campaigns and that the specific factors responsible for behavior change be identified.

Although people can adopt a healthy lifestyle at any age, many prevention strategies target young people, many of whom are vulnerable to social pressure to engage in unhealthy and unsafe behaviors. Many high school students, for example, engage in behaviors such as smoking cigarettes, using smokeless tobacco, drinking alcohol, smoking marijuana, using cocaine and other drugs, eating unwisely, and shunning vigorous physical activity—all of which may contribute to long-term health problems. Table 12.3 shows the percentage of 9th to 12th graders by gender and ethnicity who participate in various health-related behaviors (Kann et al., 1995). These figures are based on a national survey plus various state and local surveys that were conducted in 1993.

Note that there are many similarities among ethnic and gender groups in these risky behaviors. However, a few notable differences are also apparent. One dramatic difference was the regular use of cigarettes and smokeless tobacco; only 9% of African American high school students were regular cigarette smokers, compared with 28% of European American students and 19% of Hispanic students; and only 2.6% of African Americans used smokeless tobacco during the month preceding the survey compared with 14.6% for European Americans and 4.9% for Hispanics. (We discuss ethnic differences in cigarette smoking in Chapter 13.) In addition, African American students were somewhat less likely than other groups to be current users of alcohol and Hispanic students were much more likely to be current users of cocaine.

This survey also showed that high school students tend to have poor eating habits. More than one-third of them were overweight; only 15% ate five or more fruits and vegetables per day; one-third thought they were overweight; two of every five were trying to lose weight; and one-third ate more than two daily servings of foods high in fat, such as hamburgers, hot dogs, sausage, french fries, potato chips, cookies, doughnuts, pie, or cake. In addition, more than one-third of high school students did not participate in vigorous physical activity for at least 20 minutes a day for 3 or more days a week.

The next four chapters address in more detail the effects of smoking, using alcohol and other drugs, unwise eating, and a sedentary lifestyle on health. They also examine strategies for preventing unhealthy behaviors and present recommendations for adopting a health-enhancing lifestyle.

CHAPTER SUMMARY

This chapter looked at ways of staying healthy and avoiding unintentional injuries and reducing chances of disease and death. Unintentional injuries are the leading cause of death among young people in the United States and about half of all fatal unintentional injuries are due to motor vehicle crashes. An important contributor to these fatalities is alcohol, although both the number of motor vehicle

Table 12.3   Percentage of high school students who participate in health-related behaviors by gender and ethnicity—United States, 1993

Ethnic group	Regular cigarette use[1]	Current alcohol use[2]	Current marijuana use[3]	Current cocaine use[4]	Eating Recommended Fruits & Vegetables[5]	Doing Vigorous Physical Activity[6]
White	28.4%	49.9%	17.3%	1.6%	16.1%	67.7%
Female	28.6	48.6	14.7	1.2	13.5	58.8
Male	28.2	51.1	19.7	2.0	18.4	75.9
Black	9.2	42.5	18.6	1.0	9.1	60.0
Female	9.1	37.1	13.0	0.5	7.2	48.8
Male	9.4	48.2	24.3	1.5	11.2	71.4
Hispanic	18.6	50.8	19.4	4.6	11.5	59.4
Female	18.3	46.9	15.7	3.0	9.8	50.0
Male	19.0	55.0	23.2	6.2	13.2	68.8
Total	24.7	48.0	17.7	1.9	15.4	65.8
Female	24.5	45.9	14.6	1.4	13.0	56.2
Male	24.9	50.1	20.6	2.3	17.6	74.7

[1] Smoked at least one cigarette every day for 30 days.
[2] Drank alcohol on one or more of the 30 days preceding the survey.
[3] Used marijuana one or more times during the 30 days preceding the survey.
[4] Used cocaine one or more times during the 30 days preceding the survey.
[5] Ate five or more daily servings of fruits and vegetables, including fruit juice, green salad, and cooked vegetables.
[6] Engaged in activities that caused sweating and hard breathing for at least 20 minutes on 3 or more days during the week preceding the survey.

SOURCE: "Youth Risk Behavior Surveillance—United States, 1993," by L. Kann, C. W. Warren, W. A. Harris, J. L. Collins, K. A. Douglas, M. E. Collins, B. I. Williams, J. G. Ross, & L. J. Kolbe, (1995). *Morbidity and Mortality Weekly Report, 44,* No. SS-1, pp. 35, 38, 41.

deaths and the percentage due to drunk driving has declined during the past decade. Alcohol is also a contributor to other unintentional fatal injuries, such as falls, fires, and even bicycle fatalities.

Strategies for reducing unintentional injuries can be aimed at changing the individual's behavior, changing the environment, or changing legislation. Change in individual behavior is included in interventions to prevent home injuries, motor vehicle injuries, and bicycle-related injuries. Programs to prevent home injuries frequently target children and elderly people, but most of these programs have not been very successful. Similarly, strategies, such as having a designated driver, that attempt to reduce motor vehicle fatalities by emphasizing individual behavior have been only marginally successful. Also, individualized approaches to increase bicycle helmet use are not very effective, but when the cost of helmets goes down and their social acceptance

goes up, adults and children are more likely to buy and use them.

Strategies to alter the environment are generally more successful than those that attempt change through individual interventions. Environmental changes include building safer cars and roads and making the home and neighborhood safer. Laws, too, can have an impact on reducing unintentional injuries. Laws requiring the use of automobile seatbelts and bicycle helmets have saved many lives and prevented thousands of serious injuries.

This chapter also discussed suicide and violence, the third and second leading causes of death among young adults in the United States. Traditional suicide hot lines have not been very successful, but a newer program called Tele-Help/Tele-Check has shown some promise in preventing suicides. Domestic violence and violence perpetrated by and against young people are serious problems in the

United States, but programs to prevent them must be multifaceted and based on the root causes of violence, which include poverty, overcrowded housing, the ready availability of weapons, and the general acceptance of violence as a means of solving interpersonal difficulties.

Health campaigns are designed to prevent illness by creating an atmosphere in which people will be motivated to adopt certain behaviors and a healthy lifestyle. Rather than being aimed at individuals, health campaigns are directed toward large communities or even an entire nation. Campaigns oriented toward disseminating information are generally ineffective and may even have a negative effect on health behaviors. Similarly, campaigns that use fear tactics seldom change behavior in the desired direction.

Recently, companies have become more interested in creating a healthy environment for their employees. Thus, many workplace wellness programs have been established to improve workers' health. Research indicates that these programs pay off financially in reduced insurance premiums, lower absenteeism, fewer accidents, and decreased employee turnover.

Communitywide programs, such as the North Karelia Project and the Stanford Five-City Project, are directed at stimulating and maintaining healthy lifestyle changes. These community-based interventions are relatively expensive and pose some ethical problems. In addition, long-term assessment tends to indicate that these programs do not have large effects, but even small changes in many people can represent changes in the health risks for the community.

Programs designed to help people adopt a healthy lifestyle must be based on a solid theoretical model, target a specific at-risk population, include a variety of interventions, be sensitive to cultural differences, and involve experts from several medical, psychological, and sociological disciplines.

SUGGESTED READINGS

Carden, A. D. (1994). Wife abuse and the wife abuser: Review and recommendations. *Counseling Psychologist, 22,* 539–582. This report reviews nearly 200 publications on wife abuse and presents theories that might explain why some people become spouse abusers. Carden also presents a profile of the abuser and suggests possible strategies to prevent domestic violence.

Kizer, W. M. (1987). *The healthy workplace: A blueprint for corporate action.* New York: Wiley. Written by the chief executive officer of a life insurance company and the founder of a wellness council, this book is a practical guide for those interested in health promotion and wellness in the workplace. Kizer argues that workplace wellness programs are cost effective because they reduce absenteeism, employee turnover, and accidents.

Susser, M. (1995). Editorial: The tribulations of trials — Intervention in communities. *American Journal of Public Health, 85,* 156–158. In this editorial, Mervyn Susser offers insightful comments on the failure of community intervention to deliver more than modest benefits, and he describes why these "failures" may be more successful than many might believe.

Williams, A. F., & Lund, A. K. (1992). Injury control: What psychologists can contribute. *American Psychologist, 47,* 1036–1039. This brief article provides some background to the injury control field and discusses the role of psychologists in injury reduction.

13 Smoking Tobacco

Lisa, a 31-year-old African American office manager, has been smoking for 9 years. Neither of her parents smoked, and as a teenager, Lisa was never tempted to try smoking. After working in an office for about 3 years, one day Lisa had a particularly unpleasant argument with a co-worker in another office. When she returned to her office, she was still angry. She asked her friend, Karen, for a cigarette. She smoked just one that day and did not inhale. About 10 days later, after another altercation with the same co-worker, she stormed back to her office and almost demanded a cigarette from Karen. Again, she smoked just one, but the next morning she stopped at a convenience store and bought a pack of cigarettes. At

first, she smoked just two a day—one at work and one in the evening after work.

Gradually, Lisa increased the number of cigarettes she smoked per day. After about a year, she was up to a pack a day, a number that she maintains at present. Interestingly, she never purchased cigarettes by the carton, reasoning that it would be easier to quit if she did not have several unused packs around her apartment. Twice Lisa has made serious attempts to stop smoking. The first time was about 2 years ago when she asked her doctor for a prescription for the nicotine patch. That procedure was partially successful—she quit for 4 months. When she began smoking again, she returned almost immediately to one pack a day. About a year later, she tried for a second time to quit—this time on her own. Once again she was partly successful, but she refrained from cigarettes for only 3 weeks. Why did she go back to smoking after wanting to quit and succeeding at doing so? Lisa says that one day she got angry at her boss, and she knew if she didn't do something to occupy her hands and mouth she might do or say something she would later regret.

When Lisa first began smoking, people were permitted to smoke in her building. When the building became smoke free, Lisa would step outside to smoke, or she would smoke while running errands between one building and another. The prohibition against smoking in her building neither reduced nor increased the number of cigarettes Lisa smokes at work.

Lisa believes that she is at greater risk for cancer than other people because she had cancer when she was 12 years old. Lisa's attitude of vulnerability is therefore different from that of most smokers who think that smoking is generally unhealthy but who nevertheless believe that other smokers are at greater risk for cancer and heart disease than they are. This chapter reports on the level of those risks, the risks for other tobacco products, the dangers of passive smoking, the prevalence of smoking in the United States, the reasons people smoke, and some methods of preventing and reducing smoking. First, though, we briefly review the functioning of the respiratory system, the body system most immediately affected by smoking.

THE RESPIRATORY SYSTEM

Through respiration, oxygen is taken into the body and carbon dioxide is expelled. The exchange of these two gases occurs deep in the lungs. To get air into the lungs, the **diaphragm** and the muscles between the ribs (intercostal muscles) contract, increasing the volume within the chest. As the space inside the chest increases, the pressure within the chest falls below atmospheric pressure, and air is forced into the lungs by that pressure.

The flow of air into the lungs is traced in Figure 13.1. The nasal passages, pharynx, larynx, trachea, bronchi, and bronchioles conduct air into the lungs. These passages have little ability to absorb oxygen, but in the process of inhalation, the air is warmed, humidified, and cleansed. Millions of **alveoli**, located at the ends of the bronchioles, are the site of oxygen and carbon dioxide exchange. Each tiny alveolus in the lungs is like a bubble, giving the lungs a spongy appearance. The alveoli have thin walls (only one cell in thickness) that allow the easy exchange of gases.

Air rich in oxygen is drawn into the lungs and reaches the alveoli. Blood that has circulated through the body travels back to the heart and then back to the lungs. This blood has a high carbon dioxide content and a low oxygen content. In the lungs, the blood circulates to the capillaries that surround each alveolus, where an exchange of carbon dioxide and oxygen occurs based on differences in diffusion pressures. The blood, now oxygen-rich, travels back to the heart and is pumped out to all areas of the body.

During exhalation, the diaphragm and the muscles between the ribs relax. The air in the alveoli is compressed, and the increased pressure forces the air out of the lungs by the same route through which

it entered. The expelled air contains a great deal of carbon dioxide and little oxygen. Not all air leaves the lungs during exhalation, and each breath mixes new air with air that remains in the lungs.

Air is an excellent medium for the introduction of foreign matter into the body. Airborne particles potentially move into the lungs with every breath. Protective mechanisms in the respiratory system, such as sneezing and coughing, expel some of the dangerous particles. Noxious stimulation in the nasal passages may activate the sneeze reflex whereas stimulation in the lower respiratory system promotes the cough reflex.

Another protective mechanism in the respiratory system is called the **mucociliary escalator.** Diffusion of gases requires a moist environment, and the respiratory system is kept moist by its mucous membrane lining. In the nasal cavity, pharynx, and bronchi, the lining of the respiratory system contains **cilia,** tiny hairlike structures. The cilia and mucous membranes form the mucociliary escalator. Mucus is secreted in the respiratory system, and the beating of the cilia moves the mucus toward the pharynx, where it is usually swallowed or coughed out. This transport mechanism cleanses the system of inhaled particles, providing an important defense against dangerous particles that may be inhaled.

Several respiratory disorders are of interest to health psychologists. All kinds of smoke, as well as other types of air pollution, increase mucus secretion in the respiratory system but decrease the activity of the cilia, thus decreasing the efficiency of the mucociliary escalator. As mucus builds up, people cough to get rid of the mucus, but coughing may also irritate the bronchial walls. Irritation and infection of the bronchial walls may damage the cilia and destroy tissue in the bronchi. The formation of scar tissue in the bronchi, irritation or infection of bronchial tissue, and coughing are characteristics of **bronchitis,** one of several chronic obstructive pulmonary diseases, which are the third leading cause of death in the United States.

Acute bronchitis is the most common form. This type of bronchitis is caused by infection and usually responds quickly to antibiotics. When the irritation persists and the mechanism underlying the illness continues, it can become a chronic problem. Cigarette smoke is the major cause of chronic bronchitis,

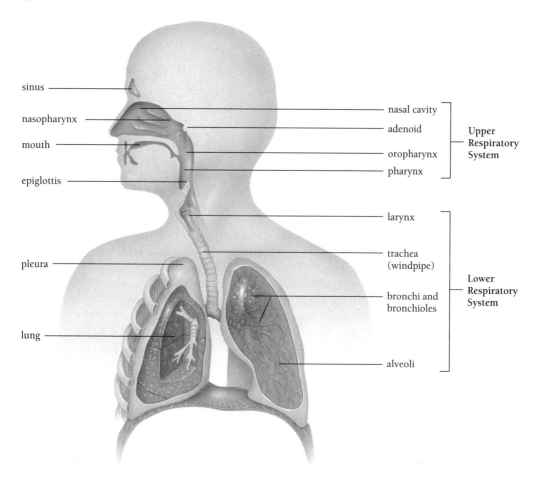

sinus

nasopharynx

mouth

epiglottis

pleura

lung

nasal cavity

adenoid

oropharynx

pharynx

Upper Respiratory System

larynx

trachea (windpipe)

bronchi and bronchioles

Lower Respiratory System

alveoli

Figure 13.1 Respiratory system. SOURCE: Ingraham & Ingraham (1995), p. 525.

but environmental air pollution and occupational hazards may also underlie chronic bronchitis.

Another chronic obstructive pulmonary disease is **emphysema,** a disorder that develops when scar tissue and mucus obstruct the respiratory passages, bronchi lose their elasticity and collapse, and air is trapped in the alveoli. The trapped air breaks down the alveolar walls, and the remaining alveoli enlarge. Both damaged and enlarged alveoli reduce surface area for the exchange of oxygen and carbon dioxide. They also obstruct blood flow to the undamaged alveoli, and so the respiratory system becomes restricted. The loss of efficiency in the respiratory system means that respiration delivers a limited amount of oxygen. People with emphysema usually cannot exercise strenuously, and even normal breathing may become impossible for them.

Chronic bronchitis, emphysema, and lung cancer are all diseases of the respiratory system associated with the inhalation of irritating, damaging particles. Cigarette smoking is of particular interest to health psychologists because it is a voluntary behavior that can be avoided; air pollution and occupational hazards, however, are a societal rather than an individual problem. The harmful effects of smoking are not limited to respiratory illnesses; far more smokers die of cardiovascular disease than all the cancers combined. The Public Health Service (USDHHS, 1995) has called cigarette smoking the largest preventable cause of death and disability in the United States and has estimated that this behavior is responsible for more than 400,000 deaths yearly—a figure that represents about 20% of all deaths in the United States.

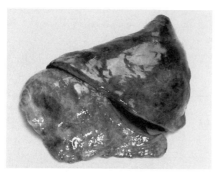 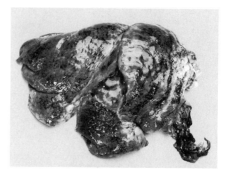

Healthy and unhealthy lungs.

A BRIEF HISTORY OF SMOKING

When Christopher Columbus and other early European explorers arrived in the Western hemisphere, they found that the Native Americans had a custom considered odd by European standards: They carried rolls of dried leaves, which they set afire, and then they "drank" the smoke. The leaves were, of course, tobacco. Those early European sailors tried smoking, liked it, and spread smoking and the cultivation of tobacco around the world.

Smoking was a habit that grew rapidly in popularity among Europeans, but it was not without its detractors. Elizabethan England adopted the use of tobacco, although Elizabeth I disapproved, as did her successor, James I. Another prominent Elizabethan, Sir Francis Bacon, spoke against tobacco and the hold it exerted over its users. Many objections to tobacco were of a similar nature—namely, that those who could not afford it still spent their money on it because of the power it gained over its users. Because of its scarcity, tobacco was expensive: In London in 1610, it sold for an equal weight of silver.

In 1633, the Turkish Sultan Murad IV decreed the death penalty for smoking. From the early Romanoff empire in Russia to 17th-century Japan, the penalties for tobacco use were severe. Still the habit spread. Smoking during Mass became so prevalent among priests in the Spanish colonies that the Catholic Church forbade it. In 1642 and again in 1650, tobacco was the subject of two formal papal bulls, but in 1725 Pope Benedict XIII annulled all edicts against tobacco—he liked to use snuff.

The form in which tobacco is used varies with time and country, but Brecher (1972) contended that no country where the people have learned to use tobacco has ever barred the habit. Columbus found the Indians smoking tobacco in pipes as well as in the form of cigars. Cigarettes (shredded tobacco rolled in paper) were not popular until the 20th century, although some appeared before the U.S. Civil War. Cigarette use was not widespread at first because it was considered rather effeminate. Ironically, cigarette smoking was not socially acceptable for women either, and few women smoked during the first part of the 20th century. It was, however, acceptable for women and men to use snuff, or ground tobacco. Taking snuff became very popular in 18th-century England after the English fleet captured a cargo of high-quality Spanish snuff. Taking snuff was widespread in all Europe as well as in America. But chewing shredded tobacco never became popular in Europe where it was considered a filthy American habit, and that habit became less popular in America after the U.S. Civil War.

The widespread adoption of cigarette smoking was aided in 1913 by the development of the "blended" cigarette, a mixture of the air-cured Burley and Turkish varieties of tobacco mixed with flue-cured Virginia tobacco. This blend provided a cigarette with a pleasing flavor and aroma that was also easy to inhale. Cigarette smoking became increasingly popular during World War I, and during the 1920s, the age of the "flapper," cigarette smoking started to gain popularity among women. It continued to increase until the mid-1960s when the dangerous consequences of smoking first became widely recognized.

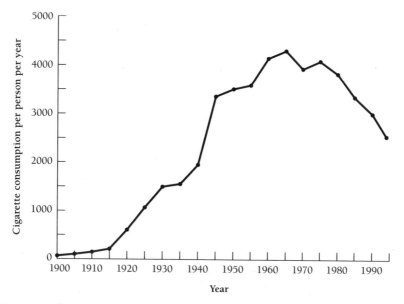

Figure 13.2 **Cigarette consumption per person 18 and over, United States, 1900–1994.**
SOURCE: "Surveillance for Selected Tobacco-use Behaviors—United States, 1990–1994," by G. A. Givovino et al., 1994, *Morbidity and Mortality Weekly Report, 43* No. SS-3, pp. 6–7.

WHO SMOKES AND WHO DOES NOT?

Currently, about 25% of the adults in the United States smoke cigarettes on a regular basis (U.S. Department of Health and Human Services [USDHHS], 1994a). This percentage represents millions of smokers, but it also means that three of every four adults in the United States are nonsmokers. Currently, about one-fourth of the adult population are cigarette smokers, one-fourth are former smokers, and one-half have never smoked (USDHHS, 1994d). This section addresses the question of who smokes and who does not; later we look at the question of why people smoke.

In 1964, the U.S. Surgeon General issued a report spelling out the adverse effects of smoking on health (U.S. Public Health Service [USPHS], 1964). Beginning in 1967 each package of cigarettes had to carry a warning of the potential danger of smoking, and in 1970 cigarette advertising was banned from television. Partially because of these warnings, smoking rates have declined in the United States. The highest rate of per capita cigarette consumption in the U.S.

was in 1966, 2 years after the first Surgeon General's report on the dangers of smoking, and since that time the per capita consumption has steadily decreased. Figure 13.2 shows the per capita consumption of cigarettes in the United States from 1900 to 1994.

Not only has per capita consumption declined since the 1964 Surgeon General's report, but the number of regular smokers has also dropped. In 1965, almost 41% of all adults in the United States smoked. Since then, the number of smokers has decreased significantly; presently only 25% of adults smoke. These numbers suggest that the Surgeon General's warning probably made a significant difference in the number of smokers in the United States.

Since 1965, both men and women have begun to smoke less, but the rate of smoking for men has declined more sharply than the rate for women. Figure 13.3 reveals a decline in the percentage of male and female smokers from 1965 to 1994. (Incidentally, beginning with 1992, the National Center for Health Statistics [1994] changed its definition of current smoker to include people who smoke only "some days." The old definition was more limiting, defining smokers as people who described themselves as current smokers and who had smoked at least 100

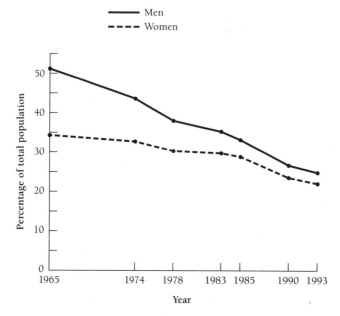

Figure 13.3   **Estimated percentages of adult male and female cigarette smokers, United States,**
1965–1993.   SOURCE: Data from *Statistical Abstracts of the United States, 1995* (115th ed., p. 143). By U.S. Bureau
of the Census, 1995, Washington, DC: U.S. Govenment Printing Office.

lifetime cigarettes. This new definition, of course, will inflate data for 1992 and all subsequent years; thus, comparisons between numbers of smokers before and after 1992 are deceptive.)

In 1965, more than half of all adult men in the United States were smokers, and about 34% of adult women smoked. During the next 28 years, the percentage of male smokers dropped dramatically while the percentage of female smokers declined at a somewhat slower rate. Several possibilities exist to explain the slower decline in smoking prevalence among women, but no single explanation has gained substantial support from the research. Some investigators (Silverstein, Feld, & Kozlowski, 1980) have sought to determine whether the availability of low-nicotine cigarettes to teenage women could be a reason for the slower decline in smoking among women. Advertising targeting young women and girls may also have contributed to the slower decline in rate of female smokers. Pierce, Lee, and Gilpin (1994) reported that the rate of smoking initiation for girls 10 to 17 increased dramatically during the mid-1960s when tobacco companies began to direct advertising toward this market. Since 1975, however, the sale of women's cigarettes has declined

slightly. Women's concern about weight gain and the women's rights movement have also been suggested as reasons for the slower decline in their rate of smoking (USDHHS, 1989), but neither hypothesis has received much research support. Another suggestion is that women have a lower quitting rate than men (Remington et al., 1985). Although some evidence exists to support the idea that women have more difficulty than men in quitting, the reason may be that female smokers who try to quit may have more obstacles to overcome. A recent study by Wendy Bjornson et al. (1995) found, as have many previous researchers, that men have higher sustained quit rates than women. However, when Bjornson et al. looked at baseline factors that might account for these differences, they found that men had more favorable predictors for quitting. At the beginning of this study, men were more likely be married, to have made a previous attempt to quit, to have made longer quit attempts, and to be heavier smokers. Women were more likely to have other smokers in the household. Each of these factors would predict a higher quit rate for men. Although these conditions probably do not totally explain differences in quit rate between men and women, they should cau-

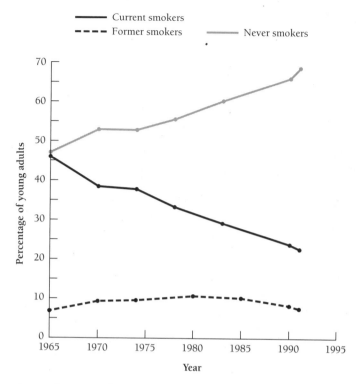

Figure 13.4 *Percentage of current, former, and never smokers among young adults, 18–24, United States, 1965–1991.* SOURCE: "Surveillance for Selected Tobacco-use Behaviors—United States, 1990–1994" by G. A. Givovino et al., 1994, *Morbidity and Mortality Weekly Report, 43*, No. SS-3 p. 9.

tion other researchers to examine baseline factors prior to studying gender differences in quitting smoking.

Daily smoking rates for both male and female adolescents declined from 1975 to 1987, but more recently that trend has been reversed, as both boys and girls have begun to smoke more. In the senior class of 1975, slightly more boys than girls smoked—27% versus 26%. By 1987, daily use had dropped to 16% for male and 20% for female adolescents, but by 1993 the rate of regular smoking for 12th graders was about 27% for both girls and boys (Kann et al., 1995) In 1993, about 28% of European American high school students smoked at least one cigarette a day, about 18.5% of Hispanic American adolescents smoked, but only about 9% of African American adolescents smoked. For all three groups, the percentages were nearly identical for boys and girls (Kann et al., 1995). Nelson et al. (1995) suggested that despite some decrease in smoking among young African Americans, it is unlikely that the United States

will achieve its national health objective to reduce cigarette smoking by children and youth to 15% by the year 2000.

For young adults 18 to 24, smoking rates are currently about half the 1965 rate. In 1965, more than 45% of young adults smoked; in 1991 that rate had dropped to less than 23%. Most of this decline is attributed to people who have never smoked; the percentage of ex-smokers among young adults gradually increased until 1980, but then, as the number of current smokers declined, the percentage of former smokers also declined. Figure 13.4 reveals a sharp decline in smoking among young adults, a gradual up and down trend for former smokers, and a relatively consistent increase in those who have never smoked.

The percentage of smokers varies greatly by educational level; the more years of school people have attended, the less likely they are to smoke. Moreover, the *rate* of decline has been steeper for college graduates than for high school dropouts. In 1974, the percentage of college graduates who smoked was about two-thirds the rate for high school drop-outs, but by 1991, the rate for college graduates was only about one-third the rate for high school drop-outs. Figure 13.5 shows not only the inverse relationship between smoking and education but also the steeper decline in more educated individuals.

Does the decline in smoking rates depend on adverse publicity? Many cultures throughout the world have not received much information about the adverse health effects of cigarettes, and worldwide tobacco sales have increased in the past 25 years (USBC, 1994). What practices and attitudes do people from these societies have with regard to smoking? In one study, Damon (1973) examined the smoking attitudes and habits of people in seven preliterate societies: four from Melanesia and three from sub-Saharan Africa. Some of the tribes had been introduced to tobacco over 100 years earlier, and one was introduced as recently as the 1960s. In these seven societies, all adults smoked as much as possible, unless it was forbidden by their religion. Their attitudes about tobacco smoking were generally positive. In five of the cultures, the people said that personal satisfaction was their main reason for smoking. In two of the cultures, the main reason for smoking was prestige. Curiously, nearly half the people in these preliterate cultures believed that smoking is harmful even though negative publicity about smoking was not available to most of them.

In summary, the number of smokers in the United States has slowly declined since the mid-1960s. The historical trend for men to smoke at a higher rate than women has begun to change, and presently only a slightly higher percentage of men than women smoke. The downward trend for men leveled off from 1990 to 1992 while the downward trend for women was reversed, with a greater percentage of women smoking in 1991 than in 1990. Rates for years subsequent to 1991 will be artificially higher because the National Center for Health Statistics has changed the definition of current smoker to include anyone who smokes only "some days." Currently, educational level has become a better predictor of smoking status than gender, with more highly educated people smoking at a much lower rate than those with less education.

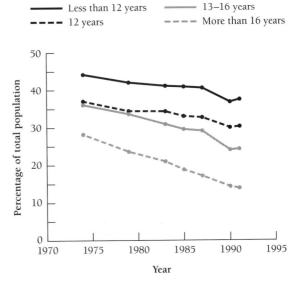

Figure 13.5 *Smoking rates by educational level, United States, 1974–1991.* SOURCE: *Health, United States, 1993*, p. 157, by National Center for Health Statistics, 1994. (DHHS, Publication No. PHS 94-1232), Hyattsville, MD: U.S. Government Printing Office.

SMOKING AND ILLNESS OR DEATH

During the past 25 years, a decreasing number of studies have concentrated on the relationship between smoking and illness or death because the link is so well established. A great deal of research has been conducted on the topic of smoking, but that research has explored other smoking-related issues. Some of the recent research has examined the relationship between health hazards and passive smoking—that is, breathing the smoke from others. We look at this research later, but first we present data on the relationship between smoking and illness, much of which is gathered by the Centers for Disease Control and Prevention (CDC).

Cigarette smoking is the leading cause of preventable illness and death in the United States. The Public Health Service reported that cigarette smoking currently accounts for about 400,000 deaths a year in the United States, a figure that translates to nearly 1,100 deaths per day (USDHHS, 1995). However this number represented a decline from

1988 when cigarettes killed 434,000 people (CDC, 1993). Currently, about one of every five deaths in the United States is related to smoking. Although most of those deaths are from heart disease, cancer, and chronic obstructive pulmonary disease, about 1,400 people die a year from fires begun by cigarettes (CDC, 1993). The combination of smoking cigarettes while drinking alcohol produces a number of fatal and nonfatal burns every year, but smoking by itself contributed more to those fires than drinking by itself (Ballard, Koepsell, & Rivara, 1992). Heavy smokers were nearly four times as likely as nonsmokers to be injured or killed in a residential fire. In addition to adults killing themselves by smoking, they also contribute to the deaths of more than 1,700 infants a year by forcing them to breathe environmental tobacco smoke (CDC, 1993).

WHAT COMPONENTS IN SMOKE ARE DANGEROUS?

The processed tobacco in cigarettes contains at least 2,550 compounds, and burning increases the number to over 4,000 (USDHHS, 1989). But which of these components in cigarette smoke might be dangerous? Nicotine is the pharmacological agent that underlies addiction to cigarette smoking (USDHHS, 1988), but is nicotine the main culprit responsible for the adverse health effects of smoking? Can nicotine cause coronary heart disease, cancer, ulcers, bronchitis, and emphysema? What does this drug do in the body?

Nicotine is a stimulant drug, an "upper." It affects both the central and the peripheral nervous systems. Research suggests that certain central nervous system receptor sites are specific for nicotine; that is, the brain responds to nicotine, as it does to many drugs. But smoking is a particularly effective means of delivering drugs to the brain. Nicotine, for example, can be found in the brain 7 seconds after having been ingested by smoking—twice as fast as via intravenous injection. The half-life of nicotine, the time it takes to lose half its strength, is 30 to 40 minutes. Addicted smokers rarely go more than this length of time between "fixes."

When nicotine is delivered to the brain, catecholamines, neurotransmitters that include epine-

phrine and norephinephrine, are released. These substances act as stimulants, increasing cortical arousal, which can be measured by an electroencephalograph (EEG). In addition, smoking releases beta-endorphins (Pomerleau, Fertig, Seyler, & Jaffe, 1983), and the pleasurable effects of smoking may be due to the release of these opiates produced by the body. Nicotine also increases the metabolic level (Perkins, Epstein, Marks, Stiller, & Jacob, 1989), and this effect explains the tendency for smokers to be thinner than nonsmokers. Cigarette smoking may also account for the finding that thinness is associated with mortality—thin smokers are at an increased risk for death, but thin people who do not smoke are not at an elevated risk (Sidney, Friedman, & Siegelaub, 1987).

The term *tars* describes the water-soluble residue of tobacco smoke condensate, which is known to contain a number of compounds identified or suspected as **carcinogens**—that is, agents that may cause cancer. Mortality from smoking-related diseases decrease with decreasing tar yields (Tang et al., 1995), but the problem in evaluating the role of tars in cigarette smoke is that tars and nicotine vary together in commercially available cigarettes. Some cigarettes are high in both, although the trend is toward cigarettes that are relatively low in both. However, currently no commercially available cigarettes are low in tars and high in nicotine, even though such a product might have advantages.

Schachter (1980) reported that low-nicotine cigarettes result in more smoking. Similarly, smokers inhale more deeply when given low-nicotine cigarettes, and inhaling more deeply exposes smokers to more of the dangerous tars (Herning, Jones, Bachman, & Mines, 1981). So low-tar and low-nicotine cigarettes may not be entirely successful in restricting the hazards involved in smoking. Maron and Fortmann (1987) also found that the lower the nicotine yield, the greater the number of cigarettes smoked, and their data failed to find any health advantage to low-yield cigarettes.

Several other by-products of tobacco smoke are suspected of being health risks. **Acrolein** and **formaldehyde** belong to a class of irritating compounds called **aldehydes**. Formaldehyde, a demonstrated carcinogen, disrupts tissue proteins and causes cell damage. **Nitric oxide** and **hydrocyanic acid** are gases generated in smoking tobacco that affect oxygen metabolism and thus could be dangerous.

In summary, several chemicals, either within the tobacco itself or produced as a by-product of smoking, have some potential to cause organic damage. Although nicotine in large doses is extremely toxic, its precise harmful effects to the average smoker are difficult to assess. This difficulty exists because the level of nicotine in commercial cigarettes varies with the level of tars, another class of substances that are potentially hazardous. Thus, determining what components of smoke connect to which sources of illness and death is difficult.

Smoking and Cardiovascular Disease

Cardiovascular disease (including both heart disease and stroke) is not only the leading cause of death in the United States but it is also the primary cause of cigarette-related deaths. More than 850,000 people die of cardiovascular disease in the United States every year, and more than one-fifth of these deaths, or 180,000 a year, are due to smoking (USDHHS, 1995). The Centers for Disease Control and Prevention (CDC, 1993) has estimated that male cigarette smokers are nearly twice as likely to die of cardiovascular diseases as male nonsmokers, and female smokers are about 1.7 times as likely as female nonsmokers to die of CVD.

What is it about smoking that might contribute to cardiovascular disease? Although scientists have yet to identify the exact pathway by which cigarette smoking leads to CVD, one possible contributor is nicotine, the principal pharmacological agent in tobacco. Nicotine has a stimulant effect on the nervous system, activating the sympathetic division of the peripheral nervous system. Under nicotine stimulation, heart rate, blood pressure, and cardiac output increase, but skin temperature decreases and blood vessels constrict. This combination of increased heart rate and constricted blood vessels places increased strain on the cardiovascular system and thus may constitute one factor that elevates smokers' risk of coronary heart disease.

Smoking and Cancer

Cancer is the second leading cause of death in the United States, and smoking plays a role in the development of several cancers, especially lung cancer.

Currently, more than one-third of smoking-related deaths are from various cancers (CDC, 1993). Although about 80% of these deaths are due to lung cancer, smoking may also be responsible for deaths from cancers of the lip, oral cavity, pharynx, esophagus, pancreas, larynx, trachea, urinary bladder, and kidney (CDC, 1993).

Cigarette smoking's relative risk of about 9.0 for lung cancer is the strongest link established to date between any behavior and a major cause of death. More than 150,000 people die each year from smoking-related cancers, and about 120,000 of these are from lung cancer (USDHHS, 1995).

During the 1990s and about 20 to 25 years after cigarette consumption began to decline (see Figure 13.3), lung cancer deaths also began to level off. However, from 1950 to 1989, lung cancer deaths rose sharply, a trend that lagged about 20 to 25 years behind the rapid rise in cigarette consumption. Could the rise in lung cancer deaths before 1990 have been due to environmental pollution or some other factor? Evidence from two prospective studies (Thun, Day-Lally, Calle, Flanders, & Heath, 1995) strongly suggested that neither pollution nor any other nonsmoking factor was responsible for the increase in lung cancer deaths from 1959 to 1988. The first of these studies examined the period from 1959 to 1965 when lung cancer mortality rates, especially for women, were relatively low; the second covered 1982 to 1988, a period of markedly increased death rates from lung cancer. For cigarette smokers, lung cancer deaths per 100,000 from Study 1 to Study 2 rose from 26 to 155 for women and from 187 to 341 for men. However, for nonsmokers during these same periods, lung cancer death rates remained stable, indicating that indoor/outdoor pollution, radon, and other suspected carcinogens had little or no effect on lung cancer mortality. These results, along with those from earlier epidemiological studies, strongly suggest that cigarette smoking is the primary contributor to lung cancer deaths.

Smoking and Chronic Obstructive Pulmonary Disease

Chronic obstructive pulmonary disease (COPD) is currently the third leading cause of death in the United states, and cigarette smoking accounts for more than four of every five deaths from this disease

(USDHHS, 1995). Chronic obstructive pulmonary disease includes a number of respiratory and lung diseases; the three most common are chronic bronchitis, emphysema, and asthma. Since 1950, mortality rates from COPD have increased faster than for any other major cause of death except HIV infection. By the early 1990s, deaths from COPD had risen to about 85,000 a year, and the death rate was nearly five times higher than it was in 1950 (USDHHS, 1994b). Reasons for this increase are not completely clear, but the risk for COPD increases with cigarette smoking (Gross, 1994).

Chronic obstructive pulmonary disease is relatively rare among nonsmokers. Only 4% of male nonsmokers and 5% of female nonsmokers receive a diagnosis of COPD (Whitemore, Perlin, & DiCiccio, 1995), with 85% of COPD mortality in men and 60% of COPD deaths among women attributable to smoking. Nonsmokers who live with spouses who smoke are at slightly increased risk for chronic obstructive pulmonary disease.

In summary, the three leading causes of death in the United States are also the three principal smoking-related causes of death. Nearly half of all deaths from cardiovascular disease, lung cancer, and chronic obstructive pulmonary disease are cigarette related, and the U. S. Public Health Service has estimated that about half of all cigarette smokers will eventually die from their habit (USDHHS, 1995).

Other Effects of Smoking

In addition to heart disease, cancer, and chronic obstructive pulmonary disease, a number of other diseases and disorders have been linked to smoking. For example, smoking is related to the recurrence of ulcers (Gugler, Rohner, Kratochvil, Branditätter, & Schmitz, 1982; Sontag et al., 1984); smoking is associated with diseases of the mouth, including periodontal disease (Ismail, Burt, & Eklund, 1983); smokers have less physical strength, poorer balance, and more impaired neuromuscular performance compared with nonsmokers (Nelson, Nevitt, Scott, Stone, & Cummings, 1994); and female smokers have about twice the chance of developing ovarian cysts than nonsmoking women (Holt et al., 1994). Cohen, Tyrrell, Russell, Jarvis, and Smith (1993) intentionally exposed people to respiratory viruses and found that smokers are at greater risk than non-

smokers for developing the common cold; and Hopper and Seeman (1994) studied female twins and found that women who smoke at least one pack of cigarettes a day throughout adulthood have a 5% to 10% deficit in bone density, sufficient to increase the risk of bone fractures. In addition to these diseases and disorders, smoking may be linked to at least two other rather unpleasant problems (see box — Would You Believe . . . ?).

Smokers are also ill more often than nonsmokers, and the effects of these illnesses are not limited to individual smokers. Society, too, pays a price. The Public Health Service estimated that smoking-related illnesses cost the nation $50 billion in 1993 in direct costs and another $47 billion in indirect costs (USDHHS, 1995). The frequency of acute illness is 14% higher for male smokers and 21% higher for female smokers than for nonsmokers. Men who smoke lose 33% more workdays than men who do not smoke, and women who smoke miss work 45% more often than women who do not smoke (USDHHS, 1989). In addition, the Centers for Disease Control and Prevention (CDC, 1994c) reported that young people who smoke are less physically fit, more prone to coughing spells, and are more likely to develop early atherosclerotic lesions than their counterparts who do not smoke. In summary, smokers have a much higher mortality rate than nonsmokers, suffer from more nonfatal illnesses, and are more likely to develop chronic illnesses that eventually kill them.

DOES QUITTING HELP?

From 1965 to 1991, the prevalence of former smokers doubled, from 24% to 48% (National Center for Health Statistics, 1994), and evidence by Fielding (1985) strongly suggests that quitting pays off. Fielding estimated that the average reduction in life expectancy for smokers is 5 to 8 years, depending on the amount of smoking. Can smokers regain some of their life expectancy by quitting? How long must ex-smokers remain abstinent before they reverse the detrimental effects of smoking?

The 1990 report of the Surgeon General summarized studies indicating that former light smokers (fewer than 20 cigarettes a day) who are able to abstain for 16 years have about the same rate of mortality as people who have never smoked (USDHHS,

WOULD YOU BELIEVE . . . ?

Smoking, Ugliness, and Impotence

Would you believe that smoking may cause ugliness in women and impotence in men? Actually, cigarette smoking may result in ugliness in both women and men, according to studies published during the past 25 to 30 years.

In 1992, Deborah Grady and Virginia Ernster published an article in the *American Journal of Epidemiology* called Does Smoking Make You Ugly and Old?" They reviewed five earlier studies that had investigated the relationship between smoking and facial wrinkles. Despite the attempt of tobacco companies to portray smokers as young, healthy, and sexually attractive, with clear, smooth skin, the reality is quite different. Ample evidence suggests that cigarettes may cause smokers to appear old, unhealthy, sexually unattractive, and with gray, wrinkled skin. Grady and Ernster cited an earlier study that had defined "cigarette skin" as pale, grayish, and wrinkled, with thick skin between the wrinkles. One study examined only women and found that 79% of smokers had "cigarette skin," but only 19% of the nonsmokers fit that description.

Some of the studies on facial wrinkling had used a 6-point scale for categorizing wrinkles (Daniell, 1971). On this scale, observers look at pictures of people's faces and rate them from 1 to 6, with higher scores indicating many wrinkles and lower scores few wrinkles. Grady and Ernster cited a study using Daniell's scale and found that smokers were five times more likely than non-smokers to have high scores. Moreover, the greater the number of cigarettes smoked per day and the more years of smoking, the more likely they were to be heavily wrinkled. This study controlled for age, sun exposure, and skin pigmentation and still found smokers to be much more likely to appear old and ugly.

European American smokers may be more susceptible to wrinkling and aging than African American smokers. One study found that European American smokers were a great deal more likely than European American nonsmokers to have crow's feet, wrinkled foreheads, and wrinkled cheeks. These differences held true even when the investigators controlled for other factors. However, the difference between African American smokers and African American nonsmokers was not significant.

Grady and Ernster hypothesized that smoking dries and irritates the skin and thus promotes wrinkling, giving smokers the appearance of being old and unattractive. They suggested that the many toxic components in cigarettes are absorbed into the body and may cause vascular changes or connective tissue damage. Also, they cited evidence that smoking decreases blood flow in the skin. In addition, smoking causes chronic squinting, leading to premature aging.

In 1995, Ernster and Grady, along with their associates (Ernster et al., 1995) reported on their own cross-sectional study of smokers and current smokers 40 years old and older. After controlling for sun exposure and body mass index, these investigators found that current male smokers were 2.3 times more likely than male nonsmokers to have moderate to severe facial wrinkling, and current female smokers were 3.1 times more likely than female nonsmokers to have substantial facial wrinkling. These investigators also found a dose-response relationship between number of lifetime cigarettes smoked and amount of wrinkling. Ernster et al. estimated that smoking added about 1.4 years of aging to the appearance of smokers. Grady and Ernster (1992, p. 92) concluded their review by saying that "American women spend more than $7 billion

per year on over 20,000 different cosmetics promoting youth and beauty." With many Americans devoted to maintaining a youthful appearance, the evidence that smoking causes aging and ugliness might be used to persuade young people not to start smoking and to motivate current smokers to quit.

Male smokers may receive a double dose of undesirable side effects from cigarettes. Smoking may make them old and less attractive in appearance and impotent in sexual performance. David Mannino, R. Monina Klevens, and W. Dana Flanders (1994) conducted a survey of U.S. Army Vietnam-era veterans to learn whether smoking was linked to sexual impotence. Participants in this survey ranged in age from 31 to 49, with a mean age of 38. The researchers found that about 2.2% of men who had never smoked were impotent whereas 3.7% of current smokers had had "persistent difficulty in getting a satisfactory erection for sexual purposes within the past year" (Mannino et al., 1994, p. 1004). This 80% greater chance of impotence among smokers dipped to 50% when the researchers adjusted to such confounds as vascular disease, psychiatric disease, hormonal factors, substance abuse, marital status, ethnicity, and age. Nevertheless, a 50% greater risk for impotence among smokers represents a significant number of men who might not have been impotent had they not been smokers. Does quitting help? In this study men who quit smoking actually had a lower rate of impotence than men who had never smoked!

The studies seem to be sending these messages: If you don't want to appear old and ugly and if you are a man who wants to retain sexual functioning, stay away from smoking!

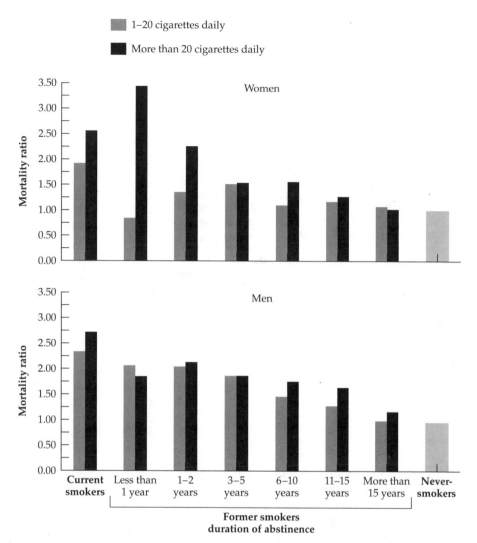

Figure 13.6 *Overall mortality ratios for current and former smokers compared with never smokers, by sex and duration of abstinence.* SOURCE: *The Health Benefits of Smoking Cessation: A Report of the Surgeon General* (p. 78) by U.S. Department of Health and Human Services, 1990 (DHHS Publication No. CDC 90-8416), Washington, DC: U.S. Government Printing Office.

1990b). This encouraging finding was true for both women and men (see Figure 13.6). For women who were heavy smokers (more than 20 cigarettes a day), the benefits of quitting were substantial, especially after the third year of abstinence. Women who were light smokers seemed to have benefited almost immediately from quitting, and by the 16th year of abstinence they had the same mortality rate as women who had never smoked. So Lisa, the smoker de-

scribed in the introduction to this chapter who smokes 20 cigarettes or fewer a day, could eventually reduce her risk of death to a level about equal to what it would have been if she had never smoked.

Figure 13.6 shows that men who are heavy smokers have a risk of death 2.73 times greater than those who have never smoked. But those who can quit show a steady reduction in mortality rate after the first year of abstinence if they have not already developed some smoking-related condition. After 16 years without smoking, men have reduced their mortality risk to about half that of current smokers and only slightly more than nonsmokers. Men who were formerly light smokers do even better after 16 years of abstinence, and they have about the same relative risk as men who have never smoked. For those with cancer, heart disease, or stroke, the benefits of quitting do not show up until 3 years of abstinence. This lack of initial improvement is probably due to the fact that many sick people quit in the years immediately before they die (USDHHS, 1990b). For relatively healthy people, however, some types of risk dissipate quickly. For example, women who stopped smoking decreased their risk of heart attack within 3 years of quitting (Rosenberg, Palmer, & Shapiro, 1990).

Long-time smokers who quit reduce their chances of dying from heart disease much more than they lower their risk of death from lung cancer. Several studies have shown that cigarette smokers who quit can eventually reduce their risk of cardiovascular disease to that of a nonsmoker, but that their risk of cancer, especially lung cancer, remains elevated. For example, men who quit smoking for 30 years had only a very slightly elevated risk of coronary heart disease, but these same men had nearly a threefold risk for lung cancer (Ben-Shlomo, Smith, Shipley, & Marmot, 1994). However, this increased risk of lung cancer for former smokers was less than one-fourth the risk of men who continued smoking. Thus, men who quit smoking for 30 years reduce their risk of both cardiovascular disease and lung cancer, but their risk for lung cancer remains substantially higher than that of men who have never smoked. Women also reduce their risks by quitting. The excess risk of stroke disappears in middle-aged women who stop smoking after 2 to 4 years of not smoking, regardless of the number of cigarettes they had smoked, the age at which they had started, or the presence of other stroke risk factors (Kawachi et al., 1993). These studies suggest that by quitting smoking, both male and female smokers can reduce their risk of cardiovascular disease to that of nonsmokers, although they may never completely erase their elevated risk of lung cancer. Never starting to smoke is healthier than quitting, but quitting can pay off. However, quitting is seldom easy. Later, we dis-

cuss several methods of quitting and evaluate their effectiveness.

CIGAR AND PIPE SMOKING

In the United States, cigar and pipe smoking are limited almost exclusively to men. In 1991, less than 0.5% of women smoked either cigars or pipes (Givovino et al., 1994) but men too have been lowering their rates for both cigar and pipe smoking. Men who quit cigarette smoking do not seem to be switching to cigars or pipes in substantial numbers. In fact, the rates for cigar and pipe smoking have declined much faster than the rate for cigarette smoking. In 1970, 16.3% of men in the United States smoked cigars; in 1991, that rated had dropped to 3.5%. The comparable rates for pipe smokers was 13.1% and 2.0% (Givovino et al., 1994).

Are cigar and pipe smoking as hazardous as cigarette smoking? The tobacco used in pipes and cigars differs somewhat from the tobacco used to make cigarettes, but pipe and cigar tobacco is similarly carcinogenic. The risk to pipe and cigar smokers, however, is not as elevated as it is for cigarette smokers because pipe and cigar smokers do not inhale smoke as much as cigarette smokers. Lubin et al. (1984) examined the relative risk of cigarette, cigar, and pipe smokers for developing lung cancer. The relative risk for those who smoked only cigarettes was 9.0, indicating that cigarette smokers were nine times more likely than nonsmokers to die from lung cancer. In comparison, those who smoked only cigars had a risk of 2.9 and those who smoked only pipes had a 2.5 elevation in their risk for lung cancer. However, the combination of cigars or pipes with cigarettes dramatically increased the relative risk for lung cancer. The combination of cigars and cigarettes yielded a rate of 6.9, whereas the combination of pipes and cigarettes raised the relative risk to 8.1, a rate nearly as high as cigarettes alone. These researchers found no elevation in risk for lung cancer for either cigar or pipe smokers who had never inhaled. In summary, cigar and pipe smoking may be less hazardous than cigarettes, but they are not safe.

PASSIVE SMOKING

Whereas few doubt that smoking contributes to a higher probability of premature death from heart disease or cancer, authorities are still somewhat divided on hazards of breathing other people's smoke. Many nonsmokers find the smoke of others to be a nuisance and even irritating to their eyes and nose. But is this **passive smoking**, also known as **environmental tobacco smoke (ETS)** or secondhand smoke, harmful to the health of nonsmokers? In the 1980s, some evidence began to accrue that passive smoking might be a health hazard. Specifically, passive smoking has been linked to lung cancer, heart disease, and a variety of respiratory problems in children.

Passive Smoking and Lung Cancer

Research on the excess risk for lung cancer for passive smokers reveals a slight but consistent relationship between nonsmokers' exposure to the smoke of others and their likelihood of developing lung cancer. In 1990, Wu reviewed earlier epidemiological studies on the relationship between passive smoking and lung cancer and found that 18 of 23 studies failed to find a significant effect. A meta-analysis by Wu (1990) revealed a statistically significant but slightly elevated relative risk of 1.34 for lung cancer in people exposed to environmental tobacco smoke.

Later studies have found either a slight risk or no additional risk for lung cancer in people exposed to environmental tobacco smoke. In a case-control study comparing female lung cancer patients with a group of controls (Brownson, Alavanja, Hock, & Loy, 1992), the cases consisted of lung cancer patients who had never smoked and former smokers who had stopped for at least 15 years. No increased risk of lung cancer appeared for women who were exposed to passive smoking as a child, but women whose adult exposure to cigarettes placed them in the highest quartile had an excess risk of lung cancer of 30%. Although any excess risk of lung cancer is too much, only those women in the top one-fourth of smoke exposure experienced that much risk. A large-scale study by Fontham et al. (1994) found a 30% excess risk for nonsmoking women 65 and older whose husbands were smokers. This study also confirmed results from earlier studies that being exposed to smoking parents during childhood was *not* significantly related to later lung cancer. A review of earlier studies (Siegel, 1993a) showed that high levels of exposure may contribute, in part, to a 50% increase in lung cancer among food-service

employees working in bars and restaurants that permit smoking, but another study (Kabat, Stellman, & Wynder, 1995) found no increased risk for lung cancer in lifetime nonsmokers exposed to environmental tobacco smoke. In addition, another recent study (Matanoski, Kanchanaraksa, Lantry, & Chang, 1995) found that nonsmokers exposed to ETS had other characteristics that may have placed them at risk for lung cancer. For example, nonsmoking wives exposed to ETS, compared with those not exposed, tended to be older, had less education, lived in a larger city, consumed more alcohol, ate less nutritious foods, and consumed fewer dietary vitamin supplements. Each of these factors carries some risk of poorer health and some may contribute to a higher risk of lung cancer.

These studies suggest that passive smoking may contribute to a slight additional risk for lung cancer, possibly as high as 30%. Relative risks of this magnitude should be interpreted with reference to the prevalence of the disease within the comparison group—in this case, nonsmokers who are not exposed to cigarette smoke. Because lung cancer in this comparison group is quite rare, an elevated risk of 30% for nonsmokers exposed to environmental tobacco smoke does not add a great number of nonsmokers to the lung cancer mortality rates. In summary, environmental tobacco smoke may contribute slightly to lung cancer rates, but evidence for any direct, independent contribution is still extremely weak.

Passive Smoking and Heart Disease

Much of the early debate on the toxicity of environmental tobacco smoke centered on lung cancer, but more recent attention has focused on heart disease, which claims many more deaths per year from passive smoking. Several studies (Helsing, Sandler, Comstock, & Chee, 1988; Humble et al., 1990) found no large excess risk of heart disease for passive smokers. However, even a small elevated risk translates into thousands of unnecessary deaths each year in the United States because a large number of people in the comparison group (which consists of nonsmokers who are not exposed to ETS) die of heart disease. This risk contrasts with the risk of lung cancer, which kills relatively few nonsmokers who are not exposed to environmental tobacco smoke.

How does passive smoking contribute to heart disease? Glantz and Parmley (1995) offered four hypotheses. First, passive smoking reduces the blood's ability to deliver oxygen to the heart, making the heart less efficient; second, passive smoking increases platelet activity; third, it increases tissue damage following ischemic heart disease or a myocardial infarction; and fourth, passive smoking may reduce people's ability to exercise. A fifth possibility was suggested by a recent study on passive smoking and healthy young adults (Calermajer et al., 1996). In this study, researchers found more early signs of artery disease in 15- to 30-year-old nonsmokers who had been exposed to environmental tobacco smoke for at least 3 years than in a comparable group of nonsmokers who had not been exposed to passive smoking. Thus, environmental tobacco smoke may have several mechanisms through which it produces cardiovascular damage.

In 1992, Steenland reviewed nine earlier studies that had investigated the relative risk of passive smoking on ischemic heart disease. Results of these individual studies were somewhat mixed, although most showed a slight but significant excess risk of heart disease for people forced to breathe the smoke of others. Of the nine studies, seven yielded positive results, one was negative, and one was positive for women but not for men. Steenland's review prompted him to speculate that environmental tobacco smoke accounts for 35,000 to 40,000 deaths from ischemic heart disease per year in the United States for those who have never smoked and for former smokers who had quit for at least 5 years. Although the relative risk of passive smoking for heart disease is about the same as it is for lung cancer (1.3 to 1.5), environmental tobacco smoke claims far more victims from heart disease than from lung cancer. Steenland (1992) estimated that passive smoking kills less than one-tenth as many people through lung cancer as it does through heart disease.

In summary, exposure to environmental tobacco smoke presents a much greater relative risk of death from heart disease than from lung cancer. With both illnesses, however, the risk from passive smoking is far less than the risk from active smoking. Sandler, Comstock, Helsing, and Shore (1989) found the increases in the all-cause mortality rates were 1.17 for men and 1.15 for women, rates that are only slightly above those of nonsmokers who are not exposed to ETS. In summarizing research on environmental tobacco smoke, Wu (1990, p. 375) stated that "the published data, when critically examined and evaluated, are inconsistent with the notion that ETS is a health hazard."

Passive Smoking and the Health of Children

Infants are possibly the people at greatest risk from environmental tobacco. The 1984 Surgeon General's report, which concentrated on chronic obstructive pulmonary diseases, cited a study that found babies of smokers to have a greater incidence of respiratory symptoms of bronchitis and pneumonia than babies in nonsmoking households (USDHHS, 1984a). More recently, Stoddard and Miller (1995) found that children whose mothers smoked had an increased risk of wheezing respiratory illness and that the risk was especially high for children younger than 2 years old. Stoddard and Miller estimated that maternal smoking is responsible for about 380,000 excess cases of childhood asthma and lower respiratory tract illnesses per year, a number that represent about 7.5% of the total of such symptoms. Moreover, the symptoms of children with existing cases of asthma are more likely to be exacerbated if their parents smoke (Chimonczyk et al., 1993). In addition to respiratory illness, environmental tobacco smoke is associated with low birth weight (Martin & Bracken, 1986), sudden infant death (Haglund & Cnattingius, 1990), and childhood cancers (John, Savitz, & Sandler, 1991). However, the negative effects of environmental tobacco smoke diminish as children pass the age of 2 years (Wu, 1990).

In summary, passive smoking has been associated with a number of respiratory problems in children under the age of two. Moreover, some evidence exists that environmental tobacco smoke may be a risk factor for other health conditions in young children.

WHY DO PEOPLE SMOKE?

Despite widespread publicity linking cigarette smoking to a variety of health problems, millions of people continue to smoke. That fact is puzzling because many smokers themselves acknowledge the potential dangers of their habit. The question of why peo-

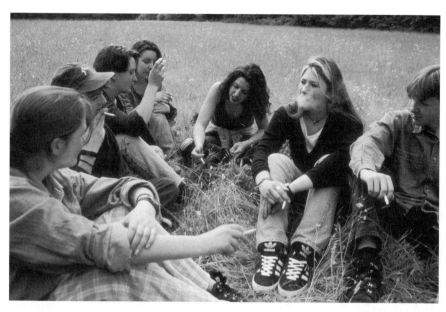

Acceptance into a social group can be a powerful source of reinforcement for adolescents, increasing the pressure to begin smoking.

ple smoke can be divided into two separate ones. Why do people begin to smoke and why do they continue? Answers to the first question are difficult because most young people are aware of the hazards of smoking. The best answer to the second question seems to be that different people smoke for different reasons, and the same person may smoke for different reasons in different situations.

WHY DO PEOPLE START SMOKING?

Most young people are aware of the hazards of smoking (Zuckerman, Ball, & Black, 1990), yet many of them begin smoking each year. Why do young people start smoking after they have learned of the dangers of this practice? One possible explanation is that most teenage smokers believe they will no longer be smoking in 5 years (USDHEW, 1979). Therefore, they do not believe that the health hazards will apply to them because those hazards are generally the results of long-term exposure. Because teenagers tend to be oriented to the present, threats about the long-term health hazards of smoking are neither an effective way to persuade them not to begin smoking nor a good strategy to convince them to stop.

Leventhal and Cleary (1980) hypothesized that teenagers may begin smoking for any one of three different reasons: tension control, rebelliousness, or social pressure. Many teenagers start smoking because cigarettes are associated with the image of rebelliousness and independence (Mittelmark et al., 1987). Another hypothesized reason for starting smoking is social pressure. Leventhal and Cleary (1980) said that some teenagers are especially sensitive to social pressure and may start smoking if they have friends who smoke. A great deal of research evidence supports this contention. Indeed, having friends who smoke is a strong predictor of experimentation with cigarettes (Mittelmark et al., 1987). In addition, the perceived smoking behavior of friends was a strong predictor of smoking onset in teenagers. Peers influence teenage smokers to continue by offering cigarettes; teenagers who smoked received 26 times more offers of cigarettes than teenagers who were nonsmokers (Ary & Biglan, 1988). One study (Stanton, Mahalski, McGee, & Silva, 1993) showed that "image" was an important reason for smoking among 11-year-olds, and that peers, relaxation, and pleasure were other reasons young adolescents gave for smoking. In addition, peer and parental smoking influences young adolescents not only in the use of tobacco but also in the use of alcohol and marijuana (Hansen et al., 1987).

Not all peer groups are equally in favor of smoking, according to Mosbach and Leventhal (1988). In their interviews, junior high school students identified four different peer groups. The "dirtballs" were boys who smoked, used other drugs, were poor students, and had other personal or school-related problems. The "hotshots" were mainly girls who were popular and successful students, and the "jocks" were mainly boys who were interested in organized sports. The last group, the "regulars," were students who did not belong to any of these groups and were typical students. Mosbach and Leventhal found that the "dirtballs" and the "hotshots" made up only 15% of their sample but accounted for 56% of the smokers. The attitudes and attractions of smoking differed in the two groups. The "dirtballs" were typically smokers before they entered junior high school and were attracted to one another and the behavior of the group because of the satisfaction of excitement and danger. The "hotshots," on the other hand, experimented with smoking during junior high school because of peer pressure and a need for acceptance and excitement. Unlike the "dirtballs," who were unconcerned with the dangers of smoking, these girls were worried about smoking's hazards. This study explored the complexities of peer pressure and peer acceptance in the initiation and maintenance of smoking in young adolescents. Its findings demonstrate that the motivations of teenagers differ with respect to smoking and suggest that smoking prevention efforts must be varied to succeed with young adolescents.

The evidence on the influence of social surroundings and smoking has led to a consensus on the importance of situational factors. The 1989 U.S. Surgeon General's report (USDHHS, 1989) suggested that situational factors are more important than personality factors in the initiation of smoking. Teenagers with smoking parents are more likely to start, although some controversy exists over which parent is more critical as an influence. Those with older siblings who smoke are more likely to start. Teenage boys who start smoking are very likely to have friends who smoke, and teenage girls who start are likely to have boyfriends who smoke.

Many young women and girls (especially Whites and Hispanics) begin smoking as a means of weight control. A survey of mostly European American, upper-middle class students in grades 7 to 10 (French, Perry, Leon, & Fulkerson, 1994) found that weight concerns were related to smoking initiation for girls but not for boys. Girls were most likely to begin smoking if they had (1) two or more eating disorder symptoms, (2) a history of attempts at weight loss during the past year, (3) a fear of weight gain, and (4) a strong wish to be thin. Girls who reported any one of these behaviors or concerns were about twice as likely as other girls to be current smokers.

Once young people begin to smoke they quickly become dependent on the habit. The Centers for Disease Control and Prevention (CDC, 1994d) surveyed young smokers 10 to 22 years old and found that nearly two-thirds of these young people who had smoked at least 100 cigarettes during their lifetime reported that "It's really hard to quit," but only a small number of young people who had smoked fewer than 100 lifetime cigarettes gave this response. In addition, nearly 90% of young people who smoked more than 15 cigarettes a day found quitting to be very hard. These results suggest that once people have smoked about 100 cigarettes or have increased their daily cigarette consumption to more than 15 per day, they have become dependent on smoking and will have great difficulty quitting.

WHY DO PEOPLE CONTINUE TO SMOKE?

Research into why people smoke suggests that no single explanation is satisfactory and that different people probably smoke for different reasons. Much of this research can be traced to theoretical work by Tomkins (1966, 1968), who hypothesized four different types of smoking behavior: habitual, positive affect, negative affect, and addictive.

Habitual smokers are those who smoke with little awareness and little reward. These smokers probably began smoking either to increase positive affect or to reduce negative affect, but they continue as a matter of habit. Often they are unaware that they have lit a cigarette. *Positive affect* smokers seek to increase stimulation, to bring about a feeling of relaxation, or to gratify sensorimotor needs. *Negative affect* smokers, on the other hand, smoke to reduce feelings of anxiety, distress, fear, guilt, and so forth. Theoretically, negative affect smokers should smoke more during periods of stress and less while relaxed.

Lisa, our case study seems to be a negative affect smoker. She started smoking as a reaction to an emotional confrontation with a co-worker, then, after quitting for 3 weeks, she relapsed when she became angry with her boss. Unlike habitual smokers, *addictive* smokers are not only aware of smoking but are also keenly conscious of the fact that they are *not* smoking. They usually know how long it has been since their last cigarette and how long it will be before their next one. Addictive smokers are those who never leave home or office without first checking their supply of cigarettes. They often keep several extra packs available in case of emergency.

Research has tended to support Tomkins's notion that types of smoking behavior are somewhat separate and distinct. In a study using factor analysis (Ikard, Green, & Horn, 1969), six rather than four types of smoking behavior appeared. In addition to habitual, addictive, and negative affect smokers, this analysis showed three kinds of positive affect smoking: pleasurable relaxation, stimulation, and sensorimotor manipulation (the fiddle factor). Only two factors, addiction and negative affect, showed any marked correlation to each other. Thus this research supported the views that there is no simple reason that people smoke and that individual differences play a role in explaining smoking behavior.

In another factor analytic study, Zuckerman, Ball, and Black (1990) identified five factors related to reasons for smoking. The first factor, *Attentive-Coping,* refers to smokers who light up when they must attend to a complicated task or help someone who is emotionally upset. *Negative Emotionality* describes people who smoke when emotionally upset, anxious, angry, or depressed. Lisa tends to smoke more when she is emotionally upset. The third strongest factor was *Alone-Relaxed,* which relates to people who enjoy smoking when they are relaxed, having a restful time alone, reading, and so forth. Factor 4, *Social Situations,* is defined by people who smoke more while at a party or with friends, especially if they are drinking alcohol. The final factor is *Heavy Smoking,* which includes people who are strongly dependent on smoking and may use cigarettes as a negative reinforcer to relieve withdrawal symptoms. These people smoke when first getting out of bed in the morning, or even before leaving their bed, and they use smoking both to increase or to decrease emotional arousal. One-third of the

smokers in a survey (Jarvik, Killen, Varady, & Fortmann, 1993) rated the first cigarette in the morning as their favorite cigarette of the day. A strong relationship also appeared between nicotine dependence and likelihood of choosing the first cigarette of the day as the favorite, a finding suggesting that nicotine-dependent smokers need a "fix" after being without cigarettes for several hours during the night.

Because smokers tend to have different reasons for smoking, Leventhal and Avis (1976) have argued that smoking cessation programs should be tailored to fit the individual smoker. Using Tomkins's original model, Leventhal and Avis identified three different mechanisms that sustain smoking behavior: pleasure-taste, addiction, and habit. In one experiment, Leventhal and Avis affected the taste of cigarettes by dipping them in vinegar, allowing them to dry, and then repackaging them. They gave these adulterated cigarettes to smokers who had scored high on the pleasure-taste scale, predicting that these smokers should be more affected by the change in taste than those who had scored high on the addiction scale. The results turned out as predicted. Pleasure-taste smokers decreased their smoking when they had to smoke the vinegar-dipped cigarettes, but the addiction smokers smoked just as many of the bad-tasting cigarettes as they did their normal brand. In addition, Leventhal and Avis identified smokers who scored high on the habit scale and contrasted their behavior with those high on pleasure-taste. To make smokers more aware of their smoking, they were asked to keep a record of when they smoked. Simply keeping a record made a difference in smoking rate for the habit smokers but not the pleasure-taste smokers. In yet another phase of the experiment, Leventhal and Avis deprived high-addiction smokers of cigarettes and found that they reported more distress than those scoring low on the addiction scale. However, the high-addiction smokers did not show a greater postdeprivation smoking rate than low-addiction smokers.

In conclusion, a combination of Tomkins's theoretical model and the factor analytic studies would suggest that people smoke for at least four or five basic reasons. Some people smoke for relaxation and pleasure; some smoke as a reaction to negative emotion; some smoke as a reaction to environmental cues, such as alcohol or other people smoking; and some people seem to be nicotine-dependent and must smoke to avoid the unpleasant symptoms of nicotine withdrawal.

MODELS TO EXPLAIN SMOKING BEHAVIOR

Several theoretical models have been proposed to explain smoking behavior. This section looks at two of these models: the nicotine addiction model and the social learning model. To be useful, these models should be able to predict who will begin to smoke and who will continue.

The Nicotine Addiction Model

The nicotine addiction model holds that people continue to smoke to maintain an adequate level of nicotine and to prevent withdrawal symptoms from occurring. The model thus offers a better explanation for maintenance of the smoking habit than for its initiation.

If the nicotine addiction model is valid, smokers should smoke a greater number of low-nicotine than high-nicotine cigarettes. Stanley Schachter (1980) tested this hypothesis by supplying heavy, long-duration smokers with cigarettes that alternately, over several weeks, were high or low in nicotine. The cigarettes all looked the same, and the participants did not know how much nicotine they would be ingesting. The different nicotine levels made a difference in smoking rates for every participant. On the average, they smoked 25% more low-nicotine than high-nicotine cigarettes. In another experiment in the series, Schachter measured the number of puffs taken from low- and high-nicotine cigarettes. Smokers took more puffs from low-nicotine cigarettes than from ones high in nicotine. Both experiments indicated that smokers are able to regulate the amount of nicotine they ingest, even when that amount is not directly related to the number of cigarettes smoked.

The nicotine addiction model does not explain why people start to smoke or why some people smoke and others do not. It also fails to explain why some people are light smokers and others smoke heavily. If nicotine were the only reason for smoking, other modes of nicotine delivery should substitute fully for smoking. Evidence, however, indicates that other delivery methods are not entirely satisfactory to smokers. Experiments with administering nicotine through the nicotine patch (Kenford et al.,

1994), intravenously (Lucchesi, Schuster, & Emley, 1967), and with nicotine chewing gum (Hughes, Gust, Keenan, Fenwick, & Healey, 1989) indicate that although smokers may decrease smoking when nicotine is available through other modes, they still have difficulty stopping smoking. Also, smokers prefer cigarettes with nicotine to those without, but if only nonnicotine cigarettes are available, smokers still will smoke them (Jarvik, 1977). Although nicotine may play a role in the maintenance of smoking, these findings indicate that something other than nicotine is involved.

The Social Learning Model

A second model of smoking is based on social learning theory. According to this model, people learn patterns of behavior (including smoking) because they are reinforced in some manner for those behaviors (Bandura, 1977; Rotter, 1982; Skinner, 1953). How can smoking become acquired behavior, given that many smokers report negative consequences of their initial attempts at smoking? One's first cigarette is often followed by coughing, dizziness, watering eyes, and even nausea. Why would anyone continue a behavior that is associated with so many negative consequences? The answer is that for those who do continue (and many do not), the reinforcement value of smoking outweighs all these negative aspects.

Most smokers begin smoking during adolescence, a time when peer pressure is often quite strong. Also, most who begin at a young age smoke their first cigarettes in the presence of peers. The positive reinforcement of being accepted or of being "cool" may easily outweigh the unpleasant aspects of one's first attempt at smoking. In addition, initial smoking may be negatively reinforcing if it removes unpleasant stimuli, such as the fear of being regarded as "nerdy" or "chicken." Also, many people do not inhale when they first begin to smoke, thus avoiding many of the aversive stimuli. In any event, the aversive effects of first inhalation of smoke are outweighed by some form of positive consequences.

With practice, the aversive consequences of smoking are lessened so that there are few, if any, immediate negative effects of smoking. This situation is potentially dangerous because beginning smokers do not feel the long-range negative effects on their health. The smoking habit is therefore maintained because it continues to relieve tension or to be reinforcing in other ways.

Social learning theory is able to explain the initiation of smoking and also offers a suitable explanation of why people continue to smoke. Once smokers become addicted, they must continue to smoke to receive the rewarding effects of a stimulant drug and especially to avoid the aversive effects of withdrawal.

The nicotine addiction model and the social learning model both offer explanations for why people begin smoking and why they continue. A combination of these two models yields a useful explanation for both the initiation and the maintenance of the smoking habit.

METHODS OF REDUCING SMOKING RATES

In view of the evidence that cigarette smoking is potentially life threatening, people should have ample motivation to refrain from smoking—either to quit or never begin. However, considering the positive and negative reinforcement offered by smoking, overcoming the temptation to start and especially breaking an established smoking habit should be quite difficult. Programs designed to reduce smoking rates can be divided into those that deter people (usually adolescents) from beginning and those that encourage current smokers to stop.

DETERRING SMOKING

As we discussed in Chapter 12, information alone is not an effective way to change behavior, and the research on smoking prevention substantiates this lack of effect. Neither the warning messages on cigarettes packages nor educational programs aimed at providing young people with information on the hazards of smoking are very effective in deterring adolescents from smoking. Adolescents pay little attention to the health warnings that appear on cigarette packages, and these legally mandated warnings are not an effective means of informing adolescents about the dangers of smoking (Fischer, Richards, Berman, & Krugman, 1989). As for information-based programs, the Surgeon General's report of 1989 con-

cluded that most educational programs are not very successful in preventing smoking, although they do solidify negative attitudes toward smoking. In addition, Thompson (1978) found that smoking prevention programs that use lectures, posters, pamphlets, articles in school newspapers, and so forth were almost universally ineffective in preventing young people from starting to smoke.

Why are these attempts at deterring smoking ineffective? Perhaps it is because many young smokers possess an *optimistic bias*—that is, a belief that negative consequences will affect others but not them (Weinstein, 1984). A study by Brannon and Papadimitriou (1985) indicated that college-age smokers tended to have an optimistic bias. Smokers in this study rated themselves as no different from the average college student for their risk of developing lung cancer and rated their risk of heart disease and bronchitis/emphysema as somewhat less likely than that of the average college student. Because smoking elevates the chances of developing all three disorders, these ratings were unrealistically optimistic. A later study with younger participants found that sixth graders also had an optimistic bias concerning several health and environmental risks, including smoking (Whalen et al., 1994).

Procedures aimed at buffering young adolescents against the social pressures to smoke have been more effective than educational programs. These techniques, usually called "inoculation" programs, are based on the same concepts as the stress inoculation programs discussed in Chapter 6. These programs use a model of social influence, referring to influences from the social environment as the source of both encouragement to begin and strength to refuse smoking. Such programs are based on the notion that young adolescents can be "inoculated" against social pressures emanating from parents, older siblings, and peers who model smoking behavior as well as from the media (including tobacco advertisements) that encourage cigarette smoking. This social pressure is analogous to a disease, and the therapy program is comparable to inoculation because it intervenes with small amounts of the disease rather than trying to cure an established disorder.

Several teams of researchers have had some success in deterring teenagers from smoking by using other young people as models. One program was developed by Richard Evans and his colleagues at the University of Houston (Evans, 1976; Evans et al., 1978; Evans et al., 1981; Evans, Smith, & Raines, 1984). Evans and his colleagues developed a multidimensional program designed to increase feelings of self-esteem, provide information on the negative aspects of smoking, increase skills for coping with social influences to smoke, strengthen feelings of self-efficacy, and reward any behavioral steps in the direction of resisting social pressure. The innovative aspect of this program, however, was the use of films in which other teenagers were depicted using persuasive communication to counter arguments in favor of smoking. In these films, the teenage models are shown encountering and resisting social pressure to smoke and also transmitting information regarding the immediate and the long-term negative consequences of smoking. Evans et al. (1981) reported promising results for this approach in a 3-year follow-up of a program conducted in the Houston public schools. Participation in the program appeared to give young adolescents the skills to be more successful at resisting urges to begin smoking.

In a similar program, Murray, Richards, Luepker, and Johnson (1987) found that a peer-led program designed to build skills to counteract social pressure to smoke was successful in restraining smoking immediately and also at a 2-year follow-up. After 4 years, some effects for the program persisted (Murray, Davis-Hearn, Goldman, Pirie, & Luepker, 1988). Also, Penty et al. (1989) found that a multicomponent community program designed to delay the onset of cigarette smoking was successful at follow-ups as long as 2 years after the termination of the program. The results from this study and others using similar programs indicate that when teenagers are buffered against possible media and peer pressure, they are more successful at resisting the temptation to begin smoking.

Although the immediate results seemed promising and follow-ups after 2 and 4 years demonstrated effectiveness for such programs, long-term follow-up data have not been so positive. Flay et al. (1989) reported on a 6-year follow-up of a smoking prevention program that used the social influence model. Although the program had produced differences during the first 2 years, the 6-year follow-up found no differences in smoking rates during the senior year in high school for children who had received the experimental intervention during the sixth grade and those who had received the regular health education program. Another program also found effects for a smoking prevention program immediately after the intervention and at a 4-year follow-up but failed to find differences in smoking after 8 years (Vartianen, Fallonen, McAlister, & Puska, 1990). Similarly, the program that demonstrated lower rates of smoking when participants were tested both 2 and 4 years afterward (Murray, Davis-Hearn, et al., 1988; Murray, Richards, et al., 1987) failed to show effects after 6 years (Murray, Pirie, Luepker, & Pallonen, 1989).

The diminishing influence of these programs may be due to changes in the social environment for young people 5 or 6 years after they participated in the program. Perhaps the skills that are effective in the sixth grade are no longer effective for juniors or seniors in high school, or perhaps the increase in positive attitudes toward smoking that occurs during early adolescence plays a role (Dinh, Sarason, Peterson, & Onstad, 1995). As Murray et al. (1989) suggested, some type of "booster" session may counteract the decline in effectiveness of these programs, or other types of interventions for older adolescents may be necessary.

John Elder and his associates in San Diego developed a more comprehensive program designed to deter junior high school students from smoking. Elder, Wildey, et al. (1993) compared the smoking rates of seventh, eighth, and ninth graders in 11 treatment schools with the rates of students in 11 control schools, which were matched for size and tobacco use. The refusal skills treatment called for students to practice responding to audiotaped offers of cigarettes and smokeless tobacco. Judges then rated the quality of their refusal skills. When Elder, Sallis, Woodruff, and Wildey (1993) looked at refusal skills alone, they found that this single intervention was mostly ineffective. The quality of refusal skills was not related to either overall tobacco use or cigarette use at any grade, and refusal training itself was effective only for seventh graders.

However, when refusal skills were embedded in a multimodal program, Elder, Wildey, et al. (1993) reported that smoking rates in the treatment schools were lower than those in the control schools and that the difference between the two became greater with the passage of time. This program, called SHOUT (Students Helping Others Understand Tobacco) used 100 undergraduate college students to help as group leaders and to conduct telephone "booster" calls. The intervention consisted of seventh graders watching videotapes on the health consequences of tobacco use, reading celebrity endorsements of abstinence, discussing the consequences of smoking in small groups, becoming familiar with tobacco products, rehearsing methods of refusing peer pressure (refusal skills), practicing decision making, writing letters to tobacco companies, and performing a skit that involved offers and refusals of tobacco. Near the end of the seventh grade, the students publicly proclaimed themselves tobacco free and received T-shirts with the SHOUT logo. In the eighth grade, these students rehearsed refusal skills, participated in community action projects, continued to receive positive reinforcement for abstinence, and learned possible methods of encouraging parents to quit smoking. During the ninth grade, students in the treatment schools received no direct intervention, but they did receive telephone and mail messages aimed at boosting their refusal skills.

Elder, Wildey, et al. found little difference in smoking rates of students in the treatment school and those in the control schools at the end of the seventh grade, but changes began to appear in subsequent years. At the end of the eighth grade there was a small difference, and by the end of the ninth grade only 14% of students in the intervention schools reported smoking cigarettes during the past month compared with 22.5% of those in the control schools.

As one would expect, the total number of smokers increased from the seventh through the ninth grades for students in both the treatment schools and the control schools. However, the *rate* of increase was less in the treatment schools than in the controls. Elder, Wildey et al. (1993) concluded that the program was cost effective and that it probably deterred as many as 8% of participants from smoking.

QUITTING SMOKING

A second method of reducing smoking rates is for current smokers to quit. Although quitting smoking is not easy, millions of Americans have done so during the past 30 years. Currently, there are about as many former smokers in the United States as there are smokers—about one-fourth of the adult population are in each category, and about one-half have never smoked (USDHHS, 1994d).

Like adolescents contemplating starting to smoke, many long-term smokers considering quitting smoking possess an optimistic bias. In a smoking cessation program with adults, Gibbons, McGovern, and Lando (1991) found that although all the participants had acknowledged the dangers of smoking, ex-smokers who remained abstinent maintained that view, whereas ex-smokers who relapsed decreased their perception of smoking's risks. Also, Brownson et al. (1992) compared the beliefs of never smokers, former smokers, and current smokers and found that current smokers were less likely than either of the other two groups to believe that smoking caused lung cancer and emphysema, or that it was generally harmful to health.

A study in Australia (Chapman, Wong, & Smith, 1993) found significant differences between smokers and ex-smokers in 11 of 14 beliefs about smoking. Smokers were more likely than ex-smokers to say that (1) quitting causes weight gain, (2) no strong evidence exists that smoking causes cancer, (3) most lung cancer is caused by other things, (4) most people smoke, (5) the hazards of smoking are not important enough for the government to take action, (6) people would have to smoke "more than me" to be at risk for disease, (7) smoking can't be bad because many smokers live a long life, (8) exercise gets rid of tar in the lungs, (9) low-tar cigarettes are safe, (10) environmental tobacco has no serious effect on nonsmokers, and (11) smoking fewer than 20 cigarettes a day is safe. Although some of these beliefs may be debatable, 2, 3, 4, 8, and 9 are all clearly false.

In addition, Chapman et al. found that smokers were less likely than ex-smokers to believe that smokers have more than their share of heart disease, stroke, lung cancer, bronchitis, poor circulation, and symptoms of cough and breathlessness. Not surprisingly, those smokers who correctly agreed that smokers were more likely than nonsmokers to get these diseases nevertheless exempted themselves from those risks. Once again, optimistic bias seems be one factor contributing to the difficulty of quitting.

Besides an optimistic bias, another factor contributing to the difficulty of quitting smoking is its addictive qualities. Most people who both smoke and drink alcohol consider smoking to be a more difficult habit to break. Kozlowski et al. (1989) asked people seeking treatment for alcohol or drug dependence who also smoked which would be most difficult to quit—their problem substance or tobacco. A majority of these people—57%—reported that cigarettes would be more difficult to quit. Those who had sought treatment for alcohol dependence were four times more likely than those who had sought treatment for drug dependence to report that their urge for cigarettes was the stronger of their urges. These results highlight the comparative difficulty of quitting smoking in a sample of participants who, because of their experience with cigarettes and some other dependence, have a good basis for comparison.

Nevertheless, a growing number of people have successfully quit smoking, which indicates that the decline in smoking rates (as shown in Figure 13.3) is due not merely to fewer people starting to smoke but in large part to increased cessation rates. Many of these people have quit on their own, but others have found assistance through formal therapy programs.

Quitting without Therapy

Most people who have quit smoking have done so on their own, without the aid of formal cessation programs. Schachter (1982) reported a survey he conducted using two populations: the psychology department at Columbia University and the resident population of Amaganset, New York. In questioning these people about their success in quitting smoking, Schachter found a success rate of over 60% for both groups, with an average abstinence length of 7.4 years. People who had been heavy smokers (defined as more than three-quarters of a pack a day) reported that they found it more difficult to quit and had more unpleasant effects from quitting than did light smokers. However, Schachter found no difference in success rates between heavy and light smokers. Surprisingly, nearly 29% of the heavy smokers who quit said they had no problems in quitting. Schachter interpreted the high success rate, even for heavy smokers, as evidence that quitting may be easier than the clinic evaluations indicate. He suggested that people who attend clinic programs are

those who have, for the most part, failed in attempts to quit on their own. In addition, he hypothesized that the clinic success rates of 20% to 30% represent success for each program, with those who fail in one program going on to another in which they may also have about a 20% to 30% chance for success.

Schachter's data suggest that those who try to quit on their own largely succeed and never attend a clinic. Thus, people who attend clinics are an atypical group, self-selected on the basis of previous failure. These people, therefore, do not represent the general population of smokers, and failure rates based on clinic populations may be spuriously high.

However, Sheldon Cohen and his colleagues (1989) contended that smokers who quit on their own were no more successful than those who had received therapy. This analysis looked at evidence from 10 prospective studies of people who had tried to quit with benefit of clinical programs. Although Cohen et al. agreed with Schachter that success rates of self-quitters cannot be evaluated on the basis of a single attempt to stop smoking, their analysis revealed that people who quit on their own are basically similar to those who enroll in smoke therapy programs. They also found that the number of unsuccessful quit attempts was not related to eventual success at stopping smoking. Also contrary to Schachter's data, Cohen et al. found that light smokers were more than twice as likely as heavy smokers to quit.

This last finding partially agrees with Coambs, Li, and Kozlowski (1992), who found that, among younger smokers 16 to 44 years old, light smokers were most likely to stop. However, for smokers 45 and older, heavy smokers were more successful at quitting. Coambs et al. hypothesized that older smokers may quit because they have experienced some serious health problems.

Multimodal Approaches

Multimodal approaches are those that combine more than one technique to control a behavior. These strategies often include behavior modification techniques, cognitive-behavioral approaches, contracts made by smoker and therapist in which the smoker agreed to stop smoking, group contact and support, "booster" sessions to prevent relapse, and other treatment approaches. During the 1970s, a rapid smoking component was sometimes used in multimodal approaches. The rapid smoking technique required a smoker to take a puff every six seconds until smoking became very unpleasant.

A meta-analysis of smoking cessation programs (Kottke, Battista, DeFriese, & Brekke, 1988) found that multimodal approaches were more successful than single techniques. They also found that the number of sessions and the duration of individual sessions both contributed to higher cessation rates. In addition, they concluded that smokers who received individualized advice on many occasions were most likely to quit.

Paul Cinciripini and his colleagues (1995) added a unique component to a multimodal treatment program: smoking on schedule. In addition to evaluating the efficacy of quitting "cold turkey" versus cutting down gradually, these researchers explored the value of adding a schedule to smokers' quit attempts. They randomly assigned people in a smoking cessation program to one of four groups: (1) smokers who were allowed to smoke only during a specified time frame and who had to gradually reduce their consumption as the interval between smoking periods became progressively longer; (2) smokers who also followed a clock but were allowed to smoke as much as they could during the specified time

frame; (3) smokers who did not follow a schedule but who had to gradually reduce consumption until they reached a quit date; and (4) smokers who did not follow a schedule and who had to quit "cold turkey" when their quit date arrived. Cinciripini et al. found that the scheduling component had a significant effect on quit rate. After 1 year, 44% of the smokers in the scheduled reduced smoking group (Group 1) and 32% in the scheduled nonreduced group (Group 2) were no longer smoking. By contrast, quit rates in the two nonscheduled groups were only 18% for Group 3 and 22% for Group 4. Thus, those who quit "cold turkey" after smoking on schedule (Group 2) had better quit rates than the two groups without schedules, suggesting that the clock component offers a promising addition to multimodal programs.

Table 13.1 compares quit rates for several types of programs. The rates are the percentages of smokers who were not smoking at 6 months and 1 year after completing various types of programs. These rates are based on an assessment of hundreds of effectiveness studies for smoking programs (Schwartz, 1987). Table 13.1 shows the range of success rates for each type of program because various assessments showed differing quit rates. The median percentage of smokers who quit at the two follow-up

Table 13.1 Summary of follow-up quit rates for various types of smoking cessation programs

Type of Program	6 months range	6 months median	1 year range	1 year median
self-help	0–33%	17%	12–33%	18%
nicotine gum	17–33%	23%	8–38%	11%
nicotine gum + behavior modification	23–50%	35%	12–49%	29%
hypnosis, individual	0–60%	25%	13–68%	19.5%
physician advice	5–12%	5%	3–13%	6%
acupuncture	5–34%	18%	8–32%	30%
rapid smoking alone	7–62%	25.5%	6–40%	21%
rapid smoking in multimodal program	8–68%	38%	7–52%	30.5%
multimodal program	18–52%	32%	6–76%	40%

SOURCE: *Review and Evaluation of Smoking Cessation Methods, the United States and Canada, 1978–1985* by J. L. Schwartz, 1987, U.S. Department of Health and Human Services, Public Health Service, National Institutes of Health (NIH Publication No. 87-2940), Washington, DC: U.S. Government Printing Office.

points gives a method of comparison for the various cessation programs. Schwartz noted that caution is required in interpreting the success rates of some of the studies and mentioned that the quit rates for hypnosis and acupuncture may be lower than these figures suggest because of poor methodology in the studies on which the rates were based. An examination of Table 13.1 reveals that the components found effective by Kottke et al. (1988) were included in the more effective programs assessed by Schwartz. Furthermore, the cessation programs that included a behavior modification component were among the most successful. Schwartz's evaluation showed that multimodal programs were quite effective, with a median success of 40% after a 1-year follow-up.

Pharmacological Treatments

Besides psychological interventions, pharmacological treatments have been used to help people stop smoking. Since 1984, nicotine chewing gum has been a frequent component in a multicomponent smoking cessation program. By itself, nicotine gum does not seem to be effective in smoking cessation (Hughes, Gust, Keenan, Fenwick, & Healey, 1989; USDHHS, 1989), but when combined with other components in a behavioral program, it may contribute to quit rates (Hall, Tunstall, Ginsberg, Benowith, & Jones, 1987). Millard, Waranch, and McEntee (1992) found that most nicotine chewing gum users reported that the gum produced fewer cravings for a cigarette and made them feel less anxious and more relaxed. However, Gottlieb, Killen, Marlatt, and Taylor (1987) suggested that nicotine chewing gum may not be the effective component in cessation programs. Their study found that the relief of withdrawal symptoms and the prevention of relapse that accompanied use of gum were largely a placebo effect rather than an effect of the pharmacological properties of the gum.

Nicotine patches have become the most common of the pharmacological treatments for smoking. The patches, which resemble large bandages, work by releasing a small, continuous dose of nicotine into the body's system. People move from larger dose to smaller dose patches until the person is no longer dependent on nicotine. Like nicotine chewing gum, the patch is available only through a physician's prescription, and it is expensive, costing about $250 for a 10-week program.

How effective is the nicotine patch? In 1992, the same year patches reached a peak in sales in the United States, a review of 11 studies (Fiore, Jorenby, Baker, and Kenford, 1992), all of which had used a placebo, double-blind methodology, revealed that the patch was 18% to 77% effective at the end of the treatment period, with a median of about 40%. These percentages indicate a somewhat higher quit rate than the 5% to 28% attained with only a placebo. After a follow-up of at least 6 months, the quit rate for people who had worn the patch dropped to 22% to 44%. These somewhat discrepant percentages were probably due to differences in the related therapy that the participants had received. For example, those whose treatment was accompanied by intensive group behavior therapy tended to have the highest cessation rates. The nicotine patches reduced some nicotine withdrawal symptoms but not hunger and weight gain.

When used alone, the nicotine patch system is only moderately successful. For example, the patches showed only about a 17% advantage over a placebo after 1 year of follow-up (Tønnesen, Nørregaard, Simonsen, & Säwe, 1991). Two double-blind, placebo-controlled studies (Kenford et al., 1994) also found only a moderate benefit for the patch over a placebo. In the first study, more than half the participants who wore a 22-mg patch for 8 weeks had quit smoking at the end of the treatment period. However, after only a 6-month follow-up, 34% of the nicotine patch group were abstinent, whereas 21% of the placebo patch group had stopped smoking. This represents a net gain of only 13 percentage points for the patch. The second study revealed similar results, and another study (Hurt et al., 1994) found that smokers who tried the nicotine patch to quit smoking had a high relapse rate, with only 27% abstinent after 1 year.

The 13% net gain for the patch also emerged from a meta-analysis by Fiore and his associates (Fiore, Smith, Jorenby, & Baker, 1994), who looked at 17 studies of the nicotine patch that had used a double-blind, placebo-controlled design with random assignment of disease-free participants, biochemical confirmation of adherence, and a duration of least 4 weeks. This meta-analysis revealed an end-of-treatment quit rate of 27% for active patch participants and 14% of people who wore a placebo patch. After 6 months, the active patch had produced a 22% quit rate, while 9% of people in placebo groups were smoke free. Fiore et al. also found that treatment beyond 8 weeks did not increase abstinence rates. In summary, the nicotine patch adds about 13 percentage points to the quit rate attained by the placebo patch. In other words, of smokers who attempt to quit through the use of a nicotine patch, about one in eight receives additional and specific help beyond that achieved by a placebo.

A third pharmacological intervention is the nicotine inhaler, a plastic tube filled with 10 mg of nicotine that smokers use 2 to 10 times a day. For each use they inhale deeply and puff about 10 times more often than they would while smoking a cigarette. Thus, the inhaler method combines some aspect of rapid smoking with the nicotine patch. A randomized double-blind, placebo-controlled trial of the nicotine inhaler (Tønnesen, Nørregaard, Mikkelsen, Jørgensen, & Nillson, 1993) administered the treatment for 3 months, followed by a tapering off period of 3 months when participants reduced by 25% the number of inhaler uses per day. After 1 year, 15% of the intervention group were still abstinent, compared with 5% of participants in the control group. Thus, the inhaler method seems to offer no improvement over the nicotine patch.

The discrepancy between the success at the end of a cessation program and at the 6-month or 1-year follow-up emphasizes the magnitude of the relapse rate. Many programs use a variety of techniques, and one of the components in some of the more effective programs is the use of "booster" sessions. This component is intended to deal with the problem of relapse by prolonging the effects of treatment. Whether people quit on their own or with the help of various therapeutic interventions, relapse remains a serious problem. Most smokers who quit relapse within 3 days (Hughes et al., 1992).

RELAPSE PREVENTION

The high rate of relapse after smoking cessation treatment prompted Marlatt and Gordon (1980) to examine the relapse process itself. For many people who have been successful in quitting, one cigarette precipitates a full relapse, complete with feelings of total failure. Marlatt and Gordon termed this phenomenon the *abstinence violation effect*. They incorporated strategies into their treatment to cope with patients' despair when they violate their intention to remain abstinent. By training patients that one "slip" does not constitute relapse, Marlatt and Gordon buffer them against a full relapse.

Given the relapse rate of between 70% and 80%, relapse prevention procedures are essential adjuncts to any smoking cessation program. However, the problem of relapse is not unique to smoking. Relapse rates similar to those for smoking have also been found in the treatment of alcohol and heroin addiction (Hunt, Barnett, & Branch, 1971), and relapse prevention techniques have also been used in these treatment programs.

Curry, Marlatt, and Gordon (1987) further explored people's reactions to a violation of abstinence and found that both cognitive and emotional factors are involved. In addition, violations of abstinence or slips reliably predict relapse, with one slip strongly relating to subsequent relapse (Baer, Karmack, Lichtenstein, & Ranson, 1989). However, Hall, Havassy, and Wassermen (1990) failed to find that the violation of abstinence goals affected people who were attempting to abstain from alcohol, opiates, or nicotine. Therefore, Marlatt and Gordon's (1980) idea that both cognitive and emotional components play a role in adherence to abstinence goals has received only mixed support. But the lack of unanimity does not negate the importance of relapse prevention in smoking cessation programs.

In a study of smokers who quit on their own, John Hughes and his associates (1992) were interested in relapse rates during the very early days and weeks after quitting. They found that two-thirds of self-quitters relapsed after only 2 days. After 1 week, only 24% were still abstinent; after 2 weeks, that percentage had declined to 22%, and at 6 months, only 8% of self-quitters were still smoke free. These investigators also reported that slips were common and that one-fourth of eventual quitters had slipped at one time or another. This study showed how difficult quitting on one's own can be.

Some evidence indicates that relapse into smoking may not be permanent; people who start smoking after a period of abstinence may also quit again. Swan and Denk (1987) studied patterns of smoking relapse and found that no "safe" point existed for smokers who had quit—relapse was possible at any time, even many years after a smoker had stopped. But Swan and Denk also found that smokers who relapsed and returned to smoking may quit a second time. Shiffman (1989) found the situations that tempted ex-smokers to smoke again varied, although these situations usually involved being around other smokers. Swan and Denk concluded that the factors affecting relapse differ from the factors prompting a return to abstinence. The results from these two studies suggest that relapse is a dynamic and complex process. One is never simply a smoker or an ex-smoker.

WHO QUITS AND WHO DOES NOT?

Another issue revolves around the question of who quits smoking and who does not. What factors relate to smoking cessation? Investigators have examined several factors that may possibly answer this question, including gender, weight concern, social support, perceived health benefits, and confidence that one can quit.

Because quit rates for men have increased more than those for women during the past 30 years, many observers have assumed that women have more difficulty quitting than men, and some research seems to confirm that assumption. For example, Flaxman (1978) found that women had worse cessation percentages when they set an immediate date for quitting as opposed to a later date. However, some research (Pirie, Murray, & Luepker, 1991) found no differences between women and men in either their attempts at quitting or their success in quitting. Similarly, women in the Framingham study were as likely to quit as men—except that women who were very heavy smokers had lower quit rates than men who were very heavy smokers (Freund, D'Agostino, Belanger, Kannel, & Stokes, 1992).

Female participants in a smoking cessation program seemed to have greater difficulty quitting than men, but the evidence was more complex than a simple count of the percentage of each gender who had quit (Fortmann & Killen, 1994). First, women were more likely to volunteer to participate in such programs—possibly they were simply going along with a friend. Second, once women expressed a genuine interest in quitting, they were as likely as men to quit. Third, although women had more difficulty during the first 24 hours, after that time they had the same quit rates as men. In summary, women may be more willing to make quit attempts, are less successful during the first 24 hours, but are equal to men in avoiding relapse once they have quit.

In a study cited earlier, Bjornson et al. (1995) found additional reasons that women seem to find quitting harder than men. In this study women had lower quit rates than men at both 12 months and 36 months, but all the differences at the 12-month follow-up and most at 36 months could be explained by baseline differences. That is, at the beginning of the study, women were less likely to be married, to have made a previous attempt to quit, to have made longer quit attempts, and to be heavy smokers. Also, women were more likely to live with other smokers. Regardless of gender, each of these factors is associated with poorer quit rates. In other words, women generally have more obstacles to hurdle in trying to quit smoking.

Social support is another factor that predicts who will quit smoking and who will not. Some studies (Coppotelli & Orleans, 1985; Mermelstein, Cohen, Lichtenstein, Baer, & Kamarck, 1986) have shown that cessation programs are more effective in maintaining abstinence when spouses of participants are trained to offer support to the partner who is trying to quit. Mermelstein et al. (1986) also found that having a greater than average number of smokers in one's social network was a hindrance to maintaining abstinence 12 months after completing a cessation program.

An additional factor that predicts smoking cessation is the perceived health benefit from quitting. Eisinger (1972) found that people who know someone whose health has been hurt by smoking were much more likely to quit than smokers who did not know anyone whose health has been affected— 27% versus 10%. Freund et al. (1992) found that recent hospitalization and recently diagnosed heart disease were both positively related to cessation rates. However, a diagnosis of cancer did not prompt people to quit, possibly because those people believed that it was too late to benefit from quitting.

Finally, smoking cessation seems to be related to smokers' level of confidence that they have the ability to do what is necessary to quit and to maintain abstinence. This perception that one is capable of performing the behaviors that will produce desired outcomes in any particular situation relates to Albert Bandura's concept of *self-efficacy*. One study (Condiotte & Lichtenstein, 1982) measured self-efficacy before, during, and after involvement in smoking control programs and found that it predicted which ex-smokers would relapse, how soon they would relapse, and in what situations relapse was likely to occur. In addition, people high in self-efficacy were more likely than inefficacious participants to reestablish abstinence following a slip.

Another study (DiClemente, 1981) found that self-efficacy scores were better predictors of smoking cessation than either demographic data or smoking history. In this study, a self-efficacy questionnaire was administered to participants who had stopped smoking through one of three procedures: an expensive behavioral management program, an even more expensive aversion program, or quitting on their own. A 5-month follow-up interview found that two-thirds of all participants were still abstaining and that a third of them had relapsed. The only significant predictor of abstinence was self-efficacy scores obtained at the beginning of the cessation programs. Participants who paid up to $500 for a clinic program were no more or less likely to be abstaining from cigarettes 5 months after quitting than were self-quitters. Other factors that did not differentiate between abstainers and recidivists were age, educational level, socioeconomic status, age at beginning smoking, cigarettes smoked per day, number of prior attempts to quit, longest previous abstinence, or number of years smoking. In this study, self-efficacy alone predicted success at quitting.

SMOKING AND WEIGHT GAIN

Smokers and former smokers generally agree that quitting smoking may mean that one will gain weight. Chapman, Wong, and Smith (1993) found the

80% of smokers and two-thirds of ex-smokers believed that quitting puts on weight. Are such concerns justified? Katherine Flegal and her colleagues (Flegal, Troiano, Pamuk, Kuczmarski, & Campbell, 1995) considered the possibility that the increase in obesity of U.S. adults might be the result of weight gain from smoking cessation. Their analysis indicated that quitting smoking does not account for the majority of the increases in overweight, but it is a factor. Former smokers tended to gain weight, and those who had quit were significantly more likely to become overweight compared to those who continued to smoke.

The weight gain associated with quitting is typically modest (Coates & Li, 1983). The estimates of average weight gains have varied between about 4 pounds (Manley & Boland, 1983) to as many as 9 pounds for men and 11 for women (Flegal et al., 1995). Women tend to be more concerned about weight gain (Pirie, Murray, & Luepker, 1991), and they also gain more weight than men after quitting smoking (Flegal et al., 1995; Williamson et al., 1991). However, little difference in weight gain appeared between men and women after a 12-month nicotine chewing gum cessation intervention (Nides et al., 1994). Both men and women gained about 12 pounds, but because the men were heavier than the women at baseline, the women's gain represented 8.4% of their baseline weight whereas the men's gain was only 6.7% of their original weight. The use of nicotine gum partially delayed weight gain, especially for women.

In a study that included only women, Pirie et al. (1992) studied cessation rates and weight gain in four treatment modes: (1) standard smoking cessation program, (2) standard program plus nicotine gum, (3) standard program plus a behavior-oriented weight control intervention, and (4) standard program plus nicotine gum plus the behavioral weight control program. Interestingly, cessation rates were highest in the second group, but Pirie et al. observed no differences in weight gain among the four treatment modalities. People who quit for 1 year gained an average of 10.6 pounds compared with a gain of 1.6 pounds for those who continued to smoke.

More optimistic findings came from a study reporting that weight gain following smoking cessation can be temporary (Chen, Horne, & Dosman,

1993). The mean body mass index was highest in ex-smokers, lowest in smokers, and intermediate in never smokers. However, for female ex-smokers, both body mass index and body weight decreased significantly with years of smoking cessation. Men experienced a nonsignificant trend in the same direction. Former smokers are heaviest about 2 years after quitting, after which time their weight matches that of never smokers. Another study (Swan & Carmelli, 1995) found that men had an average weight gain of only 8 pounds after 16 years of not smoking, although 13% of their sample gained 25 pounds or more. In this study, men who gained the most were younger and from a lower socioeconomic level. The inclusion of fraternal and identical twins in the study allowed the conclusion that weight gain after smoking cessation may be influenced by genetic factors, because identical twins were more alike than others in amount of weight gain.

Williamson et al. (1991) conducted a long-term follow-up of a national sample of former smokers that controlled for level of physical activity and illness due to smoking. They found that women who stopped smoking gained about eight pounds more than women who continued, and men put on about six extra pounds. People who had the most trouble with weight gain were African Americans (both men and women), heavy smokers, smokers under age 55, and women with children. However, major weight gain (30 pounds or more) occurred in only about 10% of the men and 13% of the women. The extra weight former smokers might gain does not negate the health benefits of smoking cessation.

A later study (Grover, Gray-Donald, Joseph, Abrahamowicz, & Coupal, 1994) reached a similar conclusion—namely, that quitting smoking is much more beneficial to health than maintaining lower weight. A diet of no more than 10% of calories from saturated fat would extend the life of the average heart disease-free man anywhere from 11 days to 3 months; for women such a diet would increase life expectancy anywhere from 3 days to about 2 months. In contrast, quitting smoking would give the average male smoker who is free of heart disease 2.6 to 4.4 additional years of life, and it would extend the life of the average heart disease-free female smoker anywhere from 2.6 to 3.7 years. Grover et al. concluded that men 30 to 59 (who generally have a higher saturated fat diet than women) could profit to some extent by adhering to a low-fat diet, but older men and women of all ages would benefit very little from such a diet. However, the benefits of quitting smoking are huge for everyone.

SMOKELESS TOBACCO

Smokeless tobacco includes snuff and chewing tobacco, forms of tobacco that were more popular during the 19th century than at the present. Currently, about 5.9% of men and 0.2% of women in the United States use smokeless tobacco (USBC, 1995). In addition to gender, other sociodemographic factors relate to the use of smokeless tobacco, including age, geographic area of residence, family income, and employment status (USDHHS, 1989). Use is heaviest among younger people, residents of the South, people who are unemployed or who work in service and blue-collar jobs, and young adults whose family income falls below the poverty level. In addition, adolescents who live in other than two-parent homes are more likely to use smokeless tobacco (Jones & Moberg, 1988).

Initiation into the use of smokeless tobacco typically occurs between the ages of 10 and 13, and peers strongly influence the use of these products (Ary et al., 1987). Not surprisingly, cigarette smoking is also associated with the use of smokeless tobacco, as is the use of other drugs such as alcohol and marijuana (Jones & Moberg, 1988). Indeed, the use of smokeless tobacco may relate to a pattern of adolescent risk taking or antisocial behavior that includes behaving delinquently, doing poorly in school, and using legal and illegal drugs. The use of smokeless tobacco is similar to cigarette smoking in terms of onset, patterns of use, social influences, and attempts to quit (Ary, Lichtenstein, Severson, Weissman, & Seeley, 1989).

Health risks of smokeless tobacco include cancer of the oral cavity, periodontal disease, and possibly high cholesterol and heart disease. In a survey of professional baseball players, Ernster et al. (1990) found that many chewed tobacco; of those, 46% had oral leukoplakia, a disorder that may develop into oral cancer. In addition, oral use of tobacco is associated with dental and periodontal problems, and these baseball players also showed evidence of a high rate of periodontal disease.

People who use smokeless tobacco are 2.5 times more likely to have high cholesterol levels than those who do not use tobacco (Tucker, 1989). Even though the study included no control for diet, the higher cholesterol levels for smokeless tobacco users is one more risk associated with the use of these products. A 12-year follow-up of male Swedish construction workers (Bolinder, Alfredsson, England, & de Faire, 1994) showed that use of smokeless tobacco more than doubled the risk of cardiovascular mortality for men 35 to 54. Cancer mortality, however, was not significantly increased by the use of smokeless tobacco. In summary, the risks of smokeless tobacco are probably not as great as those of cigarette smoking; nevertheless, chewing tobacco has significant health hazards.

CHAPTER SUMMARY

Ten questions concerning cigarette smoking have attracted attention, and this chapter deals with each of them: (1) Who smokes and who does not? (2) What are the health effects of smoking? (3) Does quitting pay off? (4) Is passive smoking dangerous? (5) Why do people start smoking? (6) Why do they continue to smoke? (7) How can smoking be prevented? (8) How can people quit smoking? (9) Does smoking cessation lead to weight gain? (10) What are the risks of smokeless tobacco?

First, who smokes? Currently, about one-fourth of all U.S. adults smoke, about one-fourth are former smokers, and about one half have never smoked. Smokers are represented in nearly every demographic category, with men and women now smoking in about equal numbers. Although the past 2 decades have seen a general decline in the number of smokers, college graduates have stopped smoking at a faster rate than less-educated smokers.

Second, smoking is the number one cause of preventable death in the United States, causing about 400,000 deaths a year. Cigarette smokers have higher rates of absenteeism than nonsmokers, suffer more illness, and have a much higher rate of mortality.

Third, stopping smoking helps, and some evidence suggests that, after smokers have quit for 16 years, their all-cause mortality rate may return to that of nonsmokers, although they may continue to have an excess risk for lung cancer mortality.

Fourth, is passive smoking dangerous? Many nonsmokers are bothered by the smoking of others, and young children have an excess risk of respiratory disease from passive smoking. Research suggests that environmental tobacco smoke does not contribute substantially to death from lung cancer, but it may be responsible for several thousand deaths a year from cardiovascular disease.

Fifth, why do people start smoking? Most smokers begin as teenagers, at a time when peer pressure is especially strong. Teenagers are as well informed as adults about the potential hazards of smoking, but many of them smoke anyway, assuming that the risks do not apply to them. Other young people recognize the dangers of smoking but do so anyway as part of a risk-taking, rebellious style of life.

Sixth, why do people continue to smoke? This question is a difficult one and has not been fully answered. However, several theoretical models have been proposed, including the nicotine addiction model and the social learning model. The first explains smoking behavior on the basis of a chemical addiction whereas the social learning model suggests that smokers begin smoking to gain peer approval or to avoid social ostracism. Once they begin, they continue in part to avoid the aversive stimuli connected with withdrawal symptoms.

Seventh, how can smoking be prevented? One successful approach to preventing young people from starting smoking is the "inoculation" method, in which teenagers are given information to buffer them against the persuasive arguments of peers and media. Multimodal approaches that include peer influence, training in refusal skills, and practice at making decisions have had some success in deterring young people from smoking.

Eighth, how can people quit smoking? Some single-component formal therapy programs are able to achieve a modest success rate, but multimodal approaches are generally more successful. In addition, millions of people have stopped smoking on their own. Many people are able to quit for 6 months to 1 year, but the problem of relapse remains serious. Some therapy programs have reported impressive cessation rates at the end of the program, but most people who quit eventually resume smoking. Programs aimed at this relapse problem can be successful.

Ninth, does quitting smoking lead to weight gain? Many smokers fear that if they stop smoking they will gain weight, but the evidence shows that the average weight gain for most men and women is relatively modest—about 8 to 10 pounds. However, for about 10% to 12% of the population, the gain may be 25 pounds or more. Nevertheless, even excessive weight gain is far less risky than continuing to smoke.

Tenth, what are the risks of smokeless tobacco use? Like cigars and pipes, smokeless tobacco is probably somewhat safer than cigarette smoking, but none of these forms of tobacco are safe. Teenagers who use smokeless tobacco tend to believe that this form of tobacco is much safer than cigarette smoking, but the use of smokeless tobacco is associated with increased rates of oral cancer and periodontal disease and may be related to coronary heart disease. Prevention of smokeless tobacco use typically occurs as part of smoking prevention programs rather than as a separate intervention.

SUGGESTED READINGS

Centers for Disease Control and Prevention (CDC). (1993). Cigarette smoking—attributable mortality and years of potential life lost—United States, 1990. *Morbidity and Mortality Weekly Report, 42,* 645–649. The Centers for Disease Control and Prevention publishes weekly reports on morbidity and mortality in the United States, and any recent report on smoking would probably be informative. This particular report includes a table with the relative risks for male and female current and former smokers for a variety of diseases.

Gilbert, D. G. (1995). *Smoking: Individual differences, psychopathology, and emotion.* Washington, DC: Taylor & Francis. In this book, Gilbert discusses the relationship between smoking and emotion, gender differences in the effects of tobacco use, and the association between personality and smoking behavior.

Koop, C. E. (1989). A parting shot at tobacco. *Journal of the American Medical Association, 262,* 2894–2895. This short article was former U.S. Surgeon General C. Everett Koop's last official denouncement of the tobacco industry. Of the several people who have held the office of Surgeon General, Koop was the most vigorous and eloquent in his opposition to smoking and in his fight to eliminate smoking.

Pomerleau, O. F. (1980). Why people smoke: Current psychobiological models. In P. O. Davidson & S. M. Davidson (Eds.), *Behavioral medicine: Changing health lifestyles* (pp. 94–112). New York: Brunner/Mazel. This review of the leading theories of tobacco use includes a summary of relevant research.

14 Using Alcohol and Other Drugs

James classifies himself as a social drinker because he drinks only in social situations and when he is out with friends. Now, his typical drinking is one drink per night, and he never drinks more than four drinks per evening. A year ago, his limit was much higher. During the time he was a member of a fraternity, James went out with his friends and drank more heavily. About two or three times a year, he would get "stupid, falling down drunk," usually as a celebration for some occasion such as the completion of mid-term exams.

Being part of a college fraternity shaped James's drinking habits. Unlike the majority of his peers in high school, James had no interest in experimenting with alcohol. In fact, he had a very negative attitude toward drinking, an attitude that started to change when he began to drink. His first experience with alcohol was just before his 18th birthday, when some friends took him out and got him drunk on beer. Although this episode resulted in a terrible hangover, James did not develop negative feelings about drinking.

As a freshman in college, James joined a fraternity, where drinking was a major part of the social life. Although he did not drink as much as many of his fraternity brothers, he began to drink at the fraternity house and at local clubs and bars. When one of the fraternity brothers had drunk too much, the other brothers would try to keep him from doing anything too embarrassing and to get him back to the fraternity house safely. Occasionally, James was the one in need of assistance, but more often, he provided assistance.

During college, James's level of alcohol consumption escalated to frequent moderate drinking combined with occasional binges. Now, as a senior, however, his drinking has decreased, partly because his fraternity has been dissolved. Another reason was his behavior during his last binge when he experienced a "blackout"; this resulted in his not remembering any of his socially embarrassing behavior, which got him thrown out of his favorite club. As a consequence of his embarrassment, he has resolved never to get drunk again. However, he continues to be a light social drinker, limiting his drinking to one drink per night on most nights and four drinks as a maximum.

James believes that his reduction in drinking was the result of a natural process of "settling down." He has also noticed that his classmates and fraternity brothers seem to be drinking less, mostly as a result of a recent change that increased the legal drinking age from 18 to 21.

Is James's assessment of his drinking patterns accurate — is he a social drinker, or does he have problems associated with alcohol? Is his drinking typical for college students? What drinking patterns present problems? This chapter includes answers to these questions, but first, we examine the history of drinking.

A BRIEF HISTORY OF DRINKING

The use of alcohol is not something that can easily be traced; it was discovered worldwide and repeatedly, dating back beyond recorded history. The yeast that is responsible for producing alcohol is airborne, and fermentation occurs naturally in fruits, fruit juices, and grain mixtures. Producing beverage alcohol requires no sophisticated technology, and there is evidence that most ancient cultures used beverage alcohol. Ancient Babylonians discovered both wine (fermented grape juice) and beer (fermented grain), as did the ancient Egyptians, Greeks, Romans, Chinese, and Indians. Pre-Columbian tribes in the Americas also used fermented products.

Ancient civilizations also discovered drunkenness, of course. In several of those countries, such as Greece, drunkenness was not only allowed but practically required on certain occasions, but these occasions were limited to festivals. This pattern resembles present-day practices in the United States, where drunkenness is condoned at some parties and celebrations. Most societies condone drinking alcohol but not drunkenness, except on certain occasions.

Distillation was discovered in ancient China, and refined in eighth-century Arabia. Because the process is somewhat complex, the use of distilled spirits did not become widespread until they were commercially manufactured. In England, fermented beverages were by far the most common form of alcohol consumption until the 18th century, when England encouraged the proliferation of distilleries to stimulate commerce. Along with cheap gin came widespread consumption and widespread drunkenness. However, intoxication from distilled spirits was confined mostly to the lower and working classes; the rich drank wine, which was imported and thus expensive.

In colonial America, drinking was much more prevalent than it is today. Men, women, and children all drank, and it was considered acceptable for all to do so. This practice may not seem consistent with our present-day image of the Puritans, but nevertheless the Puritans did not object to drinking. Rather, they considered alcohol one of God's gifts. Indeed, in those years alcohol was often safer than unpurified water or milk, so the Puritans had a legitimate reason to condone the consumption of alcoholic beverages. What was not acceptable to them was drunkenness. They believed that alcohol should, like all things, be used in moderation. Therefore, the Puritans established severe prohibitions against drunkenness but not against drinking.

The 50 years following U.S. independence marked a transition in the way early Americans thought about alcohol (Critchlow, 1986; Levine, 1980). An adamant and vocal minority came to consider liquor a "demon" and to totally abstain from its use. Similar attitudes arose in Britain (McMurran, 1994). This attitude was mostly limited to the upper and upper-middle classes. Later, abstention came to be an accepted doctrine of the middle class and people who aspired to join the middle class. Intemperance in drinking alcohol thus became associated with the lower classes, and "respectable" people, especially women, were expected not to be heavy drinkers.

Temperance societies proliferated throughout the United States during the mid-1800s. However, the term is a misnomer: The societies did not promote *temperance* — that is, the moderate use of alcohol. Rather, they advocated *prohibition,* the total abstinence from alcohol. Temperance societies held that liquor weakened inhibitions; loosened desires and passions; caused a large percentage of crime, poverty, and broken homes; and was powerfully addicting, so much so that even an occasional drink would put one in danger. Figure 14.1 shows a dramatic decrease in per capita alcohol consumption in the United States after 1830, a decrease due directly to the spread of the temperance (prohibition) movement.

In response to the growing temperance movement, both the demographics and the location of drinking changed. Drinking became associated with the lower and working classes. Rather than being consumed in a family setting, alcohol became increasingly confined to the saloon. Popham (1978)

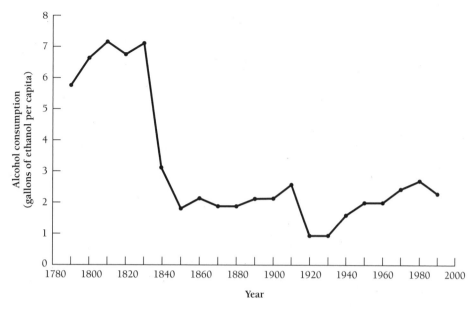

Figure 14.1   **U.S. consumption of all alcoholic beverages, 1790–1989, ages 15 and older.**
SOURCE: From *The Alcoholic Republic: An American Tradition* (p. 9) by W. J. Rorabaugh, 1979, New York: Oxford University Press. Copyright 1979 by Oxford University Press. Reprinted by permission. Also from *Fifth Special Report to the U.S. Congress on Alcohol and Health* (DHHS Publication No. ADM 84-1291), p. 2 by National Institute on Alcohol Abuse and Alcoholism (NIAAA), 1983, Washington, DC: U.S. Government Printing Office. *Seventh Special Report to the U.S. Congress on Alcohol and Health* (DHHS Publication No. ADM 90-1656), by NIAAA, 1990, Washington, DC: U.S. Government Printing Office. *Eighth Special Report to the U.S. Congress on Alcohol and Health* by NIAAA, 1993, Washington, DC: U.S. Government Printing Office.

drew a distinction between taverns and saloons, characterizing taverns as family places and saloons as urban establishments patronized largely by industrial workers. Portrayed by the temperance movement as the personification of evil and moral degeneracy, saloons served as a focus for growing Prohibitionist sentiment.

Prohibitionists were finally victorious in 1919 with the ratification of the 18th Amendment to the Constitution of the United States. This amendment outlawed the manufacture, sale, or transportation of alcoholic beverages and lowered per capita consumption drastically (as shown in Figure 14.1). This amendment was not popular and created a large illegal market for alcohol. The growing unpopularity of Prohibition resulted in the 21st Amendment, which repealed the 18th Amendment and ended Prohibition in 1934. Figure 14.1 shows that after the repeal of Prohibition, alcohol consumption rose sharply. Although the current per capita consumption of alcohol is considerably higher than during Prohibi-

tion, it is less than half the rate reached during the first 3 decades of the 19th century.

THE PREVALENCE OF DRINKING TODAY

Currently, more than 60% of the adults in the United States drink alcoholic beverages, at least occasionally (U.S. Department of Health and Human Services [USDHHS], 1993a). More specifically, nearly 40% of adults in the U.S. describe themselves as nondrinkers; another 38% are light drinkers; and the remaining are moderate or heavy drinkers, divided into 17% moderate and 6% heavy drinkers (see Figure 14.2). During the past 10 years the percentage of current, weekly, and binge drinkers has gradually declined (Midanik & Clark, 1994). These findings are consistent with data indicating that per capita consumption of alcohol has dropped since 1980 (see Figure 14.1). Consumption, of course, is

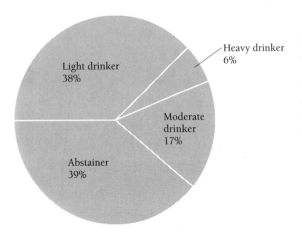

Figure 14.2 Alcohol consumption by type of drinker, adults, United States, 1990.
SOURCE: *National Economic, Social, and Environmental Data Bank* [Electronic database] (May 22, 1995), Hyattsville, MD: National Center for Health Statistics [Producer and Distributor].

not equally distributed within the population. The U.S. Department of Health and Human Services reported that most of the drinking is done by a small number of drinkers and that half the alcohol consumed is drunk by about 10% of the population.

The acceptability of alcohol use, frequency of drinking, and prevalence of heavy drinking is not equal for all demographic groups in the United States. Rather, drinking varies by ethnic background and by age. Adult European Americans tend to have higher rates of drinking and more positive attitudes toward drinking than members of other ethnic groups. In a study of junior high and high school students (Roberts, Fournet, & Penland, 1995), Asian American students showed the highest rate of alcohol use and Hispanic American students the lowest rate, with African American and European American students reporting intermediate levels of use. Young adult European Americans tend to drink more heavily than young adults from other ethnic groups, and they also experience more alcohol-related problems (Bucholz, 1992). For those who have received treatment for problem drinking, European American women were less likely to abstain and more likely to binge drink than African American and Hispanic American women (Caetano,

1994). Although educational level and social environment play a significant role in drinking, ethnic background has some relationship to alcohol use.

Consumption of alcohol is related not only to ethnic background but also to age; young and middle-aged adults drink more than either older people or young adolescents (USDHHS, 1994c). About 90% of adolescents have used alcohol by the time they become seniors in high school (Johnston, O'Malley, & Bachman, 1994a; National Institute of Alcohol Abuse and Alcoholism [NIAAA], 1983; USDHHS, 1994c). Even among high school seniors, the percentage of current drinkers has declined significantly—from 72% in 1978, to 64% in 1988 (Johnston, O'Malley, & Bachman, 1989), and to 51% in 1993 (Johnston et al., 1994a).

One pattern of drinking that is especially common among young people is binge drinking, usually defined as having five or more drinks on one occasion. James's drinking to get drunk is an example of binge drinking. This pattern of drinking can be particularly dangerous (especially for inexperienced drinkers), leading to intoxication, poor judgment, and impaired coordination. Certain situations promote binge drinking, and college students are at particular risk. James chose to binge drink on "special occasions," such as homecoming or after mid-term and final exams. Corcoran (1994) studied drinking at a college festival and found that binge drinking was common and that legal drinking age had little impact on binge drinking among these college students. Women under age 21 and men over age 21 showed the strongest tendencies toward binge drinking. In addition, Corcoran and Kisler (1994) found that college women who rated themselves as more likely to binge drink were also more likely to minimize the seriousness of this practice. Indeed, heavy drinkers tend to hold an optimistic bias (Hansen, Raynor, & Wolkenstein, 1991), believing that their drinking is not likely to cause them problems.

Binge drinking is a risky pattern of alcohol use, but the rate of episodic binge drinking among high school students has declined. In 1982, 41% of high school students reported that they had consumed five or more drinks on some occasion within 2 weeks of the survey. By 1988, this number had dropped to 35% (USDHHS, 1990a), and by 1993 the number had declined to 30% (Kann et al., 1995).

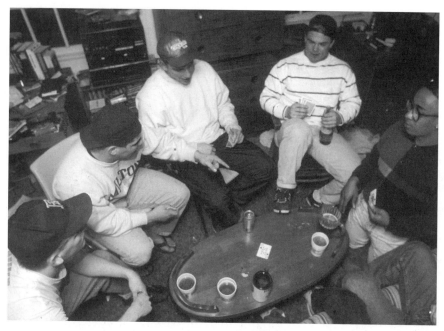

College social gatherings may encourage binge drinking.

Why are young people drinking less? One possibility is that they are replacing alcohol with illicit drugs, but the data do not support this view. Instead, statistics show a parallel decrease in both drug and alcohol use among high school seniors (Johnston et al., 1994a). An alternative possibility is that more high school students have come to believe that alcohol use is hazardous. Indeed, a report by Johnston and his colleagues (1994a) found that the seniors of the early 1990s expressed more negative attitudes toward drinking than the seniors during the prior 2 decades. A large majority of secondary school students disapproved of drug use, including alcohol and tobacco, holding negative attitudes even about experimental use of these substances.

Alcohol consumption rates are lowest among older adults, but the reasons are not clear. Studies have consistently shown relatively low levels of drinking as well as alcohol dependence among people over 60 (USDHHS, 1990a; USDHHS, 1994c). One hypothesis for this observation is that people who drink heavily tend to die before they reach age 65, thus leaving mostly abstainers and moderate drinkers in that age category. Although this explanation accounts for some of the decline, it does not account for all of it. Some studies that have followed the same people over time (NIAAA, 1988; Stall, 1986) have found only a small decrease in alcohol consumption as people become older, but other research (Chen & Kandel, 1995; Fillmore, 1987a, 1987b) has shown a decrease in both drinking and illicit drug use after age 29. James's belief that he is "settling down" may be correct, although he is still several years younger than 29.

THE EFFECTS OF ALCOHOL

As Goodwin (1976) pointed out, essentially the same thing happens to alcohol when you drink it as when you do not—it turns to vinegar. In the body, two enzymes turn alcohol into vinegar, or acetic acid. The first enzyme, **alcohol dehydrogenase,** is located in the liver and has no other known function except to metabolize alcohol. Alcohol dehydrogenase breaks down alcohol into aldehyde, a very toxic chemical. **Aldehyde dehydrogenase** converts aldehyde to acetic acid.

The process of metabolizing alcohol produces at least three health-related outcomes: (1) an increase in lactic acid, which correlates with anxiety attacks; (2) an increase in uric acid, which causes gout; and (3) an increase of fat in the liver and in the blood.

The specific alcohol used in beverages is called **ethanol**. Like other alcohols, ethanol is a poison. But cases of alcohol poisoning are rare and almost always involve inexperienced drinkers who have drunk a bottle of distilled liquor in a very short time, often on a "dare." James reported that "funneling," putting a funnel in someone's mouth and pouring beer into the funnel, was sometimes practiced at his fraternity. This method of drinking can provide so much alcohol so rapidly that it can be dangerous. Otherwise, ingesting beverage alcohol is self-limiting: Intoxication usually yields to unconsciousness, preventing lethal poisoning.

Men and women are not equally affected by drinking alcohol. One factor is the difference in body weight; a 120-pound person will be more strongly affected by three ounces of alcohol than a 220-pound person. Research (Frezza et al., 1990) has also indicated that women are more strongly affected by alcohol because of differences in the absorption of alcohol into the blood. These differences may make women more vulnerable to the effects of alcohol regardless of body weight.

Among the problems associated with drinking are alcohol's ability to produce tolerance, dependence, withdrawal, and addiction. Although these concepts can be applied to many drugs, a consideration of the relevance to alcohol is necessary in evaluating alcohol's potential hazards.

Tolerance is a term applied to the effects of a drug when, with continued use, more and more of the drug is required to produce the same effect. Drugs with high tolerance potential are dangerous because people who build up tolerance need to take more of the drug to produce the effect they want and expect. If this amount is progressively larger, any dangerous effects or side effects of the drug will become more of a hazard. Alcohol is not a drug with a high tolerance potential. For some people, heavy use of alcohol for an extended period is required before noticeable tolerance begins to develop. For others, tolerance can develop within a week of moderate daily consumption. With increased tolerance comes an increased risk of damage.

Dependence is separate from tolerance, and it too is a term that can be applied to many drugs. Dependence occurs when a drug becomes so incorporated into the functioning of the body's cells that it becomes necessary for "normal" functioning. If the drug is discontinued, the body's dependence on that drug becomes apparent and **withdrawal** symptoms develop. These symptoms are the body's signs that it is adjusting to functioning without the drug. Dependence and withdrawal are physically determined and are manifested in physical symptoms. Generally, withdrawal symptoms are the opposite of the drug's effects. Because alcohol is a depressant, withdrawal from it produces symptoms of restlessness, irritability, and agitation.

The combination of dependence and withdrawal is often described as **addiction**. Addictive drugs are those that produce dependence and when discontinued, result in withdrawal. Many drugs produce notoriously unpleasant withdrawal, and alcohol is one of the worst. How difficult the process will be depends on many factors, including the length of use and the degree of dependence. In some cases, withdrawal from alcohol can be life threatening, with mortality rates estimated as high as 5% to 10% (Lerner & Fallon, 1985). Usually the first symptom to appear is tremor, the "shakes." Sleep difficulties are also common. In those severely addicted, **delirium tremens** occurs, with hallucinations and disorientation. Convulsions may also occur during withdrawal, a process that usually lasts between 2 days and a week. The physical dangers are so severe that the process is often completed in a special facility devoted to alcohol treatment.

Tolerance and dependence are independent properties. A drug may produce tolerance but not dependence; also, a person can develop dependence on a drug that has little or no tolerance potential. In addition, some drugs have both a tolerance and a dependence potential. Some research (Zinberg, 1981, 1984) even indicates that tolerance and dependence are not inevitable consequences of taking drugs. Not everyone who drinks alcohol does so with sufficient frequency and in sufficient quantity to develop a tolerance, and most drinkers do not become dependent.

Some people speak of "psychological" dependence, but this term has little scientific meaning beyond the notion that some activities, including drinking alcohol, become part of one's habitual manner of responding. Giving up the activity is accomplished only through much difficulty because the person has become habituated to it. Psychological dependence could be extended to many behaviors that are difficult to change, such as gambling, overeating, jogging, or even watching television.

HAZARDS OF ALCOHOL

Alcohol produces a variety of hazards, both direct and indirect. *Direct hazards* are all those harmful physical effects due to alcohol itself, exclusive of any psychological, social, or economic consequences. *Indirect hazards* include all those harmful consequences that result from psychological and physiological impairments produced by alcohol.

Direct Hazards

Although alcohol affects almost every organ system in the body, liver damage is the main health consideration for the long-term, heavy drinker. With heavy drinking (more than five or six drinks a day), fat accumulates in the liver, resulting in its enlargement. If this level of drinking continues, blood flow through the liver becomes blocked, liver cells die, and a form of hepatitis develops. The next stage is **cirrhosis**, the accumulation of nonfunctional scar tissue in the liver. Cirrhosis, an irreversible condition, is a major cause of death among alcoholics, yet not all alcoholics develop it. Moreover, people with no history of alcohol abuse may also develop liver cirrhosis (Gordon & Kannel, 1984), but cirrhosis is significantly associated with heavy alcohol use (Klatsky & Armstrong, 1992) and is the tenth leading cause of death in the United States (USBC, 1995). For reasons not yet clearly understood, mortality from cirrhosis has steadily declined since 1973.

Chronic alcohol abuse is also a factor in developing and dying from respiratory distress. In studying cases of critically ill patients, Marc Moss and his colleagues (Moss, Bucher, Moore, Moore, & Parsons, 1996) found that critically ill patients who were chronic alcohol abusers were more than twice as likely to develop potentially fatal respiratory distress

than those who had no history of alcohol abuse. In addition, the patients with a history of drinking problems were more likely to die if they developed this disorder.

Prolonged, heavy drinking has also been implicated in the development of neurological damage. Alcohol becomes intoxicating when it reaches the brain in sufficient quantity to affect the brain's complex chemistry. Long-term, heavy alcohol use is also related to a specific brain dysfunction called **Korsakoff syndrome** (also known as Wernicke-Korsakoff syndrome). This disorder is characterized by chronic cognitive dysfunction, severe memory problems for recent events, disorientation, and an inability to learn new information. Alcohol is related to the development of this syndrome through its interference with the absorption of thiamine, one of the B vitamins (Martin, Adinoff, Weingarter, Mukherjee, & Eckardt, 1986). Heavy drinkers can experience thiamine deficiency, which is worsened by their typically poor nutrition. Alcohol accelerates the progression of thiamine-related brain damage, and when this process has started, vitamin supplements do not reverse the progression. Most alcoholics do not receive treatment until the process is at an irreversible stage.

Another possible direct hazardous effect of alcohol is cancer. Research evidence on this issue is not entirely clear due to the confounding effects of cigarette smoking in many heavy alcohol users (Popham, Schmidt, & Israelstam, 1984), but prolonged drinking seems to be implicated in cancer of the liver, esophagus, nasopharynx, and larynx (Driver & Swann, 1987). In the Framingham study, deaths from all cancers were only slightly related to heavy consumption of alcohol in men and not at all related in women (Gordon & Kannel, 1984). No evidence from that study showed that light or moderate drinking significantly increased the chances of dying from cancer.

The evidence of alcohol as a risk for breast cancer is also unclear. Some research has suggested that alcohol may increase a woman's risk for breast cancer by about 30% to 50%, with higher levels of consumption leading to increasing risk (van den Brandt, Goldbohn, & van 't Veer, 1995; Willett, Stampfer et al., 1987b). However, several studies

(Feinstein, 1988; Lowenfels & Zevola, 1989) have failed to find a consistent relationship between alcohol consumption and breast cancer, leaving the relationship in question.

Alcohol also affects the cardiovascular system, but the effects may not all be negative. (The next section looks at the possible positive effects of moderate alcohol consumption on cardiovascular functioning.) Heavy, chronic drinking, however, does have a direct and harmful effect on the cardiovascular system. In large doses, alcohol reduces oxidation of fatty acids (the heart's primary fuel source) in the myocardium. The heart directly metabolizes ethanol, producing fatty acid ethyl esters that impair functioning of the energy-producing structures of the heart. Alcohol also can depress the myocardium's ability to contract, which can lead to abnormal cardiac functioning. In addition, large doses of alcohol may have harmful effects on the vascular system, and heavy drinking seems to be responsible for high blood pressure in some individuals. Klatsky (1987) estimated that 5% to 24% of all hypertension is associated with alcohol and that the prevalence of high blood pressure for European Americans who consume more than six drinks a day is twice that of a comparison group of abstainers. Drinking binges have also been associated with stroke, hemorrhage, and other intracranial bleeding (Altura, 1986). These cerebrovascular conditions sometimes occur within 24 hours of a drinking binge. Thus, heavy consumption of alcohol has been linked to nearly all aspects of cardiovascular functioning.

Alcohol has a direct and hazardous effect on pregnancy and the developing fetus. Drinking may affect pregnancy in two basic ways. First, very heavy alcohol consumption reduces fertility (Greenwood, Love, & Pratt, 1983). Several possible reasons exist for infertility in women who are chronic, heavy users of alcohol. For one, excessive alcohol consumption produces amenorrhea, cessation of the menstrual cycle. This effect may be caused either by cirrhosis or by a direct effect of alcohol on the pituitary or the hypothalamus. Another possibility for infertility is vitamin deficiency, especially a lack of thiamine (Greenwood et al., 1983).

The second direct, hazardous effect of excessive drinking during pregnancy is that it increases the risk of **fetal alcohol syndrome (FAS)**. FAS affects

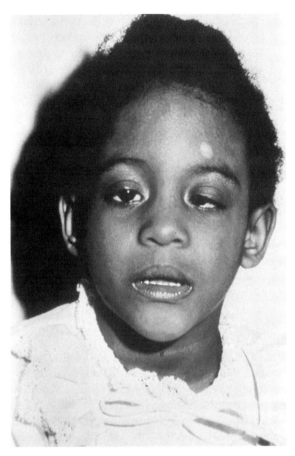

Facial abnormalities, growth deficiencies, central nervous system disorders, and mental retardation are symptoms of fetal alcohol syndrome.

many infants of mothers who drank excessively during pregnancy. This syndrome includes specific facial abnormalities, growth deficiencies, central nervous system disorders, and mental retardation. The disorder has increased during recent years, climbing from an incidence of 1.0 per 10,000 births in 1979 to 6.7 per 10,000 births in 1993 (CDC, 1995d). Although heavy drinking is the main contributor to fetal alcohol syndrome (Pratt, 1980, 1982), heavy smoking, stress, and poor nutrition are also involved. Combinations of these factors are not unusual in heavy drinkers.

Reducing alcohol consumption during pregnancy can help reduce the chances of fetal alcohol syndrome. One study (Ouellette, Rosett, Rosman, & Weinen, 1977) found that heavy drinkers—five or more drinks per occasion—had a good chance of delivering normal infants if they significantly decreased their level of drinking before becoming pregnant. Such a decrease may not be likely. According to one survey (CDC, 1995a), over 45% of women who had become pregnant and completed their pregnancies had drunk during the 3 months before they became pregnant, and over 20% continued to drink after they learned they were pregnant.

What about moderate and even light drinking during pregnancy? Light to moderate drinking is not likely to cause fetal alcohol syndrome (USDHHS, 1990a), but significant decreases in cognitive functioning have been observed in children of mothers who drank 3 or more drinks per day during pregnancy (Larroque et al., 1995). More than a decade ago, the U.S. Surgeon General warned pregnant women and women who were trying to become pregnant not to drink (Public Health Service, 1981). Children born to women who average two drinks a day have a lower average birth weight, and this condition, although not itself a danger, is related to many risks for newborns. Also, women who drink as little as four drinks a week show an increased risk of spontaneous abortion. Children of women who drank moderately during pregnancy showed somewhat slower reaction times and greater distractibility (Streissguth et al., 1986). Even small amounts of alcohol, especially during the early months of pregnancy, have a direct and hazardous effect on the developing fetus, at least for many women (Coles, Smith, Lancaster, & Falek, 1987).

Indirect Hazards

In addition to the direct physiological dangers of alcohol consumption, several indirect effects pose further (and more common) risks, not only for the drinker but for others as well. These dangers arise from alcohol's effects on coordination and from effects on the processes of aggression, judgment, and attention. Alcohol affects coordination and alters cognitive functioning in ways that may be hazardous. Alcohol diminishes the ability to perform tasks requiring complex attention and decision making (Damkot, Kirk, & Huntley, 1983). Large doses of alcohol may reduce the ability to assess a task's importance, so that poor performance becomes more acceptable to the drinker (Damkot et al., 1983).

These effects are most prominently and obviously related to driving ability, but they also influence decision making in sexual situations. Problem drinkers (Avins et al., 1994) and nonproblem drinkers (Stall, McKusick, Wiley, Coates, & Ostrow, 1986) both tend to be less likely to use safe sex procedures when they use alcohol. Unsafe sexual practices are also associated with drug use, especially cocaine and marijuana. Lowry et al. (1994) gathered information on 9th- to 12th-grade students and found that those who used alcohol, compared with those with no substance use, were somewhat more likely to have had four or more sexual partners and less likely to have used a condom in their last sexual encounter. In contrast, high school students who used cocaine were 10 times more likely and those who used marijuana were 6 times more likely to have had four or more sexual partners and not to have used a condom during their last sexual event.

Both laboratory experiments and crime statistics have shown a relationship between alcohol and aggression. In a review of laboratory studies, Taylor and Leonard (1983) concluded that moderate and high doses of alcohol produce aggression in about 30% of drinkers. In a nonlaboratory situation, Taylor, Gammon, and Capasso (1976) found that both a threat of harm and actual physical injury can prompt aggression among heavy drinkers. In addition, people exposed to others who urge aggression (as opposed to restraint) are more likely to act aggressively (Taylor & Leonard, 1983). Aggression, therefore, is not an inevitable or a simple consequence of the pharmacological effects of alcohol but rather a response that may occur in certain situations and with certain individuals.

An early study (Wolfgang, 1957) on the relationship between alcohol and crime indicated that either the victim or the offender or both had been drinking in two-thirds of the homicides studied. A later study (Mayfield, 1976) substantiated those earlier results, indicating that in only one-third of homicides was neither offender nor victim using alcohol. Not only are people who commit homicides likely to be drinking, but consuming alcohol also increases the chances of being a crime victim. These relationships, however, do not demonstrate a *causal* relationship between alcohol and crime. In addition, the majority of crimes are committed by people who are *not* alcohol dependent, and the majority of alcohol abusers do *not* commit crimes.

Alcohol also increases the likelihood of accidents, the fourth leading cause of death in the United States and the leading cause of death for people under age 45 (USBC, 1995). Anda, Williamson, and Remington (1988) found a strong relationship between the number of drinks consumed per occasion and the incidence of fatal injuries. People who consumed five or more drinks per occasion were twice as likely to die from accidents as people who drank fewer than five drinks per occasion. People who reported drinking nine or more drinks were 3.3 times as likely to die from injuries. Li, Smith, and Baker (1994) found that people who drank five or more drinks per occasion were 50% more likely to die of injuries of all kinds than light or nondrinkers, but Brewer et al. (1994) found people with a history of drunkenness were at least four times more likely than other people to die in an automobile crash.

These risks were relevant to James and his fraternity brothers who were binge drinkers. They tried not to drive while drunk and to take care of each other, but they did not designate a nondrinking driver. Instead, the designated driver role fell to the least intoxicated person. The fraternity members were not exempt from hazards; one member was killed in an automobile crash and one committed suicide while drinking and playing Russian roulette. James says that these tragedies did not slow the rate of drinking in the fraternity.

Alcohol also increases the incidence of nonfatal injuries as well as the use of medical services. Blose and Holder (1991) studied utilization of medical services for injury in a group of problem drinkers compared to a matched group of nonproblem drinkers. They found that the drinkers had 1.6 times more incidents of medical care utilization (and three times the cost) compared with those without drinking problems. These increased risks and costs applied to both women and men and to all the age groups studied.

In summary, alcohol is a risk factor for many types of violence, both criminal and accidental. The level of alcohol consumption necessary to increase the risk is not so high as the level necessary to produce legal intoxication; any amount of drinking increases the risk. However, the relationship is dose related: People who drink heavily are more likely to be involved in accidents and violent crimes than are light or moderate drinkers.

BENEFITS OF ALCOHOL

Is it possible that drinking might be *good* for you? This question was raised as a result of several early studies (Room & Day, 1974; Stason, Neff, Miettinen, & Jick, 1976) that reported a U-shaped or J-shaped relationship between alcohol consumption and mortality. In other words, light to moderate drinkers (one to five drinks per day) had the best prospects for good health, whereas nondrinkers and heavy drinkers had the greatest risk. Later evidence from several longitudinal studies supported the findings that light or moderate drinking was positively related to both reduced mortality and lower risk of disease. These early studies have prompted further research, which has consistently found some health benefits for light to moderate levels of alcohol consumption.

Reduced Mortality

A group of researchers (Klatsky, Friedman, & Siegelaub, 1981) at the Kaiser Permanente health facility conducted a longitudinal study of alcohol and mortality. This study followed more than 2,000 European American and African American men and women for 10 years and charted their mortality rates in relation to their drinking habits. The participants were divided into four groups: (1) nondrinkers, (2) those reporting two or fewer drinks per day, (3) those reporting three to five drinks per day, and (4) those reporting more than six drinks per day. Light drinkers (those reporting two or fewer drinks per day) had the lowest mortality rate. Nondrinkers had a mortality rate comparable to that of moderate drinkers, and both had mortality rates 50% higher than those of the light drinkers. Heavy drinkers (people who reported drinking over six drinks per day) fared worst, with a mortality rate double that for light drinkers. Cancer, cirrhosis, accidents, and respiratory conditions all contributed to this increase in mortality.

Additional research has confirmed the results that drinking can be beneficial, in studies of both the general population and selected populations. The Alameda County study (Berkman, Breslow, &

Wingard, 1983), the Framingham study (Friedman & Kimball, 1986; Gordon & Kannel, 1984), the Albany study (Gordon & Doyle, 1987), a population-based study of European Americans in the United States (Coate, 1993), and a study conducted in Australia (Cullen, Knuiman, & Ward, 1993) found that moderate-drinking men had a survival advantage, although the relationship for women was not so clear. However, a later study of female nurses (whose drinking habits were similar to those of U.S. women in general) showed that compared with nondrinkers, women who consumed 3 1/2 to 18 drinks per week had a reduced risk of death, especially from cardiovascular disease (Fuchs et al., 1995). Women who drank more than 18 drinks per week, however, had an increased risk of death from other causes, such as breast cancer and cirrhosis. Yet another study (Scherr et al., 1992) extended the benefits of drinking to both men and women over the age of 65. This study found that older people who drank moderately had both lower mortality and lower cardiovascular risk than nondrinkers.

The decrease in mortality associated with drinking seems to be due to lowered coronary heart disease (CHD) (Gordon & Doyle, 1987). Although non-CHD death rates for drinkers and nondrinkers differed little, abstainers were significantly *more* likely to die of coronary heart disease than were drinkers. This and other reports strongly suggest that moderate consumption of alcoholic beverages can reduce one's risk of death, especially from cardiovascular disease (Klatsky, 1987; Lange, & Kinnumen, 1987; Stampfer, Colditz, Willett, Speizer, & Hennekens, 1988). Furthermore, the type of alcoholic drink may make a difference for mortality risk. Grønbaek et al. (1995) found that, among adult drinkers in Denmark, wine decreased mortality risk, distilled spirits increased risk, and beer made no difference in risk. Because other studies have found no differences relating to type of alcohol, this study's results may be due to the location or to some socioeconomic or behavioral differences among those who drank various types of alcoholic beverages.

What factors could account for this negative relationship between light to moderate levels of drinking and cardiovascular mortality? Several suggestions have been made, but the most likely explanation involves high-density lipoprotein (HDL). Specific sub-fractions of high-density lipoprotein known as HDL_2 and HDL_3 are negatively associated with coronary heart disease. If consumption of alcohol contributes specifically to the elevation of HDL_2 and HDL_3, then moderate or heavy drinking should offer protection against heart disease. Several reports (Avogaro, Cazzolato, Belussi, & Bittolo Bon, 1982; Gaziano et al., 1993; Linn et al., 1993) have indicated that drinking is related to elevations of these HDL subfractions and to decreased risk for heart attack.

More recent research has suggested that increases in HDL are not the only means by which alcohol consumption protects against heart disease. Jackson, Scragg, and Beaglehole (1992) found that even recent consumption of alcohol tends to protect against heart attack; that is, people who had consumed alcohol during the past 24 hours had a lower risk of both fatal and nonfatal heart attack than those who had not drunk alcohol. Because HDL levels cannot increase so rapidly, this finding indicated that some other mechanism also contributes to alcohol's protective qualities. Ridker, Vaughan, Stampfer, Glynn, and Hennekens (1994) explored an additional factor: plasma concentration of tissue-type plasminogen activator, a substance in the blood that relates to clotting. They compared this factor in healthy men and found a direct, significant correlation between alcohol consumption and plasma levels of this substance. They interpreted their findings as evidence that alcohol may protect against the formation of blood clots, thus guarding against heart attacks. Furthermore, this protective factor changes quickly, providing some protection against heart attack within hours of consumption

In summary, the reduced mortality associated with light to moderate levels of drinking is largely attributable to decreased coronary heart disease fatalities, which offsets other sources of mortality, such as cirrhosis and accidents. The decrease in CHD mortality seems to be due to increases in high-density lipoprotein and possibly to decreased tendency to form internal blood clots.

Other Benefits of Alcohol

If moderate drinking has a beneficial effect on mortality rates, could it also be related to better health? Investigators in the Alameda County study (Camacho & Wiley, 1983) found that moderate alcohol consumption (17 to 45 drinks per month) was most closely associated with good health scores. Abstention was negatively related to subsequent health, and heavy drinkers, especially women, reported somewhat lower health scores than the average, but these people were not as unhealthy as the nondrinkers.

People who drink may also have better mental health than those who abstain due to the buffering effects of drinking on stress. Lipton (1994) studied depression, stress, and drinking and found that drinkers who were under stress were less likely to be depressed than abstainers under similar stress. As in the studies that have related physical health and drinking, Lipton found a U-shaped relationship between drinking and depression in which those who do not drink and those who drink heavily showed higher levels of depression than light and moderate drinkers.

In addition, alcohol may increase bone mineral density in both women and men and thus provide some protection against bone fractures. As part of the Framingham study, Felson, Zhang, Hannan, Kannel, and Kiel (1995) studied alcohol consumption in a group of elderly people and found that women who drank seven or more ounces of alcohol per week had higher bone mineral density than women who were light drinkers or nondrinkers. For men, consumption of 14 ounces or more per week was associated with higher bone mineral density, although the difference for men was not as great as it was for women. Felson et al. reported that lesser amounts of alcohol intake did not improve levels of bone mineral density.

The conclusion that drinkers not only have a lower mortality rate than abstainers but are sick less often, are less depressed, and have stronger bones is controversial (see box — Would You Believe . . . ?).

WHY DO PEOPLE DRINK?

Those trying to understand drinking and alcohol abuse have proposed several models to explain behavior related to alcohol. These models go beyond the pharmacological effects of alcohol and even beyond the research findings to integrate and explain drinking. To be useful, a model for drinking behavior must address at least three questions. First, why do people start drinking? Second, why do most people maintain moderate rather than excessive drinking levels? Third, why do some drink so much as to develop serious problems?

As we discussed in the section "A Brief History of Drinking," alcohol use has varied across time and culture. Until the 19th century in the United States and Europe, drinking was well accepted but drunkenness was unacceptable under most circumstances. This attitude makes drinking the norm, thus requiring no explanation for it, but leaves drunkenness unexplained. McMurran (1994) described how the need to explain drunkenness led to the development of two views of drinking problems: the moral model and the disease model.

The moral model appeared first, holding that people have free will and choose their behaviors, including excessive drinking. Those who do so are, thus, either sinful or morally lacking in the self-discipline necessary to moderate their drinking. The moral model of alcoholism began to fade in the late 19th century, when the medical model started to gain prominence. Unacceptable behaviors that were formerly seen as moral problems became medical problems and, thus, subject to scientific explanation and medical treatment. The medical model of alcoholism conceptualized problem drinking as symptomatic of underlying physical problems, and the notion that alcoholism is hereditary grew from this view. The first form of this hypothesis took the view that a "constitutional weakness" ran in families and that this weakness produced alcoholics.

Today, the concept of constitutional weakness has taken the form of a genetic component for alcoholism. Several methods of addressing the genetics of alcoholism are possible, but most research has concentrated either on twins or adopted children. Twin studies ordinarily involve measuring the degree of agreement between pairs of identical twins, with comparisons in the amount of agreement between pairs of fraternal twins. If identical twins are more similar to each another than fraternal twins are, the difference is assumed to be due to genetics. Deitrich and Spuhler (1984) reviewed five studies using this method. One found a 54.2% agreement between pairs of identical twins compared to only a 31.5% agreement between fraternal twins, when alcoholism was defined as a pathological desire for alcohol, physical dependence on alcohol, and blackouts. This greater concordance between identical

WOULD YOU BELIEVE . . . ?

What Your Doctor Never Told You about Alcohol

Would you believe that drinking may be good for you, but health care professionals are reluctant to admit it? Addiction authority Stanton Peele (1993) contended that medical investigators, public health officials, and health educators are uneasy about research findings concerning alcohol's beneficial health effects. He suggested that the United States has been so influenced by what he called the "temperance mentality" that medical authorities have trouble accepting their own findings about alcohol. "A cultural preoccupation with alcoholism and the negative effects of drinking works against frank scientific discussions in the United States of the advantages for the cardiovascular system of alcohol consumption" (Peele, 1993, p. 805).

Medical authorities have spent so much time in forming arguments for the negative effects of alcohol that they have trouble acknowledging that it might also have positive effects. For example, Shari Linn and her colleagues (1993) studied a representative sample of the U.S. population to determine the relationship between high-density lipoprotein (HDL) and alcohol consumption. They found such a relationship for both European Americans and African Americans even after controlling for other factors that influence HDL. These researchers were left with the finding that drinking increases HDL, which has been shown to relate to lowered cardiovascular risk. However, they did not conclude that people at risk for heart disease should increase their alcohol consumption. Instead they said, "Even if there is a causal association between alcohol consumption and higher HDL cholesterol levels, it is suggested that efforts to reduce coronary heart disease risks concentrate on the cessation of smoking and weight control" (Linn et al., 1993, p. 811). In making these conclusions, they ignored their own findings.

Peele contended that the negative effects of alcohol dominate discussions at professional conferences and meetings. Researchers, despite the research findings, are eager to condemn and reluctant to recommend drinking, an obvious bias among these scientists. No official medical organization in the United States has made a recommendation concerning the positive effects of drinking alcohol. Peele pointed out that the benefits of light to moderate drinking are similar to those obtained by following a low-fat diet in decreasing the risk for coronary heart disease, yet many medical groups have made official statements concerning the wisdom of adopting a low-fat diet, and none have recommended moderate drinking.

The first official statement about the benefits of light drinking came in 1996 from a joint committee of the Agriculture Department and the Department of Health and Human Services (Burros, 1996). The acknowledgment that light drinking may lower the risk of heart disease appears in the latest version of the *Dietary Guidelines for Americans,* but these guidelines continue to caution against drinking other than with meals and more than one drink per day for women and two for men.

The potential for danger from heavy drinking is a continuing theme in the *Guidelines* as it is in the recommendations from medical groups. The reason for this hesitation to recommend drinking despite the evidence of its cardiovascular benefits may be the inherent conservatism of medical groups and the fear that some people may take the recommendation to drink as permission to overindulge. Peele, however, believes that the history of the Temperance movement has resulted in a widespread reluctance to acknowledge alcohol's positive effects, perhaps to the detriment of those who could benefit from such recommendations.

---

twins supports the idea of at least some genetic component in alcohol abuse, but the other studies in the review were less clear in implicating heredity in problem drinking.

A stricter test of a hereditary factor in alcohol abuse is the study of adopted children. Adoption studies investigate the frequency of alcohol abuse in adoptees whose biological parent was alcoholic, and the most widely publicized of these studies have been conducted in Denmark by Donald Goodwin and his colleagues (Goodwin, Schulsinger, Hermansen, Guze, & Winokur, 1973). Despite Goodwin's interpretation of results from these studies as clear support of a hereditary component for alcoholism, questions concerning the definition and diagnosis criteria have resulted in less than clear support.

C. Robert Cloninger has conducted studies in Sweden with adopted men (Cloninger, Bohman, & Sigvardsson, 1981) and adopted women (Bohman, Sigvardsson, & Cloninger, 1981). By dividing participants into groups with combinations of environmental and genetic risks and diagnoses of different levels of drinking problems, these researchers were able to conclude that men with both types of risk had the greatest likelihood of developing drinking problems. The small differences between those men with either social or genetic risks suggest that both factors contribute to the development of both mild and severe drinking problems. For the moderate problem category, however, a different picture developed: Genetics was clearly more influential than social factors. Men with only a genetic risk had a 16.9% chance of developing moderate alcoholism whereas men at risk socially had a 4.1% chance. Men with both risks had only a 17.9% likelihood, thus indicating that the social environment added very little to the contributions of heredity.

These studies suggest that understanding the relative influence of heredity and environment for alcoholism is a complex problem, with few clear-cut answers. Both factors play a role in the development of alcohol abuse, and the people most likely to become alcoholics are those who have both a genetic and an environmental risk. Peele (1993) warned against accepting a simple version of hereditary influences on drinking by saying:

> Whatever people may inherit that heightens susceptibility to alcoholism operates over years as a part of the long-term development of alcohol dependence. Moreover, a large majority of children of alcoholics do not become alcoholic, and the majority of alcoholics do not have alcoholic parents. (p. 809)

THE DISEASE MODEL

The disease concept of alcoholism is a variation of the medical model, holding that people with problem drinking have the disease of alcoholism. Over the past 50 years, this model has been the most influential. In psychiatric and other medically oriented treatment programs in the United States, the disease model still predominates, but it is less influential in psychologically based treatment programs and in treatment programs in Europe and in Australia.

Throughout history, isolated attempts have been made to describe alcohol intoxication as a disease brought about by the physical properties of alcohol, but not until the late 1930s and early 1940s did this view begin to become popular. Room (1972) has argued that advocacy of the disease model was based

not so much on scientific evidence but on the desire to free the alcoholic from the stigma of sin and debauchery.

The disease model of alcoholism was elevated to scientific respectability by the pioneering work of E. M. Jellinek (1960), who identified several different types of alcoholism and described various characteristics of these types, such as loss of control and inability to abstain. More recently, Jellinek's disease model has been replaced by the alcohol dependency syndrome.

The Alcohol Dependency Syndrome

The alcohol dependency syndrome (Edwards, 1977; Edwards & Gross, 1976; Edwards, Gross, Keller, Moser, & Room, 1977) grew out of some dissatisfaction with the term *alcoholism* and the traditional concept of alcoholism as a disease. The word *syndrome* adds flexibility to the disease model by suggesting a group of concurrent behaviors that accompany alcohol dependence. The behaviors need not always be observed in an individual, nor do they need to be observable to the same degree in everyone who is alcohol dependent. Edwards and his colleagues modified several of Jellinek's concepts, including the notion that alcoholics experience loss of control. Rather, the alcohol dependency syndrome holds that those who are alcohol dependent have *impaired control*, suggesting that people drink heavily because, at certain times and for a variety of reasons, they do not exercise control over their drinking.

Edwards and Gross (1976) described seven essential elements of the alcohol dependency syndrome. First is a *narrowing of drinking repertoire*. Second is a *salience of drink-seeking behavior*, meaning that drinking begins to take priority over all other aspects of life. A third element of the alcohol dependency syndrome is *increased tolerance*. As noted earlier, alcohol does not produce as much tolerance as some other drugs do, but some drinkers gradually become accustomed to going about their daily routine "at blood alcohol levels that would incapacitate the non-tolerant drinker" (Edwards & Gross, 1976, p. 1059).

A fourth element of the alcohol dependency syndrome is *withdrawal symptoms*. As previously mentioned, the severity of withdrawal depends on length and amount of use. Those who are alcohol dependent

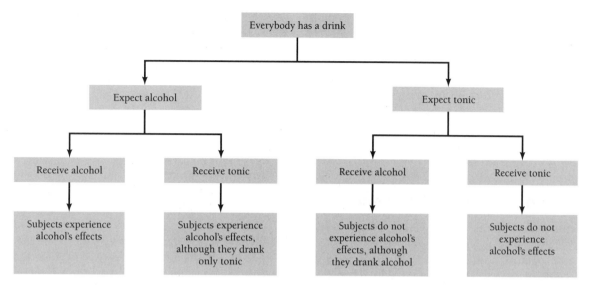

Figure 14.3   Balanced placebo design.

avoid withdrawal symptoms by further drinking, the fifth characteristic of the alcohol dependency syndrome. A mildly dependent person might relieve the morning "blues" by having a drink with lunch, but some drinkers use the strategy of avoiding withdrawal symptoms by maintaining a steady alcohol level.

The sixth element is the *subjective awareness of the compulsion to drink.* The final element of the alcohol dependency syndrome is *reinstatement of dependence after abstinence.* Edwards and Gross believe that time of reinstatement is inversely related to the degree of dependence. Moderately dependent people may not reinstate drinking for months, whereas severely dependent patients may resume full dependence in as little as 3 days.

Evaluation of the Disease Model

Despite the continuing popularity of the disease model of alcoholism, the concept has serious limitations, failing to address our first two questions: "Why do people begin to drink?" and "Why do some people continue to drink at a moderate level?" The disease model is limited to explaining why some people drink too much, but only limited empirical evidence supports the disease model.

One key concept in the disease model is loss of control or impaired control—the inability to stop or moderate alcohol intake once drinking begins.

Research has not supported this key concept. G. Alan Marlatt and his colleagues (Marlatt, Demming, & Reid, 1973; Marlatt & Rohsenow, 1980) have conducted experiments suggesting that many effects of alcohol, including impaired control, are due more to expectancy than to any pharmacological effect of alcohol. Their experimental design, called the *balanced placebo design,* included four groups, two of which expect to be given alcohol and two of which do not. Two groups actually received alcohol, and two did not. Figure 14.3 shows all four combinations.

Using the balanced placebo design, several studies (Marlatt et al., 1973; Marlatt & Rohsenow, 1980) showed that people who think they have received alcohol behave as though they have (whether they have or not). Even for those who had been in treatment for problem drinking, expectancy appeared to be the controlling factor in the craving for alcohol and in the amount consumed. These findings suggest that loss of control and craving for alcohol results from expectancy rather than from some physical property of alcohol. The difference between severely dependent drinkers and moderately dependent drinkers (Stockwell, Hodgson, Rankin, & Taylor, 1982) suggests some possible differences between those whose dependence is severe and those with less serious drinking problems. Although this study did not provide strong support for the disease model of alcoholism, it is one of the few well-controlled studies to have found any support for the model.

Some investigators (Alexander, 1988; Marlatt, 1987; McMurran, 1994) have criticized the disease model of alcohol, arguing that it does not adequately consider environmental, cognitive, and affective determinants of abusive drinking; that is, in its emphasis on the physical properties of alcohol, the disease model neglects the cognitive and social learning aspects of drinking.

COGNITIVE-PHYSIOLOGICAL THEORIES

Alternatives to the disease model exist, several of which emphasize the combination of physiological and cognitive changes that occur with alcohol use. Rather than hypothesizing that alcohol use and misuse are based only on the chemical properties of alcohol, these models contend that alcohol use also depends on the cognitive changes experienced by drinkers.

The Tension Reduction Hypothesis

As the name suggests, the tension reduction hypothesis (Conger, 1956) holds that people drink alcohol because of its tension-reducing effects. This hypothesis has much intuitive appeal because alcohol is a sedative drug that leads to relaxation and slowed reactions.

However, alcohol's effects on physiological processes are not simple (Levenson, Sher, Grossman, Newman, & Newlin, 1980). Moderate doses of alcohol stimulate some responses (such as heart rate); other responses (such as pulse wave velocity, a measurement that relates to the heart muscle's ability to contract) become slower, and yet other responses (such as skeletal muscle tension) remain unaffected. Such a complex pattern of physiological responses does not support a simple version of the tension reduction hypothesis.

Studies that have manipulated tension or anxiety to observe their effects on a participants' readiness to consume alcohol have yielded contradictory results. Higgins and Marlatt (1973) found no relationship between the threat of a painful shock and subsequent amount of alcohol consumed, but a later study by these same investigators (Higgins & Marlatt, 1975) found that male participants who expected to be evaluated by a woman on the basis of their looks (and thus were considered to be anxious) drank more than those participants who expected no such evaluation.

A longitudinal study (Rohsenow, 1982) of men who were heavy social drinkers found social anxiety to be negatively related to drinking; that is, the *less* socially anxious the participants were, the more they drank. This study also found that men who had social support for their drinking were the ones who tended to drink most heavily. Thus, men may drink to attain a positive mood rather than to avoid a negative state of tension.

Wilson (1987) reviewed some of these same studies and concluded that they do not support the tension reduction hypothesis. He cited studies that show alcohol may increase, decrease, or have no effect on tension in both social drinkers and problem drinkers. In addition, situational variables other than the alcohol itself may reduce tension. For example, men may feel less shy about approaching women when they are drinking, but this strategy may not be successful because women who drink often act more defensively in a sexual setting. Wilson concluded that one's social learning history may determine the degree of relaxation in many social situations.

Although the original version of the tension reduction hypothesis has found little support, a reformulation of this view seems to be more viable. A group of researchers at Indiana University (Levenson et al., 1980; Sher, 1987; Sher & Levenson, 1982) discovered that high levels of alcohol consumption decrease the strength of responses to stress. They labeled this decrease the **stress-response-dampening (SRD) effect**. People who had been drinking did not respond as strongly as nondrinking participants to either physiological or psychological stressors. Interestingly, people whose personality profile suggested a high risk of developing problem drinking showed the strongest SRD effect, and those whose profile indicated a low risk showed a weaker effect (Sher & Levenson, 1982). These results suggest that rather than reducing tension, alcohol may cause some people to avoid tension.

The Self-Awareness Model

A second approach, proposed by Jay Hull, is based on social psychological theories of self-awareness

(Hull, 1981, 1987; Hull & Bond, 1986). Hull built a model of drinking behavior on the observation that alcohol consumption indirectly affects behavior through changes in cognitive processes. He then hypothesized that alcohol can interfere with cognition to make thought more superficial and to decrease negative self-feedback. Negative self-feedback consists of statements such as "I can't do anything very well" or "I shouldn't be such a coward." By making cognition more superficial, alcohol enables people either to reduce or to avoid these kinds of tension-producing self-statements and thus to think better of themselves than when they are not drinking.

Hull's explanation of drinking is therefore based on changes in self-awareness. By inhibiting the use of normal, complex information-processing strategies, such as memory and information acquisition, drinking makes people less self-aware. Decreased self-awareness leads to decreased monitoring of behavior, resulting in the disinhibition that commonly occurs among drinkers.

This model also proposes that drinkers become less self-critical as they become less self-aware because they fail to process information that reflects badly on them. Hull (1987) hypothesized that this effect may be the reason that some people consume alcohol—to avoid self-awareness. Reduced self-awareness might also be rewarding through decreased self-censure for inappropriate (but personally attractive) social behavior. Therefore, loss of self-awareness can offer some rewards, which explains why people drink and why some people drink unwisely. What this model fails to elaborate is who will fall into each category.

Alcohol Myopia

Claude Steele and his colleagues (Steele & Josephs, 1990) have developed a model of alcohol use and abuse based on alcohol's psychological and physical properties. This model hypothesizes that alcohol use creates effects on social behaviors that produce a kind of *alcohol myopia*, a type of shortsightedness in which alcohol blocks out insightful cognitive processing and alters thoughts related to the self, stress, and social anxiety. That is, "Alcohol makes us the captive of an impoverished version of reality in which the breadth, depth, and time line of our understanding is constrained" (Steele & Josephs, 1990, p. 923).

Part of alcohol myopia is drunken excess, the tendency for those who drink to behave more excessively. This tendency appears as increased aggression, friendliness, sexiness, and many other exaggerated behaviors. Steele and Josephs contended that tendencies to behave in such extreme ways are usually inhibited, but when people drink, they experience less inhibition, and their behavior becomes more extreme.

Another aspect of alcohol myopia is self-inflation, a tendency to inflate self-evaluations. Banaji and Steele (1989) studied self-inflation by asking people to rate the importance of 35 trait dimensions for their real and ideal selves. They found a difference between responses for participants when they were drunk and when they were sober. When drunk, participants rated themselves higher on traits that were important to them and on which they had rated themselves low when sober. Thus, drinking allowed participants to see themselves as better than they did when they were not drinking.

Steele and Josephs (1990) described a third aspect of alcohol myopia as "drunken relief" (p. 928). They contended that people who drink tend to worry less; that is, they pay less attention to their worries. Thus, alcohol can have stress-relieving properties. Steele and Josephs argued that alcohol alone is not sufficient to reduce stress unless consumed in large quantities, but combined with distracting activity, lower levels of alcohol become a powerful stress reducer. Steele, Southwick, and Pagano (1986) demonstrated the combined effect of alcohol and distraction by presenting people with either alcohol, a pleasant and distracting activity, both, or neither. They found that participants who received both were the only ones who experienced significant anxiety relief. Therefore, drunken relief is not entirely an effect of alcohol but of alcohol in combination with other factors in the social environment that provide distraction.

THE SOCIAL LEARNING MODEL

Many psychologists accept the social learning model as the most useful explanation for why people begin to drink, why they continue to drink in moderation, and why some people drink in a harmful manner (Abrams & Niaura, 1987). Social learning theory conceives of drinking as learned behavior, acquired in the same manner as other behaviors.

People begin to drink, according to social learning theory, for at least three reasons. First, the taste of alcohol and its immediate effects may bring pleasure (positive reinforcement); second, a person may decide earlier that drinking alcohol is consistent with personal standards (cognitive mediation); and third, the person may learn to drink through observing others (modeling). Any one or a combination of these factors is sufficient to initiate and guide drinking behavior. Social learning was a prominent feature of drinking for James. He began to drink with his friends and continued to drink in the company of fraternity brothers who also drank. Now that he is not around his fraternity friends so much, he drinks less.

As the social learning model would predict, culture affects the expectations for pleasant effects of alcohol. By questioning people from eight countries, Lindman, Sjöholm, and Lang (1994) found significant national differences in beliefs about alcohol's effects. Participants from the United States had the most and those from Spain the least positive expectations for drinking. U.S. participants responded that alcohol increases the pleasure of social interactions, interpersonal warmth, and optimism whereas people from Belgium, Poland, France, Italy, and Finland believed less strongly in these positive effects, and participants from Panama and Spain said that drinking decreased these pleasurable effects.

The social learning model also offers several explanations for why people drink too much. Lang and Marlatt (1982) suggested that excessive drinking may serve as a coping response. Although alcohol acts as a depressant, the initial effect of small doses is often interpreted by drinkers as enhancement of their ability to cope. This response gives drinkers a sense of power and also a feeling of avoiding responsibility or minimizing stress. People will then continue to drink as long as they perceive that alcohol has desirable effects.

Modeling also provides an explanation for heavy drinking. Ample evidence indicates that people who observe a heavy-drinking model will consume more alcohol than those who observe a light-drinking model or no model at all. Caudill and Marlatt (1975), for instance, found that heavy-drinking college men

(social drinking), when exposed to no model or to a light-drinking model consumed less than participants who were exposed to a heavy-drinking confederate. In a similar study, Lied and Marlatt (1979) found that observing a heavy-drinking model increased consumption in drinkers with a prior history of heavy drinking; but when light drinkers observed a heavy-drinking model, they increased their consumption only slightly. Thus people are not compelled to imitate a heavy-drinking model, a finding that offers some support for the assumption that personal standards play a role in shaping behavior.

A third explanation for excessive drinking offered by the social learning model is based on the principles of negative reinforcement. Most heavy drinkers have learned that they can avoid or reduce the painful effects of withdrawal symptoms by maintaining blood alcohol concentrations at a particular level. As this level begins to drop, the alcohol addict feels the discomfort of withdrawal. These symptoms can be avoided by ingesting more alcohol; thus, negative reinforcement increases the probability that heavy drinking will continue.

Social learning theory provides an explanation for why people start drinking, why some continue to drink in moderation, and why others become problem drinkers. In addition, social learning theory also suggests a variety of treatment techniques to help people overcome excessive drinking habits. Because drinking behavior is learned, it can be unlearned or relearned, with either abstinence or moderation as a goal of therapy.

QUITTING DRINKING

Despite a recent and steady decline in the percentage of drinkers in the United States, an increasing number of people seek help for problem drinking, with over half a million people receiving treatment on any given day (Weisner, Greenfield, & Room, 1995). During the 1980s private, for-profit treatment facilities proliferated at a much higher rate than nonprofit and public facilities. In addition, the number of workplace substance abuse treatment programs and drunk driver campaigns have increased during the past 15 years.

Although the number of people who seek treatment for alcohol abuse has grown, their demographic characteristics have remained much the same. People between ages 25 and 44 years are the most likely to seek treatment, and men outnumber women by a ratio of 8 to 1 (Weisner et al., 1995). However, the prevalence of women who seek treatment may be partially shielded by their greater tendency to seek help in non-alcohol-specific settings, such as mental health treatment services (Weisner & Schmidt, 1992). Most people receive outpatient rather than inpatient treatment, although private, for-profit facilities emphasize inpatient treatment. Inpatient programs are eight times more costly than outpatient treatment (Hayashida et al., 1989), and existing evidence shows no differences in outcome among inpatient, outpatient, partial hospitalization, and day clinic settings (USDHHS, 1987). In addition to the various treatment settings, a majority of alcoholics are able to quit drinking without formal treatment (McMurran, 1994).

CHANGE WITHOUT THERAPY

Some problems (and even some diseases) disappear without formal treatment, and problem drinking is no exception. When a disease disappears without treatment, the term **spontaneous remission** is used to describe the cure. Many authorities in the field of problem drinking do not accept the term *spontaneous remission;* they prefer the term *unassisted change* to describe a switch from problem to nonproblem drinking (McMurran, 1994). Even the term *unassisted change* may be misleading because people who change their drinking patterns may have the help and support of many people among their family, employers, and friends. It would be accurate to say that some people change from problem to nonproblem drinking without formal treatment.

Many people have stopped drinking without entering treatment, and others fluctuate among problem drinking, light drinking, and abstinence. Clark and Cahalan (1976) found substantial fluctuation in drinking behavior among problem drinkers, who at times drink at problem levels and then change to a nonproblem level of drinking.

Researchers have investigated change in problem drinking status for a number of years. In 1976,

Smart reviewed nine earlier studies and found that improvement rates ranged from 4% to 42%, thus indicating considerable variability in the likelihood that drinkers will quit on their own. Another early study (Imber, Schultz, Funderburk, Allen, & Flanner, 1976) calculated an average remission rate of 19%, which suggests that some problem drinkers can improve on their own. However, the majority do not.

TREATMENTS ORIENTED TOWARD ABSTINENCE

All treatment programs for alcohol abuse have abstinence as their short-term goal, but this goal is not always achieved. Hayashida et al. (1989) reported that 95% of inpatients but only 72% of outpatients completed detoxification. Although all treatments seek immediate abstinence, some programs, especially in England, Australia, and Canada, include controlled drinking as an ultimate goal for some patients. The possibility of some alcohol abusers returning to controlled, moderate drinking is explored later. This section examines several treatment programs aimed at total and permanent abstinence.

Alcoholics Anonymous

Alcoholics Anonymous (AA) is one of the most widely used alcohol treatment programs, and it is often a component in other treatment programs. Founded in 1935 by two former alcoholics, AA has become the best known of all approaches to problem drinking. The organization follows a very strict version of the disease model and combines it with quasi-religious meetings that are designed to bring the problem drinker into the group. To adhere to the AA doctrine, a person must maintain total abstinence from alcohol. Part of the AA philosophy is that those who are in need of joining AA can never drink again and that problem drinkers are addicted to alcohol and have no power to resist it. According to AA, alcoholics never recover but are always in the process of recovering. They will be alcoholics for a lifetime, even if they never take another drink.

AA and other 12-step programs have become increasingly popular, attracting large numbers of people. A survey of U.S. adults (Room & Greenfield, 1993) revealed that 9% had attended an AA or other

12-step-type meeting, but only a third of those went to receive help with their own problems. This survey also revealed that nearly 5% of adults had sought help at some time during their lives for drinking problems, and for those who had sought help, 60% of the men and 80% of the women had attended AA meetings (Weisner et al., 1995).

Despite AA's long history and widespread popularity, little research has been reported on its effectiveness. The anonymity offered to those who attend AA meetings presents serious barriers to researchers wishing to conduct follow-up studies of members. However, several studies have used questionnaires passed out at AA meetings. According to one survey (AA, 1987), 29% of regular attenders (four meetings per week) reported that they had been sober for more than 5 years; 38% had been sober 1 to 5 years; and 33% had been sober less than 1 year. These percentages, however, are not an indication of AA's effectiveness or ineffectiveness. Only experimental studies with adequate control groups can yield valid effectiveness data.

In one of the few controlled experimental studies, Brandsma, Maultsby, and Welsh (1980) included (1) an AA group, (2) an insight therapy group, (3) a behavior therapy group conducted by a professional, (4) a behavior therapy group conducted by a paraprofessional, and (5) a no-treatment control group. The AA group showed the highest dropout rate: 68% versus 57% for the other treatment groups. In addition, the AA participants were most likely to binge drink during the 3 months of the study. This study indicated that AA is no more effective than alternative treatments and is possibly less so.

Other research on AA has indicated that it may be more effective for some problem drinkers than for others. Men with lower educational levels who have high needs for authoritarianism, dependence, and sociability may be good candidates (Miller & Hester, 1980). AA also seems to work better for people who need to give as well as to receive help (Maton, 1988).

Psychotherapy

Nearly as many psychotherapeutic techniques have been used to treat alcohol abuse as there are psychotherapies. Every approach from psychoanalysis (Blum, 1966) to behavior modification (Wallace, 1985), from psychodrama (Blume, 1985) to assertive-

ness training (Materi, 1977), has been used with alcoholic patients. This variety should not be surprising because a variety of psychiatric and behavioral problems often accompany alcohol abuse. Whether these personality disorders are the cause or the effect of heavy drinking, the immediate goal of all treatment approaches should be sobriety (Zimberg, 1985a). No psychotherapy is successful with intoxicated patients. For this reason, psychotherapeutic approaches are often combined with detoxification, AA, or some form of chemical treatment aimed at stopping drinking.

In terms of setting, treatment may be centered in Veterans Administration hospitals, care units in other hospitals, private treatment clinics, offices of psychiatrists and psychologists, halfway houses, or one of a variety of other treatment facilities. In terms of form, psychotherapeutic treatment can be divided into group procedures and individual therapy, with patients frequently participating in both within a single treatment regimen.

Group therapy for alcoholics has both advantages and disadvantages. Observing others who have successfully stopped drinking can raise expectancies for achieving the same goal, and patients within a group setting are more likely to receive praise and recognition from other group members for staying away from problem drinking. Another advantage for group treatment is the opportunity that groups provide to allow the patient a chance to give help. As Maton (1988) found, the experience of being helpful is, itself, often therapeutic. For example, when AA members reach the final step of their program, they sponsor a new member. This type of responsibility can be beneficial to both persons.

Individual psychotherapy offers its own set of advantages. The therapist obviously can give more personal attention to a single patient. Zimberg (1985b) pointed out that group therapy is often superficial in its ability to deal effectively with personal conflicts and that individual therapy "permits . . . a much greater understanding of the patients' defenses and conflicts and therefore makes the probability of successful interventions or lack of interventions much greater" (p. 55).

How effective are the various psychotherapeutic programs for alcohol abuse? Unfortunately, reports of success are frequently exaggerated, with some private treatment centers claiming a greater than

90% recovery rate (Hunter, 1982). Well-controlled studies, however, usually yield somewhat lower success rates, depending on the type of treatment (multimodal programs typically report higher rates than single-approach treatments); the sample composition (healthy, middle-social class, married, employed alcoholics have the highest improvement rates); the definition of success (abstinence versus improved); and the interval before follow-up (longer periods before follow-up report lower success rates) (Emrick & Hansen, 1983). The percentage of successes ranges from 4% to 42%, with perhaps 19% to 20% being the median. Even these rates are subject to decline as a result of relapse in the months and years following treatment (Armor, Polich, & Stambul, 1976; Brownell, 1982; Wiens & Menustik, 1983).

Chemical Treatments

Many treatment programs for problem drinking include the administration of drugs that interact with alcohol to produce a range of unpleasant effects. The most commonly used of these drugs is **disulfiram** (Antabuse). The unpleasant effects include flushing of the face, chest pains, a pounding heart, nausea and vomiting, sweating, headache, dizziness, weakness, difficulty in breathing, and a rapid decrease in blood pressure. These effects do not occur unless disulfiram and alcohol are both ingested. Disulfiram does have side effects of its own, including skin eruptions, fatigue, drowsiness, headache, and impotence. As with all side effects to drugs, these vary from person to person, and some individuals have few or none.

A major problem with disulfiram therapy is patient compliance (Fuller et al., 1986; Kofoed, 1987): People are not eager to take a drug that will make them sick if they drink. Because disulfiram must be taken at least twice weekly, patients are frequently hospitalized to ensure compliance, but this strategy is not practical for long-term treatment. Noncompliance, of course, lowers the effectiveness of this treatment because low levels of the drug may not cause the unpleasant effects after a person drinks alcohol. Despite the extremely unpleasant effects of drinking while on disulfiram, research does not show it alone to be any more effective than alternative treatments (see Fuller et al., 1986; Miller & Hester, 1980).

Aversion Therapy

Drugs like disulfiram, which produce nausea when combined with alcohol, are intended to produce an aversion to drinking or to act as a punishment for drinking. Thus they would technically be considered aversion therapies. However, the term **aversion therapy** is more commonly applied to the classical conditioning technique of using an electric shock, an emetic drug, or some other aversive stimulus to countercondition the patient's response to alcohol. In the classical conditioning paradigm, the unconditioned stimulus (shock or the emetic drug) is paired one or more times with the conditioned stimulus (sight, smell, taste, or image of alcohol) so that it will elicit the unconditioned response (aversion or withdrawal from alcohol). Through this process, drinking should come to be associated with an aversive condition and thus be avoided.

Miller and Hester (1980) reviewed therapy programs that used aversive shock therapy. Such programs vary according to level of shock and type of exposure to alcohol. Higher levels of shock produce higher dropout rates but not lower drinking rates. The type of exposure to alcohol makes little difference, with holding, sniffing, or drinking alcohol equally effective. However, real alcohol must be present. Studies that used pictures of drinks or of drinking did not work well.

Rather than relying on electric shock, many alcohol treatment programs use **emetine**, a drug that induces vomiting as the aversive stimulus. The use of this drug dates back to the 1930s, and the procedure pairs emetine with the sight, smell, taste, and thought of alcohol. In evaluating the effectiveness of emetine treatment, Wiens and Menustik (1983) found that 63% of patients were not drinking at the end of a year, and 31% were abstinent after 3 years. This relapse rate indicates that emetine aversion therapy, like many other treatment programs for alcohol and drug abuse, loses much of its effectiveness after a moderately long time.

Aversion conditioning has also been used in programs oriented toward moderation in drinking. Indeed, Miller and Hester (1980) cited a number of studies indicating that aversion therapy may be more useful in inducing controlled drinking among problem drinkers than in inducing abstinence, even when abstinence is the goal.

CONTROLLED DRINKING

Until the late 1960s, all treatments were aimed at total abstinence. Then something quite unexpected happened. In 1962 in London, D. L. Davies found that 7 of the 93 recovered alcoholics whom he studied were able to drink "normally" (defined as consumption of up to three pints of beer or its equivalent per day) for at least a 7-year period following treatment. These moderate drinkers represented less than 8% of those Davies studied, but this finding was still remarkable because it opened up the possibility that diagnosed alcoholics could successfully return to nonproblem drinking. All seven of the controlled drinkers had been completely abstinent for at least a few months following treatment, yet all had been able to resume "normal" drinking without relapsing into a heavy, harmful pattern of drinking.

STUDIES WITH ABSTINENCE AS THE GOAL

As expected, the interest generated by Davies's paper spurred others to investigate the phenomenon of controlled drinking, and several other investigators were able to confirm his findings. The most significant study to support Davies's findings was a study by Armor, Polich, and Stambul (1976) sponsored by the Rand Corporation of Santa Monica, California. Data on the participants in this study came from different Alcoholism Treatment Centers throughout the United States with a variety of treatment programs, but all had a treatment goal of abstinence. An 18-month follow-up study on a random sample of patients from eight selected facilities showed that a small but significant number (about 12%) of former alcoholics were able to drink moderately.

This report drew an immediate wave of criticism, not because its findings were new but because the report through the popular media drew widespread attention. Due to the criticism and some limitations of the study, the research group (Polich, Armor, & Braiker, 1980) planned a more extended follow-up that would address some of the methodological issues concerning the adequacy of the first follow-up and the validity of its self-reports. The result was a

4-year follow-up study of a random sample of almost 1,000 male participants. After extensive tests and interviews concerning drinking behavior over the previous 6 months, the researchers found that 18% of the patients were drinking without problems. Studies with longer follow-ups also revealed controlled drinking (Helzer et al., 1985).

The percentage of reported controlled drinkers was quite small, ranging from 3% to about 20%, and no clear pattern emerged that would reliably differentiate alcoholics who could successfully resume normal drinking from those who would need to abstain completely. These studies brought up a new question: Could the number of successful controlled drinkers be increased if treatment programs were designed specifically to teach heavy drinkers to drink safely?

STUDIES WITH CONTROL AS THE GOAL

In 1970, two Australian psychologists, S. H. Lovibond and Glenn Caddy, published a report on the first study designed explicitly to train problem drinkers to become nonproblem drinkers. These authors found considerably more controlled drinkers than did earlier studies, where moderate drinking was merely an incidental outcome of a total abstinence program. Lovibond and Caddy's follow-up data revealed that 59% of the 28 experimental participants were reported to be drinking moderately, a substantial gain over earlier studies.

Since 1970, a number of researchers have investigated the effectiveness of controlled drinking programs. Almost all have found that the success rate is at least as high in programs where moderate drinking is explicitly planned as it is in treatment approaches where total abstinence is the goal. The most famous and controversial of these controlled drinking studies was conducted by Linda Sobell and Mark Sobell at Patton State Hospital in San Bernadino, California, during the late 1960s and early 1970s (Pattison, Sobell, & Sobell, 1977; Sobell, 1978; Sobell & Sobell, 1973, 1976, 1978, 1982).

These researchers divided male inpatient volunteers who had been diagnosed as experiencing serious drinking problems into two major treatment groups, one whose goal was controlled drinking (controlled drinking group) and the other whose goal was abstinence (nondrinking group). This division was not random, and those participants who had requested one or the other type of treatment were accommodated. Next, participants within each major group were randomly assigned to an experimental or a control subgroup. In all, the study included four groups consisting of controlled drinking versus abstinence and a control comparison group for each.

After 2 years, the controlled drinker experimental group had significantly more days of functioning well (85%) than did the controlled drinker control group (42%). A 3-year follow-up study by an independent team (Caddy, Addington, & Perkins, 1978) essentially confirmed the Sobells's findings, although many of the differences between these two groups were not as large as in the previous follow-ups. Nevertheless, Caddy et al. found that participants in the controlled drinker groups continued to function well after 3 years.

Although the Sobell studies have been sharply criticized by some (Pendery, Maltzman, & West, 1982), they have also been defended by some of the leading scholars in the field (Brownell, 1984a; Heather & Robertson, 1983; Marlatt, 1983; Miller, 1983; Peele, 1984). Despite criticisms, legitimate and otherwise, these studies showed promise that controlled drinking might be a viable alternative to total abstinence programs.

Abstinence-oriented programs usually teach that the urge to drink will always be present and that if it is indulged even for a single drink, total relapse is inevitable. In contrast, controlled drinking programs do not have such a self-fulfilling prophecy built into them. Instead, they emphasize moderating patients' behavior and finding environmental supports that will reinforce moderation. They teach patients to monitor their intake, set weekly goals for total consumption, intersperse nonalcoholic drinks with alcoholic ones, and dilute drinks. In addition, behaviorally oriented controlled drinking programs train patients in a variety of human relations skills so they can modify all their self-destructive behaviors (Alden, 1988).

Despite potential advantages, treatment centers in the United States resisted controlled drinking programs until quite recently (Neimark, Conway, & Doskoch, 1994). Therapists and treatment centers are beginning to realize that traditional treatments work for less than half of alcoholics and that matching patient to treatment can offer a higher success rate. In Britain, nearly all treatment centers accept the principle of controlled drinking treatment (McMurran, 1994; Robertson & Heather, 1982).

According to Pukish and Tucker (1994), controlled drinking is a more likely outcome for problem drinkers who quit on their own than for those who enter treatment. Rosenberg (1993) reviewed the factors that related to success in controlled drinking but found no single characteristic that consistently predicted success. Several, however, were related to positive outcomes, including low severity of dependence and belief in the possibility of controlled drinking. The amount of drinking that problem drinkers can handle without problems will always be limited, with men allowed no more than 16 drinks and women 12 drinks per week (Sanchez-Craig, Wilkinson, & Davila, 1995). However, some evidence (Bullock, Reed, & Grant, 1992) indicates that alcoholics who can maintain abstinence cut their mortality risk.

None of the findings in favor of controlled drinking programs should be interpreted as evidence that moderate drinking is indicated for *all* alcohol abusers. No responsible proponent of controlled drinking would advocate such a course of action. One cannot state too strongly that *controlled drinking is not for everyone*. Some former alcohol addicts must abstain completely, and even those drinkers who are candidates for controlled drinking must apparently undergo at least 1 month of complete abstinence to allow the toxic effects of excessive drinking to diminish.

The best candidates for controlled drinking are people under age 40 who have not had long histories of problem drinking and serious alcohol-related physiological damage. In addition, married people do better than unmarried people, and people who attribute their drinking to situational factors are better candidates than those who believe they are physically dependent on alcohol. Also, people with regular employment are more likely to succeed than those who are frequently out of work.

THE PROBLEM OF RELAPSE

Problem drinkers who successfully complete either an abstinence-oriented or a moderation-oriented treatment program do not necessarily maintain their goals. As we saw with smoking, people who complete a treatment program usually improve quite a bit, but the problem of relapse is often substantial. Hunt, Barnett, and Branch (1971) indicated that the time course and rate of relapse was similar for those who have completed treatment programs for smoking, alcohol abuse, or opiate abuse. Most relapses occur within 90 days after the end of the program. At 12 months after the end of treatment, only about 35% of those completing the programs are still abstinent.

Since the early 1970s, treatment programs have improved, and relapse rates have declined. Studies obviously vary in success rate, depending on such factors as severity and duration of the drinking problem, age of the drinker, type of treatment, and definition of success. Amid this diversity of contributing factors, generalizations are difficult. However, a reasonable estimate is that with some relapse or "booster" training, roughly two-thirds of those treated for alcohol abuse show some improvement after 1 year; about a third are still improved (either abstinent or drinking in a controlled manner) after 3 years; and about a sixth are still improved after 5 years. These figures, of course, are rough estimates. Furthermore, some studies, especially those using abstinence as the criterion for success, show much lower success rates. The Rand Report (Polich et al., 1980), for example, found that only 7% of treated alcoholics did not drink at all in the 4 years following treatment, and Vaillant (1983) reported that after a 40-year follow-up, only 5% remained abstinent. Although complete abstinence may be too strict a standard to impose, relapse following treatment for alcohol abuse remains a serious problem.

Most behavior-based treatment regimens include training for relapse prevention (Marlatt & Gordon, 1980). As discussed in Chapter 13, relapse prevention training is aimed at changing cognitions so that the addict comes to believe that one slip does *not* equal total relapse. Programs that incorporate relapse prevention into their regimen have reported some success in avoiding complete relapse. For example, a study by Annis and Davis (1988) used coping skills, including enhancement of self-efficacy, to train alcoholic patients in relapse prevention. At intake, participants averaged 46 drinks per week. Three months after treatment they averaged fewer than two drinks a week. After 6 months, the average rose to fewer than six drinks, an indication that most patients had not totally relapsed. In addition to significant decreases in alcohol consumption, these participants reported marked improvement in self-efficacy in a broad range of personal and social skills.

OTHER DRUGS

In recent years, illicit drugs have created many serious problems in the United States. The problems, however, are mainly social and not related to physical health. Compared with alcohol and nicotine, few people die from the effects of illegal drugs. Clarke (1988) cited a *Time* magazine story of July 1986 titled "Drugs and Death," which implied that cocaine deaths had reached epidemic levels. The story predicted a rise in deaths from cocaine from 560 in 1985 to 580 in 1986. Clarke pointed out that 580 deaths in 1 year was equal to the number of alcohol-related deaths that occurred in the United States from midnight on New Year's Day of 1986 until midday of January 3. Another comparison would be that more people died from cigarette smoking between midnight on New Year's Eve and the kickoff of the Rose Bowl on January 1 than from cocaine in all of 1986. Even one death from illicit drugs, of course, is too many, but compared to smoking cigarettes, drinking alcohol, eating unwisely, and failing to exercise, health problems involving illicit drugs are a minor problem in the United States. Table 14.1 shows the rates of use of various drugs, including alcohol.

HEALTH EFFECTS

Both legal and illegal drugs pose potential health hazards. However, illegal drugs present certain risks not found with legal drugs, regardless of pharmacological effects. Illegal drugs may be sold as one drug when they are actually another; buyers have no insurance as to dosage; and illegally manufactured

Table 14.1 Lifetime, past year, and past month use of various drugs, persons aged 12 years and older

Drug	Lifetime Use	Use during Past Year	Use during Past Month
Sedatives	3.4%	0.8%	0.3%
Tranquilizers	4.6	1.2	0.3
Heroin	1.1	—	0.1
Alcohol	83.6	66.5	49.6
Stimulants	6.0	1.1	0.3
Cocaine	11.3	2.2	0.6
Crack cocaine	1.8	0.2	0.1
Marijuana	33.7	9.0	4.3
Anabolic steroids	0.4	—	0.1

SOURCE: *National Household Survey on Drug Abuse: Population Estimates 1993,* by U.S. Department of Health and Human Services, 1994, DHHS Publication No. (SMA) 94-3017, Rockville, MD: Substance Abuse and Mental Health Services Administration.

drugs may have impurities that can be dangerous chemicals themselves. In addition, the sources of illegal drugs can be dangerous people. Legal drugs are free from these risks, but they are not always safe or harmless. For any drug to have an effect, it must intervene in biological processes. For example, psychoactive drugs produce their effects by crossing the blood-brain barrier and changing the brain's chemistry. Such actions are not without risks.

All drugs have potential hazards, but drugs termed safe are tested by the federal Food and Drug Administration (FDA) and defined as safe. The FDA considers a drug safe if its potential benefits outweigh its potential hazards. Many drugs, such as antibiotics, have been approved although they produce severe side effects in some people. The more potentially beneficial a drug, the more likely it is to be labeled safe despite unpleasant side effects.

The FDA classifies drugs into five categories, based on their potential for abuse and their potential medical benefits. Schedule I includes drugs judged to be high in abuse potential and with no accepted medical use. Included in this category are heroin, LSD, and marijuana. Schedule II includes drugs that have high abuse potential, capable of causing severe psychological or physical dependence but having some medical use. In this category are most opiates, some barbiturates, amphetamines, and cocaine. Schedule III consists of drugs judged to produce moderate or low physical dependence or high psychological dependence but with accepted medical uses, such as some opiates and some tranquilizers. Schedule IV drugs, such as phenobarbital and most tranquilizers, are judged to have low abuse potential, limited dependence properties, and accepted medical uses. Schedule V contains drugs with less abuse potential than those in Schedule IV.

Drugs in Schedule V do not require a prescription and are available over the counter in drug stores, drugs in Schedule I are not legally available, and those in Schedules II, III, and IV are available only by prescription. As Avorn (1995) pointed out, this classification has evolved over the past 100 years as part of the social history of the United States and represents legislative and social convention rather than scientific findings. Indeed, recent legislation has changed some drugs from one schedule to another, making a wider variety of drugs available without prescription.

Sedatives

Sedatives are drugs that induce relaxation and sometimes intoxication by lowering the activity of the brain, the neurons, the muscles, and the heart, and even by slowing the metabolic rate. In low doses, these drugs tend to make people feel relaxed and even euphoric. In high doses, they cause loss of consciousness and can result in coma and death due to their inhibitory effect on the brain center that controls respiration. Sedatives include barbiturates, tranquilizers, opiates, and methadone, but the most commonly used drug in this category is alcohol.

Depressant effects are a major problem with sedative drugs, and these effects are additive when sedatives are taken in combination. The effect of mixing two or more of these drugs can be depression of the respiratory system to a dangerously low level. Some people mix alcohol with tranquilizers or other depressants, providing a potentially lethal combination. Furthermore, sedatives and stimulants have opposite effects, but these effects do not cancel each other; instead, both sets of effects occur. For example, caffeine (the stimulant drug in coffee) will not sober a person intoxicated on alcohol (a sedative). Rather, caffeine merely makes a drunken person more alert and less sleepy—not less drunk.

Barbiturates are synthetic drugs used medically to induce sleep. Taken recreationally, barbiturates produce effects similar to alcohol: relaxation and intoxication in small doses, drunkenness and unconsciousness in larger doses. Because they are ingested in pill form, barbiturate overdoses are more common than alcohol overdoses. Barbiturates produce both tolerance and dependence, although the tolerance properties are difficult to assess. Many people can take barbiturates in the form of sleeping pills over an extended time without increasing the dose whereas others rapidly escalate their dosage to dangerous levels. People who use barbiturates as sleeping pills on a regular basis are not able to sleep without them, and they manifest withdrawal symptoms when they stop taking them—two definite indications of dependence. Withdrawal is similar to that from alcohol, lasting up to a week and including tremor, nausea, vomiting, sweating, sleep disturbances, and sometimes hallucinations and deliriums.

Tranquilizers are relatively recent, dating only to the 1960s. The most prominent variety of these chemical compositions are those of the *benzodiazepine* group. Like barbiturates, tranquilizers induce depression, but they are less likely to produce sleep and more likely to suppress anxiety. During the 1970s, a single class of tranquilizers, *diazepam,* accounted for more visits to hospital emergency rooms than any other drug (Julien, 1978). Recognition of the dangers of this class of drug has led to decreased prescriptions and fewer problems.

Benzodiazepines produce both tolerance and dependence, but only over an extended period. Neither tolerance nor dependence is particularly severe if the drug is taken in small or even moderate amounts. In large amounts, however, these drugs not only produce tolerance and dependence but also cause disorientation, confusion, and even rage, a paradoxical effect for a tranquilizer.

Another category of depressants is the **opiates,** drugs derived from the opium poppy. Opium can also be refined into *morphine,* which can be further chemically treated to produce *heroin.* Synthetic compounds, including *meperidine* and *methadone,* are chemically similar to the opiates and produce similar effects.

Opium has been used for centuries for both medical and recreational purposes. It can be ingested by swallowing, sniffing, smoking, or injecting under the skin, into a muscle, or intravenously, making it one of the most versatile drugs for transmission into the body. In the 19th century in the United States, physicians prescribed opiates frequently and for a variety of conditions. Today, the principal medical use of opiates is to relieve pain. Because they act on the central nervous system and the digestive system, opiate drugs are also prescribed for cough and for diarrhea. Opiates cross the blood-brain barrier and attach to receptors in the brain, altering the interpretation of pain messages. The physical condition responsible for the pain is not halted, of course, but the person's subjective experience of pain diminishes. Opiate drugs, therefore, have important medical uses.

Opiates produce both tolerance and dependence after only a brief time, sometimes as little as 24 hours, thus making opiates like heroin easily abused. However, heroin use is not common in the United States (see Table 14.1). Johnston et al. (1994a) reported little change in the annual prevalence of heroin use among high school seniors, college students, and young adults from 1979 to 1993. For seniors, heroin use was 0.5% at both points in time; for young adults and college students, the rate has remained constant, at about 0.1% to 0.2%. Use of other sedatives, including illicitly obtained tranquilizers, has also declined among young people.

Stimulants

Stimulant drugs tend to make some people feel more alert and energetic, more able to concentrate, and more able to work long hours. They make others feel jittery, anxious, and unable to sit still. More specifically, stimulants tend to produce alertness, reduce feelings of fatigue, elevate mood, and decrease appetite. They are synthetic but are similar in chemical structure to norepinephrine, the neurotransmitter identified as the brain's main excitatory chemical.

Amphetamines are one type of stimulant drug that is often abused. In addition to having a mood altering effect, amphetamines produce such physical symptoms as increased blood pressure, slower heart rate, increased respiration, relaxation of bronchial muscles, dilation of pupils, increased EEG activity, and increased blood supply to the muscles. These effects can be dangerous to the cardiovascular system, especially for people who have heart problems or other cardiovascular diseases. Amphetamines can also produce psychological effects, including hallucinations and paranoid delusions. High energy levels combined with paranoid delusions can make amphetamine users dangerous to society. In addition to these physical, psychological, and social effects, amphetamines produce both tolerance and dependence. Thus, they are undesirable as diet pills, despite their appetite suppressant effects.

Since 1982, the nonmedical or illicit use of amphetamines has declined in the United States. Johnston et al. (1989, 1994a, 1994b) surveyed a nationwide sample of high school seniors, college students, and young adults on their use of amphetamines and found a significant decrease in annual prevalence (defined as one or more uses during the previous 12 months) in all three age categories. For high school seniors, the annual prevalence dropped from 20% in 1982 to 8.4% in 1993. Annual use among college students declined even more, from 21% to 4.2%. Table 14.1 shows that the overall rate of stimulant use is even lower, 1.1%. At the same time, however, high school seniors increased their use of over-the-counter *stay-awake pills,* which usually contain caffeine as their active ingredient. The percentage of seniors who had used these drugs within the month prior to the survey rose from 5.5% in 1980 to 7.0% in 1993. Increases also occurred among college students and young adults. These findings suggest that young people in the United States have, to some extent, replaced illicitly obtained amphetamines with legally purchased stimulants.

Another stimulant drug, **cocaine**, is extracted from the coca plant, which grows in the Andes Mountains in South America. In the 1880s, several European physicians, including Sigmund Freud, discovered that cocaine was capable of blocking neural transmission at the site of application and therefore was useful for **anesthesia**. For a time, cocaine was used as an anesthetic for surgery, especially eye surgery. In the 1890s, it became a popular drug in America and was widely available in tonics, wines, and soft drinks. Soon, however, people began to recognize the dangers of cocaine, and the passage of U.S. federal drug laws restricted its use. Today the medical uses of cocaine are quite limited because more effective anesthetics have been developed.

Cocaine acts as a stimulant to the nervous system, and the strength and duration of its action depend

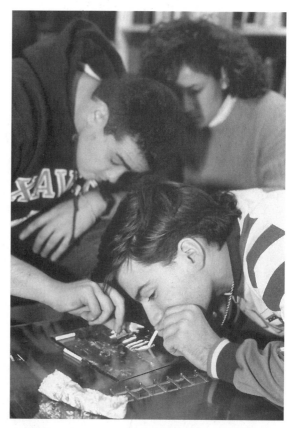

Cocaine use can pose serious problems in users' lives, but cocaine use has decreased in recent years.

not only on dose but also on mode of administration. Although South American Indians take cocaine orally by chewing the coca leaves, this method is seldom used elsewhere. Instead, cocaine is snorted through the nasal passages, smoked or "freebased," or injected intravenously. The stimulant effects of cocaine are short, lasting only 15 to 30 minutes. During this time, the user often feels a powerful euphoria, a strong sense of well-being, and heightened attention. But when the effects wear off, the user frequently feels fatigued, sluggish, and anxious and is left with a strong craving to repeat the experience. Frequently the user will increase the dose in a futile effort to make the euphoria last longer the next time. The stimulant effects of increased doses of cocaine can endanger the cardiovascular system.

The tolerance and dependence properties of cocaine are still debated. Nevertheless, nearly all authorities agree that people who use cocaine repeatedly eventually stop getting the "high" they initially felt (Brecher, 1972; Grinspoon & Bakalar, 1976; Julien, 1978). With heavy use, many people experience frequent anxiety, insomnia, depression, and irritation of the nose. Even heavy users suffer few withdrawal symptoms, the main criterion for determining physical dependence. However, most heavy users who quit suffer serious depression, coupled with a strong desire to continue taking the drug. The term *psychological dependence* may seem appropriate, but this term is a problem because it can be applied to many habitual behaviors, both drug and nondrug, good and bad. Cocaine can become an important part of the lives of users, and these people tend to have problems as a result of their cocaine use.

A group of neuropharmacology researchers have discovered that cocaine and alcohol interact in the body to form a third chemical, *cocaethylene.* Hearn et al. (1991) found that cocaethylene produces or enhances the euphoria that cocaine users experience. However, the mixture of cocaine and alcohol is potentially lethal and accounts for a higher death rate and a greater rate of emergency room admissions than either drug alone.

Crack cocaine has become a serious social problem in the United States, partially because this form of cocaine is cheap and widely available. Crack, a form of freebase cocaine, is ingested by smoking. The use of crack among high school seniors, college students, and young adults has declined since the 1980s. A national survey by Johnston et al. (1994a) reported that the use of crack cocaine among 1993 high school seniors has dropped. In 1988, 3.1% of high school seniors, 1.4% of college students, and 3.1% of young adults had used crack during the past year (Johnston et al., 1989), but in 1993 the percentages were 1.5%, 0.6%, and 1.3%, respectively (Johnston et al., 1994a). The use of both cocaine and crack cocaine is quite low in the general population (see Table 14.1).

For cocaine in any form, including crack, the decline in use began in 1987 and continued to 1993, when the annual prevalence rates were 3.3% for seniors, 2.7% for college students, and 4.7% among young adults. Johnston et al. (1994a) suggested that the decline in use of cocaine among young people corresponds to an increase in the number who regard cocaine as harmful. In 1980 only 31% of 19- to 22-year-olds saw cocaine as harmful if tried once or twice. By 1993, this number had risen to 79%, a clear indication that young people had become more convinced of the dangers of cocaine.

Marijuana

The most commonly used illegal drug in the United States is *marijuana.* Its potential for serious health consequences is still debated, but few authorities regard it as a major health risk. If smoked as frequently as cigarettes, however, marijuana would be at least as harmful to the respiratory system as tobacco.

Marijuana is composed of the leaves, flowers, and small branches of *Cannabis sativa,* a plant that flourishes in almost every climate in the world. The intoxicating ingredient in marijuana, delta-9-tetrahydrocannabinol (THC), comes from the resin of the male plants and especially the female plants. The most reliable physiological effect of THC is increased heart rate, which occurs with the consumption of heavy doses. Although a rapid heartbeat may present health hazards to users with coronary problems, no evidence exists that marijuana in small or moderate doses causes any organic damage. Nevertheless, any drug used chronically and in heavy doses poses a danger to health, so marijuana, like nicotine, alcohol, or aspirin, has some potential to impair health.

Marijuana has been used medically to treat glaucoma and to prevent the vomiting and nausea associated with chemotherapy. During the 1970s, controlled studies (Sallan, Zinberg, & Frei, 1975) demonstrated that orally administered THC in gelatin capsules was capable of reducing nausea and vomiting in cancer patients treated with chemotherapy. At about the same time, Hepler and Frank (1971) noticed that healthy young marijuana smokers experienced a lessening of pressure within their eyes, decreasing glaucoma. In 1992, however, the Drug Enforcement Administration rejected all pleas for reclassifying marijuana to Schedule II. Nevertheless, marijuana continues to be used illegally for nausea, glaucoma, muscle relaxation, and as an appetite stimulant for AIDS patients (Grinspoon & Bakalar, 1995).

The desired psychological effects of marijuana are euphoria, a sense of well-being, feelings of relaxation, and heightened sexual responsiveness, and these are usually attained by experienced smokers who expect to attain them. On the negative side, marijuana also has an effect on short-term memory, judgment, and time perception. Ferraro (1980) reviewed the literature on the effects of marijuana on memory and cognition and concluded that both cognition (speaking, thinking, attending) and memory (short-term recall) are affected, although the impairment is usually slight. Even small deficits, however, may be hazardous when a person is operating an automobile. Possibly the greatest immediate danger of the social use of marijuana is its influence on the judgment and perception of drivers. Long-term negative consequences may also exist; heavy use is associated with the development of schizophrenia (Thornicroft, 1990).

Marijuana does not seem to produce physiological dependence, and no withdrawal symptoms accompany the cessation of marijuana use. One study (Miller & Cisin, 1983) reported that nearly 75% of adults ages 26 and older who had been marijuana users stopped taking the drug. Also, marijuana does not seem to create tolerance; regular users are not ordinarily compelled to escalate dosage in order to achieve the same effect. The psychological effects of marijuana, like those of alcohol and other drugs, seem to depend partially on setting and expectation.

Unlike the use of most other illicit drugs, marijuana use among young people has recently increased in the United States, and marijuana remains the most widely used illicit drug (see Table 14.1). Marwick (1995) reviewed the latest figures showing that the percentage of high school seniors who had smoked marijuana during the past year rose from 22% in 1992 to nearly 31% in 1994 and that the rate of increase was even greater for 9th graders. College students and young adults have also shown some increase in marijuana use (Johnston et al., 1994a), but the percentage of younger users appears to be rising faster than the percentage of college students and young adults who had smoked marijuana during the past year.

The attitudes among adolescents and young adults concerning marijuana use have shown changes over the past 15 years (Johnston et al., 1994a, 1994b). Young people have always considered marijuana the least dangerous of the illicit drugs, but its perceived risks have varied over time. During the late 1970s and early 1980s, a majority of young people did not believe that marijuana use was a threat, but from the mid-1980s until the early 1990s, the perception of

its risks grew, and marijuana use decreased. In 1993, about two-thirds of young people believed that regular marijuana use was dangerous, but the perception of danger has decreased slightly, leading Johnston et al. (1994b) to predict that marijuana use may increase.

Anabolic Steroids

During the past 25 years, many athletes have used **anabolic steroids** (AS) to increase their muscle bulk and to decrease body fat. Steroids can be either endogenous (manufactured by the body) or synthetic. Endogenous steroids are produced by the adrenal glands, which secrete cortisone, and by the ovaries and testes, which secrete estrogen and testosterone. The effects of anabolic steroids include thickening of vocal cords, enlargement of the larynx, increase of muscle bulk, and decrease of body fat. These last two properties make AS attractive to athletes, bodybuilders, and people who wish to alter their appearance.

Anabolic steroids have some medical uses, including reduction of inflammation and control of some allergic reactions, but their side effects make them potentially dangerous. They can upset the chemical balance in the body, produce toxicity, and shut off the body's production of its own steroids, leaving the person more susceptible to stress and infection and altering reproductive functioning. In addition, steroid use has the effect of depressing levels of high-density lipoprotein (HDL), thus leading to an unfavorable ratio of total cholesterol to HDL (Hurley et al., 1984; Moffatt, Wallace, & Sady, 1990) and an increased risk of cardiovascular disease.

Anabolic steroids do not seem to produce tolerance or dependence. However, some authorities (Shroyer, 1990) have argued that the use of steroids often leads to psychological dependence. This argument is based on the observation that the effects of steroid use—bulky muscle development and increased athletic performance—are secondary reinforcers. Thus, some people have a strong motivation to maintain steroid use and may suffer loss of self-esteem when the drugs are discontinued.

How widespread is the use of anabolic steroids? Table 14.1 shows a very low rate of steroid use in the general U.S. population, but, as with other drugs, young people are more frequent users than older adults. Until 1988, incidence and prevalence were poorly documented, but in that year Buckley and his associates (1988) conducted a nationwide survey of male high school seniors. Their data revealed that 6.6% of 12th-grade male students were either using or had used AS. Of those who were users, two-thirds had begun at age 16 or younger; a fifth got the drug from a health professional, 60% through the black market (coaches, gym officials, older athletes), and about 10% through mail-order catalogs. The 1993 seniors in the Johnston et al. (1994a) survey reported a lower rate than Buckley et al. had found, with only 3.5% of the male and 0.6% of the female seniors indicating that they had ever used AS.

When asked their main reason for taking the drug, nearly half the young men in the Buckley et al. survey responded that they took steroids to improve their athletic performance, 27% said they wished to improve their appearance, and 11% reported that they took it to prevent injuries—despite a lack of medical evidence that steroids can protect against injuries. If anything, anabolic steroids are more likely to produce injuries, both to the person taking them and to others coming into physical contact with that person.

A study of monkeys (Rejeski, Brubaker, Herb, Kaplan, & Koritnik, 1988) suggested that steroid use can increase both aggression and submission. Dominant subjects fought with each other and with the most submissive subjects. Animals that lost fights became more submissive, displaying behaviors much like those Seligman (1975) described as learned helplessness. These submissive subjects thus became vulnerable to injuries, in part because of their increased levels of steroids. The authors found similarities between the increased aggression of their monkeys and anecdotal reports of human athletes' behaviors. Although rates of steroid use are low, this drug presents more direct health hazards than other illicit drugs, and indirect health effects are also a potential risk.

DRUG MISUSE AND ABUSE

Most people believe that some drugs are acceptable and even desirable because of the medical benefits they confer. But all *psychoactive* drugs—drugs that cross the blood-brain barrier and alter mental functioning—are potentially harmful to health. Most

have the capacity for tolerance or dependence (see Table 14.2). Even drugs that are not psychoactive have the potential for unpleasant side effects. For example, penicillin can cause nausea, vomiting, diarrhea, swelling, and skin eruptions. In addition, people who have allergies to penicillin can die from ingesting it. Also, caffeine, a commonly found drug in coffee and cola drinks, can produce effects that meet the DSM-IV criteria of substance dependence. For example, Strain, Mumford, Silverman, and Griffiths (1994) found that a high percentage of people who believed that they were dependent on caffeine had been unsuccessful in quitting or cutting down, showed withdrawal symptoms when denied caffeine, and continue to use the drug despite knowledge that its use may cause persistent or recurrent physiological and psychological problems. Therefore, even a drug that is safe for most people will not be without substantial risks for some.

Almost all drugs that have potential medical or health benefits also have the potential for misuse and abuse. The moderate use of alcohol, for instance, is related to decreased cardiovascular mortality. The *misuse* of alcohol, defined as inappropriate but not health-threatening levels of consumption, can result in social embarrassment, violent acts, and accidents. And abuse of alcohol, defined as frequent, heavy consumption to the point of addiction, can lead to cirrhosis, brain damage, heart attack, and fetal alcohol syndrome.

TREATMENT FOR DRUG ABUSE

Treatment for the use and abuse of illegal drugs is similar to the treatment of alcohol abuse, both in the philosophy and the administration of treatment. The goal of treatment for all types of illegal drug use is total abstinence. In many cases, the programs that treat drug abusers often coexist physically with treatment programs for alcohol abuse, and patients who are receiving treatment for their drug problems participate in the same therapy as those who are receiving therapy for their alcohol problems. The philosophy that guides Alcoholics Anonymous led to the development of Narcotics Anonymous, an organization devoted to helping drug users abstain from using drugs.

The reasons for entering drug abuse treatment programs are often similar to those for entering treat-

Table 14.2 Summary of the characteristics of psychoactive drugs

Name	Source	Medical use	Mode of ingestion	Effects	Duration of effects	Tolerance	Dependence
Stimulants							
Caffeine	Natural (tea, coffee, etc.)	Antidepressant	Swallowed	Increases alertness reduces fatigue	1–2 hrs.	Yes	No
Cocaine	Natural (coca plant)	Local anesthetic	Swallowed, injected, sniffed	Produces euphoria, suppresses appetite	15–30 mins.	?	?
Amphetamines	Synthetic	Appetite suppressant	Swallowed, injected	Produces alertness, reduces fatigue	4 hrs.	Yes	Yes
Nicotine	Natural (tobacco plant)	None	Smoked, sniffed chewed	Elevates blood pressure	30 mins.	Yes	Yes
Depressants							
Barbiturates	Synthetic	Sedative	Swallowed	Relaxes, intoxicates	Varies depending on type	Yes	Yes
Tranquilizers	Synthetic	Reduces anxiety	Swallowed	Relaxes, intoxicates	3–4 hrs.	Yes	Yes
Opiates	Natural (opium poppy) semisynthetic	Analgesic	Swallowed, sniffed, smoked, injected	Produces euphoria, sedates	4–6 hrs.	Yes	Yes
Methadone	Synthetic	Treatment for heroin addiction	Swallowed	Prevents heroin withdrawal	12–24 hrs.	Yes	Yes
Alcohol	Natural (fruits, grains)	External antiseptic	Swallowed	Relaxes, intoxicates	1–2 hrs.	Yes	Yes
Marijuana	Natural (cannibis)	Treatment for glaucoma, antiemetic	Smoked	Relaxes, intoxicates	2–3 hrs.	?	No
Steroids	Natural, synthetic	Agent for reducing inflammation and rashes	Swallowed, injected, applied to skin	Builds muscles, increases blood pressure, reduces immune system functioning	7–14 days	Yes	No

ment for alcohol abuse. These reasons are primarily social. The abuse of illegal drugs leads to legal, financial, and interpersonal problems, as does alcohol abuse. Like alcohol, most illegal drugs produce impairments of judgment that lead to accidents, making accidental injury the leading health risk for drug abuse. Unlike alcohol abuse, the abuse of illegal drugs does not often directly damage health. However, when health problems occur, these prob-lems are likely to be major and life threatening. Such crises may precipitate a person's decision to seek treatment or lead family members to enforce treatment.

Inpatient treatment programs for drug abuse are strikingly similar to those designed to treat alcohol abuse, but they do differ from programs for alcohol abuse in several minor ways. The detoxification phase of inpatient hospitalization is typically shorter and less severe for most types of drug use than it is for alcohol, for which withdrawal can be life threatening. Alcohol is a depressant drug, as are barbiturates, tranquilizers, and opiates. Therefore, all these drugs have similar symptoms during withdrawal, including agitation, tremor, gastric distress, and possibly perceptual distortions. Stimulants such as amphetamines and cocaine produce different withdrawal symptoms, namely lethargy and depression. These differences necessitate different medical care during detoxification.

Another difference between the treatment for alcohol abuse and the treatment for other types of drug abuse is the existence of disulfiram (Antabuse). Patients who take disulfiram can be restrained from drinking, but no equivalent chemical deterrent exists for other types of drug abuse. Therefore, treatment for drug abuse consists of detoxification followed by therapy oriented toward self-exploration and insight into the reasons for drug taking.

One similarity between drug and alcohol abuse treatment is the high rate of relapse. As Hunt et al. (1971) discovered, alcohol, smoking, and opiate treatment all share a high rate of relapse, and the first 6 months after treatment are critical. To ameliorate this problem, drug treatment programs, like alcohol treatment interventions, typically include some aftercare or "booster" sessions. Frequently, this continued care comes from joining a support group such as Narcotics Anonymous. However, evidence exists that more comprehensive psychosocial services boost the effectiveness of drug treatment (McLellan, Arndt, Metzger, Woody, & O'Brien, 1993).

PREVENTING AND CONTROLLING DRUG USE

Chapter 13 presented information on attempts to decrease smoking in children and adolescents by various interventions aimed at discouraging their experimentation with cigarettes and smokeless tobacco. Similar efforts have been applied to the use of other drugs (Botvin, Baker, Dusenburg, Botvin, & Diaz, 1995), but programs aimed at children and adolescents are not the only approach to controlling drug use.

A more common control technique is the limitation of availability. This strategy is common in all Western countries through the existence of laws that limit the legal access to drugs. The assumption underlying this strategy is that legal drugs will be more widely used than illegal drugs, and the history and present use of drugs confirms this assumption: More people use legal than illegal drugs. However, legal restriction of drugs has a number of side effects, some of which create other social problems (MacCoun, 1993; Robins, 1995). For example, when the United States legally prohibited the manufacture and sale of alcohol, illegal manufacture and distribution flourished, creating a huge criminal enterprise, huge profits, loss of tax revenue, and corruption among law enforcement agencies. Therefore, the limitation of availability has negative as well as positive consequences, and MacCoun is representative of those who urge an examination and reformulation of drug control policies.

The prevention attempts aimed at keeping children and adolescents from experimenting with drugs are intended to inhibit initiation, with the goal of eliminating the use of drugs completely (McMurran, 1994). As with the efforts at preventing smoking (see Chapter 13), those aimed at preventing drug use do not have an impressive success rate. Some programs have been counterproductive, increasing drug use (Stuart, 1974) or increasing adolescents' beliefs that drug use is more prevalent than it is (Donaldson, Graham, Piccinin, & Hansen, 1995). As with smoking prevention programs, drug prevention programs that rely on scare tactics, moral training, factual information about drug risks, and boosting self-esteem generally are ineffective (Donaldson et al., 1995). Indeed, a meta-analysis of the effectiveness of Project DARE (Drug Abuse Resistance Education), a widely used school-based drug education program, showed that this popular intervention is not very effective, even in the short term (Ennett, Tobler, Ringwalt, & Flewelling, 1994).

Some types of prevention programs are more effective than others. By conducting a meta-analysis of drug prevention programs aimed at adolescents, Tobler (1986) found that peer programs were most successful. Such programs involve adolescents rather than adults as counselors and typically involve developing social skills necessary for avoiding initiation due to social pressure. In addition, research (Chilcoat, Deshion, & Anthony, 1995) has demonstrated that parental monitoring of children's activities and whereabouts decreased the risk for drug involvement among children of elementary school age.

The attempts to prevent initiation into drug use has succeeded with some individuals but not for all participants and not for society as a whole. Indeed, Des Jarlais (1995, p. 10) argued that "the nonmedical use of psychoactive drugs is inevitable in any society that has access to such drugs." Acceptance of this view necessitates alternative control strategies.

One alternative control strategy is the control of harm (Des Jarlais, 1995; McMurran, 1994). This new strategy involves the assumption that people will use psychoactive drugs, sometimes unwisely, but that reduction of the health consequences of drug use should be the first priority. Rather than taking a moralistic stand on drug use, this strategy takes a practical approach to minimizing the dangers of drug use. An example of the harm reduction strategy is to help injection drug users exchange used needles for sterile ones and thus slow the spread of HIV infection. The controversy surrounding such programs is representative of the debate over the harm reduction strategy.

CHAPTER SUMMARY

This chapter examined several questions concerning the consumption of alcohol. First, what are the effects of alcohol? Prolonged, heavy drinking of alcohol is a major health hazard, often leading to cirrhosis of the liver and other serious health problems, such as heart disease and brain dysfunction. However, some evidence suggests that moderate drinking may have certain long-range health benefits in reduced heart disease. Scientists are still not certain of all the mechanisms through which alcohol consumption buffers against mortality and morbidity from heart disease, but part of the answer seems to lie in alcohol's ability to increase HDL. However, increases in HDL do not account for all of alcohol's protective benefits, and reduction of blood clotting is an additional possibility.

Second, why do people drink? More specifically, why do they start, continue in moderation, or drink

to excess? Models for drinking behavior seek to answer these three questions. The *disease model* assumes that people drink excessively because they have the disease of alcoholism. Cognitive-physiological models, including the *tension reduction hypothesis*, the *self-awareness model*, and *alcohol myopia*, propose that people drink because alcohol produces alterations in cognitive function that allow people to escape tension and negative self-evaluations. *Social learning theory* assumes that people acquire drinking behavior in the same manner that they learn other behaviors—that is, through positive or negative reinforcement, modeling, and cognitive mediation.

The third question asks how people can quit drinking to excess. About one person in five may be able to quit without therapy. Traditional alcohol treatment programs have been oriented toward abstinence, but most have had only moderate success. The effectiveness of the AA programs are difficult to assess because members are anonymous. The drug disulfiram has been used for some time to curb alcohol consumption, but its drastic effects hinder its usefulness. Electric shock and emetine have been used as aversive stimuli with some success.

Controlled drinking might be a reasonable goal for a substantial minority of all problem drinkers. However, many medically oriented therapists do not consider controlled drinking a viable alternative to abstinence, but attitudes toward alcohol treatment are undergoing changes, and controlled drinking may become a more accepted goal.

Relapse is common among heavy drinkers who have quit, although many are able to maintain abstinence or to drink in a controlled manner. Most relapses occur during the first 3 months. After a year, about 65% of all successful quitters have resumed drinking in a harmful manner.

Other drugs—including depressants, stimulants, cocaine, marijuana, and anabolic steroids—have had some medical use, but they also are potentially harmful to health. Currently, however, the principal problems from most of these drugs are social, not physical. Treatments for drug abuse are similar to those for alcohol abuse, and programs aimed at prevention are similar to those aimed at preventing smoking. A new strategy called harm reduction aims at decreasing the social and health risks of taking drugs by changing drug policies.

SUGGESTED READINGS

Gross, L. (1983). *How much is too much? The effects of social drinking*. New York: Random House. This is a very readable report on the effects of social rather than heavy drinking. It is an important little book for anyone wanting to know how much is too much.

Heather, N., & Robertson, I. (1990). *Problem drinking* (2nd ed). Oxford, England: Oxford University Press. The authors present evidence that problem drinking is not a disease but a learned behavior disorder and should be treated as such. This edition is directed at both the general public and professionals in the field of alcohol treatment.

McMurran, M. (1994). *The psychology of addiction*. London: Taylor & Francis. Mary McMurran is a British psychologist whose background is in treatment of drug and alcohol problems. Her book is an interesting review of the history, legislation, theory, treatment, and prevention of drug use. Writing in Great Britain, she offers a different view of substance abuse from that of most U.S. therapists and theorists.

Neimark, J., Conway, C., & Doskoch, P. (1994, September–October). Back from the drink. *Psychology Today, 27*, 46–49. This article in a popular magazine offers a short, readable review of current statistics and trends on alcohol use and abuse. The review highlights the critical factors for successful quitting and includes tips for moderating your own drinking.

15 Eating to Control Weight

Elise was a senior in high school who had always been an excellent student. She made good grades and was involved in many school-related activities, but like many high school girls, she was unhappy with her weight. Elise wanted to weigh less than 100 pounds, a weight she felt was reasonable for her 5'2" frame, but she weighed over 120 pounds. She began eating less—not eating at all during the day, missing dinner due to school-related activities, and fooling her family into thinking that she was eating. She tended to wear baggy clothing, so at first her family and friends did not notice her weight loss. Elise found fasting difficult and did not feel like exercising as a way to lose weight, so she began to vomit as a way to compensate for eating. Soon she added laxatives as an additional technique. She kept both practices secret from her family, who would have tried to stop her.

It was not her disordered eating that resulted in her receiving treatment but signs of depression—she cried easily, was always tired, and didn't seem to enjoy anything. Elise's family insisted that she go to a psychiatrist, who recognized her eating problems and tried to get Elise to recognize them, too. Elise's psychiatrist gave her a copy of Hilde Bruch's *The Golden Cage* (1978) and asked her to read it. The book describes **anorexia nervosa**, an eating disorder that involves self-starvation and distorted body image. Elise read the book, but at that time rejected the possibility that she was anorexic. She listened to her psychiatrist and trusted her, forming a positive relationship, but she resisted any acceptance of her behavior as an eating problem.

Not only did Elise deny her eating problems, but she also continued to vomit and abuse laxatives as ways to lose weight. By the time she graduated from high school, she had lost more than 15 pounds (but still weighed 104 pounds, 5 pounds away from her goal). Her weight began to be an issue with her family and friends, who told her that she was too thin and that she looked terrible. Despite the amount of weight she had lost, she did not meet the criteria to be diagnosed as anorexic according to the *Diagnostic and Statistical Manual of Mental Disorders* (American Psychiatric Association [APA], 1987, 1994). Those criteria include weight loss to the point that the person is 15% below ideal weight, which Elise was not. However, she exhibited the distorted body image, fear of gaining weight, and **amenorrhea** (cessation of menstrual periods) that are symptoms of anorexia.

Her diagnosis was **bulimia**, an eating disorder consisting of binge eating followed by some method to compensate for the binge, such as fasting, excessive exercising, or purging through either vomiting or using laxatives. Elise exhibited these symptoms, forcing herself to vomit and abusing laxatives, even when the amount of food she had eaten was not excessive.

Elise's eating problems got worse when she began college. She purged by both vomiting and using laxatives. But the more laxatives she consumed, the less effective they became. So she increased the dosage to the point that she took 45 tablets in less than 2 days. This precipitated a medical crisis, resulting in her being hospitalized and receiving psychotherapy. Her therapist tried to convince Elise to accept a reasonable body image, to eat reasonably, and to stop purging.

Her therapy continued over the next 5 years, but so did her distorted body image and purging behavior. She spent much time and energy making sure that she had sufficient laxatives to take care of any eating that she might consider excessive, and she gained a lot of satisfaction from throwing up. Unlike many bulimics, Elise was not completely secretive about her behavior, and several of her friends knew of her habit of throwing up when she felt that she had eaten too much.

Elise tried hard to get better, but several factors complicated her recovery. Despite her good relationship with her therapist, the two lived in different cities, so appointments were a logistical problem. Nor did Elise feel that her mother was helpful. They had never gotten along well, and Elise felt that her mother did things to make her feel guilty. For example, her family was aware of the expense of her treatment, and Elise felt guilty about the financial burden she had created for them.

Although Elise is still unhappy with her weight, she continues to work on her recovery. She remains sensitive about her weight and eating, reacting strongly to situations that most people would find routine, such as being weighed at the doctor's office and being fitted for a bridesmaid's dress. She no longer purges and says that the urge to do so has decreased.

Like millions of Americans, Elise has an **eating disorder**. An eating disorder is any serious and habitual disturbance in eating behavior that produces unhealthy consequences. This definition excludes starvation resulting from the inability to find suitable food supplies and also unhealthy eating resulting from inadequate information about nutrition. Also excluded are disturbances in eating behavior

such as pica, or the eating of nonnutritive substances like plastic and wood, and the rumination disorder of infancy — that is, regurgitation of food without nausea or gastrointestinal illness. Neither of these latter disorders presents serious health problems to adults, and they are of relatively minor importance in health psychology. This chapter examines in detail the three major problems of eating — overeating and dieting, anorexia nervosa, and bulimia — each related to certain difficulties in weight maintenance. To put these in context, we first consider the organs and functions of the digestive system.

THE DIGESTIVE SYSTEM

The human body can digest a wide variety of plant and animal tissues, converting these foods into usable proteins, fats, carbohydrates, vitamins, and minerals. The digestive system takes in food, processes it into particles that can be absorbed, and excretes the undigested wastes. The particles that are absorbed through the digestive system are transported through the bloodstream so as to be available to all body cells. These molecules nourish the body by providing the energy for activity as well as the materials for body growth, maintenance, and repair.

The digestive tract is a modified tube, consisting of a number of specialized structures. Also included in the digestive system are several accessory structures connected to the digestive tract by ducts. These ducted glands produce substances that are essential for digestion, and the ducts provide a way for these substances to enter the digestive system. Figure 15.1 shows the digestive system.

In humans and other mammals, some digestion begins in the mouth. The teeth tear and grind food, mixing it with saliva. Several **salivary glands** furnish the moisture that allows the food to be tasted. Without such moisture, the taste buds on the tongue do not function. Saliva also contains an enzyme that digests starch, and so some digestion actively begins before food particles leave the mouth.

Swallowing is a voluntary action, but once food is swallowed, its progress through the **pharynx** and **esophagus** is largely involuntary. **Peristalsis** propels food through the digestive system, beginning with

The mixture of food particles and gastric juices moves into the small intestine a little at a time. The high acidity of the gastric juices results in a very acidic mixture, and the small intestine cannot function in high acidity. To reduce the level of acidity, the pancreas secretes several acid-reducing enzymes into the small intestine. These **pancreatic juices** are also essential for digesting carbohydrate and fats.

The digestion of starch that begins in the mouth is completed in the small intestine. The upper third of the small intestine absorbs starch and other carbohydrates. Protein digestion, initiated in the stomach, is also completed when proteins are absorbed in the upper portion of the small intestine. Fats, however, enter the small intestine almost entirely undigested. **Bile salts** produced in the **liver** and stored in the **gall bladder** break down fat molecules into a form that is acted on by a pancreatic enzyme. Absorption of fats occurs in the middle one-third of the small intestine. The bile salts that aid the process are reabsorbed later in the lower third of the small intestine.

Large quantities of water pass through the small intestine. In addition to the water that people drink, digestive juices increase the fluid volume. Of all the water that passes into the small intestine, 90% is absorbed. This absorption process also causes vitamins and electrolytes to pass into the body at this point.

From the small intestine, digestion proceeds to the large intestine. As with other portions of the digestive system, movement through the large intestine occurs through peristalsis. However, the peristaltic movement in the large intestine is more sluggish and irregular than in the small intestine. Bacteria inhabit the large intestine and provide another function: They manufacture several vitamins. Although the large intestine has absorptive capabilities, it typically absorbs only water, a few minerals, and the vitamins manufactured by its bacteria.

Feces consist of the materials left after digestion has taken place. Feces are composed of undigested fiber, inorganic material, undigested nutrients, water, and bacteria. Peristalsis carries the feces through the large intestine, through the **rectum**, and finally through the **anus**, where they are eliminated.

Digestion starts with eating, and hunger is a factor. Hunger, however, does not originate within the

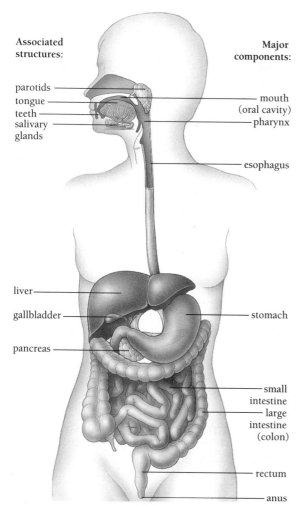

Associated structures:

parotids
tongue
teeth
salivary glands

liver
gallbladder
pancreas

Major components:

mouth (oral cavity)
pharynx

esophagus

stomach

small intestine
large intestine (colon)

rectum

anus

Figure 15.1 The digestive system.

the esophagus. Peristaltic movement is the rhythmic contraction and relaxation of the circular muscles of structures in the digestive system. In the stomach, rhythmic contractions mix the food with **gastric juices** secreted by the stomach and the glands that empty into the stomach. The major digestive activity of the stomach is that of proteins, initiated by the action of the enzyme **pepsin**. Little absorption of nutrients occurs in the stomach; only alcohol, aspirin, and some fat-soluble drugs are absorbed through the stomach lining. The major function of the stomach is to mix food particles with gastric juices, preparing the mixture for absorption in the small intestine.

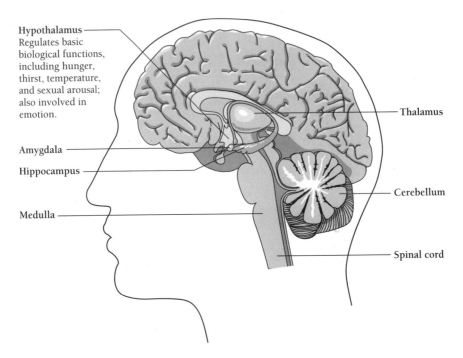

Figure 15.2 **Hypothalamus and other brain structures.**

digestive system. A brain structure, the **hypothalamus** (see Figure 15.2), contains centers that control both hunger and satiation. Surgical experimentation using rats has allowed an understanding of the various centers in the hypothalamus and how they relate to eating. Both the **lateral hypothalamus** and the **ventromedial hypothalamus** are involved in hunger. Direct stimulation of the lateral hypothalamus prompts the initiation of feeding whereas direct stimulation of the ventromedial hypothalamus causes eating to cease. Damage to these centers interferes with eating, producing either enormous overeating (ventromedial damage) or voluntary starvation (lateral damage) (Teitelbaum, 1955). Although the effects of stimulation and damage to the rat hypothalamus are well established, the extension of rat studies to human disorders such as obesity and anorexia nervosa should be made only with caution.

The digestive system is plagued by more diseases and disorders than any other body system. Many digestive disorders are not of active concern to health psychology, but several, such as obesity, anorexia nervosa, and bulimia have important behavioral components.

FACTORS IN WEIGHT MAINTENANCE

A stable weight is maintained when the calories absorbed from food equal those expended for body metabolism plus physical activity. However, this balance is not a simple calculation. Caloric content varies with foods, with fat having more calories per volume than carbohydrates or proteins. The degree of absorption depends on how rapidly food passes through the digestive system and the composition of the foods. The body turns dietary fat into body fat more easily than other types of fuels (Rodin, 1992), putting those who eat a high-fat diet at higher risk for obesity than those whose diet is lower in fat (Tremblay, Plourde, Després, & Bouchard, 1989). Furthermore, large differences exist in people's metabolic rates, and an individual's metabolism can vary from time to time. Activity level is another source of variability, with greater activity requiring greater caloric expenditures. To understand the complexities of weight loss through reducing food intake, consider an extreme example, an experiment in which participants were systematically starved.

EXPERIMENTAL STARVATION

More than 50 years ago, Ancel Keys and his colleagues (Keys, Brozek, Henschel, Mickelsen, & Taylor, 1950) developed an interest in the physical effects of starvation. They had an opportunity to study conscientious objectors during World War II, men who volunteered to be part of a study on starvation as an alternative to military service.

For the first 3 months of the project, the 36 volunteers ate regularly and participated in various tests. In most ways the participants were quite normal young men; their weights were normal, their IQs were in the normal to bright range, and they were emotionally stable. All held religious convictions that forbade fighting. After the 3 months of normal eating and establishing caloric requirements, the men were put on half their previous rations, with the goal of reducing their body weight to 75% of previous levels. Although the researchers cut the participants' caloric intake in half, they were careful to give them adequate nutrients so that the men were never in any danger of actually starving.

At first these men lost weight rapidly, although they were constantly hungry. The initial pace of weight loss, however, did not last. To continue losing weight, the men had to consume even fewer calories, which led to a few dropping out of the experiment. However, most stayed with the project through the whole 6 months, and most met their goal of losing 25% of their body weight.

The behaviors that accompanied the semistarvation were quite surprising to Keys and his colleagues. At the beginning the men were optimistic and cheerful, but these feelings soon vanished. The men became irritable, aggressive, and began to fight among themselves, behavior that was completely out of character. Although the men continued this bellicose behavior throughout the 6 months of starvation, they also became apathetic and avoided as much physical activity as they could. They become neglectful of their dormitory and their own physical appearance. Also uncharacteristic was their apparent loss of interest in sex (Keys et al., 1950).

The men were, of course, hungry, and they became increasingly obsessed with thoughts of food. Mealtimes became the center of their lives, and they tended to eat very slowly and to be very sensitive to the taste of their food. At the beginning of the period

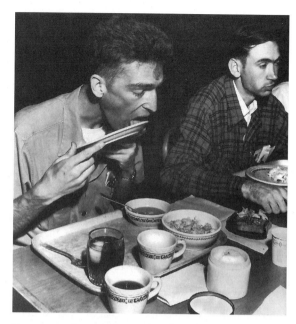

Experimental starvation produced an obsession with food and a variety of negative changes in the behavior of these volunteers.

of caloric reduction, no physical restrictions had been imposed to prevent the men from cheating on their diets. But about 3 months into the starvation, restrictions became necessary. The men felt that they would be tempted to cheat if they left the dormitory alone. As a result, they were allowed to go out only in pairs or in larger groups. These dedicated, polite, normal, stable young men had become abnormal and unpleasant under conditions of semistarvation.

Obsession with food and continued negative outlook characterized the refeeding phase of the project. During this phase, the plan was for the men to regain the weight they had lost. This phase was to have lasted 3 months, with food introduced at gradually increasing levels, but the men objected so strongly that this phase was accelerated. As a result, the men ate as much and as often as they could, some as many as five large meals a day. By the end of the period of refeeding, most men had regained their preexperimental weight. In fact, many were even slightly heavier. About one-half were still preoccupied with food, and for many, their prestarvation optimism and cheerfulness had not completely returned.

EXPERIMENTAL OVEREATING

Whereas a study in experimental starvation does not seem attractive to volunteers, an experiment on overeating might sound like fun to many people. Ethan Allen Sims and his associates (Sims, 1974, 1976; Sims et al., 1973; Sims & Horton, 1968) found a group of people who should have been especially interested and appreciative—prisoners. Inmates at the Vermont State Prison volunteered to gain 20 to 30 pounds as part of an experiment on overeating. Sims's interest was analogous to Keys's: an understanding of the physical and psychological components of overeating. Special living arrangements were made for these prisoners, including plentiful and delicious food. In addition, the experiment included a restriction of activity to make weight gain easier.

Did these men gain weight? With an increase in calories and a decrease in physical activity, weight gain was nearly assured. At first they gained fairly easily. But soon the rate of weight gain slowed, and the participants had to eat more and more to continue gaining. As with the men in the starvation study, these men needed about 3,500 calories to maintain their weight at normal levels, but many had to double that amount to continue gaining. Not all the men were able to attain their weight goals, regardless of how much they ate. One man did not reach his goal even though he ate over 10,000 calories per day.

Were the overeating prisoners as miserable as the starving conscientious objectors? No, but they did find overeating unpleasant. Food became repulsive to them, despite the excellent quality and preparation. They had to force themselves to eat, and many considered dropping out of the study.

When the prisoners were no longer required to eat, they cut down their food intake dramatically and lost weight. Not all lost as quickly as others, and two had some trouble returning to their original weight. An examination of these men's medical backgrounds revealed some family histories of obesity, although the men themselves had never been overweight. These results indicate that normal-weight people have trouble increasing their weight substantially and that, even if they do, the increased weight is difficult to maintain.

THE CONCEPT OF SETPOINT

The findings from the Keys et al. study on experimental starvation and the Sims et al. studies on experimental overeating indicate that deviations from normal weight in either direction are achieved only with effort and suffering. One interpretation of these findings is the existence of a **setpoint** for weight maintenance. In this formulation, setpoint is a type of internal thermostat that works on the basis of fat. Losing fat throws off the setpoint, spurring the body to take corrective action. Part of that action includes slowing the metabolic process to require fewer calories, and the body becomes more conservative in its energy expenditures. With conditions of prolonged and serious starvation, this slowed metabolism is expressed behaviorally as listlessness and apathy—both of which were exhibited by Keys's starving volunteers.

This metabolic slowdown is the reason Keys's conscientious objectors stopped losing weight before reaching their goal, even with severely restricted caloric intake. It is also the reason that people on diets find continued weight loss increasingly difficult: Their bodies are fighting against a further depletion of fat supplies. Beller (1978) interpreted this mechanism as a great advantage in times of uncertain food supply because it can buffer the effects of famine. As an anthropologist, she found it reasonable that those humans with the tendency not only to store fat but also to metabolically protect those fat stores would be at a substantial advantage in most situations in human history.

Increased hunger is the body's other corrective action when fat supplies fall below setpoint. Again, this mechanism seems to be consistent with the results of the Keys et al. study on starvation. The men who dieted to 75% of their normal body weight became miserable and hungry, and they stayed that way until they were back to their original weight. During the entire time they were below their normal weight (which would be below setpoint), they were obsessed with food. When they were allowed to eat, they preferred the high-calorie foods that tended to increase their fat stores most rapidly. This preference is consistent with setpoint theory.

Does the experiment on overeating also fit with setpoint theory? Bennett and Gurin (1982) claimed

WOULD YOU BELIEVE . . . ?

Good Taste May Be Fattening

Would you believe that good taste may be fattening? Research on both humans and rats has found that taste and weight gain are related.

Surgery to the hypothalamus of rats stimulates them to overeat to the point of enormous obesity. But without such surgery, laboratory rats do not readily overeat or become obese. However, an eating program called the "supermarket diet" will induce rats to gain weight (Sclafani & Springer, 1976). This "supermarket" diet consists of a variety of goodies— chocolate chip cookies, salami, cheese, bananas, marshmallows, chocolate, peanut butter, sweetened condensed milk, and fat. Rats given seven of these foods on a frequently changing menu combination gained 269% more weight than a control group of rats that ate lab chow.

Although Sclafani and Springer speculated that the variety of food contributed to the rats' eager eating, a later study (Ackroff & Sclafani, 1988) found that rats offered a varied diet gained less weight than rats offered lab chow plus sucrose (sugar). As chocoholics would guess, a diet with a combination of sugar and fat produced a greater weight gain than a diet of sugar or fat or lab chow. Lucas and Sclafani (1990) also found that the combination of saccharine and fat was not as appealing as the combination of sugar and fat, suggesting that sugar substitutes may not be good substitutes for sugar; that is, artificially sweetened foods may not satisfy junk food cravings.

Susan Schiffman (1983; Schiffman, Musante, & Conger, 1978) has found that obese humans also crave both flavor and variety in their food and that their preferences bear a resemblance to the "supermarket diet" that readily fattens rats. Perhaps obese people have spontaneously followed such a diet, contributing to their weight problem.

Schiffman observed that taste may be a factor in dieting because many reducing diets are bland and monotonous, depriving dieters of both flavor and variety. In order to create a diet that can be maintained, Schiffman advised people to eat a variety of flavorful foods, a recommendation that may tempt anorexics to return to a more normal eating pattern. However, both dieters and anorexics should probably avoid foods with the sugar and fat combination that was so tempting to the fattened rats.

that it does, pointing out that the prisoners who tried to gain more than their normal weight were fighting their natural setpoint. According to the setpoint concept, the bodies of the overfed prisoners should have sent messages that they had enough fat stored already and did not need more. This message should have translated into something like "Stop eating," which seems to have happened because the prisoners found eating unpleasant.

Bennett and Gurin discussed some evidence, mostly from animal studies, suggesting a metabolic mechanism that also aids in preventing upward deviations from setpoint. Such a mechanism would increase the metabolic process, the opposite of the mechanism that follows severe caloric restriction. Such alterations in metabolic rate may be possible so that setpoint is normalized. Research by several teams (Campfield, Smith, Guisez, Devos, & Burn, 1995; Halaas et al., 1995; Pelleymounter et al., 1995) has demonstrated that a protein hormone named *leptin* is capable of altering weight in genetically obese mice. When they were injected with leptin,

normal-weight mice were not strongly affected, but mice that had been fed to the point of obesity experienced weight loss and increase in activity (Campfield et al., 1995). The treated mice decreased their food intake, increased their activity level, and lost 30% of their body weight, all of it in fat. When the leptin injections were discontinued, however, the mice started to regain the weight they had lost. Further research on the effects of leptin (Tartaglia et al., 1995) has determined that leptin is part of a complex signaling system to the brain that includes the hypothalamus. This research provides evidence that is consistent with the setpoint model concerning the regulation of body weight. Furthermore, it suggests that adipose tissue produces a factor that circulates throughout the body and affects the brain in such a way as to regulate feeding behavior and activity.

The setpoint hypothesis also received support from a study of how people adjust to weight loss and weight gain. Leibel, Rosenbaum, and Hirsch (1995) underfed obese men and women until they lost 10%

to 20% of their baseline body weight. They also overfed normal weight men and women who had never been obese until these participants gained 10% of their baseline body weight. Participants who lost weight also lost energy, expending 15% less than before they were underfed whereas participants who gained weight increased their total expenditure of energy. Like Keys's conscientious objectors, the people who lost weight became increasingly hungry, and this hunger along with decreased energy made it very difficult for them to maintain weight loss. On the other hand, the reduced energy and decreased hunger of the overfed participants hampered their ability to maintain weight gain. Bennett (1995) interpreted these findings as evidence for a setpoint for body fat and speculated that the mechanism for it is in the brain but not confined to the hypothalamus. He also interpreted these results as suggesting that there is no easy solution to weight loss for obese people.

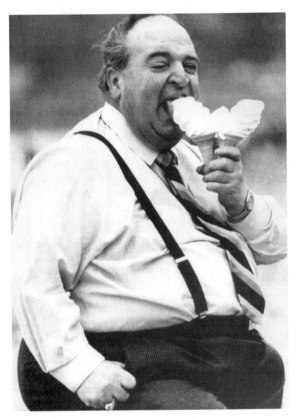

The weight maintenance equation is complex, but overeating is a cause of obesity.

OVEREATING AND OBESITY

Many people assume that overeating is the sole cause of obesity, but the weight maintenance equation is not a simple one. Not all obese people eat a great deal, and many overweight people eat less than normal-weight people and possibly even less than some thin people. As the studies on experimental starvation and overeating show, metabolic level changes with food intake as well as with energy output.

In addition, individual variations in body metabolism allow some people to burn calories faster than others; this means that two people who eat the same amount may have different weights. Certainly, these findings are not true of all obese people, some of whom are fat because they eat a lot, do too little physical activity, or engage in a combination of these two factors (Blair, 1993; Bray, 1992). Before examining the health consequences of obesity, we look at the meaning of obesity and consider the question of why some people are overweight.

WHAT IS OBESITY?

What is obesity? Answers to this question vary by personal and social standards. Should obesity be de-

fined in terms of health? Appearance? Body mass? Percentage of body fat? Weight charts? Total weight? No definition of obesity would consider only body weight, because some individuals have a small skeletal frame and others are more muscular. Muscle tissue and bone weigh more than fat, so some people can be heavier yet leaner than normal, as athletes often are. Therefore, an accurate measure of percentage of body fat is a better index of obesity than total weight.

Determining percentage and distribution of body fat is not as easy as consulting a chart, and several different methods exist to assess body fat (Lukaski, 1987). Many of the new technologies for imaging the body—computer tomography, ultrasound, and magnetic resonance imaging—can be applied to assessing fat content, but these methods have the drawbacks of being very expensive and relatively inaccessible. Simpler methods are less accurate but more accessible. The skinfold technique involves measuring the thickness of a pinch of skin. Although this method is relatively easy and inexpensive, it is not very accurate (Bray, 1992). The water immersion technique in which a person is lowered into water to determine the amount of displacement is awkward and moderately expensive. Although this technique accurately records the percentage of body fat, it does not measure the distribution of body fat. However, the waist-to-hip ratio method does, and Bray (1992) recommended this measurement as preferable to other methods when estimating body fat and its distribution.

Another method is the **body mass index (BMI)**, defined as body weight (in kilograms) divided by height (in meters) squared, that is, BMI $= kg / m^2$. Bray (1992) suggested that the BMI was the preferred estimate of obesity and proposed categories of obesity based on BMI and the approximate health risk for each category (see Table 15.1). Although BMI does not consider a person's age, gender, or body build, Williamson (1993) has argued that this index can provide a standard for measuring obesity, which he defined as a BMI of 27.8 or more for men and 27.3 or more for women. (A 5'10" man with a BMI of 27.8 would weigh 194 pounds, and a 5'4" woman with a BMI of 27.3 would weigh 159.) These numbers are approximately 20% above the weights in the 1983 Metropolitan Life Insurance Company's height-weight charts for people with a medium frame.

Most people (and many researchers) continue to rely on the charts that provide normal weight ranges for various heights and body frame sizes. The charts

published by the Metropolitan Life Insurance Company are based on statistics from the Society of Actuaries and thus reflect weight ranges with the lowest mortality. Table 15.2 shows both the 1959 and the 1983 charts, and a comparison shows that being overweight has been redefined in an upward direction.

Overweight is often defined in terms of social standards, and such definitions usually have little to do with health. Both Beller (1978) and Bennett and Gurin (1982) discussed how the criteria for physical attractiveness have changed during human history. During the times when food supply was uncertain (the case throughout most of history), carrying some supply of fat on the body was a type of insurance and was thus considered attractive. Fat could also be considered a mark of prosperity; fat advertised to the world that a person could afford an ample supply of food. Only in very recent history has this standard changed. Before 1920, thinness was considered unattractive, possibly due to the association between thinness and diseases or perhaps its association with poverty (Bennett & Gurin, 1982).

Thinness is no longer considered unattractive. In fact, today it is as highly desirable as plumpness was in the previous centuries, especially for women. A study by Garner, Garfinkel, Schwartz, and Thompson (1980) examined the changes in ideal weights by measuring changes in the body weight of *Playboy* centerfolds and also Miss America candidates from 1959 to 1978. They found that weights for both groups had decreased relative to average weight of the general population. A follow-up study (Wiseman, Gray, Mosimann, & Ahrens, 1992) examined the same relationship from 1979 to 1988. During that time, Miss America contestants became significantly thinner, indicating that the socially ideal weight for women dropped during both decades. Clearly, obesity, like beauty, is in the eye of the beholder.

Women's actual weight has not decreased during the past 2 decades. In fact, weight for both women and men in the United States has recently increased, but women's relative weight gain has been greater than that of men (Kuczmarski, 1992), and women have become more conscious of their weight and dissatisfied with even normal weight. A national survey by Biener and Heaton (1995) revealed that

Table 15.1 Categories of obesity and health risks based on body mass index (BMI)

Category	BMI Range	Risk
0	20–25	Not obese; No increased risk
I	25–30	Low risk
II	30–35	Moderate
III	35–40	High risk
IV	40+	Very high risk

SOURCE: Based on G. A. Bray, (1992), "Pathophysiology of Obesity," *American Journal of Clinical Nutrition, 55*, 488S–494S.

Table 15.2　Metropolitan Life Insurance Company's desirable weights for the years 1959 and 1983

Height	Small frame		Medium frame		Large frame	
	1959	1983	1959	1983	1959	1983
Women						
4 ft. 10 in.	92– 98 lb.	102–111 lb.	96–107 lb.	109–121 lb.	104–119 lb.	118–131 lb.
4　11	94–101	103–113	98–110	111–123	106–122	120–134
5　0	96–104	104–115	101–113	113–126	109–125	122–137
5　1	99–107	106–118	104–116	115–129	112–128	125–140
5　2	102–110	108–121	107–119	118–132	115–131	128–143
5　3	105–113	111–124	110–122	121–135	118–134	131–147
5　4	108–116	114–127	113–126	124–138	121–138	134–151
5　5	111–119	117–130	116–130	127–141	125–142	137–155
5　6	114–123	120–133	120–135	130–144	129–146	140–159
5　7	118–127	123–136	124–139	133–147	133–150	143–163
5　8	122–131	126–139	128–143	136–150	137–154	146–167
5　9	126–135	129–142	132–147	139–153	141–158	149–170
5　10	130–140	132–145	136–151	142–156	145–163	152–173
5　11	134–144	135–148	140–155	145–159	149–168	155–176
6　0	138–148	138–151	144–159	148–162	153–173	158–179
Men						
5 ft. 2 in.	112–120 lb.	128–134 lb.	118–129 lb.	131–141 lb.	126–141 lb.	138–150 lb.
5　3	115–123	130–136	121–133	133–143	129–144	140–153
5　4	118–126	132–138	124–136	135–145	132–148	142–156
5　5	121–129	134–140	127–139	137–148	135–152	144–160
5　6	124–133	136–142	130–143	139–151	138–156	146–164
5　7	128–137	138–145	134–147	142–154	142–161	149–168
5　8	132–141	140–148	138–152	145–157	147–166	152–172
5　9	136–145	142–151	142–156	148–160	151–170	155–176
5　10	140–150	144–154	146–160	151–163	155–174	158–180
5　11	144–154	146–157	150–165	154–166	159–179	161–184
6　0	148–158	149–160	154–170	157–170	164–184	164–188
6　1	152–162	152–164	158–175	160–174	168–189	168–192
6　2	156–167	155–168	162–180	164–178	173–194	172–197
6　3	160–171	158–172	167–185	167–182	178–199	176–202
6　4	164–175	162–176	172–190	171–187	182–204	181–207

SOURCE: From "New Weight Standards for Men and Women" by Metropolitan Life Insurance Company, 1959, *Statistical Bulletin, 40*, p. 1. Copyright 1959, 1983 by The Metropolitan Life Insurance Company. Adapted by permission.

many women of normal weight are unwisely concerned that they weigh too much. In this survey, nearly half of European American women and one-fourth of African American women with a body mass index under 25 (see Table 15.1) were currently trying to lose weight. Interestingly, these dieters stated that their primary motive was to improve their health. However, Biener and Heaton found that the dieters had a history of 50% more weight fluctuation than the nondieters, and research discussed in Chapter 9 suggests that frequent changes in weight are associated with greater risk for coronary heart disease. Biener and Heaton also reported that 13%

of their sample (or 2 million women in the United States) were using unhealthy strategies to lose weight, such as fasting, vomiting, using diet pills, and taking laxatives.

WHY ARE SOME PEOPLE OBESE?

Just as there are several definitions of obesity, there are several models that attempt to explain why some people are obese. These models, which should be able to explain both the development and the maintenance of obesity, include the psychodynamic model, the social learning model, and the setpoint model.

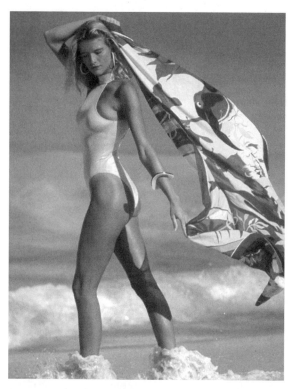

Once considered unattractive, thinness is now considered the ideal.

The Psychodynamic Model

Psychodynamic theories rest on the assumption that many human motives are unconscious attempts to minimize anxiety and to deal with conflicts, many of which originate during childhood. The psychodynamic model of obesity sees failure to maintain normal weight as the result of an unconscious conflict (Slochower, 1983), but psychodynamic theorists do not agree among themselves on the nature of this unconscious conflict. For example, Kaplan and Kaplan (1957) discovered 27 different psychodynamic theories of obesity, each of which viewed overeating as a symptom of an emotional conflict, but these theories differed widely as to what constituted the source of that conflict.

Slochower (1983) reported several studies supporting the view that overeating represents a response to anxiety. Her experiments involved both anxiety produced in a laboratory by providing false information about heart rate and the naturally oc-

curring anxiety of final examinations. In both types of anxiety situations, Slochower's obese participants ate significantly more than her normal-weight participants. However, not all anxiety-producing situations induced overeating, a finding that clouds the hypothesis that overeating is a response to anxiety.

Until the 1960s, virtually all psychological treatment for obesity took a psychodynamic approach. The goal of psychodynamic treatment is to discover the unconscious conflict that is the basis of overeating. In theory, once the conflict has been discovered, the motivation to overeat will gradually disappear. Although this model is no longer widely accepted, some evidence exists that psychodynamic treatment can be effective. Rand and Stunkard (1983) found that obese patients who received psychodynamic-oriented treatment not only lost weight but also maintained the loss after therapy and developed more positive body images. Because the therapists did not specifically treat obesity, these results were unexpected. The researchers were in doubt as to why the patients lost weight. Although the study does not confirm the psychodynamic explanation for obesity, the findings suggest that obese patients who develop a better body image and improve their overall functioning as the result of psychotherapy may also lose weight, even though weight loss is not the goal of therapy.

The Social Learning Model

Eating is a biologically based reinforcement, but eating is also a social activity. When, where, what, and even how much to eat is socially regulated, so one might expect that obese people should eat not only more but also differently from the nonobese. Has research provided support for these contentions?

Stanley Schachter and his colleagues (Schachter, Goldman, & Gordon, 1968) found that physiological hunger was less important in eating for the obese than for those of normal weight. Schachter had suspected this relationship because in an experiment by Stunkard and Koch (1964), obese participants had reported less agreement between hunger and stomach contractions than normal-weight individuals. Schachter demonstrated the relative unresponsiveness of obese people to physiological hunger by experimenting on obese and normal-weight participants who ate crackers when they had either skipped lunch or had been fed lunch as part of the experiment. The obese participants showed their unresponsiveness to hunger by eating about the same number of crackers regardless of whether they had eaten lunch. Why should obese people have trouble listening to their bodies' hunger signals?

In 1972, Nisbett made an observation that suggested an answer, noting that obese people behaved rather like the starving conscientious objectors in the Keys et al. (1950) study on starvation. Could obese people be perpetually hungry? The answer to this question has come through the research efforts of Jane Polivy and C. Peter Herman.

In 1983, Polivy and Herman published a summary of their extensive research on eating and obesity, which replicated and extended Schachter's work. The Polivy and Herman research did not use obese participants as a group; instead they studied dieters. Their reasoning was that following Nisbett's suggestion, the behavioral peculiarities found by Schachter and his colleagues might be the result of constant food deprivation—that is, dieting—rather than to obesity itself. They also guessed that these effects would not be unique to the obese but would extend to that huge group of dieting people who feel they must diet to maintain a socially ideal weight. Polivy and Herman developed the concept of *restrained eating* and a scale that measures factors relating to the constant awareness and restriction of food. Using this scale, they were able to divide people into restrained and unrestrained eaters and found that restrained eaters were more responsive to taste and ate by the clock, regardless of their weight.

Polivy and Herman discovered that dieters are like lapsed alcoholics in some ways, with one dietary slip precipitating a relapse to overeating. In one of their studies, participants identified as either restrained or unrestrained eaters were fed either none, one, or two milkshakes. Thus, the experiment involved six combinations of eating style and number of milkshakes. Each participant had to eat ice cream as part of a disguised taste test. A reasonable prediction was that the restrained eaters would eat less ice cream if they had drunk one milkshake as opposed to none and that they would eat even less if they had been required to drink two milkshakes. After all, these people were dieting and had indicated by their responses to the restrained eating scale that they

were constantly aware of their eating and were trying to eat less than they wanted.

Contrary to this expectation, the restrained eaters who had been required to drink two milkshakes ate *more* ice cream than the restrained eaters who had drunk none. Nor was this finding an anomaly; Polivy and Herman have seen this effect in a number of studies. They described it as the "what the hell" effect, hypothesizing that dieters say "what the hell" after being forced to lapse from their diets. This effect occurs only when the food tastes good. If it does not, dieters can reimpose restraint immediately. However, the tendency among restrained eaters who have lapsed is not to attempt to climb back on the dieting wagon until the next day and to enjoy their lapse. Dieters, then, behave in a way similar to some alcohol abusers, trying once more to return to abstinence following a binge precipitated by a slip.

Although later research has revealed that other factors influence eating in restrained eaters, research has generally confirmed the difference in eating patterns between restrained and nonrestrained eaters. Self-esteem is one factor that interacts with restraint: Restrained eaters with low self-esteem are most subject to the disinhibiting effects of a milkshake preload (Polivy, Heatherton, & Herman, 1988). Also, the placebo effect influences how much restrained eaters consume (Heatherton, Polivy, & Herman, 1989). Restrained eaters who believed that the "vitamin" they swallowed would make them feel full ate less than restrained eaters who believed that their "vitamin" would make them feel hungry. Thus, social learning theory offers one explanation for why obese people maintain their weight, but it does not fully explain why some people are restrained eaters and others are nonrestrained eaters.

The Setpoint Model

The setpoint model holds that when fat levels rise or fall below a certain level, physiological and psychological mechanisms are activated that encourage a return to setpoint. The setpoint theory explains obesity as the norm for some people, with some people's setpoint fixed at high levels. Individuals have different setpoints; some people are thin, others are heavier, and some are fat. Women, for example, have a higher percentage of body fat than men and therefore higher setpoints. Attributing individual and gender differences to an internal mechanism, however, does not explain why those differences occur. Why do some people have a higher setpoint than others?

Bennett and Gurin (1982) hypothesized that both heredity and environment contribute to the establishment and maintenance of setpoint. The evidence for a hereditary component in weight maintenance has come from studies of adopted children (Stunkard et al., 1986) and from studies of identical twins reared together or apart (Stunkard, Harris, Pedersen, & McClean, 1990). The study of adopted children found a close relationship between their weight and that of their biological parents but no relationship between their weight and that of their adoptive parents. The study of identical twins indicated that the correlations between weights of twin pairs were high, even when the twins had not been reared together. Stunkard (1989) claimed that gender differences exist in the heritability of obesity, with obesity more heritable in women than in men, and subsequent research (Allison, Heshka, Neale, Lykken, & Heymsfield, 1994) has substantiated this claim.

Another twin study (Bouchard et al., 1990) involved experimental overfeeding of twin pairs to determine their similarities in weight gains and fat distribution. This study indicated that although genetic factors are involved in weight gain, they are even more important in *fat distribution*. In general, studies on genetic contributions to weight have found that approximately 60% to 70% of the variability of weight is attributable to genetic factors. Although this proportion sounds so large as to be the determinant of weight, Allison et al. (1994, p. 364) cautioned against such an interpretation:

> Although genes are quite influential in determining relative weight, genes make proteins, not fat. Thus, the genotype must influence the accumulation of adiposity indirectly through energy intake and expenditure. Psychological and physiological approaches both will be needed to study the genetics of energy intake and expenditure.

Keesey (1980) claimed that the human setpoint is less precise in its regulation than the setpoints for other species and hypothesized that the setpoint acts to keep weight within a range rather than at a precise point. However, the reasons some people have high setpoints and others low setpoints remains unexplained. Nor do most of its advocates believe that it explains all cases of weight deviation (Bennett & Gurin, 1982; Keesey, 1980; Nisbett, 1972; Polivy & Herman, 1983). These researchers have hypothesized that metabolic and behavioral factors regulate weight, preventing deviations in either an upward or downward direction. Even advocates of the setpoint model concede that deviations from setpoint are possible. People can become obese through overeating, or they can keep their weight lower than setpoint through constant efforts to restrain their eating.

For many people who are heavier than they would like to be, the setpoint model is a mixed blessing. On the positive side, the model explains their great difficulty in losing weight and why weight loss often leads to personality changes and misery. On the negative side, this model suggests that resetting the setpoint can be done in only minor ways and then with great difficulty because the setpoint is biologically determined. This model is especially disturbing to those who believe that obesity constitutes a serious health problem. However, the relationship between obesity and health is not a simple one.

IS OBESITY UNHEALTHY?

The question of obesity's effect on health is complicated. The answer depends on the method of measuring obesity, degree of obesity, distribution of weight, and history of weight cycling. In general, being moderately overweight may not be an independent risk factor for heart disease or for all-cause mortality. However, being severely obese, having a history of weight losses and gains, and having a high waist-to-hip ratio place a person at an elevated health risk.

Recent evidence shows that obesity carries an added risk, at least for some people and for some diseases. Moreover, the risk increases with levels of obesity. Kannel and Cupples (1989) found that the risk associated with obesity was especially strong for nonfatal cardiovascular disease and for gallbladder disease; people who were 20% or more above their ideal weight had a doubled risk for gallbladder disease. Sjöström (1992b) confirmed the risk for cardiovascular disease and obesity, extending the risk to fatal heart disease and stroke. He also reported that obesity raises the risk for death from diabetes and raises the overall mortality approximately twofold.

When factors such as smoking history, weight-related illness, age, and stability of weight are not considered, the very thinnest and the heaviest people seem to be at greatest risk for all-cause mortality and death from cardiovascular disease. However, when Manson et al. (1995) controlled for smoking and stability of weight in middle-aged women, they found a direct and consistent relationship between body mass index and all-cause mortality. Compared with very thin women, the relative risk of death steadily increased as body mass index increased. Women with a body mass index of 32 or higher had a double risk for all-cause mortality and more than a fourfold risk of death from cardiovascular disease. This study found that very lean women did not have an excess mortality rate when smoking and weight

stability were taken into consideration, and that each increase of body mass index adds to the risk of death, especially from cardiovascular disease.

Similar findings apply to middle-aged and older men (Rimm et al., 1995). A complex of weight-related characteristics, such as weight gain since age 21, body mass index, waist-to-hip ratio, and short stature, were each associated with coronary heart disease. Men who were thin at age 21 and remained thin had the lowest risk of all the participants. For men younger than 65, the higher their body mass index, the greater was their risk for coronary heart disease. Men with a body mass index of 33 or more were 3.4 times as likely to develop heart disease as were thin men, a risk that compares to the 4.1 for middle-aged women (Manson et al., 1995). Other studies have also found that distribution of fat relates to health problems (see box—Would You Believe . . . ?).

WOULD YOU BELIEVE . . . ?
A Big Butt Is Healthier Than a Fat Gut

Would you believe that a big butt is better than a fat gut, at least in terms of health risks? An increasing body of evidence indicates that not all fat is equal as a health risk: Abdominal fat creates more of a risk than fat in the thighs and hips. In a study of obese women (Hartz, Rupley, & Rimm, 1984), fat distribution related to the development of disease. Women whose waist measurements were large compared to hip measurements had an elevated risk of diabetes, hypertension, and gallbladder disease. These findings apply to men as well as to women (Sjöström, 1992b), and the location of fat on the body is a better predictor of mortality than the amount of fat.

Although the risks apply to both women and men, the likelihood of having the risky pattern is not equal. Men are more likely to have the central pattern of fat distribution with accumulated fat around the middle, whereas women are more prone to develop large hips and thighs. Indeed, the gender-related differences

in patterns of obesity may relate to gender differences in mortality. Studies by Lars Sjöström (1992a, 1992b) and Xavier Pi-Sunyer (1993) investigated the relationship between central versus peripheral fat distribution and found that the central pattern of adiposity constitutes a specific risk for the diseases that tend to be associated with obesity.

Weight around one's middle may be a better predictor of all-cause mortality than body mass index. A study of a large group of Iowa women (Folsom et al., 1993) found that the larger their waist-to-hip ratio, the higher was their death rate. This dose-response relationship remained after controlling for BMI, smoking, educational level, marital status, estrogen use, and alcohol consumption, leading to the conclusion that waist/hip ratio is a better predictor of death in older women than body mass index.

However, the health risk of a big gut may not be equal for all people. Examining the distribution of body

fat and its relation to heart disease in African American and European American men and women revealed that, consistent with other studies, fat around one's middle is related to ischemic heart disease, but not in African American women (Freedman, Williamson, Croft, Ballew, & Byers, 1995). The relative risk for African American men and European American men was essentially identical, and the risk for European American women was highest of all. However, African American women with weight distributed around the middle had no extra risk of heart disease. Some evidence (Biener & Heaton, 1995; Williamson, Serdula, Anda, Levy, & Byers, 1992) indicates that African American women are less concerned about losing a lot of weight than European American women, and results from the Freedman et al. study indicate that this reduced concern may be justified. For other subgroups, however, a fat gut is more dangerous to health than a big butt.

Table 15.3   The relationship between weight and disease or death

Study	Sample	Results
Manson et al., 1995	middle-aged women	Each increase in body mass index (BMI) adds to risk for all-cause mortality.
Manson et al., 1995	middle-aged women	Heaviest women have a fourfold risk for cardiovascular disease.
Rimm et al., 1995	middle-aged and older men	Large BMI and waist/hip ratio add to risk for coronary heart disease (CHD).
Rimm et al., 1995	men 65 and older	BMI is a weak predictor of CHD, but waist/hip ratio is a strong predictor.
Borkan et al., 1986	men with history of weight cycling	Weight cycling is associated with hypertension and high cholesterol levels.
Lee & Paffenbarger, 1992	middle-aged men	Weight gain and weight loss are each related to all-cause mortality and CHD death.
Lissner et al., 1991	Framingham men and women	Weight change is more risky than obesity.
Folsom et al., 1993	middle-aged men	Waist/hip ratio is a better predictor than BMI of all-cause mortality.
Freedman, Byers, Barrett, Stroup, & Monroe-Blum, 1995	African American women	Central fat does not predict heart disease.
Freedman et al., 1995	All other groups	Central fat predicts heart disease.

Weight cycling, or yo-yo dieting, may also be an obesity-related health risk. One study (Borkan, Sparrow, Wisniewski, & Vokonas, 1986) found that weight changes alone were associated with the risk factors for coronary heart disease. In this study, men with a 15-year history of weight changes (either increases or decreases) were more likely to have hypertension, high cholesterol, and other coronary risk factors. A report from the Framingham study (Lissner et al., 1991) indicated that people with a history of weight cycling had a significant increase in risk for all-cause mortality, heart disease, and cancer. This study also found that fluctuation in weight carried more of a risk than obesity itself.

In addition, Lee and Paffenbarger (1992) followed Harvard alumni and found that men who either lost or gained weight had a higher death rate from all causes and from coronary heart disease than men with stable weight. They found, however, that changes in weight were not related to death from cancer. In a review of the research on weight cycling, Brownell and Rodin (1994b) concluded that this pattern of weight loss and gain is associated with increased cardiovascular and all-cause mortality.

In conclusion, obese people have heightened risks of developing certain health problems, especially diabetes and cardiovascular disease. Table 15.3 summarizes studies showing that obesity, changes in weight, and fat distributed around the waist all relate to increased mortality rates, especially from heart disease.

DIETING

The frequency of dieting, defined as attempts to lose weight through food restriction, differs somewhat with age, gender, and social class. Young people, women, and middle- and upper-class people are most likely to diet. The trend toward dieting has become more severe in the past few decades. During the mid-1960s, only 10% of the overweight adults were dieting (Wyden, 1965), but during subsequent years, those percentages steadily increased; currently, as many as 70% of high school girls are either dieting to lose weight or to keep from gaining weight (see Table 15.4). Rosen and Gross (1987) found that attempts at losing weight were not limited to obese or overweight adolescents. Similarly, Dwyer, Feldman, and Mayer (1967) reported that only half of dieting high school girls were overweight. In addition, 80% of all the girls surveyed by Dwyer et al.

Table 15.4   Changing trends in dieting to lose or not gain weight, United States, 1965 to 1995

Study	Year	Sample	Percent trying to lose	Percent trying not to gain
Wyden	1965	overweight adults	10%	
Dwyer et al.	1967	overweight high school girls	50%	
Dwyer et al.	1967	overweight high school boys	6%	
Rosen & Gross	1987	adolescent girls	65%	
Rosen & Gross	1987	adolescent boys	16%	
Serdula et al.	1993	high school girls	44%	26%
Serdula et al.	1993	high school boys	25%	15%
Serdula et al.	1993	adult women	38%	28%
Serdula et al.	1993	adult men	24%	28%
Levy & Heaton	1993	adult women	33%	
Levy & Heaton	1993	adult men	20%	
French, Story, Downes, Resnick, & Blum	1995	adolescent girls*	62%	
French et al.	1995	adolescents boys*	21%	

*Had dieted at some time during their life

indicated that they would like to lose weight. The situation among teenage boys was different in that a higher percentage of the boys were obese (19%) but only 6% of them were dieting, and only 20% of the boys wanted to lose weight. Among adolescent boys, in fact, more are trying to gain than to lose weight. However, most high school students, whether they are trying to gain or lose weight, are already of normal weight (Dwyer, et al., 1967; Rosen & Gross, 1987; Serdula et al., 1993).

A survey of adolescents and adults (Serdula et al., 1993) showed that more than two-thirds of female high school students and more than one-third of male high school students were either trying to lose or to avoid gaining weight. For adults, two-thirds of the women and more than half the men were either trying to lose or not gain more weight, figures consistent with those of Levy and Heaton (1993). These rates reflect only those who were dieting at the time of the survey. When considering lifetime dieting, 72% of women and 44% of men have dieted at some time in their lives (Serdula et al., 1993), making weight loss attempts common experiences to a majority of people in the United States. Table 15.4 shows the changing trends in dieting during the past 30 years.

APPROACHES TO LOSING WEIGHT

Best-seller book lists usually contain at least one diet book and frequently more than one, with the proposed diets varying greatly. Millions of people, it seems, are interested in knowing what kind of diet works best. Despite the title of the 1961 best-seller *Calories Don't Count*, by Herman Taller, most authorities acknowledge that they do count. To be effective, all reducing diets must reduce the number of calories metabolized or increase the number of calories used by the body. This information is familiar to those who want to lose weight, and 25% of women and 17% of men who try to lose weight count calories (Levy & Heaton, 1993). Most diets reduce the amount of food eaten, but some programs alter the combination or proportion of nutrients, and some substitute special nutrient mixtures for food.

Restricting Types of Food

Restricting certain types of foods is one way to diet. Because a variety of foods is necessary for adequate nutrition, however, severely restricting or eliminating a food category may be nutritionally unwise.

Maintaining a diet consisting of a variety of foods with smaller portions is a reasonable and healthy strategy, but many people find it difficult simply to eat less. Therefore, the approach of restricting types of foods has been a popular dieting strategy.

Restricting carbohydrates has been a popular approach, possibly because low-carbohydrate diets often allow high-fat foods (which most people find tasty). Taller's 1961 diet book allowed as much fat as the dieter wanted but severely restricted carbohydrates. *Dr. Atkins' Diet Revolution* (1972) by Robert Atkins took basically the same approach: a low-carbohydrate, high-fat diet. Both books made the best-seller list, and thousands of people tried these programs. However, low-carbohydrate diets are open to severe criticism for being both ineffective and potentially dangerous. Evidence of ineffectiveness comes from research indicating that eating fat tends to increase fat intake rather than induce satiety (Tremblay et al., 1989). Thus, high-fat diets tend to be counterproductive in helping people lose weight. Such diets also produce fatigue and depression as frequent side effects, which some people develop after a few days on such diets. The primary danger of a high-fat diet is the increases in serum cholesterol. People who lose weight on such diets do so for the same reason that people on any diet lose weigh: They consume fewer calories.

High-carbohydrate, low-fat diets have also had their advocates (Ornish, 1993). These diets strive to increase the amount of foods with "complex" carbohydrates while lowering fat intake. Complex carbohydrates are found in fruits, vegetables, and whole-grain cereals, but not in sugar. Fats come from animal and vegetable fats such as oils and butter, but many meats contain a high proportion of fats. Therefore, low-fat, high-carbohydrate diets are often vegetarian or modified vegetarian diets. Some dieters find these programs easy to follow because they allow a greater volume of food (carbohydrates are lower in calories per volume, so a person can eat more). However, for some dieters, the food choices are not their favorites, and the feeling of constantly being deprived of preferred foods often leads to "cheating" and failure. Nutritionally, high-carbohydrate diets are safe and effective programs for controlling weight.

Some diets are more extreme, restricting the dieter to a limited group of foods or even a single food.

All-fruit diets, egg diets, and even the pound cake diet fall into this category. Of course, such diets are nutritional disasters. They produce weight loss by restricting calories; dieters get tired of the monotony of one food and eat less than they would if they were eating a variety. "All the hard-boiled eggs you want" turns out to be not many!

Taking monotony a step further are the liquid diets, which exist in a variety of forms and under various brand names. Fifteen percent of women and 13% of men use this approach (Levy & Heaton, 1993). Liquid diets have the advantage of being nutritionally more balanced than most restricted food diets and are also convenient, requiring little or no preparation. For those who do not want a totally liquid diet, some manufacturers make equivalent-calorie meals in pudding or bar form. Still, all these meals have the disadvantage of being monotonous and repetitive, and they tend to be low in fiber. Some people find them convenient, and others find them boring. These diets, like all others, work by restricting calorie intake.

In conclusion, any diet must be viewed as a life-long eating pattern. Diets low in animal fats and high in fruits, vegetables, and whole grain cereals will generally produce weight loss and promote health. To be effective, however, any diet must be one that a person will be able to maintain throughout life.

Behavior Modification Programs

Although dieting should be seen as a permanent modification in one's eating habits, such a change is a difficult task. People who advocate a behavior modification approach to eating behaviors tend to treat eating problems directly rather than viewing overeating as a symptom of some other problem.

The behavior modification approach toward treating obesity was originated by Richard Stuart (1967), who reported a much higher success rate than with previous approaches. Most behavior modification programs use a broad assortment of techniques. Some of the early programs used aversive conditioning in which eating certain kinds of foods or eating at certain times was followed by punishment. This method has proven to be undesirable (American Medical Association Council on Scientific Affairs, 1987), not only because such procedures are unpleasant but also because the development of food aversions encourages not eating, an unhealthy practice that can lead to eating disorders. Today, most behavior modification programs focus on eating in a particular situation, at a particular time, and in association with particular feelings. Patients often keep eating diaries to focus their awareness on the types of foods they eat and under what circumstances as well as to provide data the therapist can use to devise a personal plan for changing unhealthy eating habits.

Early behavior modification programs tended to reinforce weight loss, but weight loss is not ensured by restricting food intake. Most contemporary programs reinforce good eating habits rather than the numbers of pounds lost. In other words, the behaviors, not the consequences, are rewarded.

Whereas Stuart's program was dramatically successful, not all behavior modification programs for weight control have been comparably effective. Wilson (1980) reviewed the outcome of many programs and concluded that the early enthusiasm may have been greater than warranted, but that behavior modification represents a treatment for mild and moderate obesity that is superior to other treatments. He concluded that most people in such programs lose a significant amount of weight, although individuals differ substantially.

White and White (1988) argued that two types of obesity exist: one with physiological causes and the other with behavioral and learned causes. They cautioned that behavior modification programs can affect weight by altering behavior and thus can be successful with some obese patients, but that not all obese people can be successful in any diet program.

Exercise

Although reducing caloric intake is the most common means of losing weight, increasing one's level of exercise is also effective. Often these two tactics are combined. In recent years, the role of exercise in weight loss has been increasingly emphasized (Tucker & Friedman, 1989). This emphasis is consistent with the observation that metabolic activity decreases when food intake is decreased.

Exercise is a feasible method of counteracting this slowdown and thus may be an indispensable part of weight-reduction programs. Indeed, exercise alone is sufficient to cause weight loss (Gwinup, 1975), and Blair (1993) argued that exercise can al-

ter fitness and the distribution of fat. (The role of exercise is more fully discussed in Chapter 16.)

In a survey of U.S. adults who were trying to lose weight, Levy and Heaton (1993) found that 71% of women and 64% of men reported that they were exercising as well as changing their diet in attempting to lose weight. The most frequent exercise choice was walking. The frequency of this choice suggests that people know the importance of exercise in a weight control program.

Drastic Methods of Losing Weight

People sometimes take drastic measures to lose weight, and physicians sometimes recommend drastic measures for severely obese patients. Even with medical supervision, some weight reduction programs present risks, sometimes to the point of being life threatening.

One approach that turned out to be more dangerous than initially believed was taking drugs to reduce appetite. In the 1950s and 1960s, diet pills were widely prescribed. These drugs were amphetamines, stimulant drugs that increase the activity of the nervous system, speed up metabolism, and suppress appetite. Unfortunately, these drugs lose their appetite-suppressing effect within a few weeks at a constant dose, so the dosage must be increased to maintain the effect. These diet pills can be effective for a short time, but for people who need to lose a considerable amount of weight and who therefore must continue taking amphetamines, dependence may become a more serious problem than obesity.

Increasing evidence of the dangers of amphetamines led to the development of other diet drugs. Most were chemically similar to amphetamines and shared their disadvantages, including the possibility of abuse. One of these alternatives, **fenfluramine**, is the preferred prescription diet drug today. However, the most commonly used diet drug is **phenylpropylalamine**, a nonprescription drug available in dozens of different diet preparations. This drug is generally safe, but when combined with caffeine, it can be dangerous for people with high blood pressure. Fourteen percent of women and 7% of men in the United States use some type of diet pills in their weight loss attempts (Levy & Heaton, 1993), and their legal availability makes over-the-counter diet drugs the frequent choice.

Fasting is another weight-loss measure that can be dangerous. Under conditions of food restriction, the body metabolizes fat and muscle tissue about equally, and some muscle tissue is present in essential organs. Thus, severe fasting can lead to the metabolism of internal organs. However, the *protein-sparing modified fast* averts this problem. In this type of program, patients eat high-protein food in very limited amounts. The protein-sparing modified fast spread in popularity in the form of the liquid-protein diet, which used a product high in protein but low in calories. A person on this type of diet would ingest only this preparation and no food. Although the regimen seemed safe under close medical supervision, a number of deaths were reported for people on liquid-protein diets without supervision. The title of the book advocating this approach, *The Last Chance Diet* (Linn, 1976), was more prophetic than the author had intended.

Other drastic measures to control obesity include several types of surgery. One procedure consists of wiring the person's jaws so that he or she is unable to chew. Caloric intake can thus be severely restricted, but such body functions as coughing can be very painful, and vomiting could be deadly. For good reason, this approach is rare.

Surgery has also been performed to remove part of the intestines, preventing food from being absorbed and cutting down on the calories metabolized (Kral, 1992). Because nutrients can no longer be fully absorbed, the person has permanent diarrhea and the potential for vitamin and mineral deficiency, but the procedure usually produces weight loss and is sometimes recommended for severely obese people who have medical conditions that are aggravated by obesity.

Surgical techniques that reduce the size of the stomach may either implant mesh that wraps around the stomach or staple part of the stomach. Both variations assume that not being able to fill the stomach will result in weight loss, and this has been true in some cases (Kral, 1992). In others, the obese people simply eat more frequently.

Another surgical approach to weight loss is to remove adipose tissue through a fat-suctioning technique called liposuction. People who undergo this procedure may gain the weight back, but the technique allows for a recontouring of the body rather than an overall weight loss. This procedure is not useful in controlling obesity (Kral, 1992); rather, it is a cosmetic procedure to change body shape. Despite the discomfort and expense of the surgery, liposuction has become the most common procedure in plastic surgery (Brownell & Rodin, 1994a).

Diets that severely restrict calories—that is, allow fewer than 1,000 calories per day—tend to be nutritional risks because of the small amount of food allowed. Most nutrition and diet experts recommend against very low-calorie diets, contending that the rapid weight loss they promote is less likely to be maintained than steady, slower weight loss. However, people often attempt such diets on their own and some supervised programs exist. Wadden, Stunkard, Brownell, and Day (1984) found that participants on a very low calorie diet, combined with behavior therapy, lost substantial weight during treatment and maintained the loss at least until a 1-year follow-up study. The women in this study were obese, and they followed a 400- to 500-calories-a-day diet. The behavior training consisted of monitoring the time and amount of eating, increased physical activity, high fees for the privilege of participating, small group therapy, nutrition instruction, relapse training, and other cognitive and behavioral strategies. One year after treatment, dieters had lost an average of 45 pounds and had regained less than 3 pounds, demonstrating that such programs can be effective in some circumstances.

The National Task Force on the Prevention and Treatment of Obesity (1993) reviewed research on very low calorie diets and concluded that such diets can be effective for some obese individuals. The task force found no advantage for programs that allowed fewer than 800 calories a day but saw little evidence of serious complications for individuals who had adequate medical supervision. However, the task force did find problems with maintenance of weight loss on such programs.

All these drastic means of losing weight can be dangerous. Although anyone can attempt a very low calorie diet or a fast without a physician's guidance, these programs are recommended only for those who are severely obese and whose obesity is an immediate health threat. For those who participate under such circumstances as well as for those who attempt a drastic diet on their own, keeping weight off is a major problem. Indeed, regardless of weight loss method, maintaining weight loss is a challenge.

Maintaining Weight Loss

The commonly quoted statistics are that 95% of people who lose weight on a diet will gain it back within 1 to 5 years. Brownell and Rodin (1994a) pointed out that these discouraging figures are based on research conducted on patients in a hospital nutrition clinic over 30 years ago and may not apply to contemporary programs or to all groups of dieters. Many of the studies during the past 30 years have confirmed the difficulty of maintaining weight loss (NIH Technology Assessment Conference Panel, 1993; Stunkard & Penick, 1979), but most of this information has come from highly selected dieters, including those who are extremely obese and those who seek professional help in losing weight. For these people, weight control should probably be treated as a chronic illness, with continued professional assistance in maintaining weight loss (Wing, 1992). The information on the long-term effectiveness of people dieting on their own is very sparse (Tinker & Tucker, 1994), yet this is the approach that most people use.

The likelihood of maintaining weight loss is generally higher for behavior therapy programs than for most diets that emphasize rapid loss and ignore eating patterns and activity level. This advantage is predictable because behavior modification programs are most effective with patients who require moderate rather than severe weight loss. Even in moderate and gradual weight reduction programs, relapse remains a problem. For this reason, Wilson (1980) recommended that weight-control programs add posttreatment sessions to help the client maintain altered eating patterns.

A study by Perri et al. (1988) indicated that Wilson's suggestions are sound. Perri et al. found that several types of posttreatment programs were effective in helping dieters maintain lost weight. The effective programs included social support, aerobic exercise, and continued contact with the therapist. Eighteen months after finishing the diet phase of the program, dieters who participated in the posttreatment programs had regained only 17% of their lost weight. Dieters who participated in only the diet phase of the program regained 67% of the weight they had lost. This study demonstrated that weight loss can be maintained and that several posttreatment techniques can help dieters keep off most of their lost weight.

The social environment may be a factor in maintaining weight loss. Tinker and Tucker (1994) studied formerly obese people who had maintained their weight loss for at least a year (and for a mean of 4.5 years). They found several factors that distinguished them from a group that remained obese. Those who had lost weight and maintained a normal weight had experienced fewer intimate relationships and more negative social events prior to losing weight, but during and after weight loss some aspects of their lives got better. They experienced an increase in positive relationships and social events, which may have reinforced their efforts to lose weight. Thus, successful weight loss seems to be enhanced by an environment that rewards these efforts.

People's motivation for dieting may also play a role in maintaining weight loss. Geoffrey Williams and his colleagues (Williams, Grow, Freedman, Ryan, & Deci, 1996) tested people who had participated in a very low-calorie diet, following their success for almost 2 years. These researchers found that the motivation to go on the diet was a significant predictor of success, not only in losing weight but also in maintaining weight loss. Those dieters who were more autonomous in their reasons for dieting were the more successful. Therefore, dieting may be more successful when it is a personal choice rather than a response to pressure from family, friends, or physicians.

In contrast to the difficulty that adults have in keeping off lost weight, obese children who lose weight are more likely to maintain that loss. Leonard Epstein and his colleagues (Epstein, Valoski, Wing, & McCurley, 1994; Epstein & Wing, 1987) conducted a program for obese children, and a 10-year follow-up (Epstein et al., 1994) demonstrated that 34% of the children decreased the degree of obesity, and 30% were no longer obese. Their program was more effective when parents and children were both involved and rewarded for weight loss and when children became involved in a more active lifestyle.

Therefore, weight maintenance is a problem for those who have lost weight, but keeping weight off may not be the problem that the often-quoted pessimistic statistics suggest. Behavior modification programs are generally more successful than other types of programs, and people whose lives change in positive ways after weight loss may be motivated to maintain their weight loss. In addition, behavior modification programs with obese children have greater success in promoting permanent weight loss than similar programs with adults.

DOES DIETING WORK?

A number of authorities in the weight control field have questioned the feasibility of dieting as a method of weight control. Those who adhere to the setpoint model (Bennett & Gurin, 1982; Polivy & Herman, 1983) believe that deviations from setpoint are extremely difficult to maintain. Those who believe that dieters suffer in their attempts to attain the unattainable body (Wooley & Garner, 1991) argue that the misery of dieting (and of failure to maintain weight loss) is not worth the effort. None of these authorities contend that people cannot lose weight, but they argue that dieters often fail to meet their weight-loss goals and that dieting is not worth the psychological and physical strain.

In addition, dieting promotes lowering of the metabolic rate, a complication that prompted Brownell and Stein (1989) to hypothesize that "dieting may make dieting more difficult" (p. 50). Brownell and Stein investigated the possibility that the metabolic slowdown persists after people discontinue their diet, thus setting the stage for a rapid weight gain. Brownell and Rodin (1994b) later amended this position, claiming that subsequent research has failed to support this contention. Although weight loss may make gain easier and subsequent loss more difficult in some people, it does not occur in all dieters.

In 1982, Stanley Schachter took a different approach to studying the question of whether dieting works. His answer was yes—at least for a substantial proportion of people. Schachter contended that his answer was different from that of most investigators because he approached the problem differently.

By studying people who had never sought formal assistance in losing weight, Schachter examined the success rate for a group of people who typically do not participate in studies on weight loss. A total of 63% of those who had dieted had attained or come within 10% of their ideal weight. An additional 10% of the obese had lost substantial weight but were still more than 10% above ideal weight. These successful dieters also did a better job than therapy participants in keeping the weight off, maintaining their loss for over 7 years.

Few studies have taken Schachter's approach. Of those that have (Orme & Binik, 1987; Rzewnicki & Forgays, 1987), some have found that the overweight people they questioned were less likely to be successful than those in Schachter's study. Other researchers (Tinker & Tucker, 1994) have found that some obese people manage to diet to normal weight on their own and to maintain that normal weight. Schachter's report of successful weight loss and maintenance may have been overly optimistic in terms of the percentage of success, but it is possible.

In some cases, dieting can result in weight loss, but dieting can also result in failure, poor nutrition, and relapse. Behavior modification programs that include posttreatment sessions are the most effective of the clinic programs for weight loss, but programs in which people attempt to lose on their own are possibly even more effective. Despite some successes, losing weight and keeping it off through changes in eating and exercise habits are difficult lifestyle changes, and they raise questions concerning the wisdom of dieting.

IS DIETING A GOOD CHOICE?

Dieters often behave like starving people: They are irritable, obsessed with food, finicky about taste, easily distractible, and hungry. Polivy and Herman (1983) argued that these behavioral abnormalities make dieting foolish, especially for dieters who are close to the best weight for their health. Brownell and Rodin (1994a) contended that dieters should be divided into two groups: those who are obese and those who are normal weight. Dieting may be a good choice for those who are sufficiently overweight to endanger their health. For those who are normal weight or even underweight, dieting is not a wise choice.

Polivy and Herman's 1983 book, *Breaking the Diet Habit,* included a number of suggestions for reestablishing what they consider to be reasonable eating habits, especially for those who are dieting for cosmetic rather than health reasons. Their main suggestions were to eat to satisfy hunger and to be comfortable with setpoint weight. They called their program the "undiet" because it is not oriented toward losing weight and does not restrict calories or types of food. Polivy and Herman concede that some chronic dieters would be heavier without constant dieting, but they claim that many others would actually be thinner if they were to stop cyclic dieting.

Ironically, weight loss may be a health risk for some people. Several studies have explored the mortality risks of weight loss. Williamson and Pamuk (1993) analyzed mortality and death rates and found an increased risk for those who lost weight. Even with previous illness factored out (Pamuk, Williamson, Serdula, Madans, & Byers, 1993), weight loss was a risk. The pattern with the lowest mortality risk was one of modest weight gain during adulthood (Andres, Muller, & Sorkin, 1993). The risk associated with weight loss may be the result of involuntary weight loss, which is a mortality risk (Meltzer & Everhart, 1995). On the other hand, some people who lose weight voluntarily benefit from their weight loss. Overweight European American women who had obesity-related illnesses decreased their mortality risk by losing weight, especially if they lost 20 pounds or more (Williamson et al., 1995), but thin women who lose weight tend to increase their risk for cardiovascular disease (Harris, Ballard-Barbasch, Madans, Makuc, & Feldman, 1993).

Do these studies mean that people should not diet, or that some people should not diet? What about the risks associated with obesity? The studies on dieting suggest that dieting may not be a good choice for many people. Those who are obese may be at heightened risk due to their weight, but losing weight may not lower their risk unless they can lose to the normal range and maintain that normal weight. Most authorities (Harris et al., 1993; Pamuk et al., 1992) now agree that people who lose and

gain weight have a higher risk for mortality than those who are slightly obese but who maintain a stable weight. Thus, weight maintenance, especially for people who are not severely obese, is a healthier pattern than weight fluctuation.

EATING DISORDERS

Both Brownell (1991, 1993) and Rodin (1992) have contended that society has come to accept the belief that people have complete control over their bodies — that by diet, exercise, or a combination of the two, people can completely control their body size and shape. Both believe that this degree of control is overstated and that people do not have complete control over body weight or shape. Both the quest for the perfect body and the belief that one can exert control over the body contribute to the development of eating problems such as anorexia and bulimia.

The term *anorexia nervosa* literally means lack of appetite due to a nervous or physiological condition; *bulimia* means continuous, morbid hunger. Neither meaning, however, is quite accurate. The patterns of eating behavior to which these labels apply are only marginally related to the literal meaning of the two terms. People with anorexia nervosa have not lost their appetite. Ordinarily, they are perpetually hungry, but they insist that they do not wish to eat. Like Elise, these people become preoccupied with losing weight, and their self-induced starvation often results in a life-threatening condition. Similarly, bulimia has come to mean more than continuous morbid hunger. The chief identifying mark of this eating disorder is repeated bingeing and purging. The bingeing involves eating huge quantities of food, usually high in calories and loaded with carbohydrates, fat, or both. The purging ordinarily takes the form of vomiting, but fasting and using laxatives and diuretics are also frequently part of the purging process.

These two eating disorders obviously have much in common, and Elise experienced symptoms of both. In fact, many authorities regard them as two dimensions of the same illness. Others see them as two separate but related illnesses. We regard neither of them as an illness; they are both unhealthy eating patterns that, along with overeating, may eventually produce physical illness. Although a person may show symptoms of both, in this section we discuss anorexia nervosa and bulimia separately, as each has a somewhat different set of behaviors and each produces its own complex of physiological disorders.

ANOREXIA NERVOSA

Anorexia nervosa is an eating disorder characterized by intentional self-starvation or semistarvation, sometimes to the point of death. Despite recent publicity on anorexia, neither the disorder nor the term is new. According to Sours (1980), the first two authentic, documented cases of intentional self-starvation were reported by Richard Morton in 1689. Morton wrote about an 18-year-old English girl who had died of the effects of anorexia some 25 years earlier and about an 18-year-old boy who had survived. Both had shown a remarkable indifference to starvation, and both had been described as sad and anxious. Over the next 2 centuries several other cases were reported, but often these were not clearly distinguished from tuberculosis or consumption.

In London, Sir William Gull (1874) studied several cases of intentional self-starvation during the 1860s. He regarded the condition as a psychological disorder and coined the term *anorexia nervosa* to indicate loss of appetite due to "nervous" causes — that is, psychological factors. From that time until about 1910, Gull's psychopathological conception pervaded the psychological and psychiatric literature. From about 1910 until the late 1930s, some medical authorities tried to link anorexia nervosa with atrophy of the anterior lobe of the pituitary gland, but this medical view soon lost favor.

During the 1940s and 1950s, speculation proliferated concerning the causes and cures of anorexia nervosa. Some psychiatrists hypothesized that the ailment was a denial of femininity and a fear of motherhood. Other theorists suggested that it represented an attempt on the part of the young woman to reestablish unity with her mother. Unfortunately, none of these hypotheses proved fruitful in expanding the scientific understanding of anorexia nervosa. The last 2 decades have seen a shift away from this sort of speculation and a turn toward the view that anorexia is a learned syndrome of behavior (Darby, Garfinkel, Garner, & Coscina, 1983). Recent emphasis has been on describing the disorder in terms of the concomitant behaviors and physiological effects, the demographic correlates, and the effective treatment procedures.

Description

This chapter opened with a description of Elise, a high school student who showed symptoms of anorexia. Although Elise was never diagnosed as anorexic, her behavior and cognitions fit the pattern of anorexia nervosa with purging behaviors. The description that follows is a composite model of hundreds of cases of anorexia nervosa, and probably no one individual fits the model in every respect.

First, anorexics are most likely to be female, young, White, outwardly compliant, and high achievers in school. They are preoccupied with food, usually like to cook for others (Elise didn't), insist that others eat their food, but eat almost nothing themselves. They lose from 15% to 50% of their body weight yet continue to see themselves as overweight. Like Elise, they are ambitious, perfectionistic, and come from high-achieving families. Their preoccupation with body fat usually leads to a strenuous program of exercise — dancing, jogging, calisthenics, or playing tennis. Excessively active and energetic behavior continues until their weight loss reaches a level that produces fatigue and weakness, making further activity impossible.

Whether the characteristics connected with anorexia precede the weight loss or are a consequence of starvation is sometimes a difficult question. For example, anorexic women often display some hostility toward their mothers. But many anorexics exhibit an increase in hostility before their excessive dieting, whereas for others the mother-daughter friction seems to revolve around the daughter's lack of concern over weight loss that the mother considers alarming. Elise and her mother had never gotten along very well, and their relationship became even more tense when Elise began to diet and became alarmingly thin.

Mothers' concern with weight and their daughters' attractiveness may be factors in the development of eating disorders. By comparing a group of adolescent girls with others who did not have eating disorders, Pike and Rodin (1991) found that the girls with eating disorders had mothers who had more eating problems themselves, believed that their daughters were less attractive, and believed that their daughters should lose weight. Not only were these mothers poor models for good eating habits, but their concerns may have influenced their daughters in the development of eating problems.

A second characteristic that may either precede or follow dieting is *amenorrhea,* cessation of the menses. Because the attainment of a given percentage of body fat is necessary for menstruation, postpubescent women develop amenorrhea if they lose enough weight. However, as Neuman and Halvorson (1983) pointed out, cessation of the menstrual cycle often precedes dieting. This somewhat puzzling finding reinforces the view that simple explanations of anorexia nervosa are inadequate and that complex factors are related to both the causes and the course of the disorder.

After substantial weight loss has occurred, individual differences tend to disappear, and accounts of the disorder itself are remarkably similar. Interestingly, most of the descriptions are also consistent with the sketch of starving conscientious objectors drawn by Keys et al. (1950). Thus, these conditions are probably an effect of starvation and not its cause. As weight loss becomes more than 25% of one's previous "normal" weight, the person loses interest in sex, constantly feels chilled, grows a soft, downy covering of body hair, loses scalp hair, and develops an unusual preoccupation with food. As starvation nears a perilous level, the anorexic becomes more hostile toward those who are seen as trying to reverse the weight loss.

Many authorities, including Hilde Bruch (1973, 1978, 1982), regard anorexia nervosa as a means of gaining control. Bruch, who spent more than 40 years studying eating disorders and the effects of starvation, reported that prior to dieting, anorexics typically are troubled girls who feel incapable of changing their lives. These young women often see their parents as overdemanding and in absolute control of their life, yet they remain too compliant to rebel openly. They try to seize control of their life in the most personal manner possible: by changing the

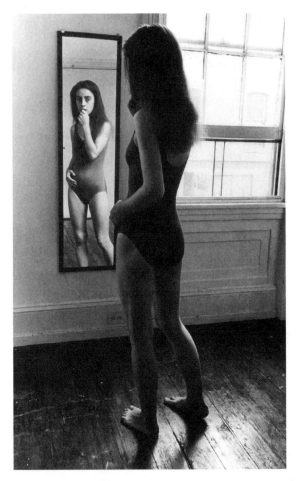

No matter how thin they get, anorexics continue to see themselves as too fat.

shape of their body. Short of force-feeding, no one can stop these young women from controlling their own body size and shape. They take great pleasure and pride in doing something that is difficult and often compare their superior willpower with that of others who are overweight or who shun exercise. Bruch (1978) stated that anorexics enjoy being hungry and eventually regard any food in the stomach as dirty or damaging.

Becky Thompson (1994) has taken a somewhat different view, holding that women often use eating as a way to cope with problems in their lives. Thompson proposed that explaining anorexia as an extension of fashion-consciousness is demeaning to women, trivializing the problems that prompt eating disorders. In interviewing and treating a variety of women from many ethnic backgrounds, Thompson concluded that physical, psychological, and sexual assaults on women are among the contributing factors to eating problems.

Demographic Correlates

Who are the people most likely to starve themselves intentionally to the point of seriously impairing their health? First, some subtle shifts in the population at risk seem to have taken place. During the early 1970s, anorexia nervosa was most common in the upper and upper-middle social classes, but then its prevalence increased among middle- and lower-class women. Garfinkel and Garner (1982), for example, noted that from 1970 to 1975, only 29% of anorexics came from the middle and lower classes but between 1976 and 1981 that number increased to 48%.

During the late 1980s and early 1990s, pursuit of thinness became more evenly distributed throughout the social classes. Whitaker et al. (1989) reported that social class was no longer a reliable predictor of anorexia and Dolan's (1991) cross-cultural review concluded that anorexia develops in all social classes and in both Western and non-Western cultures.

Anorexia nervosa, then, is no longer confined to upper-middle-class and upper-class White women in North America and Europe. Does this mean that its incidence is on the increase? Almost all clinicians and researchers working in this area are of the impression that anorexia nervosa has become more common in the United States than it was 35 years ago. However, evidence on this question is still somewhat scarce. Hsu (1990) reviewed seven studies that attempted to trace the increase of anorexia nervosa, but varying definitions of the disorder have complicated the conclusions.

Among the general population, anorexia nervosa is still a very rare disorder. Hoek (1993) estimated that anorexia appears at a rate of about 8 for every 100,000 people per year. However, among some populations the incidence rates are much higher, and the rates have increased over the past 50 years (Lucas, Beard, O'Fallon, & Kurland, 1991). Young women between the ages of 15 and 19 are at ele-

vated risk (Hsu, 1990; Lucas et al., 1991), and young women who attend private or professional schools such as ballet or modeling academies are at especially high risk. Crisp, Palmer, and Kalucy (1976) found about 0.2% of public school girls in England to be anorexic, but girls in private schools in England had a rate that was five times higher, or about 1%. Garner and Garfinkel (1980) reported that 6.5% of dance students and 7% of modeling students met the diagnostic criteria for anorexia nervosa, and the majority of them had developed the disorder in the competitive, weight-conscious atmosphere of their professional schooling. Athletic competition is also a risk for anorexia, and athletes with eating disorders can be found in programs for all sports, even those that do not emphasize appearance or an overly thin body (Thompson & Sherman, 1993). In addition, Beglin and Fairburn (1992) contended that women who decline to participate in studies about eating disorders are more likely to have such disorders, and their absence lowers the frequency estimates below the actual number. Analyzing a number of studies that used different methodologies, Hsu (1990) concluded that the prevalence of anorexia nervosa in all women in the United States and Western Europe is between 0.7% and 2.1%.

Attitudes about eating underlie the increased incidence of anorexia. Huon, Brown, and Morris (1988) surveyed young people concerning their attitudes and beliefs about abnormal eating patterns and found that these young men and women knew about anorexia but did not view the pursuit of slimness as either very abnormal or very uncommon. This study may offer the strongest evidence that anorexia has become more common: The pathological pursuit of thinness is no longer regarded as disturbingly abnormal.

Over the years anorexics have tended overwhelmingly to be women, and research and treatment have focused on women. Garfinkel and Garner (1982) and others have consistently reported that men make up about 5% to 10% of all anorexics. This estimate — that 90% to 95% of all anorexics are women — has remained constant over a period of years, but it is based mostly on clinical impressions and incomplete empirical data.

Crisp and Burns (1990) contrasted male and female anorexics and found few significant differences in social class and family configuration, symptoms, treatment, and prognosis as well as in the behaviors and personality characteristics before the onset of anorexia. Woodside, Garner, Rockert, and Garfinkel (1990) also found few differences between men and women with eating problems, but they found that the men were less likely than women to receive a diagnosis. Both sets of researchers found that gay men were slightly overrepresented among the anorexics in their studies, but they speculated that sexual orientation is probably not an important factor in anorexia among men.

Treatment

Anorexia nervosa remains one of the most difficult behavior disorders to treat because most anorexics see nothing wrong with their eating behavior, resent suggestions that they are too thin, and resist any attempt to change their eating. Because of these attitudes, parents and friends have great difficulty motivating anorexics to seek treatment. Threats, pleas, and criticisms are likely to have a negative effect (Szmukler, Eisler, Russell, & Dare, 1985). Short of force, family and friends have few options. The one aspect of the environment that anorexics can control is their own body. As long as they refuse to eat, their control remains sovereign.

As starvation continues, anorexics eventually reach the point of fatigue, exhaustion, and possible physical collapse. At that point some sort of treatment is usually forced on them. Elise's parents forced her into treatment when her roommate reported that she was unconscious in her dorm room. Although she was not dangerously thin, her laxative abuse may have put her into immediate physical danger. Elise is still unhappy with their decision. She feels that she was an "unsuccessful anorexic" who did not reach her unrealistic weight goal. Despite her knowledge that this attitude is unhealthy, she believes that if she had been allowed to diet to below 100 pounds, she would have been "better." This continued pathological attitude reflects the distorted thinking that is typical of anorexia, an attitude that is difficult to combat.

The immediate aim of almost any treatment program for anorexia is medical stabilization of any danger due to physical symptoms of starvation (Goldner & Birmingham, 1994). Then, anorexics need to work toward restoration of normal weight, healthy eating, and good body image. Recommendations concerning the methods of achieving these goals are not universally accepted. Some believe that hospitalization is required, especially for medical stabilization and restoration of weight, but others have found little evidence to support the need for inpatient treatment (Browning & Miller, 1968; Hsu, 1990; Palazzoli, 1974). Weight restoration is an important step in the treatment of anorexia, but anorexics resist attempts to get them to eat. Tube feeding and intravenous feeding can provide methods of forcing nutrient intake, but Hsu (1990) noted that force-feeding may be undesirable because it deprives the patient of control and may impede the growth of a trusting relationship between therapist and patient.

Weight restoration is a step in therapy but is not a cure for anorexia nervosa, and anorexics need to change their body image as well as their eating habits. As Goldner and Birmingham (1994, p. 139) put it:

> In order to recover, anorexic individuals will have to confront those things they fear most and will have to surrender the feelings of accomplishment gained by weight control. A therapeutic alliance is needed to catalyze and nurture the anorexic individual's motivation for recovery.

Bruch (1978) recommended that both family therapy and individual therapy should accompany weight-gain programs, and subsequent recommendations are consistent with those of Bruch (Bloom, Kogel, & Zaphiropoulos, 1994; Goldner & Birmingham, 1994). These recommendations for family therapy seem sound because both psychopathology (Kog & Vandereycken, 1985) and sexual abuse (Hall, Tice, Beresford, Wooley, & Hall, 1989; Thompson, 1994) are common in family experience of anorexics. For these reasons, most treatment programs are designed to change the anorexic's social environment, her attitude toward herself, and her distorted view of her body. In the past, these goals have been sought through the use of psychoanalysis (Wilson, 1983), drug therapy (Halmi, 1982; White & Schnaulty,

1977), family therapy (Minuchin, Rosman, & Baker, 1978), nutritional counseling, and a variety of other procedures.

Behavior modification has also been used to promote weight gain (Hsu, 1990), but this procedure is not often oriented toward changing the maladaptive cognitions that accompany anorexia. Since the mid-1970s, cognitive behavior therapy has become increasingly popular as a treatment for anorexia nervosa, and it has shown some success in both changing eating behavior and changing cognitions. Practitioners of behavior therapy have recognized that the pleasure and gratification derived from the effects of self-starvation act as potent reinforcers for anorexic eating habits (Garner, Garfinkel, & Bemis, 1982). They have attempted to change anorexics' faulty thinking patterns and their erroneous beliefs, which extend beyond matters of weight and body image. Cognitive behavior therapists attack these irrational beliefs while maintaining a warm and accepting attitude toward patients. Anorexics are taught to discard the absolutist, all-or-none thinking pattern expressed in such self-statements as "If I gain one pound, I'll go on to gain a hundred." Patients are also encouraged to stop centering all attention on themselves and to realize that others do not have the same high standards for their behavior that they do. Finally, therapists need to point out the errors in superstitious food beliefs such as "Any sweet is instantly converted into fat" or "Laxatives prevent the absorption of calories" (Thompson & Sherman, 1993). When patients understand the superstitious nature of these beliefs, they can become more realistic about the effects of food on body composition.

In general, cognitive behavior therapy has been more successful with anorexia nervosa than psychoanalytic approaches. Indeed, therapists who use a psychoanalytic framework need to be careful to avoid the sexist bias that often accompanies this approach (Bloom, Kogel, & Zaphiropoulos, 1994). However, no treatment offers a high rate of success. A number of studies (Eckert, 1983; Eckert, Goldberg, Halmi, Casper, & Davis, 1979; Garfinkel, Moldofsky, & Garner, 1977) have found some long-term benefits of cognitive behavior therapy, especially when benefit is defined in terms of weight gain.

Relapse always remains a possibility. Some patients gain weight while hospitalized but have no intention of retaining it subsequent to release. As Hsu (1990) pointed out, anorexics who have attained normal weight may not have attained normal attitudes toward food and eating. Many hospitalized patients gained weight because they knew that doing so was a prerequisite for hospital discharge (Agras & Werne, 1977). Pertschuk (1977) found that although 25 of 29 patients gained weight while in the hospital, only 2 of the 27 participants contacted after release were eating normally, maintaining near-normal weight, and functioning well. Twelve of the patients had required rehospitalization: four for attempted suicide, two for depression, and six for weight loss. In addition, 10 of these patients did what Elise did: they developed bulimia.

Several reviews (Goldner & Birmingham, 1994; Hsu, 1990; Schwartz & Thompson, 1981) have indicated that Pertschuk's findings were representative. In addition, a review of the outcomes for male and female anorexics showed a striking degree of similarity (Burns & Crisp, 1990). These reviews have found that anorexics often gain enough weight during treatment to be in the normal weight range, but about 50% relapse or develop other psychological or eating-related problems. About 20% remain underweight despite extensive treatment. In addition, about 5% of anorexics die. Those anorexics whose eating disorders have persisted for 4 years or longer have a poor prospect of recovery, and death becomes a more likely outcome.

After being hospitalized, Elise formed a therapeutic relationship with her psychiatrist. She began a weight-restoration program but has never given up her ideal, overly thin body image. Although her weight is normal, she continues to see herself as fat. Consistent with Bruch's predictions, she experienced symptoms of depression both before and after she developed eating problems, and her psychiatrist has recently prescribed antidepressant drugs for her.

It is difficult to separate the effects of anorexia from those of bulimia in Elise. Like anorexics, she stopped having menstrual periods, and she worries about permanent effects on her fertility. In fact, her concerns about not being able to ever have children were important in convincing her to start eating.

She has suffered severe and possibly permanent damage to her intestinal tract due to her laxative abuse, but this effect is related to her bulimia.

BULIMIA

Bulimia is often regarded as a companion disorder to anorexia nervosa. Like anorexia, bulimia affects mostly women and often centers around maladaptive attempts at weight control. Unlike anorexics, who rely mostly on strict fasts to lose more and more weight, bulimics binge, eating huge quantities of food in an uncontrolled manner. As defined by the fourth edition of the *Diagnostic and Statistical Manual of Mental Disorders (DSM-IV)* of the American Psychiatric Association (APA, 1994), bulimia nervosa involves recurrent episodes of binge eating, a sense of lack of control over eating, and inappropriate, drastic measures to compensate for the binge. Some bulimics fast or exercise excessively, but most use self-induced vomiting to maintain a relatively normal weight.

Binge eating may occur without any attempts to purge, but this pattern does not meet the criteria for bulimia. Although the DSM-IV includes a category for binge-eating disorder, it places it in an appendix as needing further study rather than including it as one of the eating disorders.

The seemingly bizarre practice of binge eating followed by purging is not new. The ancient Romans sometimes indulged in very similar eating rituals. Friedländer (1968) reported that, after the Romans had feasted on great quantities of rich food, they would retire to the vomitorium, empty their stomachs, and then return to eat some more. The ancient Romans were neither the first nor the last to binge and purge, but theirs was perhaps the only society to have elevated this practice to such a refined state. Today, millions of women (and a smaller number of men) continue this custom of bingeing and purging as a means of controlling weight.

Description

In many ways, Elise is not typical of people with bulimia, but in other ways she is. Like most other bulimics, she began purging as part of a diet. The common pattern for bulimia involves binge eating compensated by fasting, with this pattern developing into one of vomiting or laxative abuse or both as

methods of purging. Unlike most bulimics, Elise's binges were never a central part of her eating problem, but her purging behavior was. Like most bulimics, Elise felt guilty about her bingeing and purging and after several years, managed to end this cycle.

Guilt and depression are frequent correlates of bulimia. Depression, in fact, is so common that some authorities question whether it is a cause or an effect of bulimia. Pope and Hudson (1984) reported that half the bulimic women they studied had been depressed for a year or more prior to the onset of bulimia. Lingswiler, Crowther, and Stephens (1987) found that binge eaters experienced greater fluctuations of anxiety and depression than people who did not binge. These findings suggest that at least for some cases, negative affect may instigate bulimia. In any event, the majority of bulimics also suffer from depression.

Perhaps as a result of depression, a substantial number of bulimics have attempted suicide. Two studies (Garfinkel & Garner, 1984; Pope & Hudson, 1984) found that between 20% and 33% of bulimics in treatment had made at least one serious suicide attempt. Because many suicide attempts are not successful, one might guess that bulimic women are not deadly serious. However, bulimia remains a largely hidden disorder, and the possibility exists that many young women who kill themselves were secretly suffering from bulimia.

Lehman and Rodin (1989) investigated disordered eating patterns and found that bulimics derive a greater percentage of their self-nurturance from food than from any other source. However, while treating themselves with food, bulimics frequently criticize themselves harshly. In addition, they tend to react more strongly to negative events and to experience sustained negative reactions that interfere with effective coping. Lehman and Rodin's study painted a picture of bulimics as people who use food for comfort. Because bulimics experience many negative feelings and have difficulty in coping with the negative experiences in their lives, their need for comfort is great.

Elise felt a lot of stress in her life when she started purging, and her life centered around controlling her eating. When she ate more than she thought she should (and her criteria were very strict), she would vomit or take laxatives. Indeed, she often took laxatives in anticipation of eating and feared her stomach being full for long. Unlike most bulimics, Elise did not plan eating sprees in advance or collect special types of food for her binges. Also unlike most bulimics, she was not completely secretive about vomiting or laxative abuse.

A history of alcohol or drug abuse is common to bulimics. Garfinkel and Garner (1982) found that 18% of their bulimic patients used alcohol on a regular basis. Cauwells (1983) estimated that as many as 40% of all bulimics abuse alcohol. Pope and Hudson (1984) reported that at least half the people suffering from bulimia are problem drinkers; Killen et al. (1987) found that binge eaters have higher rates of drunkenness, marijuana use, and cigarette use than the population at large, and Holderness, Brooks-Gunn, and Warren (1994) found that bulimics were more likely than anorexics to show substance abuse problems. These studies indicate that alcohol abuse — and possibly other drug abuse — is higher among bulimics than among the general population. Like many college students, Elise's alcohol use was not always wise, but her drinking never got her into serious trouble, and she did not use alcohol or drugs (except laxatives) regularly.

The high incidence of alcohol and other psychoactive substance abuse among bulimics has led some researchers to wonder whether they might be describing an "addictive personality," one that simply has problems with impulse control in a variety of situations (Cauwells, 1983; Pope & Hudson, 1984). In reviewing research on this model, Wilson (1993) confirmed that people with alcohol and cocaine abuse are significantly more likely to binge eat, but this association, contended Wilson, does not mean that binge eating fits into the framework of an addictive disorder.

Impulsivity may be a common factor in binge eating and substance abuse. In a related vein, many bulimic women are **kleptomaniacs,** compulsively stealing items that they neither need nor intend to use. Garfinkel and Garner (1984) found that 1 bulimic in 6 had engaged in stealing, whereas less than 1 in 100 anorexics had stolen. Pyle, Mitchell, and Eckert (1981) found that two-thirds of the bulimics had engaged in stealing behaviors. Most of these patients stole food and laxatives, but several took such items as alcohol, clothing, cosmetics, and jewelry. In other words, although bulimia is an expensive habit and some bulimics steal to obtain food, a disproportionate number seem to take items that have no relationship to food or to their bingeing.

In summary, the disorders of anorexia and bulimia are both characterized by a preoccupation with body weight and a pathological concern with the maintenance of desired body shape. However, bulimics and anorexics differ in their relationship with food. Also, bulimia is a more common disorder than anorexia.

Demographic Correlates

In at least one way the population of bulimics is nearly identical to that of anorexics: Both eating disorders appear far more often in women than in men. Cauwells (1983) estimated that about 90% to 95% of all bulimics are women, a percentage nearly identical to that estimated for anorexics.

In other ways, however, the two populations differ. Although anorexia nervosa is spreading to all social classes and ethnic groups, upper-middle- and upper-class Whites are still overrepresented. Bulimia, however, is a more democratic disorder. Its prevalence seems to be about equally spread throughout the various social classes, although firm evidence for this assumption is still lacking.

How prevalent is bulimia? Is its incidence increasing or decreasing? Answers to these questions are difficult because the definition of bulimia has changed over the last three editions of the APA's *Diagnostic and Statistical Manual of Mental Disorders* (DSM). The 1980 edition of the DSM (DSM-III) failed to include purging as an essential feature of bulimia, yielding high estimates of its frequency based only on the criterion of bingeing. Two surveys of college students (Halmi, Falk, & Schwartz, 1981; Pyle et al., 1983) found that between 8% and 13% of women met the DSM-III criteria for bulimia and that 1.4% of the men were bulimic. Surveying shopping mall patrons yielded an estimate of 10.3% of women with binge eating and a fear of loss of control over eating (Pope, Hudson, & Yurgelun-Todd, 1984).

Although bingeing may be fairly common, bulimia is not widespread according to the definitions in DSM III-R (1987) and DSM-IV (1994). These stricter definitions, which include fasting, excessive exercising, or purging as methods of compensating for bingeing, have generally led to decreased estimates of the prevalence of the disorder. Schotte and Stunkard (1987) found that only 1.3% of the women and 0.1% of the men in a large university in the eastern United States were bulimic. Hoek (1993) estimated that the incidence of bulimia is 11.4 per 100,000 people per year, with 1% of young women exhibiting symptoms of this disorder. Drewnowski, Hopkins, and Kessler (1988) looked at a national sample of college students and found a similar estimate for young women—1%. They estimated that 0.2% of the men were bulimic. However, in a survey of 10th-grade girls, Killen et al. (1987) found that 10.3% met the criteria for bulimia and an additional 10.4% reported using purging as a means of weight control.

Table 15.5 indicates the widely different rates of bulimia that different investigators have found. These differences are not entirely attributable to the differences in definition but do relate to the population studied. For example, Fairburn, Hay, and Welch

(1993) noted several studies that have found not only higher rates of bulimia in younger women but also higher lifetime occurrence. That is, women born after 1960 are at higher risk to have ever been bulimic than women born before 1950, indicating that the prevalence of bulimia is increasing. Fairburn et al. estimated that between 0.5% and 1.0% of young adult women are bulimic, but they acknowledged that these figures may be underestimates.

Most of the studies on bulimia have concentrated on college student populations, which have a high prevalence of bulimia, and some evidence exists that bulimia may be "contagious." Boskind-White and White (1983) contended that as recently as the late 1970s, most bulimics were unaware that their eating practices were shared by others, but Crandall (1988) studied the women in two sororities for evidence of contagion and bulimia. The results indicated that the prevalence of binge eating changed over the academic year in accordance with the social norms of the two sororities. Crandall concluded that

Table 15.5   Prevalence of bulimia nervosa

Study	Sample	DSM-III criteria	Weekly purging and bingeing
Pyle et al. (1983)	575 first-year college women	7.8%	4.5%
Pyle et al. (1983)	780 first-year college men	1.4%	0.4%
Halmi et al. (1981)	355 male and female summer school students	13.0%	—
Pope & Hudson (1984)	287 female students (women's college)	12.6%	10.0%
Pope & Hudson (1984)	102 female students (coeducational university)	18.6%	12.9%
Pope & Hudson (1984)	47 male students (coeducational university)	0.0%	0.0%
Pope et al. (1984)	300 suburban shopping mall women (ages 12–65+)	10.3%	3.0%
Pope et al. (1984)	suburban shopping mall women (ages 13–20)	17.7%	5.1%
Killen et al. (1987)	646 10th-grade girls	10.3%	0.02%
Schotte & Stunkard (1987)	994 women at private university	—	1.3%
Schotte & Stunkard (1987)	942 men at private university	—	0.1%
Drewnowski et al. (1988)	1,007 male and female students	—	0.2% 1.0%
Hoek (1994)	women 15–24 years old	1%	

binge eating is an acquired behavior under the control of modeling and social influence.

Is Bulimia Harmful?

To many people, bingeing and purging may seem to be an acceptable means of controlling weight. To others, comfort derived from eating is important to their coping with stress and anxiety, making bingeing and purging a pattern they cannot relinquish (Rodin, 1992; Thompson, 1994). Although guilt is a nearly inevitable part of bulimia, the question remains: Is bulimia harmful to health? Unlike anorexia nervosa, which has a mortality rate of 2% to 15% (Sours, 1980), bulimia is very seldom fatal. Nevertheless, there are serious detrimental consequences to both bingeing and purging.

Binge eating is harmful in several ways. First, the intake of large quantities of sweets can result in **hypoglycemia,** or a deficiency of sugar in the blood. This may seem paradoxical because the typical binge eater consumes huge amounts of sugar. High intake of sugar, however, activates the pancreas to release excessive amounts of insulin, and insulin drives down blood sugar levels. Low blood sugar results in dizziness, fatigue, and depression. The low blood sugar level frequently produces cravings for more sugar, which in turn prompt the person to eat more cake, candy, ice cream, and other sweets. Second, binge eaters seldom eat a balanced diet. They usually lack sufficient fatty acids, a major energy source, and consequently they may experience lethargy and depression. Third, binge eating is expensive. Bulimics can spend more than $100 a day on food, and this expense can lead to other problems, such as poverty or stealing. Also, binge eaters are almost invariably preoccupied with food. They nearly constantly think of the next binge and have little time or energy for other activities. Cauwells (1983) reported that this obsession sometimes leads to the loss of a job and more frequently to disinterest in sex and other social activities.

Purging also leads to several injurious outcomes. One of the most common consequences of frequent vomiting is damaged teeth; hydrochloric acid from the stomach erodes the enamel that protects the teeth. Many long-time bulimics need expensive dental work, and thus dentists are sometimes the first health care professionals to suspect bulimia. Hydrochloric acid is also implicated in damage to other parts of the digestive system, particularly the mouth and esophagus. Unlike the stomach, they are not naturally protected against hydrochloric acid. Bleeding and tearing of the esophagus are not uncommon among bulimics, and many long-time sufferers report reverse peristalsis, a spontaneous regurgitation of food. Boskind-White and White (1983) reported that many of their participants had lost the ability to control vomiting and would regurgitate food even when they had eaten moderately.

Besides damage to teeth, mouth, and esophagus, other potential dangers of frequent purging include anemia, electrolyte imbalance, and alkalosis. **Anemia,** a reduction in the number of red blood cells, leads to generalized weakness and a lack of vitality. **Electrolyte imbalance** is caused by the loss of such body minerals such as sodium, potassium, magnesium, and calcium and leads to muscle cramps and weakness. **Alkalosis,** an abnormally high level of alkaline in the body tissues due to the loss of hydrochloric acid, results in generalized fatigue and frequent headaches. In addition, purging through excessive use of laxatives and diuretics may lead to kidney damage, dehydration, and a spastic colon, or the loss of voluntary control over excretory functions. In summary, bulimia is not a benign eating practice but a serious disorder with a multitude of harmful consequences.

Treatment

In one important respect, the treatment of bulimia has a critical advantage over therapy programs for anorexia nervosa. Unlike anorexics, who cling to their eccentric eating behaviors, bulimics usually do not approve of their own eating habits and would like to change. Unfortunately, this motivation does not guarantee that bulimics will seek therapy. Furnham and Kramers (1989) offered interesting evidence concerning a possible impediment to treatment. They assessed anorexics, bulimics, and people with normal eating habits to study the perception of normal eating. They found that both anorexics and bulimics judged the eating patterns of normal people to be at great variance from their own eating, but this perception was incorrect. Normal people have a wide variety of eating patterns, and these patterns deviate greatly from the standards that anorexics and bulimics perceive as ideal. Furnham and Kramers believed that this misperception may be one factor that prevents people with eating disorders from seeking treatment; that is, they have an unrealistic perception of the eating pattern they must achieve to be normal.

The immediate aim of treatment for bulimics is a change in eating patterns, but other long-term goals must also be included. For example, Marlene Boskind-White and her husband William C. White (1983) have developed a therapy program that aims to change clients' attitudes toward themselves and their eating habits. Their therapy relies heavily on intensive group therapy, with the emphasis on helping their clients gain control over their whole life, not just their eating habits. Boskind-White and White advocate reasonable goals rather than idealistic ones. Most bulimics set a goal of "never again," but this goal is a near guarantee of failure because slips are likely to occur. The "what the hell" effect is relevant to bulimia (as well as to dieting, abstaining from alcohol, giving up tobacco, and getting off drugs). Total bingeing often follows one lapse, especially for perfectionists who set an unrealistic goal of complete abstinence.

In addition to group therapy, cognitive behavior therapy is common in the treatment of bulimia (Agras, 1993). Cognitive behavior therapists can suggest a variety of techniques to their clients, such as keeping a diary on the factors related to bingeing and on their feelings after purging; monitoring their caloric intake and purging; eating slowly; eating regular meals; clarifying their distorted views of eating and weight control; and undergoing a procedure they call exposure plus response prevention. In exposure plus response prevention, therapists require bulimics to eat a great deal but then prevent them from vomiting. Some researchers (Hsu, 1990; Wilson, 1989) advocate the use of exposure plus response prevention, but others (Agras, Schneider, Arnow, Raeburn, & Telch, 1989; Leitenberg, Rosen, Gross, Nudelman, & Vara, 1988) have found that this technique does not increase the effectiveness of cognitive behavioral programs, which have been highly successful in changing the binge-purge cycle. Garner, Fairburn, and Davis (1987) reviewed 19 studies on cognitive behavioral treatment for bulimia and found that their average reduction of binge frequency was 79%, an unusually high percentage of success for any type of therapy.

More recently, Patricia Kaminski and Kathleen McNamara (1996) demonstrated that a combined educational and cognitive psychology program could be effective in treating women who were at risk for bulimia. These researchers recruited college women who showed potential for serious eating disorders — that is, they had low self-esteem, poor body image, a strong need for perfectionism, a history of repeated dieting, and other dysfunctional eating behaviors or attitudes. Kaminski and McNamara randomly assigned participants to either a treatment group or a control group. The treatment group received educational information about realistic weights and healthy eating habits and were given cognitive strategies for enhancing self-esteem, challenging negative thinking styles, improving body image, and combating social pressures for thinness. At the end of the 7-week session, participants in the treatment group showed significantly greater improvement in self-esteem and body satisfaction than those in the control group. In addition, they manifested fewer destructive dieting practices and less need for perfectionism. Results of this study suggest intervention can change the attitudes and risky behaviors that are symptomatic of bulimia before the appearance of the disorder.

Striegel-Moore, Silberstein, and Rodin (1986) analyzed bulimia from a developmental framework, the same approach used by interpersonal psychotherapy to understand and treat bulimia. Interpersonal psychotherapy is a nonintrospective, short-term therapy that was originally applied to depression but which has also been used successfully in treating bulimics (Agras, 1993). It focuses on present interpersonal problems and not on eating, taking the approach that eating problems tend to appear in late adolescence when interpersonal issues present major developmental challenges. In this view, eating problems represent maladaptive attempts to cope. The success rate of interpersonal therapy is comparable to cognitive behavioral therapy (Agras,

1993), but it may not provide additional help for people with binge eating disorder who failed to respond to cognitive behavioral therapy (Agras et al., 1995),

Drugs, especially antidepressants, have been used for some time in the treatment of bulimia (Pope, Hudson, Jonas, & Yurgelun-Todd, 1983). Controlled studies using these drugs tend to show decreases in frequency of binges, but Mitchell and de Zwaan's (1993) review indicated that although antidepressant drugs can add to the effectiveness of psychotherapy, drugs are not a substitute for psychotherapy for most patients.

CHAPTER SUMMARY

Weight maintenance depends largely on two factors: the number of calories absorbed through food intake and the number expended through body metabolism and physical activity. The absorption of calories through food intake occurs in the digestive tract, beginning in the mouth, where food is broken down into small particles and mixed with saliva. The stomach furthers the digestive process, but the small intestine is the site of most of the absorption of nutrients. Weight gain occurs when more nutrients are present than are required for maintenance of body metabolism and physical activity. Weight loss occurs when insufficient nutrients are present to furnish the necessary energy for body metabolism and activity.

In a study on *experimental starvation,* loss of too much weight led to irritability, aggression, apathy, lack of interest in sex, and preoccupation with food. Many of these negative personality changes persisted even after weight was regained. Surprisingly, gaining weight can be as difficult as losing weight. Initial weight gain may be relatively easy, but not all the volunteer inmates in one study were able to attain their goals for weight gain. The demonstrated difficulty of either losing or gaining weight has led several investigators to adopt the notion of a natural setpoint for weight maintenance.

Overeating and obesity are by no means identical. Many people overeat but do not get fat; others are obese but eat only moderate amounts or even less. Nevertheless, a strong relationship exists between overeating and obesity, and several theoretical models attempt to explain why some people become obese. The *psychodynamic model* sees obesity as stemming from unconscious conflict; *social learning theory* views overeating as being acquired in a social environment; and *setpoint theory* holds that psychological and physiological mechanisms work to restore fat tissue when the body loses a given amount of weight.

Obesity is associated with increased mortality, heart disease, adult-onset diabetes, and digestive tract diseases, and the risks increase with the amount of obesity. However, this relationship is complicated by a number of other factors, including one's distribution of fat. People whose excess weight is around their waist rather than hips are at an increased risk of death from several causes.

The near obsession with thinness in our culture has led to a plethora of *diets,* many of which are neither safe nor permanently effective. Most diets will produce some initial weight loss in response to the restriction of caloric intake, but maintaining the reduced weight levels is a matter of lifelong changes in basic eating habits.

Some people begin a weight-loss program that seemingly gets out of control and turns into an almost total fasting regimen. This eating disorder, called *anorexia nervosa,* is most prevalent among young, high-achieving, compliant women. A related disorder called *bulimia* is characterized by uncontrolled binge eating, usually accompanied by guilt and followed by vomiting or other purgative methods.

A variety of *treatment programs* have been used for both anorexia nervosa and bulimia. The success rates for anorexia have not been high, particularly when measured in terms of changes in both eating habits and self-image. Treatment for bulimia has been more successful, partly because of bulimics' greater motivation to change. Among the more successful programs for eating disorders are those that include cognitive behavioral techniques, which seek to change not only eating patterns but also the pathological concerns about weight and eating that characterize both anorexia nervosa and bulimia.

SUGGESTED READINGS

Bennett, W., & Gurin, J. (1982). *The dieter's dilemma: Eating less and weighing more.* New York: Basic Books. This book presents the setpoint hypothesis and evidence that supports it, along with a review of approaches to dieting. The authors combine a presentation of evidence with advice to those interested in losing weight for a readable and often entertaining book.

Bruch, H. (1978). *The golden cage: The enigma of anorexia nervosa.* Cambridge, MA: Harvard University Press. Written by one of the leading authorities on anorexia nervosa, this nontechnical book describes anorexia and suggests methods of treating this eating disorder.

Polivy, J., & Herman, C. P. (1983). *Breaking the diet habit: The natural weight alternative.* New York: Basic Books. Written by two psychologists, this book reviews research by the authors and by others who have tried to solve the problems of eating and weight control. Their approach is not a traditional one, but their book presents a provocative interpretation of the research, along with advice to dieters.

Rodin, J. (1992). *Body traps.* New York: William Morrow. Judith Rodin is one of the leading researchers in the field of eating, obesity, and eating disorders. In this popular book, she summarizes her work and that of other researchers in her analysis of the ways that people can become trapped by body concerns, food, and dieting.

16 Exercising

When Jim Fixx was 35 years old, he was 50 pounds overweight, smoked two packs of cigarettes a day, and except for an occasional game of tennis or touch football, generally lived a sedentary existence as a magazine editor. But at that point, his life changed dramatically. By his account, the impetus for this transformation was a pulled leg muscle he incurred while playing tennis (Fixx, 1977). To rehabilitate his leg and avoid another muscle pull, Fixx began a modest running program. Painfully he jogged half a mile or so three or four times a week. Gradually he increased both his distance and his speed, and running began to play an increasingly important role in his life. This exercise slowly altered both his physical appearance and his attitude toward his health. He lost weight, stopped smoking, felt physically rejuvenated, and came to believe strongly in the preventive and curative powers of running. Perhaps too much so. On a warm July day in 1984, Jim Fixx died while returning from his afternoon run. The cause of death was listed as sudden **cardiac arrhythmia** due to coronary artery disease.

The death of Jim Fixx spotlighted several questions that had long been asked about the benefits and dangers of vigorous exercise. Does exercise reduce heart disease? Does it contribute to longevity? Can exercise protect against cancer? Does it enhance personal well-being and psychological health? How much exercise is necessary to maintain good health? How much is too much? Can it be a health hazard? This chapter examines the available evidence on these issues and attempts to reach some conclusions regarding the health effects, if any, of both moderate and strenuous exercise.

A final question that has no definitive answer is this: Did exercise hasten the death of Jim Fixx, or did it prolong his life? Because Fixx, like some other runners, died during or immediately after exercising, some may conclude that exercise is hazardous to health. Others, however, might argue that Fixx would have died earlier if he had not become a runner. Pietschmann (1984), for instance, writing for *Runner's World,* noted that Fixx had a family history of heart problems; his father had suffered a heart attack at age 35 and had died of another one at 43. Fixx, then, outlived his father by 9 years—so perhaps his 17 years of long-distance running produced more benefits than risks.

TYPES OF EXERCISE

Currently, about 70% of adults in the United States engage in some form of leisure-time physical activity (Siegel, Brackbill, & Heath, 1995), but most of them do not exercise in a way that enhances their health. Although exercise can include hundreds of different kinds of physical activity, ranging from bowling to sky diving, physiologically there are only five different types of exercise: isometric, isotonic, isokinetic, anaerobic, and aerobic. Each has different goals, different activities, and different advocates, but only aerobic exercise contributes to cardiorespiratory health.

Isometric exercise is performed by contracting muscles against an immovable object. Although the body does not move in isometric exercise, muscles push hard against each other or against an immovable object and thus gain strength. Pushing hard against a solid wall is an example of isometric exercise. Because joints do not move, it may not be apparent that exercise is occurring, but the contraction of muscles produces gains in strength — and little else. Kuntzleman (1978) reviewed various types of exercise and fitness programs and concluded that isometric exercise, because it affects only muscle strength, does not rate well as an overall conditioning procedure.

Isotonic exercise requires the contraction of muscles and the movement of joints. Weight lifting and many forms of calisthenics fit into this category. Programs based on isotonic exercise can improve muscle strength and muscle endurance if the program is sufficiently lengthy and strenuous. Body-building programs that rely on weight training are based on isotonic exercises, but they are mostly oriented toward improving the appearance of the body rather than toward improving fitness and health.

Kuntzleman (1978) rated isotonic exercise in the form of weight lifting as good for developing strength but more expensive than calisthenics, which can also be effective in this respect. Neither, however, provides a comprehensive exercise program.

In **isokinetic exercise**, exertion is required for lifting, and additional effort is required to return to the starting position. This type of exercise requires specialized equipment, such as a Nautilus machine, that adjusts the amount of resistance according to the amount of force applied. Research by Pipes and Wilmore (1975) has indicated that isokinetic exercise is superior to both isometrics and isotonics in promoting muscle strength and muscle endurance. The main disadvantage to isokinetic exercise is the inconvenience and expense of its elaborate equipment.

Anaerobic exercises include short-distance running, some calisthenics, softball, and other exercises that require short, intensive bursts of energy but do not require an increased amount of oxygen. Such exercises improve speed and endurance, but they do not increase the fitness of the coronary and respiratory systems. Moreover, anaerobic exercises may be dangerous for people with coronary disease.

The term **aerobic exercise** refers to any type of exercise that requires dramatically increased oxygen consumption over an extended period of time. One of the most common forms of aerobic exercise is jogging, although many other physical activities can be performed aerobically, including walking, cross-country skiing, dancing, rope skipping, swimming, and cycling.

The important characteristics of aerobic exercise are intensity and duration. Exercise must be of sufficient intensity to elevate the heart rate into a certain range, which is computed from a formula based on age and the maximum possible heart rate. The heart rate should stay at this elevated level for at least 12 minutes, and preferably 15 to 30 minutes for the aerobic benefits to accrue. This type of program requires elevated oxygen use and provides a workout for both the respiratory system, which furnishes the oxygen, and the coronary system, which pumps the blood.

Kenneth Cooper (1968, 1970, 1982, 1985, 1994) has provided guidelines for implementing a personal program of aerobic training, and his books have done much to popularize aerobic exercise. Of the various approaches to fitness, aerobics is superior to other types of exercise in developing cardiorespiratory fitness, provided a person engages in some aerobic exercise at least three times a week.

Although Cooper is a strong advocate for aerobics, his program takes a cautious approach in several respects. First, he believes that potentially dangerous coronary abnormalities can exist without any apparent symptoms and therefore he recommends a medical examination before beginning a program of aerobic exercise. Second, he advocates the use of an exercise electrocardiogram, known as a *stress test,* to detect any abnormal cardiac activity during exercise. Any abnormality in heartbeat or insufficiency in blood supply signals some coronary problem, which may indicate a need for further testing to pinpoint the source. If no problem is indicated, exercise can probably be done with safety. Third, Cooper (1982) has been more conservative than others with respect to the distance and frequency of exercise that is necessary to produce health benefits. Many exercise adherents, including Jim Fixx advocated running long distances 6 or 7 days a week. Cooper maintained that jogging or running three miles a day for 5 days a week confers an optimum level of cardiovascular fitness. He contended that more frequent exercise or more distance is not beneficial to fitness and may increase the chances for injuries. In a later section of this chapter, we examine the question of how much exercise is enough and how much is too much.

REASONS FOR EXERCISING

People who exercise regularly report a variety of reasons for their physical activity. Surveys (Carmach & Martens, 1979; Koplan, Powell, Sikes, Shirley, & Campbell, 1982) have revealed answers such as "Exercise helps people become physically fit," "I want to lose weight," "It strengthens my heart," "Exercise helps people live longer," "I don't feel so depressed when I exercise," "I just feel better," "I'm addicted to it." This chapter looks at evidence relating to each of these reasons as well as to other benefits and potential hazards of physical activity.

PHYSICAL FITNESS

First, does exercise help people become physically fit? The effects of exercise on fitness depend both on the duration and intensity of the exercise and on the definition of fitness. To most exercise physiologists, fitness is a complex condition consisting of muscle strength, muscle endurance, flexibility, and cardiorespiratory (aerobic) fitness. Each of the five types of exercise can contribute to these four different aspects of fitness, but no one type fulfills all the requirements.

In addition, fitness can be considered in terms of organic and dynamic fitness (Kuntzleman, 1978). *Organic fitness* is the capacity for action and movement that is determined by inherent characteristics of the body. These organic factors include genetic endowment, age, and health limitations. *Dynamic fitness,* which is determined by experience, is probably what most people think of in connection with the term *fitness.* Dynamic fitness is affected by exercise whereas organic fitness is not. A person can have a good level of organic fitness yet be "out of shape" and perform poorly. Another person may train and improve dynamic fitness but still be unable to win races because of relatively poor organic fitness. Athletes who want to be champions need to have been very selective about their biological parents so they would have inherited a high level of organic fitness. Aspiring champions also need to train to gain the dynamic fitness necessary for optimal athletic performance. The following discussion is concerned almost exclusively with dynamic fitness and its components because this type of fitness can be modified through exercise.

Muscle Strength

How strongly a muscle can contract is a measure of muscle strength. This type of fitness can be achieved through isometric, isotonic, isokinetic, and, to a lesser extent, anaerobic exercise. All these types of exercises have the capability to increase muscle strength because they contract muscles. One study (Thistle, Hislop, Moffroid, & Lowman, 1967) found that isokinetic exercise was somewhat better than isotonic exercise in increasing strength and that both were considerably better than isometric exercise.

Muscle Endurance

Muscle endurance differs from muscle strength in that it requires continued performance. Some amount of strength is necessary for muscle endurance, but the opposite is not true: A muscle may be strong but not have the endurance to continue its performance. Exercises that improve strength require greater exertion for limited repetitions; exercises that improve endurance require less exertion but are performed many times. Both muscle strength and muscle endurance are improved by similar types of exercises, including isometric, isotonic, and isokinetic.

Flexibility

Flexibility is the range of motion capacity of a joint. The types of exercises that develop muscle strength and muscle endurance generally do not improve flexibility. Moreover, flexibility is specific to each joint, so that exercises designed to develop flexibility tend to be quite varied. In addition to being a component of fitness, flexibility also decreases the likelihood of injury in other types of exercise.

Flexibility is best attained through slow, sustained stretching exercises. Fast, jerky, bouncing movements are not recommended because they can cause soreness and injury (Allsen, Harrison, & Vance, 1976). Also, flexibility training should not be as intense as strength and endurance training. Kuntzleman (1978) recommended that exercises to increase flexibility be incorporated into the warm-up and cool-down phases of any fitness program, but flexibility training alone is not an adequate fitness program.

Aerobic (Cardiorespiratory) Fitness

Of all the types of physical activity, only aerobic exercise builds cardiorespiratory fitness. This sort of exercise greatly increases the body's requirement for oxygen, thereby causing the respiratory system to work harder and the heart to pump blood at a higher rate. Cooper (1968) stated that aerobic exercise must be of sufficient intensity and duration to increase heart rate to at least 60% and possibly as much as 85% of the maximum.

Research by Lakka et al. (1994) supported Cooper's notion that vigorous physical activity improves cardiorespiratory fitness and also protects against the risk of heart attack. These investigators obtained baseline measures on a large group of healthy middle-aged men. After controlling for several possible confounding factors, a 5-year follow-up revealed that men with high aerobic fitness, compared to those with low fitness, were only about one-fourth as likely to have heart attacks.

Additional studies have confirmed the benefits of fitness to decrease mortality risk. A study in Norway (Sandivk et al., 1993) found that physically fit middle-aged men had an all-cause mortality rate of less than half that of physically unfit men. Similarly, Blair et al. (1995) administered a treadmill test to adult men from Cooper's clinic in Dallas at two different times, nearly 5 years apart, and then tracked them for an additional 5 years. At the end of follow-up, men who were high in cardiorespiratory fitness

at both the first and the second treadmill examinations were only one-third as likely to have died as men who were unfit at both tests. A more important finding, however, was that men who increased their cardiorespiratory fitness from the first testing to the second reduced their all-cause mortality risk by 44%. This latter finding demonstrates that changes in cardiorespiratory fitness affect risk of mortality. Blair et al. calculated that each minute gained on the treadmill corresponded with a 7.9% decrease in all-cause mortality.

What special benefits does aerobic fitness provide? Pollock, Wilmore, and Fox (1978) listed several cardiorespiratory changes resulting from aerobic training, including an increase in the amount of oxygen that can be used during strenuous exercise and an increase in the amount of blood pumped with each heartbeat. Both the resting heart rate and the resting blood pressure decrease with gains in aerobic fitness. These changes indicate increased efficiency of the cardiorespiratory system. Thus, aerobic fitness is an important contributor to physical health and well-being.

WEIGHT CONTROL

Does physical activity contribute to weight control? Many people exercise to lose weight or to sculpt a more ideal body by improving their body composition—that is, the percentage of fat tissue on the body or the ratio of fat to muscle. Exercise increases muscle tissue and can therefore change this ratio.

Of greater interest, however, is the effect of exercise on fat itself. Wood et al. (1988) found that exercise is at least equal to dieting in controlling weight and much better than dieting in changing the ratio of fat to muscle tissue. In this study, sedentary men who were 120% to 160% above their ideal weight were randomly assigned to one of three groups: dieters, runners, or controls. The dieters did not exercise, the runners did not diet, and the controls did neither. After a year, the running group and the dieting group had both lost weight whereas people in the control group had not. However, some important differences emerged in comparing the dieters and the runners. Although both groups had lost an equal amount of weight, the dieters lost both fat and lean tissue, whereas the runners lost only fat tissue and retained more lean muscle tissue.

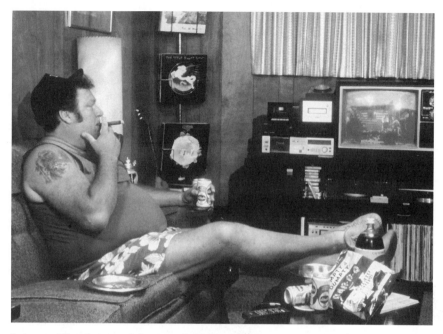

Sedentary lifestyle is a risk for several chronic illnesses.

Exercise does not produce much weight loss through burning calories. For example, more than 30 minutes of tennis is required to work off the calories in two doughnuts, but sitting and eating doughnuts is a risk for obesity in two ways—the sitting and the eating. Ching et al. (1996) found that sedentary men were 50% more likely than active men to be overweight. These researchers found that the number of hours spent watching television was related to risk of obesity; those who watched a lot of TV were much more likely to be overweight than those who watched little TV. Therefore, the weight loss associated with exercise may come in part through spending time on activities that burn calories but also in avoiding sedentary activities that may lead to consuming calories—such as snacking while watching TV.

The weight loss associated with exercise comes mostly through the elevation of metabolic rate, the rate at which the body metabolizes calories. Bennett and Gurin (1982) suggested another possibility for the role of physical activity, speculating that physical activity may lower a person's *setpoint*. As Chapter 15 explained, the setpoint model holds that the body works to keep fat levels relatively fixed, so dieters cannot lose (or gain) much weight unless the set-

point is adjusted. Moderate levels of physical activity may be capable of producing such adjustments. Thus, exercise may be capable of increasing metabolic rate and adjusting setpoint, both of which would produce changes in weight that exceed the number of calories spent in any activity.

How much exercise is enough to bring about weight loss? Gwinup (1975) reported that daily walks were sufficient to cause weight loss and Epstein and Wing (1980) found that four or more aerobic exercise sessions a week contributed to weight loss but less frequent exercise did not. Epstein, Wing, and their associates (Epstein, Valoski, Wing, & McCurley, 1994; Epstein et al., 1995) confirmed the benefits of physical exercise in weight control, finding that simply reinforcing physically active behaviors in overweight children was an effective treatment for childhood obesity. Thus, it seems that even moderate amounts of exercise will bring about weight loss for many overweight children and adults.

Is exercise helpful for people who are already thin, or will it make them too thin? Forbes (1992) looked at earlier studies of both humans and other animals and found that if people have low body mass at the beginning of an exercise program, they may have a tendency to lose some lean body weight.

However, thin exercisers can maintain lean body mass through proper diet. Also, moderate-weight exercisers who do not decrease total weight often increase lean body weight. This review suggests that even when exercisers fail to lose weight, they increase lean body mass and decrease body fat.

In summary, research suggests that overweight people can lose weight through physical activity, highly active thin people can maintain lean body mass through proper diet, and people of moderate weight can increase lean body weight without an overall weight gain.

CARDIOVASCULAR BENEFITS OF EXERCISE

More important than physical fitness or weight control is the issue of exercise and cardiovascular health. Does regular exercise reduce the chances of heart disease? During the earlier years of the 20th century, physicians often advised patients with heart disease to avoid strenuous physical activity, based on the belief that too much physical activity could damage the heart and threaten a person's life. In more recent years, however, evidence has suggested that exercise can protect against heart disease.

EARLY STUDIES

The history of the positive cardiovascular effects of physical activity began in England during the early 1950s and involved London's famous double-decker buses. Jeremy Morris and his colleagues (Morris, Heady, Raffle, Roberts, & Parks, 1953) discovered that physically active male conductors differed from less active bus drivers on the incidence of heart disease. This study, however, did not prove that physical activity decreases the chances of coronary heart disease (CHD) because workers may have been selected for jobs on the basis of body type, personality, or some other factor that is associated with a high or low risk of CHD.

Similar studies by Taylor et al. (1962) and Kahn (1963) examined the death rates among sedentary versus active employees and found differences in deaths from CHD. Kahn's study suggested that the potential benefits from past activity are lost after a few years. When he looked at former mail carriers who had switched to more sedentary clerical jobs, Kahn found that after more than 5 years of working as a clerk, former carriers had an incidence of death from CHD equal to that of men who had always been clerks. This finding suggests that exercise should be incorporated into one's lifestyle on a continuing basis.

These studies seem to imply that workers who are physically active have a reduced risk of coronary heart disease. However, the problem of self-selection clouds any conclusion about exercise benefits. Furthermore, none of the studies measured the workers' activity levels off the job. Most of these issues have been addressed in more recent studies, including a series of investigations by Ralph Paffenbarger, a professor of epidemiology at the Stanford University School of Medicine, who has investigated the relationship between physical activity and health in two large populations of participants: San Francisco longshoremen and Harvard alumni.

In the early 1970s, Paffenbarger and his associates (Paffenbarger, 1972; Paffenbarger, Gima, Laughlin, & Black, 1971; Paffenbarger & Hale, 1975; Paffenbarger, Laughlin, Gima, & Black, 1970) published several reports of a study involving nearly 3,700 San Francisco longshoremen whom they had followed since 1951. In general, they found that CHD death rates were more than 80% higher for low-activity workers than for the highly active ones. In these studies the problem of initial self-selection was not a major factor because all workers in both the high- and low-activity groups had begun their employment with at least 5 years of strenuous cargo handling. From these and other studies, Paffenbarger concluded that high-intensity exercise produces a training effect that provides protection against coronary heart disease.

THE HARVARD ALUMNI STUDY

In 1978, Paffenbarger, Wing, and Hyde published a landmark epidemiological investigation that avoided most of the flaws found in earlier studies. Paffenbarger et al. found extensive medical records of former Harvard University students dating back to 1916. They then sent detailed questionnaires to the men who were still living and received replies from nearly 17,000.

To measure the weekly total energy expenditure of these men, the investigators used a composite

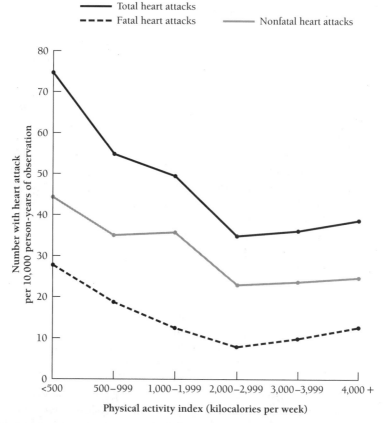

Figure 16.1 Age-adjusted first heart attack rates by physical activity index in a 6– to 10–year follow-up of male Harvard alumni. SOURCE: Adapted from "Physical Activity as an Index of Heart Attack Risk in College Alumni" by R. S. Paffenbarger, Jr., A. L. Wing, and R. T. Hyde, 1978. *American Journal of Epidemiology, 108,* p. 166. Copyright 1978 by The Johns Hopkins University School of Hygiene and Public Health. Adapted by permission of the publisher and Dr. Ralph Paffenbarger.

physical activity index that took into account all activity, both on and off the job. By asking these men how many flights of stairs they climbed, how far they walked, and what sports they played and for how long, the investigators were able to arrive at an estimate of energy expenditure per week, measured in kilocalories (kcal). For example, walking up one flight of 10 stairs per day was equated to 28 kcal per week, light sports such as golf or softball were rated at 5 kcal per minute, and strenuous sports such as running, skiing, or swimming were rated at 10 kcal per minute.

Paffenbarger et al. then divided the Harvard alumni into high- and low-activity groups. Of those men whose energy levels could be determined, about 60% expended fewer than 2,000 kcal per week and were

thus placed in the low-activity group; the 40% who expended more than 2,000 kcal made up the high-activity group. Note that 2,000 kcal of energy is approximately that expended in 20 miles of jogging or its equivalent.

Paffenbarger et al. (1978) reported that the least active Harvard alumni had a "64 per cent increased risk of heart attack over their more energetic classmates" (p. 165). However, 2,000 kcal per week seemed to be the breaking point, beyond which increased exercise paid no dividends in terms of reduced risk of fatal or nonfatal heart attacks. Figure 16.1 shows a steady reduction in the number of heart attacks as the amount of energy expended increases from 500 to 2,000 kcal per week. Exercise beyond that point was related to a slight, insignificant trend toward greater risk of coronary heart disease.

Does exercise reduce the risk of heart attack in men who smoke or who have a history of hypertension? Paffenbarger et al. (1978) also addressed this question in their study of Harvard alumni and found that physically active nonsmokers with no history of hypertension had 26.2 first heart attacks per 10,000 person-years of observation (see bottom figure, fourth column, Table 16.1). As the lowest rate in the table, this figure was given a relative risk index of 1.00. The top figure indicates that inactive smokers with a history of hypertension were 7.70 times more likely to have a heart attack than active nonsmokers with no history of hypertension. However, active men who smoked and who also had a history of hypertension had a relative risk of heart attack less than half the top figure—down to 3.03. This figure suggests that men with other coronary risk factors can reduce their risk of a first heart attack through physical activity.

Paffenbarger and his associates have continued to publish reports on these same Harvard alumni men that addressed the question of longevity and exercise. In 1984, Paffenbarger, Hyde, Wing, and Steinmetz reported that only hypertension carried a heavier risk of CHD than inactivity, with high activity (more than 2,000 kcal a week) more beneficial than moderate activity (500 to 1,999 kcal per week) and moderate activity more beneficial than inactivity

(less than 500 kcal per week). In 1986, Paffenbarger, Hyde, Wing, and Hsieh found an inverse relationship between the amount of exercise and all-cause mortality, although physical activity above 3,500 kcal per week did not continue to contribute to lower death rates.

In 1993, Paffenbarger et al. reported that men who initiate a moderately vigorous physical activity program during middle age or older had a 23% lower risk of death from all causes than men who did not begin such a program. More recently, Lee, Hsieh, and Paffenbarger (1995) found that both total expenditure of energy and expenditure from vigorous exercise related inversely to all-cause mortality. This study, however, failed to find a significant relationship between nonvigorous activity and longevity.

In summary, studies by Paffenbarger and his associates of Harvard alumni suggest that men who expended 2,000 kcal or more per week can expect an average increase in longevity of about 2 years. A cynic might criticize this finding by pointing out that a person would need to jog a total of about 2 years between the ages of 20 and 80 to increase longevity by 2 years. Why live another 2 years if one spends that time jogging? Paffenbarger et al. (1986) contended that physical activity does not merely extend the life span 2 years at the end, but it adds quality years throughout a person's life. They concluded that exercise not only protects against disease and death but contributes to enhanced health in all age groups.

Table 16.1 Relative risks of first heart attacks among Harvard male alumni in a 6- to 10-year follow-up, by specific combinations of high physical activity, cigarette smoking, and history of hypertension

Physically active (more than 2,000 kcal/week)	Cigarette smoker?	History of hypertension?	Number with heart attack per 10,000 person-years of observation	Relative risk of heart attack
No	Yes	Yes	201.9	7.70
No	Yes	No	65.5	2.50
No	No	Yes	102.3	3.90
Yes	Yes	Yes	79.5	3.03
No	No	No	35.1	1.34
Yes	Yes	No	50.1	1.91
Yes	No	Yes	41.8	1.59
Yes	No	No	26.2	1.00

SOURCE: Adapted from "Physical Activity as an Index of Heart Attack Risk in College Alumni" by R. S. Paffenbarger, Jr., A. L. Wing, and R. T. Hyde, 1978, *American Journal of Epidemiology, 108,* p. 172. Copyright 1978 by The Johns Hopkins University School of Hygiene and Public Health. Adapted by permission of the publisher and Dr. Ralph Paffenbarger.

All studies on the cardiovascular effects of exercise discussed to this point have one important limitation—their exclusive use of men. To complete the picture of the health benefits of exercise, the records for women as well as men should be examined.

THE FRAMINGHAM HEART STUDY

One study that did include women was the Framingham Heart Study (Dawber, 1980), a 24-year follow-up study of a sample of more than 6,500 residents of Framingham, Massachusetts. Even though both men and women participated in this investigation, the study was limited by the fact that nearly all participants reported relatively similar levels of activity. As a result, when the investigators looked at the coronary benefits of activity for all participants, they found very few. However, when they compared extremely inactive participants with the maximally active, they found differences in coronary heart disease for both men and women. Sedentary men had an incidence of both CHD and myocardial infarction about three times higher than that of the most active men. For women, the ratios were about 2.5 to 1. For both men and women, few differences showed up between the moderately active and the most active, but clear patterns emerged when sedentary men and women were compared to either moderately active or maximally active people.

A 32-year follow-up of the Framingham study (Kiely, Wolf, Cupples, Beiser, & Kannel, 1994) looked at both middle-aged and older men and women and found no protective effect of physical activity for stroke among women. However, middle-aged men who exercised moderately or vigorously significantly reduced their risk for stroke, and older men who were physically active were less than half as likely to have a stroke as inactive older men.

EXERCISE AND STROKE

The Framingham Heart Study is not the only major study to find that exercise can help prevent stroke. Wannamethee and Shaper (1992) found that physical activity offered some protection against stroke for British middle-aged men, and Abbott, Rodriguez, Burchfiel, and Curb (1994) found similar results for men in the Honolulu Heart Program. As with the Framingham study, the Honolulu Heart Program found inactive middle-aged men to have a slightly higher risk for stroke than active men of the same age, but older sedentary men were three to four times more likely to have a stroke than older physically active men. This study also found that the benefits of exercise for stroke are lost for men who smoke cigarettes.

In summary, physical activity seems to offer some protection against stroke for middle-aged men. Because stroke is far less common than coronary heart disease among middle-aged men, exercise does not have as dramatic an impact on stroke as on heart disease. However, as men become older and more prone to stroke, the benefits of physical activity become more dramatic: Older men who exercise regularly have greatly reduced chances of stroke.

EXERCISE AND CHOLESTEROL LEVELS

How does exercise protect against cardiovascular disease? Some evidence, from both human and animal studies, suggests that exercise may increase high-density lipoprotein (HDL), the so-called "good" cholesterol. In addition, a program of regular physical activity may actually lower LDL, the "bad cholesterol." If both processes occurred, total cholesterol might remain the same but the ratio of total cholesterol to HDL would become more favorable and the risk for heart disease would be reduced.

Studies with humans have generally found that even moderate levels of exercise, with or without dietary changes, can bring about a favorable ratio of total cholesterol to HDL. An early study by Laporte, Brenes, and Dearwarter (1983) found a dose-response relationship between amount of physical activity and HDL, with marathon runners having very high rates of good cholesterol and thus very low ratios of total cholesterol to HDL. In another early study, Wood et al. (1988) assigned overweight, sedentary men to a diet group, an aerobic exercise group, or a control group. After 1 year, both the exercisers and the dieters raised HDL levels without changing LDL, but the controls did not. By raising HDL while keeping LDL constant, the aerobic exercisers (as well as the dieters) improved their ratio of total cholesterol to HDL.

As part of the Zutphen Study in Holland, Caspersen, Bloemberg, Saris, Merritt, and Kromhout (1991) investigated coronary risk factors in elderly men, 65

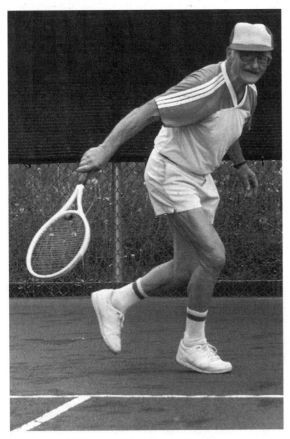

Even moderate levels of exercise can be beneficial to the elderly.

to 84. They found that even moderate exercise, such as walking and gardening, were associated with increased HDL and decreased total cholesterol. In a study of middle-aged men in Eastern Finland, Lakka and Salonen (1992) found that both leisure activity and occupational activity were associated with increases in HDL. In addition, total, occupational, and leisure time activity were all negatively related to **triglycerides** (one component of total cholesterol that has been linked to atherosclerotic plaques), and leisure activity was negatively associated with LDL. Each of these findings would result in a favorable ratio of total cholesterol to HDL for physically active middle-aged men.

Women, too, can improve their total cholesterol to HDL ratio by beginning a regular physical activity program. As part of the Stanford Five-City Project, Young, Haskell, Jatulis, and Fortmann (1993) looked

at coronary risk factors for both men and women who had changed their levels of physical activity. Physically active men increased their HDL, lowered their body mass, and decreased their coronary heart disease risk score. Physically active women also increased their HDL while lowering their resting pulse rate. Although the association between physical activity and HDL was not quite as high for women as it was for men, these findings suggest that both men and women who begin a regular exercise program can increase their HDL and lower their risk for heart disease.

A study by Raitakari et al. (1994) extended the lipid profile benefits of exercise to male and female children and young adults. These authors studied active and inactive 12-, 15-, and 18-year-olds for 6 years and found differences in lipid profiles of the physically active and the physically inactive. Physically active young men had lower triglycerides, higher HDL, and a lower total cholesterol to HDL ratio, and physically active young women had lower triglyceride concentrations and lower body fat than their inactive peers. Finally, Slyper (1994) reviewed earlier studies and concluded that both exercise and diet can lower LDL and that long-distance runners tend to have low levels of both LDL and very low density lipoprotein. These studies suggest that regular aerobic exercise may protect against heart disease by increasing HDL and by improving the ratio of total cholesterol to HDL.

Some investigators have conducted experiments on animals to determine the effects of exercise on cholesterol and atherosclerosis. Several of these studies (Kobernick, & Niwayana, 1960; Link, Pedersoli, & Safanie, 1972; Myasnikov, 1958) have found that exercise mitigates experimentally induced atherosclerosis in pigs, rabbits, ducks, geese, and other animals. In addition, Kramsch, Aspen, Abramowitz, Kreimendahl, and Hood (1981) demonstrated that exercise can have a beneficial effect on the cardiovascular system of monkeys fed an *atherogenic* diet — that is, a diet high in cholesterol and designed to induce atherosclerosis. Compared with sedentary monkeys, physically active monkeys had significantly higher HDL levels, lower LDL levels, less narrowing of arteries, and fewer sudden deaths. The authors suggested that exercise begun before the initiation of an atherogenic diet has significant cardiovascular benefits. These results, of course, do not mean that people can eat high-fat diets and then rely on exercise to protect them against coronary heart disease, but they do suggest that regular physical activity may raise HDL without raising total cholesterol and provide some protection against cardiovascular disease.

OTHER HEALTH BENEFITS OF EXERCISE

Besides contributing to physical fitness, weight control, and cardiovascular health, regular exercise confers several other health benefits, including protection against some kinds of cancer, prevention of bone density loss, and control of diabetes. In addition, regular physical activity has been shown to be related to some psychological benefits.

PROTECTION AGAINST CANCER

Although most people who exercise do so for physical fitness, weight control, or cardiovascular health, several studies have indicated that physical activity is associated with reduced chances of some cancers in men. For example, a prospective study (Vena et al., 1985) compared the lifetime occupational physical activity of three different groups: men with colon cancer, men with rectal cancer, and men who had neither a digestive disease nor any type of cancer. Interestingly, the risk of colon cancer increased as occupational physical activity decreased, but no relationship of any kind appeared between physical activity and rectal cancer. This study showed that the more sedentary the job and the longer the time spent with such a job, the greater the risk for colon cancer. In a study (Blair et al., 1989) that included both men and women, physical activity and all-cause mortality showed a consistent inverse relationship between levels of activity and cancer mortality for both men and women.

Can exercise protect men against prostate cancer? Research on this question has produced somewhat contradictory findings. Evidence concerning the lifetime occupational physical activity of older men showed that those who spent most of their working life in sedentary or relatively inactive jobs had a somewhat lower chance of developing pros-

tate cancer (Le Marchand, Kolonel, & Yoshizawa, 1991). However, this study did not assess leisure-time activity. In a study that did account for total physical activity (Lee, Paffenbarger, & Hsieh, 1992), physically active Harvard alumni were only 12% as likely to develop prostate cancer as their more sedentary cohorts. Lee et al. hypothesized that exercise moderates the production of testosterone, a potential risk for prostate cancer.

Finally, can men lower their risk of cancer deaths in general through exercise? Exercise protected middle-aged British men from cancer in general, but especially from lung cancer and cancers of the digestive tract (Wannamethee, Shaper, & Macfarlane, 1993). Looking at such activities as walking, cycling, playing golf, swimming, playing tennis, and running, Wannamethee et al. observed an inverse relationship between level of physical activity and cancer deaths as well as between physical activity and all noncardiovascular diseases. Although these studies have largely found that physical activity can lessen men's risk of several kinds of cancer, they have not addressed the question of exercise and cancer in women.

Does exercise also protect women against cancer? By studying both men and women, controlling for diet, and accounting for both leisure-time and work-related physical activity, Slattery, Schumacher, Smith, West, and Abd-Elghany (1990) found that physical activity protected against colon cancer and that the relationship was even more pronounced for women than for men. These authors concluded that physical activity may modify some of the harmful effects of a high-fat, high-protein diet. Although more research is needed in this area, these results provide some promise that exercise may protect against colon cancer, one of the leading causes of cancer death for both women and men.

How does exercise relate to breast cancer? Evidence on this question is not consistent. Some studies (Dorgan et al., 1994) have found that exercise may moderately increase risk of breast cancer, but other studies (Paffenbarger, Hyde, & Wing, 1987) have found no association between breast cancer and earlier physical activity. Still other studies (Bernstein, Henderson, Hanisch, Sullivan-Halley & Ross, 1994; Frisch et al., 1985; Vena, Graham, Zielezny, Brasure, & Swanson, 1987) have found that physical activity decreases the risk for subsequent breast cancer. Bernstein et al. found that women who had exercised at least 4 hours per week since early adolescence had a 50% reduction in incidence of breast cancer compared to less active women. The greatest protection appeared in women who were very physically active and who had given birth. Light and moderate physical activity was protective for women who had given birth, and high levels of activity offered some protection for women who had not given birth. Lee (1994) has called for more research on the connection between exercise and all cancers, especially those such as breast cancer that are more common in women.

PROTECTION AGAINST LOSS OF BONE DENSITY

Exercise has also been recommended to women as a protection against **osteoporosis**, a disorder characterized by a reduction in bone density due to calcium loss, resulting in brittleness of bones. Is this recommendation valid? An 1989 review of existing research (Harris, Caspersen, DeFriese, & Estes, 1989) concluded that physical activity offers strong protection against osteoporosis in postmenopausal women but is less effective in preventing this disorder in premenopausal women. Since this review, evidence has accrued suggesting that physical activity can protect women both during and after menopause and may even help prevent loss of bone mineral density in older men.

For example, a retrospective study (Greendale, Barrett-Connor, Edelstein, Ingles, & Halle, 1995) asked a group of older men and women to recall their level of physical activity as teenagers, at age 30, and at age 50. They found that both men and women with a history of physical activity had more bone mineral density than the more sedentary people but about the same number of bone fractures. In a study of menopausal women, Zhang, Feldblum, and Fortney (1992) found a dose-response relationship between physical activity during high school and current levels of bone mineral density, suggesting that perimenopausal women who exercised regularly continued to add bone mineral density. A similar study (Jagal, Kreiger, & Darlington, 1993) asked two groups of postmenopausal women to recall their levels of physical activity at ages 16, 30, and

50. One group consisted of women who had suffered a hip fracture and the other was a group of controls who had not suffered any recent bone fractures. When the researchers looked at both past and present levels of activity, they noted some interesting findings. Past physical activity — both moderate and vigorous — protected women ages 55 to 84 from hip fracture, and present moderate activity was also protective. However, present vigorous physical activity showed a slightly positive relationship to hip fractures. The message from this research is that older women should continue with moderate activity, but highly active older women should perhaps slow down a little.

Starting an exercise program may help older women to retain bone mineral density. Nelson et al. (1994) introduced a comprehensive program to previously sedentary women, ages 50 to 70, and compared them with women in a control group who remained sedentary. Women in the exercise group preserved their bone mineral content while those in the sedentary control group experienced a decrease in bone mineral density. Moreover, the exercise group increased muscle mass and muscle strength. This body of research suggests that both men and women should start exercising while young and continue into old age as a possible protection against a variety of disorders, including loss of bone mineral density and osteoporosis.

CONTROL OF DIABETES

Recent research has also found that physical activity may be a useful weapon in the control of diabetes. A study that followed male University of Pennsylvania alumni over a 15-year period (Helmrich, Ragland, Leung, & Paffenbarger, 1991) showed a direct relationship between leisure time physical activity and incidence of diabetes; that is, men who were the most physically active had the lowest rates of adult-onset diabetes. This relationship remained when the investigators controlled for obesity, blood pressure, and parental history of diabetes. In fact, men at greatest risk for diabetes — those with high body mass index, parental history of the disease, and hypertension — received the greatest protective effect.

A prospective study (Manson et al., 1992) also found that physical activity offers some protection against the development of adult onset diabetes. This investigation of 22,000 male physicians reported an inverse dose-response relationship between amount of exercise and incidence of diabetes; that is, the more days per week these men exercised, the less likely they were to develop noninsulin-dependent diabetes. After the investigators controlled for smoking, hypertension, and other coronary risk factors, the negative relationship between amount of exercise and incidence of diabetes persisted. Specifically, men who exercised once a week had a relative risk (RR) of 0.77, those who exercised 2–4 times weekly recorded a RR of 0.62, and physicians who exercised five or more times a week had a RR of only 0.58.

Another study (Moy et al., 1993) followed insulin-dependent mostly European American male and female children and adolescents and found that sedentary male diabetics were three times more likely to die than more active male diabetics. However, the trend for female diabetics was not as pronounced. These studies found only a modest protective benefit for physical activity and do not suggest that exercise is a panacea for the control of diabetes. Nevertheless, they do indicate that physical activity can be a useful adjunct in the treatment of insulin-dependent diabetes and can offer some protection against the development of noninsulin-dependent diabetes.

PSYCHOLOGICAL BENEFITS OF EXERCISE

The physiological benefits of physical activity are well established, but what about the psychological benefits? Can exercise lessen depression, reduce anxiety, lower stress levels, or increase self-esteem? Harris (1981) found that people who exercised listed psychological reasons nearly as often as physiological ones when asked about the benefits they receive from exercise. Does the evidence support these claims?

Decreased Depression

People who exercise regularly are generally less depressed than sedentary people. When groups of exercisers are compared to groups of sedentary people on different inventories measuring depression, highly active people are usually less depressed. In addition, aerobic exercise has been used as a therapeutic tool with patients suffering from depression. This section examines the effects of exercise as a preventive measure for depression in normal people and also as

a therapeutic intervention for clinically depressed individuals.

Does exercise reduce depression in normal, nonclinical individuals, or are depressed people simply less motivated to exercise? A brief look at the research reveals some evidence supporting the view that physical activity can, indeed, lower depressive moods in a variety of people. Koniak-Griffin (1994) found that a regular exercise program lowered depression in young pregnant women from ethnically diverse backgrounds; Ruuskanen and Parkatti (1994) explored physical activity among male and female nursing home residents ages 66 to 97 and found that a physically active lifestyle was associated with lower levels of depression. Studying a representative sample of people in Alameda County, Camacho, Roberts, Lazarus, Kaplan, and Cohen (1991) found that those who reported high levels of physical activity were less depressed than sedentary individuals. A report by Wilson, Morley, and Bird (1980) revealed that marathon runners were less depressed than joggers, and that joggers were less depressed than those who did not exercise. In addition, Joesting (1981) found that both male and female runners were significantly less depressed than nonrunners.

Physical activity need not be aerobic in order to reduce depression. Both aerobic exercise (swimming) and nonaerobic physical activity (weight training) were equally effective in lowering depression among college students (Stein & Motta, 1992). In addition, circuit weight training led to significant decreases in depression (Norvell & Belles, 1993). These and other studies indicate that various types of physical activity can lessen depression in individuals with nonclinical depression.

If exercise lowers depression in normal individuals, could it also be an effective technique for helping clinically depressed patients? Either alone or as an adjunct to other forms of therapy, aerobic exercise may be a useful tool for the clinician. Several studies have attempted to assess the effectiveness of running in reducing clinical depression (Simons, McGowan, Epstein, Kupfer, & Robertson, 1985).

One pioneer in running therapy is John Greist, who, along with his associates (Greist, 1984; Greist, Eischens, Klein, & Linn, 1981; Greist & Greist, 1979; Greist et al., 1978, 1979), has found tentative evidence supporting the use of running as a treatment for depression. In a pilot study, Greist et al. (1978)

assigned moderately depressed men and women patients either to a running group or to one of two kinds of individual psychotherapy—time-limited or time-unlimited. Patients in the running group received no conventional psychotherapy and were not permitted to talk about their depression during running therapy. Initially, they ran with a running leader in small groups for an hour three or four times a week. Later they ran less with the leader and more on their own, but they were encouraged to run at least three times a week. As a whole, patients who received the running treatment were somewhat less depressed after treatment than those in either the time-limited or the time-unlimited therapy group.

Since this early study, several other investigators have examined the usefulness of running as a psychotherapeutic tool. Buffone (1980) studied the effects of a program of running therapy combined with cognitive-behavioral therapy on a group of clinically depressed patients and found positive results. In a more tightly controlled study, Rueter and Harris (1980) randomly assigned clinically depressed college students to either a running and counseling group or to a counseling-only group and found that patients in the running and counseling group became significantly less depressed than those who received only counseling.

Also, Greist (1984) randomly assigned depressed patients to one of three treatment groups: aerobic exercise, Benson's (1975) relaxation training, or group psychotherapy. At the end of 12 weeks, all three groups were less depressed. But at the end of a 3-month follow-up, only the exercise and relaxation groups continued to show improvement. Patients who had received group therapy showed some regression toward original levels of depression. Later, Bosscher (1993) randomly assigned depressed inpatients to either a short-term running program or to a treatment-as-usual program, which included both physical and relaxation exercises. Patients in the running program increased their self-esteem and lowered their depressive symptoms whereas patients in the treatment-as-usual group showed no significant improvements.

Can clinical depression be lessened by any type of exercise, or is aerobic training necessary? Doyne et al. (1987) attempted to answer this question in a study that compared the therapeutic effects of running to those of weight lifting and found that the two exercise groups showed equally significant reductions in depression compared to the control group. Because the runners and the weight lifters showed the same results, the authors concluded that an aerobic effect was not necessary for exercise to have a therapeutic effect on depression.

Results of these studies indicate that both aerobic and nonaerobic exercise can reduce depression in normal and clinical populations alike. However, few health psychologists possess the training in exercise physiology and cardiovascular medicine to supervise exercise programs without the aid of physicians, athletic trainers, or others trained in this area.

Reduced Anxiety

Many people report that they exercise to feel more relaxed and less anxious. Does exercise play a role in anxiety reduction? The answer may depend on the type of anxiety. **Trait anxiety** is a general personality characteristic or trait that manifests itself as a more or less constant feeling of dread or uneasiness. **State anxiety** is a temporary, affective condition that stems from a specific situation. Feelings of worry or concern over a final examination or a job interview are examples of state anxiety. This type of anxiety is usually accompanied by physiological changes, such as increased perspiration and heart rate.

Among the first to investigate the effects of exercise on anxiety was William P. Morgan, a professor of physical education at the University of Wisconsin. In an early study, Morgan (1973) found that a program of strenuous physical activity reduced state anxiety for both men and women.

This finding inspired Bahrke and Morgan (1978) to compare anxiety levels in two different groups: people who exercise (an arousal state) and those who meditate (a relaxation state). They randomly assigned adult male volunteers who exercised regularly to an exercise group, a meditation group, or a control group. As expected, anxiety levels dropped for both the exercise group and the meditation group, but anxiety levels also declined for people in the control group who had merely rested in a recliner. This finding suggests that any one of several interventions may decrease state anxiety and that the crucial factor may simply be a change of pace.

In a later review of the literature, Morgan (1981) discussed studies that had used other procedures to reduce anxiety, including biofeedback, transcendental meditation, "time out" therapy, and even beer drinking in a pub atmosphere. Each of these interventions provides a change of pace and all have been demonstrated to be associated with reduced levels of state anxiety.

Both a change of pace and changes in body composition may contribute to reductions in anxiety. Norvell and Belles (1993) investigated the possible psychological and physical benefits of 4 months of weight training on law enforcement personnel and found that participants in a weight training group, compared with those in a control group, had significantly fewer psychological symptoms, including lower levels of anxiety. Norvell and Belles concluded that nonaerobic weight training can result in better overall psychological health and hypothesized that the changes in body appearance as well as the distraction from stressful work provided by weight training may have contributed to these psychological benefits.

In a review of the literature on the psychological benefits of running, Hinkle (1992) found that a program of aerobic exercise can be used in conjunction with therapeutic interventions to alleviate depression, decrease anxiety, and improve self-esteem. Additional research indicates that both aerobic and nonaerobic exercises are effective means of coping with anxiety, at least for some people. These benefits apply to older adults, and even a single exercise session can have positive effects and alleviate depression, fatigue, and anger (Pierce & Pate, 1994).

Although any one of a variety of interventions that break into a stressful daily routine may help relieve anxiety, physical activity seems particularly suitable. From a practical standpoint, walking and jogging have several advantages over most other forms of treatment: They can be done by almost anyone, nearly anywhere, and with very little expense.

Buffer against Stress

Can exercise reduce stress? More importantly, can it protect people against the harmful effects of stress? Research on the first question has generally produced an affirmative answer. For example, many people view exercise as the most effective strategy for reducing tension and eliminating a bad mood (Thayer, Newman, & McClain, 1994).

Answers to the second question are more difficult because a direct causal link between stress and subsequent illness has not yet been firmly established. Thus, no conclusive evidence exists for exercise's buffering effects. For example, some research (Sinyor, Golden, Steinert, & Seraganian, 1986) failed to find much stress-buffering benefit for exercise in healthy young men who began an aerobic exercise program or a weight-lifting intervention.

Other researchers have found some support for the hypothesis that exercise produces a buffering effect against stress-related effects. Exercise can moderate the effects of laboratory stressors, such as video games or mental arithmetic tasks, on cardiovascular reactivity in mildly hypertensive people (Perkins, Dubbert, Martin, Faulstich, & Harris, 1986). Under conditions of high stress, adolescents who exercise regularly had fewer physical illnesses than those who rarely exercised (Brown & Lawton, 1986). In addition, Roth and Holmes (1985) found that physically fit people reported fewer stress-related health problems and also fewer depressive symptoms than less active college students. For low-stressed students in this study, physical fitness had little buffering effect, largely because these students reported very few illnesses anyway. Thus, the combination of high stress and low fitness left college students vulnerable to becoming sick whereas low stress and high fitness resulted in better physical and psychological health.

Finally, Brown and Siegel (1988) and Brown (1991) found support for the hypothesis that physical activity provides benefits for people experiencing stressful life events. Using a prospective design, Brown and Siegel measured stressful life events, levels of exercise, and symptoms of such physical illness as sore throat, diabetes, and cancer in adolescent girls, grades 7 through 11. Their analysis revealed that physical illness symptoms declined as exercise levels increased. In other words, regular exercise buffered these adolescents against stress-related illnesses, a finding consistent with Brown's later research with college women. Brown's (1991) research revealed that, although life stress was strongly related to illness among women with low physical fitness, it had little harmful effect among women who had relatively high levels of fitness.

Exercise can also buffer women against the increases in blood pressure and heart rate that accompany stress. According to an experimental study (Rejeski, Thompson, Brubaker, & Miller, 1992), aerobic exercise can buffer the effects of stress in both European American and African American women.

These studies suggest that exercise is at least as powerful as personal hardiness (see Chapter 4) in buffering the negative effects of stress. Although evidence does not overwhelmingly favor the idea that exercise has protective effects, no study has shown that physical activity lowers one's resistance to stress or places one in greater jeopardy of developing physical symptoms.

Increased Self-Esteem

A fourth psychological factor that may relate to exercise is self-esteem. Do people who exercise regularly feel better about themselves? Do they have more self-confidence and improved feelings of self-worth? In the previous sections, we saw that exercise is associated with decreases in both depression and anxiety and that it may have some ability to buffer stress. This section considers the possibility that exercise might be related to increases in self-esteem.

Robert Sonstroem (1984) has provided an excellent review of the literature dealing with the relationship between exercise and self-esteem. Of the studies he examined, the majority found a significant positive relationship between self-esteem and exercise, but few had employed rigorous experimental designs. Although these studies suggest that exercise raises self-esteem, their methodological limitations prevent this conclusion. Even the experimental designs reviewed by Sonstroem cannot certify that exercise was the sole variable responsible for gains in self-esteem. Other possible factors in the treatment situation might include achievement of a goal, feelings of physical well-being, a sense of control over one's body, improved physical health, social interaction with fellow exercisers, experimental attention, or reinforcement from significant others. However, exercise advocates contend that it is not necessary to know the precise variables responsible for improved self-esteem as long as increased feelings of self-worth and self-confidence are associated with an exercise program.

People who regularly exercise often have better feelings about their body shape and physical health, feelings that may contribute to self-esteem. King, Taylor, Haskell, and DeBusk (1989) studied healthy, sedentary, middle-aged men and women who were randomly assigned to either a 6-month aerobic training group or a control group. Results showed that aerobically trained individuals were more satisfied with their level of fitness, weight, and body shape although they had not yet acquired increased levels of self-confidence. A study by Hogan (1989), however, found that fitness is related to feelings of self-confidence and self-discipline, and Ross and Hayes (1988) found that regular exercise improved subjective physical health, which in turn enhanced feelings of psychological well-being. As Sonstroem (1984) suggested, exercise may not be the direct cause of enhanced feelings of self-esteem, but it may contribute indirectly through weight loss, improved appearance, increased levels of physical energy, and greater self-discipline.

Evidence from these studies tends to support the hypothesis that regular exercise results in enhanced feelings of self-esteem. At the least, participation in an exercise program is strongly associated with feeling good about oneself.

SUMMARY OF EXERCISE BENEFITS

During the past 30 years, research has accumulated in support of the hypothesis that physical activity is associated with both cardiovascular health and improved psychological functioning. This section examined that research.

First, the evidence from numerous studies suggests that a sedentary lifestyle is dangerous to health. Berlin and Colditz (1990) found that the risk of death from coronary heart disease was nearly double for people engaged in sedentary occupations and the lack of physical activity off the job also contributed to premature death. Lissner and her colleagues (Lissner, Bengtsson, Björkelund, & Wedel, 1996) found that sedentary lifestyle contributed to mortality in women. They conducted a 20-year longitudinal study and found that women who were initially sedentary and those who decreased their activity level had higher mortality rates than active women

Table 16.2 Reasons for exercising and research supporting these reasons

Reasons for Exercising	Findings	Principal Source(s)
"Exercise helps people become physically fit."	Exercise improves several kinds of physical fitness, including cardiovascular fitness.	Lakka et al. (1994) Sandivk et al. (1993)
"I want to lose weight."	Exercise is a slow way to burn calories, but it may change setpoint.	Epstein et al. (1994, 1995) Bennett & Gurin (1982)
"It strengthens my heart."	Both the heart and the cardiovascular system benefit from exercise.	Kramsch et al. (1981)
"Exercise helps people live longer."	Exercise may increase longevity by 2 years or more.	Lee et al. (1995) Paffenbarger et al. (1993)
"I don't feel so depressed when I exercise," and "I just feel better."	Exercise can reduce anxiety, stress, and depression, as well as increase self-esteem.	International Society of Sports Psychology (1992) Sonstroem (1984)
"I'm addicted to it."	Exercise is not physiologically addictive, but some people become dependent on it.	McMurray, Sheps & Guinan (1984)

who maintained their activity levels. Interestingly, well-controlled studies have shown even greater benefits of regular exercise. Berlin and Colditz (1990, p. 626) concluded that "lack of physical activity is a potentially modifiable risk factor for coronary heart disease that should receive greater emphasis in the current efforts to reduce the impact of disease on society."

Harris, Caspersen, DeFriese, and Estes (1989) also reviewed the evidence on the role of physical activity in preventing coronary and other diseases in healthy adults and reported that exercise was a beneficial prophylactic for coronary heart disease, hypertension, obesity, noninsulin-dependent diabetes, and psychological well-being. In addition, the International Society of Sport Psychology issued a position statement delineating the benefits of physical activity on both short-term and long-term personal well-being and self-esteem. The Society also suggested that physical activity can reduce anxiety and stress and has a positive effect on hypertension, osteoporosis, and adult-onset diabetes. Moreover, regular exercise is as effective as any form of psychotherapy in lessening depression.

An earlier section of this chapter examined several reasons people exercise. Table 16.2 lists some of these reasons, summarizes research evidence, and cites at least one study pertaining to each reason.

In summary, regular physical activity contributes to several kinds of health, but it should not be viewed as a sole therapeutic strategy, especially for heart disease. As Gregory Curfman (1993a, p. 575) stated: "At the very least, exercise can improve functional work capacity and control body weight, benefits sufficient in themselves to encourage regular physical activity." However, Curfman also advised that "although the hypothesis that regular exercise can prevent coronary disease and prolong life is supported by many observational studies, it has not yet been unambiguously proved" (p. 575).

HAZARDS OF EXERCISE

Although exercise produces physiological and psychological benefits, it is also associated with some potential dangers. This section looks at the possible hazards of physical activity and examines the chances

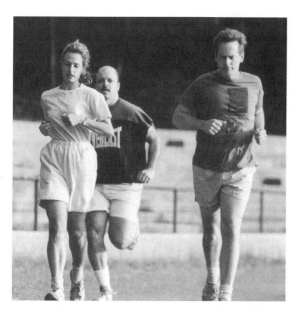

Exercise has health benefits, but it also provides risks.

the evidence is not clear. Certain research (Klonoff, Annechild, & Landrine, 1994; McMurray et al., 1984) raises doubt that endorphin levels increase in response to exercise. Other research (Pierce, Eastman, Tripathi, Olson, & Dewey, 1993) showed increases in beta-endorphin levels after exercise but failed to show that these increases have any relationship with exercise dependence.

Exercise can result in what some call *psychological addiction*—it can become a habitual behavior that is extremely resistant to extinction. Although the term *psychological addiction* is not universally accepted, William Glasser (1976) used this concept to describe several positive habits, including running and meditation. Glasser termed these habits *positive addictions* and argued that running and meditation are opposites of those habits usually considered negative addictions, such as taking drugs.

Even without evidence of a clear-cut neurochemical basis, some writers (Morgan, 1979; Sachs, 1981; Sachs & Pargman, 1979) have accepted the notion of running addiction. Sachs and Pargman (1979) even provided a definition of running addiction equivalent to the classic concept of addiction—that is, in terms of psychological and physiological mechanisms, regular usage, and withdrawal symptoms on cessation. Sachs (1982) discussed these withdrawal symptoms, such as anxiety, guilt, restlessness, tension, and irritability, maintaining that most were psychological. He also reported that runners can develop a strong commitment (addiction) to running in as little as 4 to 6 months. In addition, Conboy (1994) found that runners can become so psychologically dependent on running that they experience withdrawal symptoms on days when they do not run.

that people may become addicted to exercise, be injured, or even die while exercising.

Earlier, we cited evidence that exercise can reduce anxiety, stress, and depression as well as increase feelings of self-esteem. However, not all people who exercise regularly are models of psychological health. Many runners, in fact, probably have some history of psychopathology. One study (Colt, Dunner, Hall, & Fieve, 1981), for instance, found a higher incidence of a history of depressive disorders in runners than in a comparable group of nonrunners. In addition, for some highly active people, exercise assumes an almost addicitive importance.

EXERCISE ADDICTION

Some people become so dependent on exercise that it interferes with other parts of their lives, but the evidence is not clear concerning the underlying physiological mechanisms for exercise addiction. In Chapter 14, we saw that addictions produce tolerance, dependence, and physiological withdrawal symptoms. For exercise to produce physical addiction, a neurochemical must be involved. Although some researchers have speculated that vigorous and prolonged aerobic exercise can increase endorphins,

Running addiction is not always a positive habit. Morgan (1979) cited injuries as one negative consequence of the reluctance or inability to stop physical activity. Many injuries sustained during running or jogging result from improper footwear, but some are due to overuse of tendons, bones, and muscles. Morgan compared the process through which overuse develops to the development of other negative addictions. Initially, the tolerance for running is low, and it has many unpleasant side effects. But persistence eases the unpleasant aspects, and the pleasure of meeting goals becomes a powerful reinforcer.

Like most social drinkers who have a casual, non-obsessive relationship with alcohol, most runners are able to incorporate running into their lives without drastic changes in lifestyle. Other runners, however, cannot. Those who continue to increase their running must make changes in their lives to accommodate the time required to exercise. Morgan (1979) called these runners *negatively addicted*. One aspect of this addiction is increased neglect of family and job responsibilities due to the time and commitment required for running. A second facet of running addiction is a progressive self-absorption, with a great deal of concentration on internal experiences.

For Morgan, a third criterion of running addiction is the continuation of running after medical orders to stop. In this respect the addicted runner behaves very much like the anorexic or the alcoholic, continuing a behavior that is harmful or even self-destructive. Addicted runners, in fact, have often been compared to anorexics. Thinness is the most obvious characteristic common to the two groups, but it is by no means the only one. A report by Yates, Leehey, and Shisslak (1983) looked at the similarity between anorexic women and addicted male runners (called "obligatory runners") and found that the two groups were alike in the need for body control, the need for mastery of the body, unusually high expectations of self, tolerance or denial of physical discomfort and pain, and a single-minded commitment to endurance. In addition, both the anorexic and the obligatory runner were preoccupied with exercise and body image.

In surveying runners, Kiernan, Rodin, Brownell, Wilmore, and Crandall (1992) found they had a preoccupation with weight; 8% of the male and 24% of the female runners showed symptoms of eating disorders. In addition, male runners showed a positive relationship between symptoms of eating disorders and mileage run per week. Indeed, physical activity may play an intimate part in the development of eating disorders. By studying women hospitalized for eating disorders, Davis, Kennedy, Ravelski, and Dionne (1994) found that 78% of the patients had engaged in excessive exercise, with 60% involved in competitive athletics. Davis et al. concluded that for a majority of women with eating disorders, exercise plays an integral role in the development and maintenance of these disorders.

Additional support for the relationship between exercising and problem behavior came from Davis, Brewer, and Ratusny (1993), who developed the Commitment to Exercise Scale, which yields an Obligatory factor and a Pathological factor. Obligatory exercisers engage in activity because they believe their well-being is dependent on their exercising, whereas Pathological exercisers continue to exercise in the face of adverse circumstances, such as injuries, or who permit their activity to take precedence over other aspects of their lives. The findings of Davis et al. were consistent with those of Yates et al. (1983) in that both showed male and female committed exercisers to be preoccupied with weight control and to have an excess of eating disorders. In addition, the men in the Davis study tended to be perfectionists, obsessive, and compulsive.

Like a drug addict, the obligatory runner is willing to endure discomfort and social neglect for the sensations obtained from the running experience. Perhaps this fanaticism can be best expressed in the words of one such runner:

> One day last spring I was having an exceptionally good run. I was running about 10 miles a day at that time and on this particular day I had decided to extend my workout. I was around the 14-mile point and I was preparing to cross a one-lane bridge when all of a sudden a large cement mixer turned the corner and began to cross the bridge. I never thought for a second about stopping and letting the truck pass. I simply continued and said to myself, "Come on you son-of-a-bitch and I'll split you right down the middle—there will be concrete all over the road!" The driver slammed on the brakes and swerved to the side as I sailed by. That was really scary afterward, but at the time I really felt good. I have felt equally strong and indestructible many times since, but never have taken on a cement truck again. (Morgan, 1979, pp. 63, 67)

INJURIES FROM EXERCISE

Excluding head-to-head challenges with cement trucks, what are the chances of experiencing injuries from running? Many people with a regular exercise program accept minor injuries and soreness as an almost inevitable component of regular exercise.

WOULD YOU BELIEVE . . . ?

Misunderstandings about Exercise

Would you believe that exercise does not increase appetite? Although some people believe that exercise makes them hungry, such a belief—like several others regarding exercise—is not based on scientific evidence.

Because exercise requires energy and energy is obtained through food, exercise should logically increase one's appetite for food. In fact, only very light, brief exercise and very heavy exercise increase appetite. Moderate, sustained exercise decreases appetite. Decrease of appetite is associated with most aerobics programs and tends to last for about as long as the exercise lasted. For this reason, Cooper (1982) advised people wishing to lose weight to do their aerobic exercise in the late afternoon so their appetite for dinner would be decreased.

Very heavy, sustained exercise, such as long-distance running, does increase appetite but not immediately after the exercise. Because such exercise uses many calories, this increase in appetite is part of the body's regulation system. But this system apparently works imperfectly. Many marathon runners must force themselves to eat adequate calories.

Some evidence suggests that exercise affects obese people and thin people differently. In a review study, Hill, Drougas, and Peters (1994) reported that obese people tend to eat less during exercise periods whereas thin people eat more. Even when the taste of food was greatly enhanced, obese women did not increase their food intake. Nor is this finding limited to humans. Hill et al. also reported on a study showing that animals will almost never take in more calories than they expend through exercise. These findings suggest that fat people should not avoid exercise out of fear of increasing their appetite and adding unwanted extra pounds.

Would you believe that exercise is not an effective method of spot reduction? Despite some exercise promoters' claims, a particular calisthenic exercise will not reduce fat in a particular part of the body. Such a belief is one of the most appealing and enduring of all exercise myths. Unfortunately, it is not true. Muscle and fat have little to do with one another, and it is possible to have both in the same spot. Gwinup, Chelvam, and Steinberg (1971) measured the amount of fat and muscle on the arms of tennis players. Not surprisingly, they found that the playing arm had more muscle than the nonplaying arm. But interestingly, the fat content of the two arms was equal. The researchers

---

However, irregular exercise produces even more injuries and more discomfort, with "weekend athletes" accounting for a disproportional number of injuries.

Several factors can decrease the probability of injury. First, proper running shoes are a necessity for running, jogging, or even exercise walking (Cooper, 1970, 1982). Second, appropriate equipment and properly fitted clothing can decrease the likelihood of injury. Also, supervised training can decrease the chances of injury by preventing improperly performed exercise or an overly ambitious program. Strenuous exercise, especially for people who have been sedentary, can be a danger. For such people and for those who have been diagnosed as being at risk for coronary heart disease, supervised exercise is a wise precaution.

Injuries, however, are common. Koplan et al. (1982) surveyed a sample of participants in a 10-kilometer race and found that about a third of the runners had sustained some sort of musculoskeletal injury during the previous year and that the proba-

bility of injury went up significantly with increases in weekly running mileage. Pate and Macera (1994) reviewed the literature on exercise and musculoskeletal injuries and reported that 35% to 65% of runners had an injury during the past year and that the farther people ran each week, the more likely they were to sustain an injury. However, contrary to expectations, injury rates among runners did not increase with age.

OTHER HEALTH RISKS

Besides muscular and skeletal injuries, avid exercisers encounter a number of other health hazards. Heat, cold, dogs, and drivers can all be sources of danger.

During exercise, body temperature rises. It can be maintained at 104°F with no danger (Pollock et al., 1978). Fluid intake before, after, and even during exercise can protect against overheating by allowing cooling through sweating. However, conditions of extremely high air temperature, high humidity, and

concluded that the concept of spot reduction is invalid because the playing arm of a tennis player is exercised vigorously but with no loss of fat.

Reduction of fat happens in some spots more than others. When weight is lost, both fat and muscle tissue are depleted. If a person exercises during weight reduction, muscle tissue is built up while fat is being lost. Spot reduction appears to be the result, because fat tends to be lost from the places where it was most abundant. Therefore, the hips, thighs, or stomach may reduce more quickly than other spots during a program of diet and exercise, but this is not due to the effect of spot reducing exercises. Most exercise physiologists believe that fat distribution on the body is under strong genetic control, so some spots may never look like the ideal.

A person's belief in spot reducing can be hazardous, both physically and financially. Certain calisthenics that have been promoted as spot-reducing aids have the potential to cause injury. These include straight-leg sit-ups, deep knee bends, and any exercise involving bouncing stretches. Such exercises should be avoided for spot reducing or any other purpose. The financial hazards come from the purchase of exercise equipment and enrollment in expensive health clubs that promise spot reduction. No exercise can cause a loss of fat in a particular spot, so equipment that promises to do so is deceptive.

Would you believe that pain and injury during exercise is nature's way of telling you to quit? Although some people believe that exercise should hurt and that injury is no reason to stop or even slow down,

this belief can be dangerous and may lead to further injuries and even to permanent disability.

Pain is a message from the body that there is something wrong. Ignoring pain messages often results in more pain and even further injury. Those who exercise regularly face a dilemma. Minor injuries often occur for people who exercise for fitness or for training. Unfortunately, their desire to retain the effects of fitness training creates a strong temptation to ignore the pain and continue to exercise. Although the wise exerciser would seek professional advice about pain, few people do, probably because they do not want to be told to stop exercising. Nevertheless, prudent advice would be to stop exercising if the pain gets worse during exercise.

sunlight can combine to raise body temperature and prevent sweat from evaporating from the skin surface. If the body is prevented from cooling itself, dangerous overheating may occur. Cooper and Cooper (1972) recommended against outdoor aerobic exercise in heat exceeding 95°F, especially when humidity is above 80%.

Cold temperatures can also be dangerous for outdoor exercising, but proper clothing can provide protection. Layered clothing for the body, gloves, hat, and even a face mask can protect against temperatures of 20°F and below (Pollock et al., 1978). Temperatures below zero, especially when combined with wind, can be dangerous even to people who are not exercising.

DEATH DURING EXERCISE

Many patients who have had heart attacks are put into an exercise program, and such programs generally include close supervision. Although these coro-

nary patients are at an elevated risk during exercise, the cardiovascular benefit they receive from exercising ordinarily outweighs the risk. Nevertheless, exercise programs for those who have been diagnosed as having coronary heart disease should be undertaken only with a physician's permission and under the supervision of specialists in cardiac rehabilitation.

What about people who have no known disease? Is it possible for a person who looks and feels well to die unexpectedly during exercise? Yes — but it is also possible to die unexpectedly while watching TV or sleeping. One study (Thompson, Funk, Carleton, & Sturner, 1982) examined the causes and frequency of sudden death during jogging as well as during nonvigorous activities. This study found that the probability of sudden death increased during exercise; the risk of dying during jogging was seven times greater than the risk of dying during nonvigorous activities. This statistic seems to be an indictment of exercise, but the causes of sudden death during exercise should first be examined.

Thompson (1982) reviewed a number of studies on sudden death during exercise and found that the majority of these deaths were due to atherosclerotic cardiovascular disease. In many cases, the people who died had known of their disease. However, the coronary arteries may narrow substantially with no apparent symptoms of cardiovascular disease. This condition would likely be diagnosed during an exercise stress test, but not all people who begin and continue an exercise program have had such tests. Testing is highly recommended for people over 40 years old who plan to start an exercise program, especially if they are overweight, smoke, or have a family history of coronary disease. The majority of cardiovascular dangers discussed by Thompson were due to either diagnosed or undiagnosed cardiovascular disease.

David Siscovick and his colleagues (Siscovick, Weiss, Fletcher, & Lasky, 1984; Siscovick, Weiss, Hallstrom, Inui, & Peterson, 1982) have also investigated the relationship between cardiac arrest and level of physical health. In agreement with data from other research, Siscovick and his colleagues found that physically active men were five times more likely to experience cardiac arrest during vigorous activity than they were at other times, assuming that they spent an equal amount of time in exercise as they did in all other endeavors. In other words, although conditioned athletes like Jim Fixx may experience cardiac arrest at any time, they are somewhat more likely to die during exercise.

In contrast to physically fit people, those with low levels of habitual exercise are much more likely to have a fatal or nonfatal heart attack during vigorous activity. Siscovick et al. (1982, 1984) found that men who do not exercise regularly were far more likely to die during exercise than physically fit men. Also, Mittleman et al. (1993) interviewed more than 1,200 patients who had very recently suffered myocardial infarction and found that 4.4% of them reported heavy exertion within 1 hour before their heart attack. However, people who had a history of exercising less than once a week were more than 40 times as likely to have a heart attack during exercise than patients who had exercised five or more times a week. Using a very similar design, Willich et al. (1993) interviewed male and female patients who had recently suffered a myocardial infarction and asked about their physical exertion at the time of their heart attack. Although 7% of these patients had been engaging in some form of physical activity at the onset of their heart attack, Willich et al. found that people who did not exercise regularly were much more likely than frequent exercisers to experience a heart attack while engaging in physical exertion.

By themselves, these findings reveal little about the benefits or hazards of regular, habitual exercise. They merely suggest that heart attacks are more likely to occur during periods of exertion than during times of inactivity. However, Siscovick et al. (1982, 1984) also reported that the overall cardiac risk for active people was only about half what it was for sedentary individuals. These findings suggest that habitually inactive people should not suddenly begin vigorous exercise, and that regular exercise protects against death from heart attack.

HOW MUCH IS ENOUGH BUT NOT TOO MUCH?

Research has indicated that some amount of exercise is inversely related to a variety of disorders and diseases and also that some amount of exercise may be hazardous. These disparate findings raise the question, How much is enough but not too much?

During the 1980s, many people, perhaps led by devoted runners and writers such as Jim Fixx, believed that they had to achieve aerobic fitness through vigorous exercise if they were to enhance their health. At the same time, Ralph Paffenbarger and his colleagues were reporting that high levels of physical activity (up to 3,500 kcal expended per week) were more beneficial than moderate levels. However, Paffenbarger counted all physical activity, not merely vigorous exercise. Also at this time, the Framingham study concluded that high-level exercise could not be justified. Other researchers have reported that walking is sufficient to produce the desired health benefits. For example, Duncan, Gordon, and Scott (1991) found that previously sedentary young women could reduce their coronary risk factors through 45 minutes of brisk walking 5 days a week.

Which is more important: intensity or frequency of exercise? Investigators are still not certain whether the intensity of exercise or the total expenditure of kilocalories is the chief contributor to a reduction in coronary risk factors. However, the length of time one has been exercising is related to improved cardiovascular health. A study by Scragg, Stewart, Jackson, and Beaglehole (1987) found that physical activity was associated with lower CHD and death rates for both men and women, but only for people who had been exercising for 5 years or more. Scragg et al. estimated that 43% of coronary events could be explained by a lack of exercise and suggested that inactivity may be as important as hypertension and cigarette smoking as a risk factor in coronary heart disease.

A report from the Multiple Risk Factor Intervention Trial (MRFIT) (Leon, Connett, Jacobs, & Rauramaa, 1987) suggested that leisure-time physical activity is associated with lower rates of CHD and sudden deaths. However, high levels of exercise were no more effective than moderate levels in preventing death from heart disease. Recall that MRFIT participants were middle-aged men at high risk for coronary heart disease at the beginning of the study. A 7-year follow-up of these men revealed that those with moderate levels of activity had only 63% as many fatal heart attacks and sudden deaths as men with the lowest levels of physical activity. Men in the highest-level exercise group also had fewer coronary events than those in the low-activity group, but high levels of leisure-time physical activity offered no advantages over moderate levels.

Is exercise beneficial or hazardous to coronary health? Physician Gregory Curfman (1993b) believes that it may be both, but he commented that "exercise performed at frequent intervals over a long time span provides protection against both the development of coronary artery disease and the triggering of myocardial infarction by strenuous exertion" (p. 1731). Citing the studies by Mittleman et al. (1993) and Willich et al. (1993), Curfman warned that sudden, heavy exertion by sedentary people may put them at risk of heart attack.

Perhaps the latest word on the question of how much is enough but not too much comes from a 20-member panel of experts who reviewed the evidence on this issue and presented its recommendations in a recent article in the *Journal of the American Medical Association* (Pate et al., 1995). This panel recommended that every adult should accumulate 30 minutes of moderate physical activity a day, or at least on most days.

These experts also suggested that sedentary people should begin a program of moderate, regular physical activity.

> If Americans who lead sedentary lives would adopt a more active lifestyle, there would be enormous benefit to the public's health and to individual well-being. An active lifestyle does not require a regimented, vigorous exercise program. Instead, small changes that increase daily physical activity will enable individuals to reduce their risk of chronic disease and may contribute to enhanced quality of life. (Pate et al., 1995, p. 406)

EXERCISE MAINTENANCE

Adherence to nearly all medical regimens is a serious problem (see Chapter 8), and exercise is no exception. In a review article, Rodin and Salovey (1989) reported that 70% of the people in the United States engage in no regular exercise and that only 30% of people who begin an exercise program continue for an average of 3.5 years. Exercise is frequently prescribed in cardiac rehabilitation and diabetes treatment. However, dropout rates for both therapies are notoriously high.

Several authorities (Dishman, 1982; Martin & Dubbert, 1985) have estimated that about half the participants in therapeutic exercise programs drop out within 6 months. Dropout rates in prescribed exercise regimens are about the same as those found in other compliance studies, and they closely parallel the relapse rates reported in smoking and alcohol cessation programs; that is, compliance rates are probably below 20% after 3 years.

PREDICTING DROPOUTS

What factors predict the exercise dropouts? Martin and Dubbert (1985) reviewed the research on this question and divided the relevant factors into participant variables, social-environmental variables, and exercise program variables.

Participant variables include preexisting psychological, behavioral, and biological factors. Interestingly, one participant variable that does not appear to relate to adherence is the person's attitude toward physical activity. Sedentary people, it seems, often report favorable attitudes toward exercise. However, low self-motivation, depression, denial of the seriousness of one's heart disease, and low self-efficacy for maintaining an exercise program all predict quitting exercise. Also, smokers, blue-collar workers, obese people, individuals with the Type A behavior pattern, and those with inactive jobs and inactive leisure-time pursuits were most likely to drop out of prescribed exercise programs.

Among the social-environmental factors Martin and Dubbert found to relate to dropout were lack of social support from spouses and others, family problems, change of job or residence, and job-related duties that conflicted with exercise. Among the exercise program factors, group exercise programs usually have lower dropout rates than individual programs.

INCREASING MAINTENANCE

Identifying the correlates of noncompliance is the first step toward reducing dropout rates in health-related exercise programs. The second step is establishing an intervention strategy for all patients, with special attention for those at greatest risk of dropping out. Behavior modification methods have had some success in reducing the rate of exercise dropouts. Behavioral programs ordinarily use a multimodal approach that relies on reinforcement, contracting, self-monitoring, instruction, modeling, goal setting, increased self-efficacy, relapse prevention, and a variety of other strategies. Most of these have been discussed in earlier chapters and need no additional elaboration here.

Reviewing the research, Martin and Dubbert (1985) found that most of these behavioral strategies have been used to improve adherence to exercise programs. In addition, they found more success with the programs that increase social support than with those that do not. Moreover, an enthusiastic therapist who also participates in the exercise program is likely to reduce dropout rates. Although these strategies have demonstrated some success, especially when used in combination, maintenance remains a serious problem in most health-related exercise programs.

CHAPTER SUMMARY

All physical activity can be subsumed under one or more of five basic categories: isometric, isotonic, isokinetic, anaerobic, and aerobic. Each of these five exercises types has advantages and disadvantages for improving physical fitness. People exercise for a variety of reasons, including muscle strength, muscle endurance, flexibility, cardiorespiratory or aerobic fitness, and weight control.

Most research on the health benefits of exercise has concentrated on the relationship between physical activity and coronary risk factors. Evidence strongly suggests a relationship between physical activity and reduced incidence of coronary heart disease, and many investigators are willing to accept the relationship as a causal one. This relationship suggests that a regimen of moderate, brisk, physical activity should be prescribed as one of several components in a program of coronary health. In addition to improving cardiovascular health, regular physical activity may protect against some kinds of cancer; it may also help prevent bone density loss and thus lower one's risk of osteoporosis.

Besides improving physical fitness, regular exercise can confer certain psychological benefits. Specifically, research has demonstrated that aerobic and nonaerobic exercises can decrease depression, reduce anxiety, provide a buffer against the harmful effects of stress, and enhance feelings of self-esteem among exercisers.

Several hazards accompany both regular and sporadic exercise. Some runners appear to be addicted to exercise, becoming obsessed with body image and fearful of being prevented from their exercise regimen. Injuries are frequent among veteran runners, but the most serious hazard is sudden death while exercising. However, people who exercise regularly are much less likely than sporadic exercisers to die of heart attack during heavy physical exertion.

Exercise is frequently prescribed as therapy, especially for coronary heart disease. Unfortunately, dropout rates are about as high for this medical recommendation as they are for others. Behavioral interventions have had some limited success in improving compliance with health-related exercise programs.

SUGGESTED READINGS

Blair, S. N. (1994). Physical activity, fitness, and coronary heart disease. In C. Bouchard, R. J. Shephard, & T. Stephens (Eds.), *Physical activity, fitness, and health: International proceedings and consensus statement* (pp. 579–590). Champaign, IL: Human Kinetics. Steven Blair reviews the literature on the effects of physical activity on heart disease and concludes that a sedentary lifestyle and poor physical fitness are important risk factors for heart disease.

Cooper, K. H. (1982). *The aerobic program for total well-being.* New York: Evans. By the author who made aerobics popular in the United States, this book stresses balance in a total fitness program.

Fixx, J. F. (1980). *Jim Fixx's second book of running.* New York: Random House. This is a well-written book by one of the people who helped popularize running and jogging. This book supplements Fixx's first book, which turned out not to be the *complete* book of running.

Forbes, G. B. (1992). Exercise and lean weight: The influence of body weight. *Nutrition Reviews, 50,* 147–161. In this review article, physician Gilbert Forbes discusses evidence that regular exercise can produce modest gains in lean body mass while reducing body fat.

McAuley, E. (1994). Physical activity and psychosocial outcomes. In C. Bouchard, R. J. Shephard, & T. Stephens (Eds.), *Physical activity, fitness, and health: International proceedings and consensus statement* (pp. 551–568). Champaign, IL: Human Kinetics. An authority on the psychosocial outcomes of exercise, Edward McAuley reviews the literature and concludes that the area still suffers from methodologically weak designs, imprecise outcomes measures, lack of sufficient follow-up, and confusion between physical fitness and physical activity.

Sacks, M. H. (1993). Exercise for stress control. In D. Goleman & J. Gurin (Eds.), *Mind/body medicine: How to use your mind for better health* (pp. 316–327). Yonkers, NY: Consumer Reports Books. Sacks takes a personal perspective in presenting the benefits of exercise as a means of stress control in this nontechnical chapter.

4 Looking toward the Future

17 Health Psychology: Growth and Future Challenges

Americans are becoming increasingly health conscious, and this concern has appeared as national policy as well as in individual behavior. On a personal level, people's interest in health and their knowledge of the harmful consequences of certain health-related behaviors have never been greater. Many people now realize that their physical well-being is not solely in the hands of medical professionals and that they have an important share of the responsibility in maintaining their own health. They are aware of the dangers of smoking, abusing alcohol, eating improperly, and not exercising regularly. They know that they should learn to cope better with stress, make and keep regular medical and dental appointments, and follow the advice of their health care professionals.

This knowledge does not always translate into action, and people have difficulty in making changes in their behavior and lifestyle. But over the past 25 years, U.S. residents have managed to make some healthy changes in their behavior. The percentage of smokers has fallen, the amount of alcohol consumed has decreased, the use of seatbelts and other safety measures has increased, and illegal drug use has declined (Johnston et al., 1994b; USDHHS, 1994b). People have started to become more conscious of what they eat and to consume more fruit and vegetables and less red meat, whole milk, butter, and sugar (USBC, 1995).

These positive changes are reflected in declining mortality for heart disease, stroke, and accidents, but unhealthy and risky behaviors continue to contribute to an increasing rate of cancer and chronic obstructive pulmonary disease. This chapter looks at future health goals and the role and status of health psychology in the health care system; it also examines some of the principal challenges facing the field.

HEALTHIER PEOPLE

An example of the influence of health-consciousness on a national policy level is the *Healthy People 2000* report (USDHHS, 1990c). The subtitle of this report was *National Health Promotion and Disease Objectives,* and the report detailed 3 broad goals, 22 priority areas, and 300 main objectives for improving the health of people in the United States. The broad goals included increasing the span of healthy life, reducing health disparities among Americans, and achieving access to preventive services for all people in the United States.

INCREASING THE SPAN OF HEALTHY LIFE

Increasing the span of healthy life is a different goal from increasing life expectancy. Rather than striving for longer lives, many people are now trying to

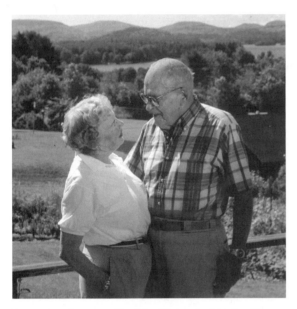

Increasing the span of healthy life is a goal for health psychologists.

increase their number of well-years. Kaplan and Bush (1982) defined a **well-year** as "the equivalent of a year of completely well life, or a year of life free of dysfunction, symptoms, and health-related problems" (p. 64). This concept has grown in acceptability since 1946, when the World Health Organization charter defined health in terms of positive states of mental and physical well-being. Both Russell (1986, 1987) and Kaplan and Anderson (1988) have advocated the well-year as the preferred unit of measurement for assessing the effectiveness of health programs.

Robine and Ritchie (1991) proposed the concept of health expectancy, defined as that period of life a person spends free from disability. These researchers found that life expectancy at age 65 is around 14 years for men and 19 years for women, but health expectancy is only 8 years for men and 10 years for women, leaving both men and women with a discrepancy that represents years of disability. This discrepancy is larger when the richest and poorest segments of the population are compared: wealthy people not only live longer but also have more years of healthy life. In addition, the disorders that shorten life are not necessarily the same ones that compromise health. For example, circulatory disor-

ders head both lists, but disorders producing restricted movement and respiratory disorders are responsible for producing lost health expectancy, and cancer and accidents are the source of lost life expectancy. Therefore, interventions aimed at increasing life expectancy will not necessarily improve health expectancy.

The need to increase the health of the elderly is important not only to improve their quality of life but also to help manage health care costs. Because of their tendency to have chronic illnesses, elderly people use health care services more heavily than younger people; the rate of physician contacts is twice as high for those over 75 as for those between ages 15 and 44 (National Center for Health Statistics, 1994). In an editorial in the *New England Journal of Medicine,* Andrew Kramer (1995) advocated a change in emphasis for health care for the elderly. Rather than concentrating on acute care delivered in hospitals, Karmer argued for the promotion of primary care and long-term care, strategies that might help improve quality of life for the elderly.

In addition, life expectancy may not continue to increase in the next century as it has in the past century. Although life expectancy has increased steadily over the past 100 years, Olshansky, Carnes, and Cassel (1993) expressed doubts that increases will continue. Without some breakthrough that changes the process of aging, life expectancy is not likely to increase much beyond 85 years. However, people's later years can include better health and thus a better quality of life, which would benefit both the individual and the health care system.

REDUCING HEALTH DISPARITIES

The goal of reducing health disparities among Americans is an imperative item on the agenda of U.S. health care. The United States does a poorer job of dispensing health care to its citizens than any other industrialized country, and this problem is reflected in many health statistics. For example, the United States ranks 21st in the world in infant mortality, 17th in life expectancy for men, and 16th in life expectancy for women (Consumers Union, 1992a).

Social and economic factors contribute to these low rankings, but the underlying reasons for the relationship between socioeconomic factors and health are complex (Anderson & Armstead, 1995). This complex relationship includes education, income, occupational status, and ethnic background, and these factors are not separate. In the United States, African Americans, Hispanic Americans, and Native Americans have lower average educational levels and incomes than European Americans and Asian Americans. Thus, the factor of ethnicity is difficult to separate from income and education, complicating the interpretation of the underlying reasons for health disparities among people of different ethnic backgrounds.

For example, African Americans, compared with European Americans, have shorter life expectancy as well as a higher infant mortality rate, more homicide deaths, increased cardiovascular disease rate, higher cancer mortality, and more tuberculosis and diabetes (USDHHS, 1995). Gorman (1991) contended that poor medical treatment and lack of health education was responsible for 60% of the disparity but that discrimination in health care provision is also a factor. She cited examples of Blacks receiving less aggressive treatment than Whites for the same conditions and symptoms.

Gorman's contention of discrimination in health care was substantiated by a study about seeking and receiving medical care for symptoms of coronary heart disease (Crawford, McGraw, Smith, McKinlay, & Pierson, 1994). No difference appeared between African Americans and European Americans in willingness to seek care when they experienced symptoms; both were equally likely to seek care. However, the African American patients were less likely to be referred to a cardiologist than were the European American patients.

Health discrepancies also exist when poor African Americans and poor European Americans are compared. Anderson and Armstead (1995) suggested that residential environments may partially explain the disadvantage of poor African Americans — poor Blacks and poor Whites tend to live in different circumstances. A majority of poor European Americans live in areas that are not classified as poverty areas whereas a small minority of poor African Americans lived outside poverty areas. Such residential isolation results in extreme segregation and concentration of African Americans in substandard housing in neighborhoods with violence and without social ties. These circumstances relate to a variety of health risks.

African Americans lack both general and special physician services (Pinkney, 1994), a condition that led *Healthy People 2000* to establish the specific goal of an increased number of ethnic minorities in the health professions. A subsequent progress report (USDHHS, 1995) indicated that the percentage of African American health care professionals has increased slightly from 5% to 5.9%, but still well short of the goal of 8%.

Low economic status and the lack of access to medical care affect Native Americans at least as strongly as African Americans. The Indian Health Service supports health care for Native Americans, but the level of funding is only half that spent on other Americans (Japsen, 1994). This situation may be a factor in the shorter life expectancy, higher mortality rate, higher infant mortality, and higher rates of infectious illness for Native Americans compared with European Americans (Grossman, Krieger, Sugarman, & Forquera, 1994).

Socioeconomic status, however, is not the only answer to the question of discrepancy between Native Americans and European Americans. One study (Cheadle et al., 1994) showed that even with socioeconomic status adjusted, Native Americans had a higher prevalence of risk-taking behaviors and poorer health status than people who were not Native Americans. Native Americans, then, are one of the groups poorly served by the current system of health care and health education in the United States. *Healthy People 2000* includes specific goals to address health problems of Native Americans.

Many Hispanic Americans also suffer from low socioeconomic status and poor education (AMA Council on Scientific Affairs, 1991; Ginzberg, 1991), but not all groups of Hispanic Americans are equally affected and their health and longevity tend to vary accordingly. Cuban Americans generally have higher education and economic levels than Mexican Americans or Puerto Ricans; thus, Cuban Americans are more likely to have jobs that include health insurance as a benefit, making them more likely to have access to regular health care and physician visits (Treviño, Moyer, Valdez, & Stroup-Benham, 1991).

For Hispanic Americans without insurance coverage, their ethnic background and geographic location

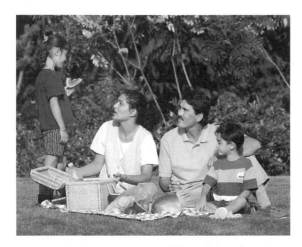

Hispanic Americans are comparable to European Americans on health and mortality measures.

may affect the health care they receive. Compared with Mexican Americans living near the U.S.-Mexican border, Puerto Ricans are more likely to live in places that offer better accessibility to Medicaid and thus more opportunity for frequent visits to physicians (AMA Council on Scientific Affairs, 1991). Puerto Ricans, however, are poorer than other Hispanic Americans (Marwick, 1991) and have higher levels of health problems (USDHHS, 1994b, 1995). Health problems of Puerto Ricans and other Hispanic Americans are the topic of over two dozen specific goals in *Healthy People 2000*.

Hispanic Americans fare about the same as or better than European Americans on health and mortality measures. Hispanic Americans have a lower death rate than European Americans (USDHHS, 1995), including death from heart disease, stroke, and lung cancer. These low death rates are puzzling, given the high rates of smoking, obesity, and hypertension among Hispanic Americans. The poor health habits of Hispanic Americans, combined with their low disease prevalence, may reflect a transition in which immigrants are adopting European American lifestyles but have not yet developed the chronic diseases typical of the United States. As Olivia Carter-Pokras of the National Center for Health Statistics (in Marwick, 1991, p. 181) said, "When Mexicans become Mexican Americans they become more like the rest of Americans," including their patterns of illness.

This same trend applies to all immigrant groups — those who adopt the lifestyle of the United States soon have the patterns of illness and death characteristic of the U.S. Asian Americans who have adopted Western habits increase their risks, but Asian Americans still have more favorable health status and life expectancy than other ethnic groups (USDHHS, 1995). Asian Americans have lower infant mortality, longer life expectancy, lower lung and breast cancer deaths, and lower cardiovascular death rates.

Low income has an obvious connection to lower standards of health care, and people without health insurance and access to a physician are at increased risk. However, universal access to health care does not remove the disparities among socioeconomic groups (Anderson & Armstead, 1995). Even in countries that have universal access to health care, health disparities between poor and wealthy people continue to exist, suggesting that factors other than receiving health care are involved in maintaining health.

Education may be one of those factors. Across ethnic groups, people who have higher educational and economic status have better health and longevity than those with lower education and income. An analysis of risk factors for chronic illness in African Americans, Native Americans, Asian Americans, and Hispanic Americans (Centers for Disease Control and Prevention, 1994b) showed that education alone is significantly related to risk factors for chronic disease. People with fewer than 12 years of education were more likely to follow unhealthy lifestyles than those with more than 12 years of schooling.

Increased risky behaviors and decreased health-protective behaviors appear to be another link between socioeconomic status and health (Anderson & Armstead, 1995). Lower socioeconomic status is related to increases in smoking and consumption of a high-fat diet and decreases in physical activity and knowledge about health. These situations have connections to a variety of disorders, which may explain at least part of the relationship between low socioeconomic status and poorer health.

Therefore, the goal of reducing the health disparities among Americans will require special efforts to serve the various ethnic and income groups that are poorly served by the U.S. health care system. Improved access to health care will eliminate some of the disparities, but changes in health-related behaviors and improved living conditions will also be necessary.

INCREASING ACCESS TO PREVENTIVE SERVICES

Most people would readily accept the notion that prevention is more effective than treatment in containing medical costs. A careful analysis, however, indicates that this is not always so. Louise Russell (1986) pointed out that "while prevention has great potential, it is neither riskless nor costless" (p. 109). Whether prevention saves money depends on the type of prevention and the target audience. *Primary prevention* consists of immunizations and programs that encourage lifestyle changes, and this type of prevention is usually a good bargain. As Leutwyler (1995) pointed out, programs that encourage people to quit smoking, eat properly, exercise, and moderate their drinking are generally low cost and have little potential to do harm. In addition, some of these targeted behaviors, such as smoking and inactivity, are risks for many health problems, and efforts oriented toward changing these behaviors can pay off by decreasing risks for several disorders (Winett, 1995). Immunizations have some potential for harm but remain good choices unless the risks from side effects of the immunization are comparable to the risk of catching the disease. Therefore, primary prevention efforts tend pose few risks and many potential benefits.

Secondary prevention consists of screening people at risk for developing a disease so as to find disease in its early and more treatable stages. Such efforts can cost more than treating people who develop the disease because many people may be at risk compared to the number who have developed the disease and who can be detected through screening. Based on the economic considerations of cost-benefit analysis—that is, how much money is spent and how much is saved—secondary prevention may not be the solution to the problem of rising health care costs (Leutwyler, 1995; Russell, 1986). Cost-benefit analyses have revealed that prevention efforts, such as control of hypertension, are no more cost effective than curative interventions, such as coronary

bypass operations, because many people who receive preventive care would not have developed heart disease. For those people who are at risk but who would not have developed heart disease, the money spent on treatment is wasted.

However, Russell (1986) argued that "good health does have intrinsic value and is worth paying for" (p. 112). By considering the benefits of good health and the economic benefits that are not directly tied to the cost of the medical procedure, she found that prevention has a clear advantage. Russell proposed that the value of health care interventions should be established on the basis of cost-effectiveness analysis rather than cost-benefit analysis. In *cost-effectiveness* analysis, all costs and benefits contribute to the evaluation, not just medical considerations.

This type of analysis, then, can incorporate the benefits of increased health as well as the benefits of avoiding pain, suffering, illness, and disability. If a program adds well-years to life, then cost-efficiency analysis can determine the cost per well-year. Such information can help individuals and policy makers decide which health programs offer the best outcomes (in terms of well-years) for the least cost. In these terms, the interventions that health psychologists provide can justify their costs (Sobel, 1995).

The *Healthy People 2000* goals, which are oriented toward prevention, incorporate both primary and secondary prevention efforts. The primary prevention goals include increasing physical activity, improving nutrition, decreasing tobacco use, decreasing alcohol and illegal drug use, increasing health education in schools and communities, increasing dental care, and increasing immunizations for a variety of childhood and adult diseases. Secondary prevention goals include testing homes for radon and lead as well as screening for a variety of other conditions. These screenings include testing newborns for genetic disorders, assessing adults (especially men) for hypertension, measuring adults for high serum cholesterol, testing women over age 40 for breast cancer, testing at-risk individuals for HIV, and assessing children and the elderly for vision and hearing problems.

The *Healthy People 2000* report set national priorities for health care and prevention. A review of progress toward these goals (USDHHS, 1995) indicated that 8% of the goals had been met or exceeded by 1994, and progress had occurred for 41% of other goals. Unfortunately, movement away from 16% of the goals has occurred, and the remaining goals show mixed patterns of change or no change from the initial levels.

These priorities not only reflect the public's increasing interest and concern over health but also provide a guide to health care professionals, including health psychologists. To become part of the future health care system, psychologists must be able to provide research and services that further these goals.

THE PROFESSION OF HEALTH PSYCHOLOGY

One important goal of health psychology is to help translate knowledge into action. The field of health psychology rests on the premise that psychology can contribute to health in four major ways: (1) accumulating more information on the correlates of health and illness, (2) helping to promote and maintain health, (3) contributing to the prevention and treatment of illness, and (4) helping to formulate health policy and promote the health care system (Matarazzo, 1982).

The first contribution—accumulating more information on the correlates of health and illness—is a necessary but not sufficient condition for improving health. Although psychology has made substantial contributions toward the body of health knowledge, much of this information is being gathered by other disciplines, such as epidemiology, immunology, dietetics, sociology, and medical anthropology. Psychology's historical involvement in changing human behavior places it in a position to contribute in two other ways: by helping with the maintenance and enhancement of health and with the prevention and treatment of illness. It does so by helping the individual eliminate unhealthy practices and incorporate healthy behaviors into an ongoing lifestyle.

The prevalence of such chronic disorders as asthma, arthritis, Alzheimer's disease, AIDS, cancer, cardiovascular disease, diabetes, headaches, and stress has created a role for psychology in the field of health. As the scientific study of behavior, psychol-ogy can contribute to disease prevention and health enhancement through the efforts of professional practitioners. The preparation of these professionals includes grounding in psychological principles and substantial training in neurology, endocrinology, immunology, public health, epidemiology, and other medical subspecialties.

PREPARATION OF HEALTH PSYCHOLOGISTS

In May 1983, a group of more than 50 leaders in health psychology met at the Arden House in Harriman, New York, to discuss standards for training future health psychologists (Stone et al., 1987). Participants at this meeting—formally known as the National Working Conference on Education and Training in Health Psychology—faced two major issues (Boll, 1987). The first was to define the core program in psychology to which health psychologists should be exposed. The second was to decide whether health psychologists should be prepared to deliver health services. If so, health psychology should establish two training tracks: one for health service providers and another for researchers and teachers.

With regard to the first issue, participants at the conference generally agreed that health psychologists should receive a solid core of training in such areas as advanced research and experimental design; methodology and statistics; the biological, cognitive, and social bases of behavior; and individual differences. They agreed that programs called *health psychology* must include this core of psychology as a minimum standard (Boll, 1987).

With regard to the second issue, participants had some disagreement. Some argued that not every health psychologist is a health care provider and therefore, not every student needs to be trained to deliver services. Other participants, however, contended that health psychologists need a strong clinical background to be employable in hospital settings. This second group of participants argued for a scientist/practitioner model based on the 1949 Boulder Conference that has guided the training of clinical psychologists. During the 1980s, about half the existing graduate training programs in health psychology required the training necessary to deliver psychological services (Istvan & Hatton, 1987), and that percentage increased slightly during the 1990s (Belar, 1996).

The participants at Arden House faced little disagreement on the issue of whether health psychologists must be trained at least to the doctoral level, but there was some disagreement over the necessity of postdoctoral training (Boll, 1987). Most leaders in the field have recommended postdoctoral training, with at least two years of specialized training in health psychology to follow a Ph.D. or Psy.D. in psychology (Belar, 1987; Friedman, 1987; Matarazzo, 1987a; Sechrest, 1987; Sheridan et al., 1988). This training might include some combination of internships and residencies in which health psychologists would learn to provide treatment in hospitals and other traditional health care settings.

Considering the expanding employment opportunities for psychologists in health care settings, Cynthia Belar (1996) has called for continuing education for psychologists so that they can develop new competencies and specializations to provide these types of services. The growing market for psychologists in health care and the shrinking, competitive market for psychologists providing traditional mental health care make practice in health psychology attractive to both new and continuing practitioners. Belar maintained that training psychologists for new specializations in health care should be a priority for the profession and warned that psychologists should be careful to be thoroughly trained before they take jobs providing health care. She also stressed the importance of training practitioners to be both researchers and clinicians, echoing the traditional emphasis on the combination of knowledge for practitioners in psychology.

JOBS OF HEALTH PSYCHOLOGISTS

Throughout this book, we have seen that health psychologists have researched many areas related to health and illness and have also devised many therapeutic interventions aimed at changing behaviors that relate to health and the development of illness. We have discovered that psychologists with many different specialties have contributed to the field of health psychology. What types of work do these health psychologists perform and in what types of settings do they work?

Health psychologists who provide services to patients usually have received their training in clinical or counseling psychology (Tulkin, 1987). The previous section discussed training programs, which have traditionally combined a scientific orientation with practical clinical skills in therapy and assessment. With the addition to this core program of a 2-year postdoctoral internship in a health care setting, the product would be a health psychologist trained for employment in health care settings, including hospitals, clinics, health maintenance organizations (HMOs), and private practice.

Clinical and counseling psychologists have traditionally provided therapy and assessment services in private practices, clinics, and hospitals specializing in behavioral disorders, but the provision of services related to physical health and the hospital setting is new for psychologists. Another aspect of providing services in health psychology involves the collaborative nature of modern health care. Stephen Weiss (1987) described the situation in which most health psychologists provide patient services:

> In most instances (including independent practice), the health psychologist will typically be working in close proximity to other health professionals as a member of a team or as a consultant specialist where his or her skills will provide information essential to the diagnostic, treatment, or planning process. (p. 67)

The services provided by health psychologists working in clinics and hospitals fit into several categories (Tulkin, 1987). One type of service provides alternatives to pharmacological treatment; for example, biofeedback might be an alternative to analgesic drugs for headache patients. Another type of service is the primary treatment of physical disorders that respond favorably to behavioral interventions, such as chronic pain and some gastrointestinal problems. Several other types of services that psychologists might provide are related to traditional clinical psychology and include ancillary psychological treatment for patients who are hospitalized, such as cardiac or cancer patients. Health psychologists employed in hospitals and clinics also help improve the rate of patient compliance with their medical regimens and provide some assessments using psychological and neuropsychological tests.

Both Weiss (1987) and Tulkin (1987) proposed that psychologists working in health settings learn to be part of a medical team because consultation with physicians and nurses is a frequent part of their work. Houston (1988) surveyed members of the American Psychological Association's Division 38 and asked about the other health care professionals with whom health psychologists work. A majority of these Division 38 members reported that they work with physicians and nurses on a regular basis. Thus, to consult effectively, psychologists must know not only the etiquette for consultation but also medical terminology. Hospitals and clinics are traditionally the province of physicians and nurses, and psychologists are only beginning to be accepted in such settings.

Tulkin (1987) also discussed a classification of health psychology services that includes prevention of disease and promotion of health-related behavior changes. Such services, Tulkin pointed out, are not likely to occur in a hospital or clinic setting because these institutions are oriented toward providing services to patients who are sick rather than helping people who want to remain well. Health psychologists who concentrate on prevention and behavior changes are more likely to be employed in health maintenance organizations, school-based prevention programs, or worksite wellness programs. All these organizations use services that trained health psychologists can perform.

Health psychologists are beginning to become members of biomedical research teams, offering specialized skills in research design and biostatistics. Weiss (1987) examined health psychology's role in both basic and applied research, pointing out that both psychology and biomedicine have long but separate histories of basic research, and few basic biomedical research teams have included psychologists. Weiss recommended that psychologists become trained in biochemistry and physiology so they can contribute to basic biomedical research. He also suggested that neither psychologists nor physicians alone can adequately address the variables that are involved with the prevention and control of disease. Success in these endeavors will require cooperation, but joint authorships — one index of collaborative efforts — have increased in recent years.

The American Psychological Association and the Centers for Disease Control and Prevention have entered into a partnership to expand behaviorally based programs (Cavaliere, 1995). In this partnership, APA members will be involved in designing and conducting prevention programs on a national level. It is consistent with the growing emphasis on prevention on a national level and compatible with the knowledge and practice of health psychology. This effort is consistent with the U.S. Congress's mandate to increase support for behavioral and social sciences, but it does not meet the congressional goal of establishing a behavioral and social science directorate at the National Science Foundation (Bennett Johnson, 1994). Involvement of health psychologists in government agencies and expansion of behavioral research in health would not only create additional jobs but would also expand health psychology's influence in health research and public health.

Most health psychologists engage in several activities. The combination of teaching and research is common among those in educational settings. Health psychologists who work in medical centers may teach medical students, conduct research, perform clinical services, or carry out some combination of these activities. Those who work in service delivery settings are much less likely to teach and do research and are more likely to spend the majority of their time providing diagnosis and therapy.

In summary, the jobs of health psychologists are similar to the jobs of other psychologists. Those employed by a university typically teach and conduct research, and those working in clinical settings are involved in assessment, diagnosis, and therapy. Health psychologists are employed in medical centers and medical schools, and their duties include collaborating with other health care professionals in providing services for physical disorders rather than for traditional areas of mental health care. Research in health psychology is also likely to be a collaborative effort that may include the professions of medicine, epidemiology, nursing, pharmacology, nutrition, and exercise physiology.

PROGRESS IN HEALTH PSYCHOLOGY

Since the founding of health psychology, the field has grown rapidly and this growth has been apparent both in the amount of research published by psychologists on health-related topics and in the growing number of psychologists who work in health care settings.

GROWTH OF HEALTH PSYCHOLOGY RESEARCH

In 1969, William Schofield published an article in the *American Psychologist* that provided a major impetus to health psychology. Analyzing the research publications in psychology that dealt with health, he found that only 19% of the research articles dealt with topics other than the traditional mental health concerns of psychology. This finding brought about a call for a wider scope of psychological services and research. The American Psychological Association (APA) appointed a task force to perform a further analysis, and this task force concluded that health was not a common area of research for psychologists (APA Task Force on Health Research, 1976). The growth of health psychology has changed the field of psychology, making health-related issues common topics in psychology journals.

According to Stone (1987), the number of articles in psychology journals concerned with health rose to about 130 per year in 1984, a rate 20 times greater than that found by the APA Task Force. The growing rate of research by psychologists on health-related topics was apparent from an examination of the number of programs sponsored by Division 38 at recent American Psychological Association conventions. At the 1994 convention, Division 38 sponsored or co-sponsored about 20 programs per day. The program index specified over 70 programs on the topics of health psychology or behavioral medicine, with another 120 programs on related topics such as exercise, HIV, or substance use and abuse. The number of paper presentations, workshops, symposia, and master lectures reflects psychologists' growing interest in the area of health.

GROWTH OF EMPLOYMENT OPPORTUNITIES

Employment opportunities have also increased for health psychologists. Altman and Cahn (1987), after surveying job announcements in the *APA Monitor* from mid-1982 to mid-1983, found an average of about 27 job announcements per month seeking psychologists for health-related positions. Altman and Cahn estimated that about 200 new jobs per year would be available for psychologists in health-related fields during the 1980s.

An examination of the *APA Monitor* in the 1990s indicated that this estimate was too conservative. In the December 1994 issue of the *APA Monitor,* more than 50 advertisements sought psychologists for positions in health settings. Several of these descriptions specifically included the term *health psychologist,* and the others included a description of the setting or the work that suggested a health-related job. These advertisements represented a wide variety of positions, including faculty appointments in universities and medical schools, postdoctoral research fellowships, predoctoral internships, and employment in hospitals, clinics, private practices, health maintenance organizations, and pain clinics.

The 1994 job advertisements were divided between positions for clinical psychologists and teaching/research psychologists. The clinical skills sought included assessment, therapy, biofeedback, stress management, and experience with chronic pain patients. Many ads mentioned that experience in behavioral medicine or in health care settings was either required or desirable. Many job descriptions, especially for jobs in hospitals and medical schools, stipulated that the person hired be part of an interdisciplinary team. Unlike Altman and Cahn's review during the early 1980s, which found most jobs concentrated in California and New York, this analysis discovered that openings were available throughout the United States. Thus, employment opportunities for health psychologists with applied or research skills expanded during the 1980s, and this trend continues during the 1990s.

ACCEPTANCE IN MEDICAL SETTINGS

For the number of health psychology jobs to increase, psychologists must be accepted in medical settings. Have psychologists gained such acceptance? A survey by Nethercut and Piccione (1984) revealed that the overall attitude of physicians was fairly favorable toward psychologists. These researchers rightly pointed out that "continued growth of opportunities for psychologists will depend on whether psychologists are seen by physicians, administrators, and other hospital staff as playing an important as well as legitimate role in patient care" (p. 176).

To determine physicians' views of psychologists, Nethercut and Piccione constructed a questionnaire, distributed it to approximately 1,000 physicians, and found both expected and surprising views. First, 60% of the responding physicians felt themselves to be inadequately trained to deal with the psychological aspects of their patients' illness, thus indicating a substantial need for psychological services. Second, physicians valued some psychological services much more than others; for example, clinical psychologists collected a favorable rating from 71% of responding physicians, whereas research psychologists received only 38% approval. Third, demographic differences existed among physicians, with women and younger physicians more likely to value psychologists' skills. Nethercut and Piccione also found that physicians on hospital staffs were more favorably disposed toward psychological services than those in private practice. Finally, psychologists' lack of medical training was of less concern to newer physicians than it was to physicians with more than 10 years of experience. This latter finding is encouraging because it indicates that younger physicians are more accepting of psychologists working in medical settings.

As successive cohorts of medical school classes are taught by psychologists, the acceptance rate should continue to increase, causing a spiraling acceptance for psychologists in medical settings. Neal E. Miller (personal communication, September 18, 1986) stated his optimism about psychology's continuation in health-related settings: "As physicians in various specialties find that psychologists can be useful to them, they will make increasing use of psychologists. Every branch of psychology will find something useful to do in the various subspecialties of medicine, dentistry and related fields."

OUTLOOK FOR HEALTH PSYCHOLOGY

Despite the growth of health psychology and its ability to contribute to health care, the field of health psychology faces several challenges. The major chal-

lenge is acceptance by other health care practitioners, an acceptance that continues to grow. As they become involved in health care, psychologists will be forced to attend to such problems as the escalating cost of medical care, which will include a justification of their own salary. Although the diagnostic and therapy techniques used by health psychologists have demonstrated effectiveness, these procedures also have costs. Health psychology must meet the challenges of justifying its costs by offering needed services in the changing health care system and in a changing society. In addition, it must be cautious in the claims it makes.

FUTURE CHALLENGES FOR HEALTH CARE

Health care in the United States faces several future challenges. Two of the more crucial ones are the changing patterns of illness and the escalating cost of health care. These two challenges are only partially interrelated. The increase in chronic illness has probably contributed less to rising health care costs than improved technology, the growth of hospitals, and the increasing specialization of physicians.

Changing Profile of Illness

Chapter 1 identified several important changes in   x-ref
the pattern of illness that have contributed to the development of health psychology. One change was a shift in the leading causes of death and disability from infectious diseases to chronic illnesses, such as cardiovascular disease (CVD) and cancer. We saw that cardiovascular disease, including heart disease and stroke, currently accounts for nearly 40% of deaths in the United States, almost twice the percentage of deaths accounted for by cancer. Research in health psychology has reflected this discrepancy; considerably more attention is paid to heart disease than to cancer. Psychologists, for example, have devoted much work to the increased risk of cardiovascular disease related to the Type A (coronary-prone) behavior pattern and have intensively investigated behavioral interventions for reducing serum cholesterol, lowering blood pressure, encouraging exercise, and promoting a heart-healthy diet. Margaret Chesney (1993) and other health psychologists have questioned this empha-

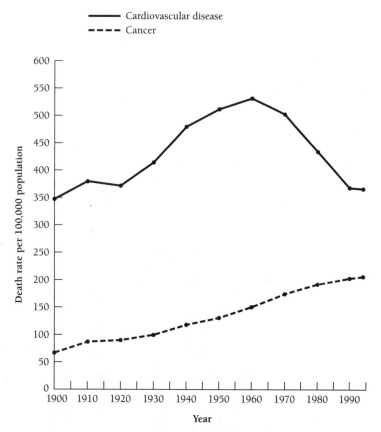

Figure 17.1   Death rates for cardiovascular disease and cancer per 100,000 population, United States 1900–1993.   SOURCE: Data from *Historical Statistics of the United States: Colonial Times to 1970,* p. 58, by U.S. Department of Commerce, Bureau of the Census, Washington, DC: U.S. Government Printing Office, and from *Statistical Abstracts of the United States, 1995,* p. 92, by U.S. Department of Commerce, Bureau of the Census, Washington, DC: U.S. Government Printing Office.

sis, which has outweighed similar efforts related to cancer.

In the coming decades, the behavioral aspects of cancer should receive more attention. First, the 2-to-1 ratio of CVD deaths to cancer deaths has changed with the decrease in CVD and the increase in cancer. Figure 17.1 shows the trends for these two causes of death since 1900. Although cardiovascular disease will probably continue to be the major cause of deaths in the United States for some time, these trends suggest that deaths from cancer will approach those from CVD during the second or third decade of the 21st century. This changing proportion of deaths is one reason cancer may receive more attention.

A second reason for an increased attention to cancer is its prominence as a cause of death among young and middle-aged adults. Figure 17.2 shows the death rates from CVD and cancer for various age groups and the tendency for younger people to be more likely to die of cancer. Efforts toward preventing or postponing this cause of death would add years of life. The third reason that cancer may attract more research is because it is easily the leading cause of death in young and middle-aged women. In 1992, cancer accounted for 38.6% of the deaths in women between the ages of 15 and 64. Coronary heart disease and stroke combined accounted for only 21.9% of their deaths (USBC, 1995). To date,

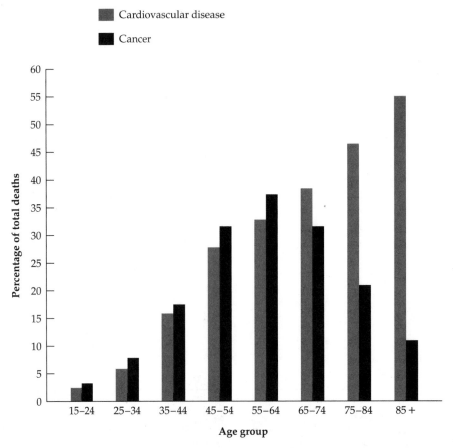

Figure 17.2 **Death rates from cardiovascular disease (CVD) and cancer by age, United States, 1991.**
SOURCE: From *Statistical Abstracts of the United States, 1994*, p. 94, by U.S. Department of Commerce, Bureau of the Census, Washington DC: U.S. Government Printing Office.

the research base for health psychology has not only emphasized heart disease over cancer but has also been slanted much more toward men than women. With an increasing emphasis on research dealing with women's health, cancer should receive increased attention, and future research on disorders that affect both women and men must include as many women as men.

Because cancer is the leading cause of death in people under 65, future health psychologists must become increasingly involved in identifying the personality and behavioral correlates of cancer and in helping people change the behaviors and lifestyles associated with this disease. In addition, they should expand their current practices of helping cancer pa-

tients manage pain and helping those patients and their families cope with the illness.

To date, American psychologists have made little progress in identifying the personality variables associated with cancer. Indeed, they have conducted scant research in this area. Friedman and Booth-Kewley (1987) reviewed the literature on personality correlates of five diseases with psychological components: asthma, arthritis, ulcers, headaches, and coronary heart disease. Cancer was not included. According to Friedman and Booth-Kewley, cancer presents certain obstacles to researchers trying to isolate a cancer-prone personality, mainly because cancer is actually a number of different diseases. Despite this obstacle, Ronald Grossarth-Maticek in Europe has identified

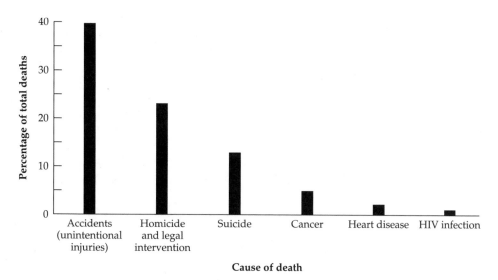

Figure 17.3 *Six leading causes of death for youth, ages 15-24, United States, 1992, by percent of total.* SOURCE: From *Statistical Abstracts of the United States, 1995*, p. 94, by U.S. Department of Commerce, Bureau of the Census, Washington DC: U.S. Government Printing Office.

a cancer-prone personality. Grossarth-Maticek and his associates (Eysenck, 1988; Grossarth-Maticek, Eysenck, Vetter, & Frentzel-Beyme, 1986) reported that people who reacted to stress with a hopeless and helpless attitude were much more likely to have died of cancer than were other people. People who adopt this helpless/hopeless attitude were also much more likely to have died of cancer than of heart disease. Although a few other studies (Greer & Morris, 1975; Shaffer, Graves, Swank, & Pearson, 1987) also reported that people who suppress emotions are more likely to develop cancer, no concerted effort has been devoted to discovering personality variables that predict cancer. This paucity of research stands in contrast to the plethora of activity surrounding the Type A (coronary-prone) behavior pattern.

However, neither coronary heart disease nor cancer is a leading cause of death for young people. For young adults 15 to 24, the principal causes of mortality have strong behavioral components, but instead of resulting from chronic illnesses, they stem from violent acts. Figure 17.3 shows that unintentional injuries, homicide and legal intervention, and suicide were the leading killers of adolescents and young adults in 1992. Most of the unintentional deaths resulted from automobile crashes, but falls,

drownings, fires, poisonings, and some firearms deaths fall into this category. Firearms are also a factor in homicide and suicide, the two other prominent causes of deaths for young people. The other three causes of death—heart disease, cancer, and HIV infection—are small compared to violent deaths for this age group. As more states passed seatbelt laws, raised the legal drinking age, and aggressively discouraged driving while drinking, deaths from automobile crashes declined (CDC, 1994g). In fact, car accidents killed fewer people in 1992 than in 1980, and the rate of automobile deaths per 100,000 decreased from 23.5 in 1980 to 16.1 in 1992 (USBC, 1995). Also, the percentage of traffic fatalities involving drunk driving has decreased for both teen-agers and adults (CDC, 1994g). As discussed in Chapter 12, psychologists have recently become involved in exploring the causes of unintentional injuries and strategies for preventing them.

The aging of the U.S. population presents an additional challenge to health psychologists. After age 65, many people develop chronic illnesses and suffer from chronic pain. As we have seen, health psychology has a role in preventing illness, promoting health, and helping people cope with pain. In old age, lifestyles can still be changed to help prevent illness, but

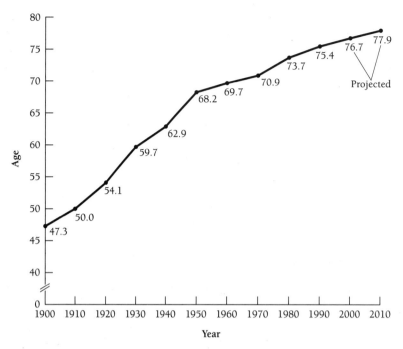

Figure 17.4 Actual and projected life expectancy, United States, 1900–2010. SOURCE: Data from *Historical Statistics of the United States: Colonial Times to 1970*, p. 55, by U.S. Bureau of the Census, 1975, Washington, DC: U.S. Government Printing Office, and *Statistical Abstracts of the United States*, p. 7, by U.S. Bureau of the Census, 1994, Washington, DC: U.S. Government Printing Office.

health psychology's alliance with gerontology will more likely produce an emphasis on promoting and maintaining health, managing pain, promoting the health care system, and formulating health care policy.

Since 1900, the number of people in the United States 65 years old or older has increased from about 3 million to more than 30 million, a tenfold growth, while the total population was increasing less than fourfold. Stated another way, in 1900, only 4% of the population was over 65 whereas in 1992, more than 12% of U.S. citizens had reached that age. During this same period, life expectancy increased from 47 years in 1900 to 76 years in 1992. The U.S. Bureau of the Census (1995) projects a life expectancy of almost 78 years by the year 2010 (see Figure 17.4). The Census Bureau also estimates that by the year 2010, the United States will have more than 18 million people, or 6.5% of the total population, over age 75. In contrast, in 1960, only 5.6 million, or 3.1% of the population, were over 75.

In the past, health psychology has been only moderately concerned with special problems of the

elderly. Gatz, Pearson, and Weicker (1987) stated that "there has been surprisingly little recognition of the natural overlap between health psychology and the psychology of the adult development and aging" (p. 303). This situation has changed, with health psychologists becoming more involved in issues of aging. One of the committees of Division 38 is concerned with issues of aging. Health-related articles appear frequently in psychology journals concerned with aging, and a journal specifically oriented to issues of health in the aging, *Behavior, Health, and Aging,* began publication in 1990. During the next few decades, as the population continues to age, psychology will play an important role in helping older people achieve and maintain healthy and productive lifestyles and adjust to the problems of chronic illness.

What will be the profile of illness and death in the 21st century? Cardiovascular disease and cancer are likely to continue for some time as the two leading causes of death in the United States. However, illnesses not yet known to be a threat to humanity

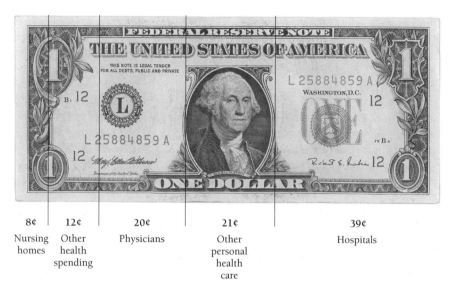

8¢ | 12¢ | 20¢ | 21¢ | 39¢

Nursing homes | Other health spending | Physicians | Other personal health care | Hospitals

Figure 17.5 Where health care dollars go.

may forge their way onto the list. Twenty years ago, AIDS was unknown, and now it is considered a major, worldwide health threat and ranks among the leading causes of death in the United States. Accurate predictions of future causes of disease and death are impossible, but health psychologists will likely be able to make some contribution to preventing and managing these disorders.

Controlling Health Care Costs

Health care costs in the United States have escalated at a higher rate than inflation and other costs of living. A number of factors have contributed, including the growth of technology, more hospitals, and a large proportion of physicians who are specialists. As Consumers Union (1992a, p. 438) described the situation:

> Medical care is totally unlike services delivered by other professionals. When clients hire an architect or a lawyer, they generally know what they need and roughly how much it's going to cost. But in medicine, physicians make virtually all the decisions that determine the cost of care. The patient, ill and uninformed, is in no position to do comparison shopping—nor motivated to, if insurance is paying the bill.

Physicians, however, do not receive the largest part of health care expenditures. Figure 17.5 shows

where health care dollars go. Hospitals receive 39% and physicians 20% of the dollars spent. Consumers Union (1992a) argued that the high cost of hospitalization is partly due to overbuilding by hospitals, resulting in the need to pay for these hospital beds by filling them. Indeed, areas of the country with more hospital beds available have higher rates of hospitalization than areas with fewer beds.

Although physicians receive only half as much as hospitals, the number of specialists adds to the cost of medical care, and the scarcity of family practitioners (and the lack of incentive for going into family practice) also plays a role in escalating health care costs. Both hospitals with expensive technology and specialist physicians who use this technology contribute to the increasing (and increasingly expensive) role of technology in medicine.

The United States is not the only country with problems associated with health care costs. Other industrialized countries such as Canada, Japan, Australia, and the countries of Western Europe and Scandinavia also have high rates of cardiovascular disease and cancer as well as aging populations, presenting similar problems for their health care systems (Caragata, 1995; Ikegami, 1992). These other countries, however, have health care systems that differ from that of the United States, and many do a better job of providing health care to a larger percentage of their residents than does the U.S. system.

In the attempt to reform the U.S. health care system, other countries' systems have been examined. Consumers Union (1992b) described the advantages of Canada's system, especially their adoption of a single payer plan for health insurance. Rather than having many insurance companies and policies purchased by individuals or employers as is the pattern in the U.S. system, Canada has only one government-funded insurance payer. This system for insurance is similar to the U.S. social security payment for retirement. All of Canada's citizens are covered by this system, regardless of employment status. Physicians, however, are not government employees; instead, they work in private offices and clinics, similar to physicians in the U.S. In Canada, however, their fees are fixed through negotiation with provincial governments, and Canadian physicians cannot charge more for their services than the fees to which they have agreed.

Does Canada's system save money? How can a system provide health care for all and still be affordable? The Canadian system is costly and requires substantial support through a variety of taxes, but health care costs are lower in Canada than in the United States (Consumers Union, 1992b). The Canadian system does not emphasize the latest technology and, unlike the United States, has decreased rather than increased the number of hospitals. The single-payer system decreases administrative costs, and such costs add significantly to U.S. health care expenditures. (See box—Would You Believe . . . ?) Victor Fuchs (1993) argued that the U.S. needs to separate health insurance from employment and limit the use of high-technology medicine. He also contended that society cannot afford to meet the demand for health care in an aging population.

The Canadian system is not without problems. The negotiations that fix physicians' fees are fierce, with physicians' associations attempting to sway public opinion with claims that health care needs are not being met (Consumers Union, 1992b). Although that system is less costly than the U.S. system, Canada is having trouble paying for its health care and is planning to cut costs (Caragata, 1995).

Insurance companies and physicians in the United States have lobbied against changes in the health care system, but many physicians are coming to accept change in their role as inevitable. Emily Friedman (1993) framed the debate over health care reform as a conflict over control of the system. She contended that health care providers have lost the power to practice medicine as they see fit, and H. Gilbert Welch and Elliott Fisher (1992) acknowledged the conflict between the goals of physicians and those of society. They recommended that physicians attempt to negotiate an arrangement that allows them to earn enough money and to practice with a minimum of interference while forming a system that provides affordable health care for all U.S. residents.

Controlling health care costs will probably require substantial changes in the U.S. health care system. Insurance companies, hospitals, and physicians will all be affected, and no system can provide a good quality of medical care for low costs. Some countries, however, do a better job than the United States, serving a larger proportion of the population and obtaining better health and longer life.

A NOTE OF CAUTION

Although health psychologists face exciting prospects, they must not allow their enthusiasm to lead to claims they cannot fulfill. Robert Kaplan (1984) warned that those within behavioral medicine and health psychology must not claim more than they can deliver. He believes that, potentially, psychology has much offer to health promotion, but he has cautioned psychologists and other behavioral scientists to be aware of "the complexities of the problems and the general absence of definitive evidence on the relationship between behavioral interventions and disease prevention." He finds "no quarrel with health promotion, only with the promotion of health promotion" (p. 763).

According to Kaplan, four assumptions underlie the field of health promotion, but he cautions that the evidence supporting each assumption is much weaker than many psychologists think. His first assumption is that specific behaviors create risks for serious illnesses, and ample evidence for this as-

WOULD YOU BELIEVE . . . ?

Affordable Health Care for Everyone

Would you believe that the United States can afford health care for all its citizens? The editors of Consumers Union (1992a) contended that the huge U.S. expenditures on health care are, at present, a bad bargain because U.S. citizens enjoy a relatively poor state of health and longevity compared to the citizens of other countries that spend less. However, the editors estimated that the level of expenditures is sufficient to provide health care for all U.S. residents.

About 20% of health care expenditures are administration costs. Restructuring the system of payment—for example, by switching to a single-payer reimbursement system—could cut administrative costs by about half (Consumers Union, 1992a).

Another area of potential cuts comes from eliminating unnecessary services and procedures. The present system allows physicians to make diagnoses and determine what procedures are appropriate, and few safeguards exist to review these decisions. Physicians can make these decisions based on what they believe is

the best course of treatment for each patient but without considering costs. Physicians also can be swayed by the availability (and even ownership) of laboratory facilities for diagnostic testing. Physicians can practice "defensive medicine" in which they perform tests and procedures that they know may be unnecessary so as to minimize the chances of malpractice lawsuits. All these strategies result in unnecessary procedures, which are not only expensive but may also endanger patients' health. For example, Consumers Union evaluated studies on unnecessary medical procedures and estimated that about half the Cesarean section deliveries, 27% of hysterectomies, 14% of laminectomy back surgeries, and 14% of heart bypass operations are unnecessary. In addition, magnetic resonance imaging may be ordered because the doctor has such equipment and will profit from its use or as a defensive test, at a cost of about $1,000 per test.

And of course, fraud in the form of billing for services that were never delivered is another factor that increases expenditures. Consumers

Union estimated that another 10% of health care costs were spent on such fraud.

Pharmaceutical companies charge U.S. residents higher prices for the same drugs that cost less in other countries, and physicians charge more for procedures that cost less in other countries. Consumers Union estimated that if these costs in the United States were brought into line with costs in other countries, the savings would help to make health care more affordable.

The editors of Consumers Union considered all these sources of waste—administrative costs, unnecessary procedures, fraud, and excessive pharmaceutical and physician charges—and estimated that the savings would be in excess of $200 billion per year. Furthermore, they contended that this figure was a conservative estimate of how much money could be saved. This magnitude of savings is sufficient to provide high-quality, technological health care for all other people in the United States who are not being served by the current system.

---

sumption exists in the form of research on smoking and excessive drinking. However, Kaplan stated that the evidence for other behavior-disease links is less persuasive.

The second assumption is that changes in risk-related behaviors will modify the incidence of disease. Kaplan conceded that the evidence clearly shows that giving up smoking will lower a person's chance of developing illnesses associated with that practice. For dietary and exercise practices, however, he claimed that the evidence is mixed. This evidence has increased since Kaplan's evaluation, but health psychologists should proceed slowly in making extravagant claims for the efficacy of their interventions.

Kaplan's third assumption concerning the field of health promotion is that behavior can be modified. Although psychologists have developed several of the most effective techniques known for modifying some health-related behaviors, health psychologists should recognize that many behaviors related to health are quite resistant to change, including drinking alcohol, smoking, and eating foods high in animal fats. We have seen that follow-up studies frequently yield success rates of about 20% to 30% for programs aimed at weight loss, smoking cessation, or alcohol abstinence. This level of effectiveness suggests some potency for behaviorally oriented programs, but much more powerful strategies are needed to ensure their inclusion in the field of health care.

The fourth assumption is that behavioral programs are cost-effective. As Russell (1986) demonstrated, prevention is not cost effective, but it is cost efficient. When the benefits of wellness are included in the analysis, prevention can be justified in terms of its costs.

Kaplan's purpose in listing these assumptions was not to discourage behavioral scientists who are searching for more effective ways of improving health but rather to caution them against making overenthusiastic claims that are not supported by close examination of all the evidence. Health psychology has grown rapidly and has ventured into health promotion, prevention, and treatment. With this rapid growth and success comes the temptation to try too much too quickly.

Pattishall (1989) proposed two rules that he deduced from examining the history of behavioral medicine. He suggested that health psychology should heed those rules to guard against inappropriate enthusiasm: "Rule 1: Don't propose more than you have data to support, and Rule 2: Don't promise more than you can deliver" (p. 44).

Health psychology has been fairly cautious in its promises of cures, and health psychologists who offer treatment are well acquainted with the difficulties of changing behavior. The temptation to promise changes in behavior is strong, but health psychologists must continue to be conservative.

CHAPTER SUMMARY

People in the United States and other industrialized countries are becoming more health conscious, and both government policy and individual behavior reflect this concern. *Healthy People 2000* stated three broad goals for the U.S. population, including increasing healthy years of life, decreasing disparities in health care delivery, and increasing access to preventive services.

Health psychology, a subspecialty of psychology, is based on the premise that physical well-being is based on psychological and social factors as well as biomedical ones. Psychology can contribute to health by (1) accumulating information on the correlates of health and illness, (2) helping to promote and

maintain health, (3) contributing to the prevention and treatment of illness, and (4) helping to formulate health policy and promoting the health care system.

Chronic illnesses have become the leading causes of death in the United States. Health psychologists have worked to change the behaviors that contribute to these diseases and to help patients cope with them. Much of that work has been in the area of cardiovascular disease. This chapter argued for a shift of emphasis and suggested that because cancer is the leading cause of premature death, more psychologically based research should be directed toward cancer. Also, cancer is by far the main cause of death for middle-aged women, but traditionally women have been underrepresented in health-related research. More research on a potential cancer-prone personality would not only identify those who are at risk but might also allow psychologists to formulate intervention strategies that can help control this disease.

The leading causes of death for young people are not chronic diseases but accidents and suicide. Alcohol is frequently implicated in both causes. In the future, health psychologists may become more involved in preventing these deaths and also in helping elderly people cope with such illnesses as asthma, arthritis, and Alzheimer's disease.

The promise of health psychology rests on the proper preparation of those entering the field. Most authorities recommend a Ph.D. in some field of psychology, followed by a two-year postdoctoral training program that adds specialized knowledge and skills in such areas as neurology, endocrinology, immunology, epidemiology, and other medical subspecialties. Health psychologists with a solid background in generic psychology and specialized knowledge in medical fields are currently employed in a variety of settings, including universities, hospitals, clinics, private practice, and health maintenance organizations.

Psychologists' expanding interest in health-related research and the growing acceptance of psychologists in medical settings indicate a robust prognosis for health psychology. However, if psychologists are to achieve even greater acceptance, they must demonstrate their worth through actions rather than enthusiastic claims.

SUGGESTED READINGS

Consumers Union. (1992, August). Wasted health care dollars. *Consumer Reports, 57,* 435–448. This article was the first in a series of three that analyzed problems in the U.S. health care system and proposed solutions to some of these difficult problems.

Kaplan, R. M. (1990). Behavior as the central outcome in health care. *American Psychologist, 39,* 755–765. Kaplan argues for considering behavioral outcomes in studies of health care and medicine. He proposes a model that includes environmental, biological, and psychological variables as predictors and mediators of health outcomes.

Sobel, D. S. (1995). Rethinking medicine: Improving health outcomes with cost-effective psychosocial interventions. *Psychosomatic Medicine, 57,* 234–244. David Sobel makes a persuasive argument for the effectiveness and cost effectiveness of the types of interventions that health psychologists have to offer.

Stone, G. C. (1984). A final word [editorial]. *Health Psychology, 3* , 585–589. The first editor of *Health Psychology* looks back over the first three volumes of the journal and outlines some of his ideas for the future direction of the profession of health psychology.

Glossary

A-beta fibers Large fibers in the spinal cord that inhibit the transmission of pain.

acetylcholine A neurotransmitter in the autonomic nervous system.

acquired immune deficiency syndrome (AIDS) An immune deficiency caused by viral infection and resulting in vulnerability to a wide range of bacterial, viral, and malignant diseases.

acrolein A yellowish or colorless, pungent liquid produced as a by-product of tobacco smoke; one of the aldehydes.

action potential An electrical discharge.

acupuncture An ancient Chinese form of analgesia that consists of inserting needles into specific points on the skin and continuously stimulating the needles.

acute pain Short-term pain that results from tissue damage or other trauma.

addiction Dependence on a drug such that stopping results in withdrawal symptoms.

A-delta fibers Small fibers that facilitate the transmission of pain.

adrenal cortex The outer layer of the adrenal glands; secretes glucocorticoids.

adrenal glands Endocrine glands that are located on top of each kidney, and that secrete hormones and affect metabolism.

adrenal medulla The inner layer of the adrenal glands; secretes epinephrine and norepinephrine.

adrenocorticotropic hormone (ACTH) A hormone produced by the anterior portion of the pituitary gland that acts on the adrenal gland and is involved in the stress response.

aerobic exercise Exercise that requires an increased amount of oxygen consumption over an extended period of time.

afferent neurons Sensory neurons that relay information from the sense organs toward the brain.

agoraphobia An anxiety state characterized by fear about or avoidance of places or situations from which escape might be difficult.

alarm reaction The first stage of the general adaptation syndrome (GAS), in which the body's defenses are mobilized against a stressor.

alcohol dehydrogenase A liver enzyme that metabolizes alcohol into aldehyde.

aldehyde dehydrogenase An enzyme that converts aldehyde to acetic acid.

aldehydes A class of organic compounds obtained from alcohol by oxidation and also found in cigarette smoke; cause mutations and are related to the development of cancer.

alkalosis An abnormally high level of alkaline in the body.

allergies An immune system response characterized by an abnormal reaction to a foreign substance.

alveoli Small, saclike structures at the end of the bronchioles; the sites of oxygen and carbon dioxide exchange.

amenorrhea Cessation of the menses.

amphetamines One type of stimulant drug.

anabolic steroids Steroid drugs that increase muscle bulk and decrease body fat but also have toxic effects.

anaerobic exercise Exercise that does not require an increased amount of oxygen.

analgesic drugs Drugs that decrease the perception of pain.

anemia A low level of red blood cells, leading to generalized weakness and lack of vitality.

anesthesia Loss of sensations of temperature, touch, or pain.

angina pectoris A disorder involving a restricted blood supply to the myocardium, which results in chest pain and restricted breathing.

angiography A method of viewing cardiovascular damage through the use of X-ray pictures and the injection of dye into the circulatory system.

angioplasty Medical intervention in which a catheter with an inflatable tip is passed into an obstructed artery in order to flatten atherosclerotic deposits of plaque.

anorexia nervosa An eating disorder characterized by intentional starvation, distorted body image, excessive amounts of energy, and an intense fear of gaining weight.

antibodies Protein substances produced in response to a specific invader or antigen, marking it for destruction and thus creating immunity to that invader.

antigens Substances that provoke the immune system to produce antibodies.

anus Opening through which feces are eliminated.

arteries Vessels carrying blood away from the heart.

arteriole A small branch of an artery.

arteriosclerosis A condition marked by loss of elasticity and hardening of arteries.

asthma A respiratory disorder characterized by difficulty in breathing.

athermatous plaques Deposits of cholesterol and other lipids, connective tissue, and muscle tissue.

atherosclerosis The formation of plaque within the arteries.

autoimmune diseases Disorders that occur when the immune system fails to differentiate between body cells and foreign cells, resulting in the body's attack and destruction of its own cells.

autonomic nervous system The part of the peripheral nervous system that primarily serves internal organs.

aversion therapy A type of behavioral therapy based on classical conditioning technique and using some aversive stimulus to countercondition the patient's response.

avoidance coping Reacting to illness by the denial of threat and the use of such strategies as overeating, taking drugs, or hoping for a miracle.

barbiturates Synthetic sedative drugs used medically to induce sleep.

B-cell A variety of lymphocyte that attacks invading microorganisms.

behavior modification Shaping behavior by manipulating reinforcement to obtain a desired behavior.

behavioral health A discipline concerned with preventing illness and enhancing health in currently healthy people.

behavioral medicine An interdisciplinary field concerned with developing and integrating behavioral and biomedical sciences.

benign Cell growth that is limited to a single tumor.

beta-carotene A form of vitamin A found in abundance in vegetables such as carrots and sweet potatoes.

bile salts Salts produced in the liver and stored in the gall bladder that aid in digestion of fats.

biofeedback The process of providing feedback information *about* the status of a biological system *to* that system.

biopsy A diagnostic procedure in which living tissue is removed from the body and examined for possible disease.

body mass index (BMI) An estimate of obesity determined by body weight and height.

bronchitis Any inflammation of the bronchi.

bulimia An eating disorder characterized by periodic bingeing and purging, the latter usually taking the form of self-induced vomiting or laxative abuse.

capillaries Very small vessels that connect arteries and veins.

carcinogen A substance that induces cancer.

carcinoma Cancers of the epithelial tissues.

cardiac arrhythmia Irregularity in the heartbeat rhythm.

cardiac catheterization A diagnostic procedure in which dye is injected into the circulatory system from a tube inserted into a vein.

cardiologist A medical doctor who specializes in the diagnosis and treatment of heart disease.

cardiovascular disease (CVD) Disease of the circulation system, including coronary heart disease and stroke.

case-control study A retrospective epidemiological study in which people affected by a given disease (cases) are compared to others not affected (controls).

case study A type of single-subject design in which one individual is studied in depth.

catecholamines A class of chemicals containing epinephrine and norepinephrine.

catharsis The spoken or written expression of strong negative emotion, which may result in improvement in physiological or psychological health.

central control trigger A nerve impulse that descends from the brain and influences the perception of pain.

central nervous system (CNS) All those neurons within the brain and spinal cord.

C fibers Small-diameter nerve fibers that provide information concerning slow, diffuse, lingering pain.

chronic diseases Illnesses that develop or persist over a long period of time.

chronic pain Pain that endures beyond the time of normal healing; frequently experienced in the absence of detectable tissue damage.

cilia Tiny, hairlike structures lining parts of the respiratory system.

cirrhosis A liver disease resulting in the production of nonfunctional scar tissue.

cluster headache A type of severe headache that occurs in daily clusters for 4 to 16 weeks. Symptoms are similar to migraine, but duration is much briefer.

cocaine A stimulant drug extracted from the coca plant.

cohort A group of subjects starting an experience at the same time.

concurrent validity The extent to which scores on a measuring instrument agree with a standard, such as another measuring instrument or ratings of experts.

construct validity The extent to which an instrument measures some hypothetical construct — that is, a construct that cannot be directly observed.

coronary heart disease (CHD) A disorder of the myocardium arising from atherosclerosis and/or arteriosclerosis.

correlational coefficient A number that expresses the strength of the relationship between two variables.

Correlation coefficients range from −1.00 to +1.00, with high values indicating a close association between the two sets of scores and scores closer to 0 indicating weaker relationship.

correlational studies   Studies designed to yield information concerning the degree of relationship between two variables.

cortisol   A type of corticoid that provides a natural defense against inflammation and regulates carbohydrate metabolism.

cross-sectional study   A type of research design in which subjects of different ages are studied at one point in time.

crowding   A person's perception of discomfort due to a high-density environment.

delirum tremens   A condition induced by alcohol withdrawal and characterized by excessive trembling, sweating, anxiety, and hallucinations.

dependence   A condition that occurs when a drug becomes incorporated into the functioning of the body's cells so that it is needed for "normal" functioning.

dependent variable   A variable within an experimental setting whose value is hypothesized to change as a consequence of changes in the independent variable.

descriptive research   A type of research that describes the relationship between variables rather than determining causation.

diabetes mellitus   A disorder caused by insulin deficiency.

diaphragm   The partition separating the cavity of the chest from that of the abdomen.

diastolic pressure   A measure of blood pressure between contractions of the heart.

diathesis-stress model   A theory of stress suggesting that some individuals are vulnerable to stress-related illnesses because they are genetically predisposed to those illnesses.

disulfiram   A drug that causes an aversive reaction when taken with alcohol; used to treat alcoholism; Antabuse.

dorsal horns   The part of the spinal cord away from the stomach that receives sensory input and that may play an important role in the perception of pain.

dose-response relationship   A direct, consistent relationship between an independent variable, such as a behavior, and a dependent variable, such as an illness. For example, the greater the number of cigarettes a person smokes, the greater is the likelihood of that person developing lung cancer.

double blind   An experimental design in which neither the subjects nor those who dispense the treatment condition have knowledge of who receives the treatment and who receives the placebo.

eating disorder   Any serious and habitual disturbance in eating behavior that produces unhealthy consequences.

efferent neurons   A motor neuron that conveys impulses away from the brain.

electrocardiogram (ECG)   A measure of electrical signals of the heart.

electrolyte imbalance   A condition caused by loss of body minerals.

electromyograph (EMG) biofeedback   Feedback that reflects activity of the skeletal muscles.

emetine   A drug that induces vomiting.

emphysema   A chronic lung disease in which scar tissue and mucus obstruct the respiratory passages.

endocrine system   That system of the body consisting of the ductless glands.

endorphins   Naturally occurring neurochemicals whose effects resemble the opiates.

environmental tobacco smoke (ETS)   The exposure of nonsmokers to the smoke of spouses, parents, or coworkers; passive smoking.

epidemiology   A branch of medicine that investigates the various factors that contribute to either positive health or to the frequency and distribution of a disease or disorder.

epinephrine   A chemical manufactured by the adrenal medulla that accounts for much of the hormone production of the adrenal glands; sometimes called *adrenalin.*

esophagus   The tube leading from the pharynx to the stomach.

essential hypertension   Elevations of blood pressure that have no known cause.

ethanol   The variety of alcohol used in beverages.

evoked potentials   Electrical signals recorded from the brain in response to sensory stimuli.

exhaustion stage   The final stage of the general adaptation syndrome (GAS), in which the body's ability to resist a stressor has been depleted.

ex post facto designs   Scientific studies in which the values of the independent variable are not manipulated but are selected by the experimenter *after* the groups have naturally divided themselves.

feces   Any materials left over after digestion.

fenfluramine   A prescription diet drug.

fetal alcohol syndrome (FAS)   A pattern of physical and psychological symptoms found in infants whose mothers drank heavily during pregnancy.

formaldehyde   A colorless, pungent gas found in cigarette smoke; it causes irritation of the respiratory system and has been found to be carcinogenic; one of the aldehydes.

gall bladder   A sac on the liver in which bile is stored.

gastric juices   Stomach secretions that aid in digestion.

gastrointestinal endoscopy   An examination of the gastrointestinal tract performed by inserting a tube through the esophagus or rectum.

gate control theory   A theory of pain holding that structures in the spinal cord act as a gate for sensory input that is interpreted as pain.

general adaptation syndrome (GAS)   The body's generalized attempt to defend itself against stress; consists of alarm reaction, resistance, and exhaustion.

glucagon   A hormone secreted by the pancreas that stimulates the release of glucose, thus elevating blood sugar level.

glucocorticoids   Hormones secreted by the adrenal cortex that increase the concentration of liver glycogen and blood sugar.

granulocytes   A type of lymphocyte that acts rapidly to kill invading organisms.

hardy personality model   The theory that suggests some people are buffered against the potentially harmful effects of stress due to their hardy personality.

health psychology   A field of psychology that contributes to both behavioral medicine and behavioral health; the scientific study of behaviors that relate to health enhancement, disease prevention, and rehabilitation.

high-density lipoprotein (HDL)   A form of lipoprotein that confers some protection against coronary heart disease.

hormones   Chemical substances released into the blood and having effects on other parts of the body.

human immunodeficiency virus (HIV)   Virus that attacks the human immune system, depleting the body's ability to fight infection; the infection that causes AIDS.

humoral immunity   Immunity created through the process of exposure to antigens and production of antibodies in the blood stream.

hydrocyanic acid   A poisonous acid produced by treating a cyanide with an acid; one of the products of cigarette smoke.

hypercholesterolemia   A generic disease characterized by abnormally high levels of cholesterol.

hypertension   Abnormally high blood pressure, with either a systolic reading in excess of 160 or a diastolic reading in excess of 105.

hypoglycemia   Deficiency of sugar in the blood.

hypothalamus   A small structure beneath the thalamus, involved in the control of eating, drinking, and emotional behavior.

identity disruption model   The notion that people with low self-esteem have their negative self-identity disrupted whenever they experience positive life events

illness behavior   Those activities undertaken by people who feel ill and who wish to discover their state of health as well as suitable remedies. Illness behavior precedes formal diagnosis.

immune surveillance theory   A theoretical model suggesting that cancer is the result of an immune system dysfunction.

immunity   A response to foreign microorganisms that occurs with repeated exposure and results in resistance to a disease.

incidence   A measure of the frequency of new cases of a disease or disorder during a specified period of time.

independent variable   A variable that is manipulated by the experimenter in order to assess its possible effect on behavior — that is, on the dependent variable.

induction   The process of being placed into a hypnotic state.

inflammation   A general response that works to restore damaged tissue.

insomnia   The inability either to fall asleep or to stay asleep.

insulin   A hormone that enhances glucose intake to the cells.

interferon   A type of protein produced by virus-infected cells that helps prevent the infection of other cells; confers nonspecific immunity.

interneurons   Neurons that connect sensory neurons to motor neurons; association neurons.

ischemia   Restriction of blood flow to tissue or organs; often used with reference to the heart.

islet cells   Part of the pancreas that produces glucagon and insulin.

isokinetic exercise   Exercise requiring exertion for lifting and additional effort for returning weight to the starting position.

isometric exercise   Exercise in which muscles are contracted against an immovable object.

isotonic exercise   Exercise that requires the contraction of muscles and the movement of joints, as in weight lifting.

Kaposi's sarcoma   A malignancy characterized by multiple soft, dark blue or purple nodules on the skin, with hemorrhages.

kleptomaniacs   People who compulsively steal items they neither need nor intend to use.

Korsakoff syndrome   A brain dysfunction found in some long-term heavy users of alcohol and resulting in both physiological and psychological impairment.

laminae   Layers of cell bodies.

lateral hypothalamus   Part of the hypothalamus involved in hunger.

learned helplessness   The learned tendency to respond with passivity to a challenging situation because past experiences have instilled the belief that this situation cannot be controlled.

lipoproteins   Substances in the blood consisting of lipid and protein.

liver The largest gland in the body; it aids digestion by producing bile, regulates organic components of the blood, and acts as a detoxifier of blood.

longitudinal studies Research designs in which one group of subjects is studied over a period of time.

low-density lipoprotein (LDL) A form of lipoprotein found to be positively related to coronary heart disease.

lymph Tissue fluid that has entered a lymphatic vessel.

lymphatic system System that transports lymph through the body.

lymph nodes Small nodules of lymphatic tissue spaced throughout the lymphatic system that help clean lymph of debris.

lymphocytes White blood cells that are found in lymph and that are involved in the immune function.

macrophages A type of lymphocyte that attacks invading organisms.

malignant Having the ability not only to grow but also to spread to other parts of the body.

mammography An X-ray technique for detecting breast tumors before they can be seen or felt.

medulla The structure of the hindbrain just above the spinal cord.

meta-analysis A statistical technique for combining results of studies when these studies have similar definitions of variables.

metastasize The process of the spread of malignancy from one part of the body to another by way of the blood or lymph systems.

migraine headache Headache pain caused by constriction and dilation of the vascular arteries.

model A set of related principles or hypotheses constructed to explain significant relationships among concepts or observations.

mucociliary escalator The mechanism by which debris is moved toward the pharynx.

myelin A fatty substance that acts as insulation for neurons.

myocardial infarction Heart attack.

myocardium The heart muscle.

myofacial pain Pain resulting from muscle tension and inflammation.

natural killer (NK) cells A type of lymphocyte that attacks invading organisms.

negative reinforcer Any painful or aversive condition that when removed from a situation, strengthens the behavior it follows.

neoplastic New, abnormal growth of cells.

neuroendocrine system The system pertaining to the influence of the neural and endocrine systems and hypothesized to be the mechanism underlying the relationship between stress and illness.

neurons Nerve cells.

neurotransmitters Chemicals that are released by neurons and that affect the activity of other neurons.

nitric oxide A colorless gas prepared by the action of nitric acid on copper and also produced in cigarette smoke; it affects oxygen metabolism and may be dangerous.

nitrosamines Powerful carcinogens that may be produced by nitrites.

nocebo effect Adverse effect of a placebo.

non-Hodgkin's lymphoma a malignancy characterized by rapidly growing tumors that are spread through the circulatory or lymphatic systems.

norepinephrine One of two major neurotransmitters of the autonomic nervous system.

nucleus raphe magnus A group of neurons in the medulla that send inhibitory signals to neurons in the spinal cord; part of the descending control system for pain.

oncologist A physician who specializes in the treatment of cancer.

opiates A group of drugs all of which are derived from the resin of the opium poppy.

osteoarthritis Progressive inflammation of the joints.

optimistic bias The belief that other people, but not oneself, will develop a disease, have an accident, or experience other negative events.

osteoporosis A disease characterized by a reduction in bone density, brittleness of bones, and a loss of calcium from the bones.

pancreas An endocrine gland located below the stomach that produces digestive juices and hormones.

pancreatic juices Acid-reducing enzymes secreted by the pancreas into the small intestine.

parasympathetic nervous system A division of the autonomic nervous system that promotes relaxation and functions under normal, nonstressful conditions.

passive smoking The exposure of nonsmokers to the smoke of spouses, parents, or co-workers; environmental tobacco smoke.

pathogen Any disease-causing organism.

pepsin Enzyme that is produced by gastric mucosa and that initiates digestive activity.

periaqueductal gray An area of the midbrain that, when stimulated, decreases pain.

peripheral nervous system (PNS) Those nerves that lie outside the brain and spinal cord.

peristalsis Contractions that propel food through the digestive tract.

phagocytosis The process of engulfing and killing foreign particles.

phantom limb pain The experience of chronic pain in an absent body part.

pharynx Part of the digestive tract between the mouth and the esophagus.

phenylpropylalamine A nonprescription diet drug.

pituitary gland An endocrine gland that lies within the brain and whose secretions regulate many other glands.

placebo effect An inactive substance or condition that has the appearance of the independent variable and that may cause subjects in an experiment to improve or change behavior due to their belief in the placebo's efficacy; a treatment that is effective because of a patient's belief in the treatment.

plasma cells Cells that are derived from B-cells and that secrete antibodies.

population density A physical condition in which a high level of population is confined in a limited space.

positive reinforcer Any positively valued stimulus that when added to a situation strengthens the behavior it follows.

posttraumatic stress disorder (PTSD) An anxiety disorder caused by experience with an extremely traumatic event and characterized by recurrent and intrusive reexperiencing of that event.

prechronic pain Pain that endures beyond the acute phase but has not yet become chronic.

predictive validity The extent to which a measuring instrument is able to predict a given condition.

prevalence The proportion of a population that has a disease or disorder at a specific point in time.

primary afferents Sensory neurons that convey impulses from the skin to the spinal cord.

primary appraisal One's initial appraisal of a potentially stressful event (Lazarus and Folkman's term).

prospective studies Longitudinal studies that begin with a disease-free group of subjects and follow the occurrence of disease in that population or sample.

punishment The presentation of an aversive stimulus or the removal of a positive one. Punishment sometimes, but not always, weakens a response.

psychoneuroimmunology A multidisciplinary field that focuses on the interactions among behavior, the nervous system, the endocrine system, and the immune system.

Raynaud's disease A vasoconstrictive disorder stemming from inadequate circulation in the extremities, especially the fingers or toes, and resulting in pain.

reactance In Brehm's theory, the angry state of reaction to loss of freedom, and the attempt to restore personal control.

reappraisal One's nearly constant reevaluation of stressful events (Lazarus and Folkman's term).

reciprocal determinism Bandura's model that includes environment, behavior, and person as mutually interacting to determine conduct.

rectum The end of the digestive tract leading to the anus.

relative risk The ratio of the incidence or prevalence of a disease in an exposed group to the incidence or prevalence of that disease in the unexposed group.

reliable The extent to which a test or other measuring instrument yields consistent results.

resistance stage The second stage of the general adaptation syndrome (GAS), in which the body adapts to a stressor.

retrospective studies Longitudinal studies that look back at the history of a population or sample.

rheumatoid arthritis An autoimmune disorder characterized by a dull ache within or around a joint.

risk factor A characteristic or condition that occurs with greater frequency in people with a disease than it does in people free from that disease.

salivary glands Glands that furnish moisture that helps in tasting and digesting food.

sarcomas Cancers of the connective tissues.

secondary appraisal One's perceived ability to control or cope with harm, threat, or challenge (Lazarus and Folkman's term).

secondary hypertension Elevations in blood pressure that are triggered by other diseases.

sedatives Drugs that induce relaxation and sometimes intoxication by lowering the activity of the brain, the neurons, the muscles, the heart, and even by slowing the metabolic rate.

self-efficacy The belief that one is capable of performing the behaviors that will produce desired outcomes in any particular situation.

self-selection A condition of an experimental investigation in which subjects are allowed, in some manner, to determine their own placement in either the experimental or the control group.

setpoint A hypothetical ratio of fat to lean tissue at which a person's weight will tend to stabilize.

shaping The conditioning of behavior by first reinforcing gross approximations of that behavior, then closer approximations, and finally the target behavior.

sick role behavior Those activities that are undertaken by people who have been diagnosed as sick and that are directed at getting well.

social contacts Number and kinds of people with whom one associates; members of one's social network.

social isolation The absence of specific role relationships.

social network Number and kinds of people with whom one associates; social contacts.

social supports Both tangible and intangible support a person receives from other people.

somatic nervous system The part of the PNS that serves the skin and voluntary muscles.

somatosensory cortex The part of the brain that receives and processes sensory input from the body.

specificity theory A physiological theory of pain that hypothesizes the existence of specific pain fibers and pathways.

spleen A large organ near the stomach that serves as a repository for lymphocytes and red blood cells.

spontaneous remission Disappearance of problem behavior or illness without treatment.

state anxiety A temporary condition of dread or uneasiness stemming from a specific situation.

stress inoculation A stress management technique in which patients are introduced to small amounts of stress and are given cognitive-behavioral strategies for dealing with those diminished levels of stress.

stress response-dampening (SRD) Decrease in strength of responses to stress, caused by consumption of alcohol.

stress test An exercise test used to diagnose coronary heart disease.

stroke Damage to the brain resulting from lack of oxygen; typically the result of cardiovascular disease.

subject variable A variable chosen (rather than manipulated) by a researcher to provide levels of comparison for groups of subjects.

substantia gelatinosa Two layers of the dorsal horns of the spinal cord.

sympathetic nervous system A division of the autonomic nervous system that mobilizes the body's resources in emergency, stressful, and emotional situations.

synaptic cleft The space between neurons.

synergistic effect The combined effect of two or more variables that exceeds the sum of their individual effects.

systolic pressure A measure of blood pressure generated by the heart's contraction.

T-cell The cells of the immune system that produce cell-mediated immunity.

temperature biofeedback Feedback concerning changes in skin temperature.

tension headache Pain produced by sustained muscle contractions in the neck, shoulders, scalp, and face.

thalamus Structure in the forebrain that acts as a relay center for incoming sensory information and outgoing motor information.

theory A set of related assumptions from which testable hypotheses can be drawn.

thermister A temperature-sensitive resistor used in skin temperature biofeedback.

thymosin A hormone produced by the thymus.

thymus An organ located near the heart that secretes thymosin and thus processes and activates T-lymphocytes.

tolerance The condition of requiring increasing levels of a drug in order to produce a constant level of effect.

tonsils Masses of lymphatic tissue located in the pharynx.

trait anxiety A personality characteristic that manifests itself as a more or less constant feeling of dread or uneasiness.

tranquilizers A type of sedative drug that reduces anxiety and induces sleep as well as depression.

transcutaneous electrical neural stimulation (TENS) A treatment for pain involving the electrical stimulation of neurons from the surface of the skin. This stimulation blocks other sensory input, providing pain relief.

transmission cells Afferent neurons that connect to other neurons; also called secondary afferents.

triglycerides A group of molecules consisting of glycerol and three fatty acids; one of the components of serum lipids that has been implicated in the formation of atherosclerotic plaque.

vaccination A method of inducing immunity in which a weakened form of a virus or bacterium is introduced into the body.

valid Accurate; the extent to which a test or other measuring instrument measures what it is supposed to measure.

veins Vessels that carry blood to the heart.

ventromedial The anterior, central region of an organ.

ventromedial hypothalamus The part of the hypothalamus involved in satiation.

venules The smallest veins.

well-year The equivalent of a year of complete wellness.

withdrawal Adverse physiological reactions exhibited when a drug-dependent person stops using that drug; the withdrawal symptoms are typically unpleasant and opposite from the drug's effects.

References

Abbott, R. D., Rodriguez, B. L., Burchfiel, C. M., & Curb, J. D. (1994). Physical activity in older middle-aged men and reduced risk of stroke: The Honolulu Heart Program. *American Journal of Epidemiology, 139,* 881–893.

Abbott, R. D., Yin, Y., Reed, D. M., & Yano, K. (1986). Risk of stroke in male cigarette smokers. *New England Journal of Medicine, 315,* 717–720.

Abraham, C., & Sheeran, P. (1994). Modelling and modifying young heterosexuals' HIV-preventive behaviour: A review of theories, findings and educational implications. *Patient Education and Counseling, 23,* 173–186.

Abrams, D. B., & Niaura, R. S. (1987). Social learning theory. In H. T. Blane & K. E. Leonard (Eds.), *Psychological theories of drinking and alcoholism* (pp. 131–178). New York: Guilford Press.

Abramson, L. Y., Garber, J., & Seligman, M. E. P. (1980). Learned helplessness in humans: An attributional analysis. In J. Garber & M. E. P. Seligman (Eds.), *Human helplessness: Theory and applications* (pp. 3–34). New York: Academic Press.

Achterberg, J., Kenner, C., & Lawlis, G. F. (1988). Severe burn injuries: A comparison of relaxation imagery and biofeedback for pain management. *Journal of Mental Imagery, 12,* 71–87.

Achterberg-Lawlis, J. (1982). The psychological dimensions of arthritis. *Journal of Consulting and Clinical Psychology, 50,* 984–992.

Ackroff, K., & Sclafani, A. (1988). Sucrose-induced hyperphagia and obesity in rats fed a macronutrient self-selection diet. *Physiology and Behavior, 44,* 181–187.

Ader, R., & Cohen, N. (1975). Behaviorally conditioned immunosuppression. *Psychosomatic Medicine, 37,* 333–340.

Ader, R., & Cohen, N. (1982). Behaviorally conditioned immunosuppression and murine systematic lupus erythematosus. *Science, 215,* 1534–1536.

Ader, R., & Cohen, N. (1993). Psychoneuroimmunology: Conditioning stress. *Annual Review of Psychology, 44,* 53–85.

Adler, N., & Matthews, K. (1994). Health psychology: Why do some people get sick and some stay well? *Annual Review of Psychology, 45,* 229–259.

Agras, W. S. (1993). Short-term psychological treatments for binge eating. In C. G. Fairburn & G. T. Wilson (Eds.), *Binge eating: Nature, assessment, and treatment* (pp. 270–286). New York: Guilford Press.

Agras, W. S., Schneider, J. A., Arnow, B., Raeburn, S. D., & Telch, C. F. (1989). Cognitive-behavioral and response-prevention treatments for bulimia nervosa. *Journal of Consulting and Clinical Psychology, 57,* 215–221.

Agras, W. S., Telch, C. F., Arnow, B., Eldredge, K., Detzer, M. J., Henderson, J., & Marnell, M. (1995). Does interpersonal therapy help patients with binge eating disorder who fail to respond to cognitive-behavioral therapy? *Journal of Consulting and Clinical Psychology, 63,* 356–360.

Agras, S., & Werne, J. (1977). Behavior modification in anorexia nervosa: Research foundations. In R. A. Vigersky (Ed.), *Anorexia nervosa* (pp.291–303). New York: Raven.

Ahlbom, A., & Norell, S. (1990). *Introduction to modern epidemiology* (2nd ed.). Chestnut Hill, MA: Epidemiology Resources.

Aiken, L. S., West, S. G., Woodward, C. K., & Reno, R. R. (1994). Health beliefs and compliance with mammography-screening recommendations in asymptomatic women. *Health Psychology, 13,* 122–129.

Ajzen, I. (1985). From intentions to actions: A theory of planned behavior. In J. Kuhland & J. Beckman (Eds.), *Action-control: From cognitions to behavior* (pp. 11–39) Heidelberg, Germany: Springer.

Ajzen, I. (1988). *Attitudes, personality, and behavior.* Chicago: Dorsey Press.

Ajzen, I. (1991). The theory of planned behavior. *Organizational Behavior and Human Decision Processes, 50,* 179–211.

Ajzen, I., & Fishbein, M. (1980). *Understanding attitudes and predicting social behavior:* Englewood Cliffs, NJ: Prentice-Hall.

Åkerstedt, T. (1988). Sleepiness as a consequence of shiftwork. *Sleep, 11,* 17–34.

Alcoholics Anonymous World Services (AA). (1987). *Membership survey.* New York: Author.

Alden, L. E. (1988). Behavioral self-management controlled-drinking strategies in a context of secondary prevention. *Journal of Consulting and Clinical Psychology, 56,* 280–286.

Alexander, B. K. (1988). The disease and adaptive models of addiction: A framework evaluation. In S. Peele (Ed.), *Visions of addiction: Major contemporary perspectives on addiction and alcoholism* (pp. 45–66). Lexington, MA: Heath.

Alexander, F. (1950). *Psychosomatic medicine.* New York: Norton.

Allison, D. B., Heshka, S., Neale, M. C., Lykken, D. T., & Heymsfield, S. B. (1994). A genetic analysis of relative weight among 4,020 twin pairs, with an emphasis on sex effects. *Health Psychology, 13,* 362–365.

Allison, S., & Wong, K. (1967). Skin cancer: Some ethnic differences. In J. Bresler (Ed.), *Environments of men.* Reading, MA: Addison-Wesley.

Alloy, L. B., & Abramson, L. Y. (1980). The cognitive component of human helplessness and depression: A critical analysis. In J. Garber & M. E. P. Seligman (Eds.), *Human helplessness: Theory and applications* (pp. 59–70). New York: Academic Press.

Allred, K. D., & Smith, T. W. (1989). The hardy personality: Cognitive and physiological responses to evaluative threat. *Journal of Personality and Social Psychology, 56,* 257–266.

Allsen, P. E., Harrison, J. M., & Vance, B. (1976). *Fitness for life.* Dubuque, IA: William C. Brown.

Alper, J. (1993). Ulcers as infectious diseases. *Science, 260,* 159–160.

Alterman, T., Shekelle, R. B., Vernon, S. W., & Burau, K. D. (1994). Decision latitude, psychologic demand, job strain, and coronary heart disease in the Western Electric Study. *American Journal of Epidemiology, 139,* 620–627.

Altman, D. G. (1995). Strategies for community health intervention: Promises, paradoxes, pitfalls. *Psychosomatic Medicine, 57,* 226–233.

Altman, D. G., & Cahn, J. (1987). Employment options for health psychologists. In G. C. Stone, S. M. Weiss, J. D. Matarazzo, N. E. Miller, J. Rodin, C. D. Belar, M. J. Follick, & J. E. Singer (Eds.), *Health psychology: A discipline and a profession* (pp. 232–244). Chicago: University of Chicago Press.

Altman, I. (1978). Crowding: Historical and contemporary trends in crowding research. In A. Baum & Y. M. Epstein (Eds.), *Human response to crowding* (pp. 3–29). Hillsdale, NJ: Erlbaum.

Altman L. K. (1995, April 4). Earliest AIDS case is called into doubt. *The New York Times,* pp. C1, C3.

Altura, B. M. (1986). Introduction to the symposium and overview. *Alcoholism, 10,* 557–559.

American Medical Association (AMA) Council on Scientific Affairs. (1987). Aversion therapy. *Journal of the American Medical Association, 258,* 2562–2566.

American Medical Association (AMA) Council on Scientific Affairs. (1991). Hispanic health in the United States. *Journal of the American Medical Association, 265,* 248–252.

American Psychiatric Association. (1980). *Diagnostic and statistical manual of mental disorders* (3rd ed.) (DSM III). Washington, DC: Author.

American Psychiatric Association. (1987) *Diagnostic and statistical manual of mental disorders* (3rd ed., rev.) (DSM III-R). Washington, DC: Author.

American Psychiatric Association. (1994). *Diagnostic and statistical manual of mental disorders* (4th ed.) (DSM IV) . Washington, DC: Author.

American Psychological Association (APA). Task Force on Health Research. (1976). Contributions of psychology to health research: Patterns, problems, and potentials. *American Psychologist, 31,* 263–274.

Amigo, I. Buceta, J. M., Becona, E., & Bueno, A. M. (1991). Cognitive behavioral treatment for essential hypertension: A controlled study. *Stress Medicine, 7,* 103–108.

Anda, R. F., Williamson, D. F., & Remington, P. L. (1988). Alcohol and fatal injuries among US adults: Findings from the NHANES I epidemiologic follow-up study. *Journal of the American Medical Association, 260,* 2529–2532.

Andersen, B. L. (1989). Health psychology's contribution to addressing the cancer problem: Update on accomplishments. *Health Psychology, 8,* 683–703.

Anderson, D., Brink, S., & Courtney, T. D. (1995). *Health risks and their impact on medical costs.* Brookfield, WI: Milliman & Robertson.

Anderson, E. A. (1987). Preoperative preparation for cardiac surgery facilitates recovery, reduces psychological distress, and reduces the incidence of acute postoperative hypertension. *Journal of Consulting and Clinical Psychology, 55,* 513–520.

Anderson, J. W., Story, J., Sieling, B., Chen, W. J., Petro, M. S., & Story, J. (1984). Hypercholesterolemic effects of oat-bran intake for hypercholesterolemic men. *American Journal of Clinical Nutrition, 40,* 1146–1155.

Anderson, N. B. (1993). Reactivity research on sociodemographic groups: Its value to psychophysiology and health psychology. *Health Psychology, 12,* 3–5.

Anderson, N. B., & Armstead, C. A. (1995). Toward understanding the association of socioeconomic status and health: A new challenge for the biopsychosocial approach. *Psychosomatic Medicine, 57,* 213–225.

Andrasik, F., Blanchard, E. B., Arena, J. G., Saunders, N. L., & Barron, K. D. (1982). Psychophysiology of recurrent headaches: Methodological issues and new empirical findings. *Behavior Therapy, 13,* 407–429.

Andrasik, F., Blanchard, E. B., & Edlund, S. R. (1985). Physiological responding during biofeedback. In S. R. Burchfield (Ed.), *Stress: Psychological and physiological interactions.* Washington, DC: Hemisphere.

Andres, R., Muller, D. C., & Sorkin, J. D. (1993). Long-term effects of change in body weight on all-cause mortality: A review. *Annals of Internal Medicine, 119,* 737–743.

Andrew, J. (1970). Recovery from surgery, with and without preparatory instruction for three coping styles. *Journal of Personality and Social Psychology, 15,* 223–226.

Aneshensel, C. S., & Pearlin, L. I. (1987). Structural contexts of sex differences in stress. In R. C. Barnett, L. Biener, & G. K. Baruch (Eds.), *Gender and stress* (pp. 75–95). New York: Free Press.

Annis, H. M., & Davis, C. S. (1988). Self-efficacy and the prevention of alcoholic relapse: Initial findings from a treatment trial. In T. B. Baker & D. Cannon (Eds.), *Assessment and treatment of addictive disorders* (pp. 88–112). New York: Praeger.

Antoni, M. H. (1993). Stress management: Strategies that work. In D. Goleman & J. Gurin (Eds.), *Mind/body medicine: How to use your mind for better health* (pp. 385–397). Yonkers, NY: Consumer Reports Books.

Antoni, M. H., Baggett, L., Ironson, G., LaPerriere, A., August, S., Klimas, N., Schneiderman, N., & Fletcher, M. A. (1991). Cognitive-behavioral stress management intervention buffers distress responses and immunologic changes following notification of HIV-1 seropositivity. *Journal of Consulting and Clinical Psychology, 59,* 906–915.

Antoni, M. H., Schneiderman, N., Fletcher, M. A., Goldstein, D. A., Ironson, G., & LaPerriere, A. (1990). Psychoneuroimmunology and HIV-I. *Journal of Consulting and Clinical Psychology, 58,* 38–49.

Antonovsky, A. (1987). *Unraveling the mystery of health: How people manage stress and stay well.* San Francisco: Jossey-Bass.

Argyle, M. (1992). Benefits produced by supportive social relationships. In H. O. E. Veiel & U. Baumann (Eds.), *The meaning and measurement of social support* (pp. 13–32). New York: Hemisphere.

Arluke, A. (1988). The sick-role concept. In D. S. Gochman (Ed.), *Health behavior: Emerging research perspectives* (pp. 169–180). New York: Plenum.

Armor, D. J., Polich, J. M., & Stambul, H. B. (1976). *Alcoholism and treatment.* Santa Monica, CA: Rand.

Armstead, C. A., Lawler, K. A., Gorden, G., Cross, J., & Gibbons, J. (1989). Relationship of racial stressors to blood pressure responses and anger expression in black college students. *Health Psychology, 8,* 541–556.

Ary, D. V., & Biglan, A. (1988). Longitudinal changes in adolescent cigarette smoking behavior: Onset and cessation. *Journal of Behavioral Medicine, 11,* 361–382.

Ary, D. V., Lichtenstein, E., & Severson, H. H. (1987). Smokeless tobacco use among male adolescents: Patterns, correlates, predictors, and the use of other drugs. *Preventive Medicine, 16,* 385–401.

Ary, D. V., Lichtenstein, E., Severson, H., Weissman, W., & Seeley, J. R. (1989). An in-depth analysis of male adolescent smokeless tobacco users: Interviews with users and their fathers. *Journal of Behavioral Medicine, 12,* 449–467.

Astemborski, J., Vlahov, D., Warren, D., Solomon, L. & Nelson, K. E. (1994). The trading of sex for drugs or money and HIV seropositivity among female intravenous drug users. *American Journal of Public Health, 84,* 382–387.

Atkins, C. J., Kaplan, R. M., Timms, R. M., Reinsch, S., & Lofback, K. (1984). Behavioral exercise programs in the management of chronic obstructive pulmonary disease. *Journal of Consulting and Clinical Psychology, 52,* 591–603.

Atkins, R. C. (1972). *Dr. Atkins' diet revolution: The high calorie way to stay thin forever.* New York: McKay.

Austin, M. A., King, M., Bawol, R. D., Hulley, S. B., & Friedman, G. D. (1987). Risk factors for coronary heart disease in adult female twins: Genetic heritability and shared environmental influences. *Americal Journal of Epidemiology, 125,* 308–318.

Avins, A. L., Woods, W. J., Lindan, C. P., Hudes, E. S., Clark, W., & Hulley, S. B. (1994). HIV infection and risk behaviors among heterosexuals in alcohol treatment programs. *Journal of the American Medical Association, 271,* 515–518.

Avis, N. E., Smith, K. W., & McKinlay, J. B. (1989). Accuracy of perceptions of heart attack risk: What influences perceptions and can they be changed? *American Journal of Public Health, 17,* 1608–1612. .

Avogaro, P., Cazzolato, G., Belussi, F., & Bittolo Bon, G. (1982). Altered apoprotein consumption of HDL_2 and HDL_3 in chronic alcoholics. *Artery, 10,* 317–328.

Avorn, J. (1995). Editorial: Drug regulation and drug information—Who should do what to whom? *American Journal of Public Health, 85,* 18–19.

Ayanian, J. Z., & Epstein, A. M. (1991). Differences in the use of procedures between women and men hospitalized for coronary heart disease. *New England Journal of Medicine, 325,* 221–225

Baer, J. S., Karmack, T., Lichtenstein, E., & Ranson, C. C., Jr. (1989). Predictors of smoking relapse: Analyses of temptations and transgressions after initial cessation. *Journal of Consulting and Clinical Psychology, 57,* 623–627.

Bahrke, M. S., & Morgan, W. P. (1978). Anxiety reduction following exercise and meditation. *Cognitive Therapy and Research, 2,* 323–334.

Ballard, J. E., Koepsell, T. D., & Rivara, F. (1992). Association of smoking and alcohol drinking with residential fire injuries. *American Journal of Epidemiology, 135,* 26–34.

Banaji, M. R., & Steele, C. M. (1989). The social cognition of alcohol use. *Social Cognition, 7,* 137–151.

Bandura, A. (1977). *Social learning theory.* Englewood Cliffs, NJ: Prentice-Hall.

Bandura, A. (1986). *Social foundations of thought and action: A social cognitive theory.* Englewood Cliffs, NJ: Prentice-Hall.

Bandura, A. (1989). Human agency in social cognitive theory. *American Psychologist, 44,* 1175–1184.

Bandura, A. (1991). Social-cognitive theory of self-regulation. *Organizational Behavior and Human Decision Processes, 50,* 248–287.

Bandura, A., O'Leary, A., Taylor, C. B., Gauthier, J., & Gossard, D. (1987). Perceived self-efficacy and pain control: Opioid and nonopioid mechanisms. *Journal of Personality and Social Psychology, 53,* 563–571.

Barber, T. X. (1969). *Hypnosis: A scientific approach.* New York: Van Nostrand Reinhold.

Barber, T. X. (1980). *Medicine, suggestive therapy, and healing: Historical and psychophysiological considerations.* Framingham, MA: Cushing Hospital.

Barber, T. X. (1982). Hypnosuggestive procedures in the treatment of clinical pain: Implications for theories of hypnosis and suggestive therapy. In T. Millon, C. J. Green, & R. B. Meagher, Jr. (Eds.), *Handbook of clinical health psychology.* New York: Plenum.

Barber, T. X. (1984). Hypnosis, deep relaxation, and active relaxation: Data, theory, and clinical applications. In R. L. Woolfolk & P. M. Lehrer (Eds.), *Principles and practice of stress management.* New York: Guilford Press.

Barefoot, J. C., Dahlstrom, W. G., & Williams, R. B., Jr. (1983). Hostility, CHD incidence and total mortality: A 25-year follow-up study of 255 physicians. *Psychosomatic Medicine, 45,* 59–63.

Barefoot, J. C., Dodge, K. A., Peterson, B. L., Dahlstrom, W. G., & Williams, R. B., Jr. (1989). The Cook-Medley Hostility scale: Item content and ability to predict survival. *Psychosomatic Medicine, 51,* 46–57.

Barefoot, J. C., Williams, R. B., Jr., Dahlstrom, W. G., & Dodge, K. A. (1987). Predicting mortality from scores on the Cook-Medley scale: A follow-up study of 118 lawyers. *Psychosomatic Medicine, 49,* 210. (Abstract)

Barnathan, E. S. (1993). Has lipoprotein 'little' (a) shrunk? *Journal of the American Medical Association, 270,* 224–225.

Barrett, J. J., Ford, G. R., Stewart, K. E., & Haley, W. E. (1994, August). *Family caregiver appraisals of stressors in senile dementia: Gender differences?* Paper presented at the American Psychological Association, Los Angeles, CA.

Basmajian, J. V. (1978). *Muscles alive: Their functions revealed by electromyography.* Baltimore: Williams & Wilkins.

Baum, A., Davidson, L. M., Singer, J. E., & Street, S. W. (1987). Stress as a psychophysiological process. In A. Baum & J. E. Singer (Eds.), *Handbook of psychology and health, Vol. 5. Stress* (pp. 1–24). Hillsdale, NJ: Erlbaum.

Baum, A., Gatchel, R. J., & Schaeffer, M. A. (1983). Emotional, behavioral, and physiological effects of chronic stress at Three Mile Island. *Journal of Consulting and Clinical Psychology, 51,* 565–572.

Baumann, L. J., Cameron, L. D., Zimmerman, R. S., & Leventhal, H. W. (1989). Illness representations and matching labels with symptoms. *Health Psychology, 8,* 449–469.

Baumann, L. J., & Leventhal, H. (1985). "I can tell when my blood pressure is up, can't I?" *Health Psychology, 4,* 203–218.

Bazargan, M. (1994). The effects of health, environmental, and socio-psychological variables on fear of crime and its consequences among urban Black elderly individuals. *International Journal of Aging and Human Development, 38,* 99–115.

Beaglehole, R., Bonita, R., & Kjellström, T. (1993). *Basic epidemiology.* Geneva, Switzerland: World Health Organization.

Beck, A. T. (1972). *Depression: Causes and treatment.* Philadelphia: University of Pennsylvania Press.

Beck, A. T. (1976). *Cognitive therapy and the emotional disorders.* New York: International Universities Press.

Beck, A. T., Ward, C. H., Mendelson, M., Mock, J., & Erbaugh, J. (1961). An inventory for measuring depression. *Archives of General Psychiatry, 4,* 561–571.

Becker, M. H. (1979). Understanding patient compliance: The contributions of attitudes and other psychosocial factors. In S. J. Cohen (Ed.), *New directions in patient compliance* (pp. 1–31). Lexington, MA: Lexington Books.

Becker, M. H., Drachman, R. H., & Kirscht, J. P. (1972). Predicting mothers' compliance with pediatric medical regimens. *Journal of Pediatrics, 81,* 843–854.

Becker, M. H., & Maiman. L. A. (1975). Sociobehavioral determinants of compliance with health and medical care recommendations. *Medical Care, 13,* 10–24.

Becker, M. H., & Maiman, L. A. (1980). Strategies for enhancing patient compliance. *Journal of Community Health, 6,* 113–135.

Becker, M. H., & Rosenstock, I. M. (1984). Compliance with medical advice. In A. Steptoe & A. Mathews (Eds.), *Health care and human behavior.* London: Academic Press.

Beecher, H. K. (1946). Pain of men wounded in battle. *Annals of Surgery, 123,* 96–105.

Beecher, H. K. (1956). Relationship of significance of wound to pain experience. *Journal of the American Medical Association, 161,* 1609–1613.

Beecher, H. K. (1957). The measurement of pain. *Pharmacological Review, 9,* 59–209.

Beglin, S. J., & Fairburn, C. G. (1992). Women who choose not to participate in surveys on eating disorders. *International Journal of Eating Disorders, 12,* 113–116.

Behrens, V., Seligman, P., Cameron, L., Mathias, C. G. T., & Fine, L. (1994). The prevalence of back pain, hand discomfort, and dermatitis in the US work population. *American Journal of Public Health, 84,* 1780–1785.

Belar, C. D. (1987). The current status of predoctoral and postdoctoral training in health psychology. In G. C. Stone, S. M. Weiss, J. D. Matarazzo, N. E. Miller, J. Rodin, C. D. Belar, M. J. Follick, & J. E. Singer (Eds.), *Health psychology: A discipline and a profession* (pp. 325–334). Chicago: University of Chicago Press.

Belar, C. D. (1996, Winter). President's column. *Health Psychologist, 18*(1), 1, 17–18.

Beller, A. S. (1978). *Fat and thin: A natural history of obesity.* New York: Farrar, Straus & Giroux.

Belloc, N. (1973). Relationship of health practices and mortality. *Preventive Medicine, 2,* 67–81.

Benca, R. M., Obermeyer, W. H., Thisted, R. A., & Gillin, J. C. (1992). Sleep and psychiatric disorders: A meta-analysis. *Archives of General Psychiatry, 49,* 651–668.

Benedetti, C., & Bonica, J. J. (1984). Cancer pain: Basic considerations. In C. Benedetti, C. R. Chapman, & G. Moricca (Eds.), *Advances in pain research and therapy: Vol. 7. Recent advances in the management of pain.* New York: Raven.

Ben-Eliyahu, S., Yirmiya, R., Liebeskind, J. C., Taylor, A. N., & Gale, R. P. (1991). Stress increases metastatic spread of mammary tumor in rats: Evidence for mediation by the immune system. *Brain, Behavior, and Immunity, 5,* 193–205.

Bennett, H. L., & Disbrow, E. A. (1993). Preparing for surgery and medical procedures. In D. Goleman & J. Gurin (Eds.), *Mind/body medicine: How to use your mind for better health* (pp. 401–427). Yonkers, NY: Consumer Reports Books.

Bennett, W., & Gurin, J. (1982). *The dieter's dilemma: Eating less and weighing more.* New York: Basic Books.

Bennett, W. I. (1995). Beyond overeating. *New England Journal of Medicine, 332,* 673–674.

Bennett, W. I., Goldfinger, S. E., & Johnson, G. T. (1987). *Your good health: How to stay well and what to do when you're not.* Cambridge, MA: Harvard University Press.

Bennett Johnson, S. (1994, Winter). Health and behavior: Getting behavioral research the attention and support it deserves. *Health Psychologist, 16*(3), 1, 25.

Ben-Shlomo, Y., Smith, G. D., Shipley, M. S., & Marmot, M. G. (1994). What determines mortality risk in male former cigarette smokers? *American Journal of Public Health, 84,* 1235–1242.

Benson, H. (1974). Your innate asset for combating stress. *Harvard Business Review, 52,* 49–60.

Benson, H. (1975). *The relaxation response.* New York: Morrow.

Benson, H., Beary, J. F., & Carol, M. P. (1974). The relaxation response. *Psychiatry, 37,* 37–46.

Berger, B. D., & Adesso, V. J. (1991). Gender differences in using alcohol to cope with depression. *Addictive Behaviors, 16,* 315–327.

Berkman, L. F. (1986). Social networks, support, and health: Taking the next step forward. *American Journal of Epidemiology, 123,* 559–562.

Berkman, L. F., & Breslow, L. (1983). *Health and ways of living: The Alameda County Study.* New York: Oxford University Press.

Berkman, L. F., Breslow, L., & Wingard, D. (1983). Health practices and mortality risk. In L. F. Berkman & L. Breslow (Eds.), *Health and ways of living: The Alameda County Study.* New York: Oxford University Press.

Berkman, L. F., & Syme, S. L. (1979). Social networks, host resistance, and mortality: A nine-year follow-up study of Alameda County residents. *American Journal of Epidemiology, 109,* 186–204.

Berlin, J. A., & Colditz, G. A. (1990). A meta-analysis of physical activity in the prevention of coronary heart disease. *American Journal of Epidemiology, 132,* 612–628.

Bernstein, D. A., & Borkovec, T. D. (1973). *Progressive relaxation training.* Champaign, IL: Research Press.

Bernstein, L., Henderson, B. E., Hanisch, R., Sullivan-Halley, J., & Ross, R. K. (1994). Physical exercise and reduced risk of breast cancer in young women. *Journal of the National Cancer Institute, 86,* 1403–1408.

Berry, D. S., & Pennebaker, J. W. (1993). Nonverbal and verbal emotional expression and health. *Psychotherapy and Psychosomatics, 59,* 1119.

Bibace, R., & Walsh, M. E. (1979). Developmental stages in children's conceptions of illness. In G. C. Stone, F. Cohen, & N. E. Adler (Eds.), *Health psychology–A handbook* (pp. 285–301). San Francisco: Jossey-Bass.

Bieliauskas, L. A. (1982). *Stress and its relationship to health and illness.* Boulder, CO: Westview.

Bieliauskas, L. A. (1984). Depression, stress, and cancer. In C. L. Cooper (Ed.), *Psychosocial stress and cancer* (pp. 37–48). Chichester, England: Wiley.

Biener, L., & Heaton, A. (1995). Women dieters of normal weight: Their motives, goals, and risks. *American Journal of Public Health, 85,* 714–717.

Biglan, A., Glasgow, R., Ary, D., Thompson, R., Severson, H., Lichtenstein, E., Weissman, W., Faller, C., & Gallison, C. (1987). How generalizable are the effects of smoking prevention programs? Refusal skills training and parent messages in a teacher-administered program. *Journal of Behavioral Medicine, 10,* 613–628.

Biglan, A., Metzler, C. W., Wirt, R., Ary, D., Noell, J., Ochs, L., French, C., & Hood, D. (1990). Social and behavioral factors associated with high-risk sexual behavior among adolescents. *Journal of Behavioral Medicine, 13,* 245–262.

Bjornson, W., Rand, C., Connett, J. E., Lundgren, P., Nides, M., Pope, F., Buist, A. S., Hoppe-Ryan, C., & O'Hara, P. (1995). Gender differences in smoking cessation after 3 years in the Lung Health Study. *American Journal of Public Health, 85,* 223–230.

Blackburn, H., Luepker, R. V., Kline, F. G., Bracht, N., Carlaw, R., Jacobs, D., Mittelmark, L. S., & Taylor, H. L. (1984). The Minnesota Heart Health Program: A research and demonstration project in cardiovascular disease prevention. In J. D. Matarazzo, S. M. Weiss, J. A. Herd, N. E. Miller, & S. M. Weiss (Eds.), *Behavioral health: A handbook of health enhancement and disease prevention* (pp. 1171–1178). New York: Wiley.

Blair, S. N. (1993). Evidence for success of exercise in weight loss and control. *Annals of Internal Medicine, 119,* 702–706.

Blair, S. N. (1994). Physical activity, fitness, and coronary heart disease. In C. Bouchard, R. J. Shephard, & T. Stephens (Eds.), *Physical activity, fitness, and health: International proceedings and consensus statement* (pp. 579–590). Champaign, IL: Human Kinetics.

Blair, S. N., Kohl, H. W., Barlow, C. E., Paffenbarger, R. S., Jr., Gibbons, L. W., & Macera, C. A. (1995). Changes in physical fitness and all-cause mortality: A prospective study of healthy and unhealthy men. *Journal of the American Medical Association, 273,* 1093–1098.

Blair, S. N., Kohl, H. W. III, Paffenbarger, R. S., Jr., Clark, D. G., Cooper, K. H., & Gibbons, L. W. (1989). Physical fitness and all-cause mortality: A prospective study of healthy men and women. *Journal of the American Medical Association, 262,* 2395–2401.

Blanchard, E. B., & Andrasik, F. (1982). Psychological assessment and treatment of headache: Recent development and emerging issues. *Journal of Consulting and Clinical Psychology, 50,* 859–879.

Blanchard, E. B., & Andrasik, F. (1985). *Management of chronic headaches: A psychological approach.* New York: Pergamon Press.

Blanchard, E. B., Andrasik, F., Neff, D. F., Arena, J. G., Ahles, T. A., Jurish, S. E., Pallmeyer, T. P., Saunders, N. L., Teders, S. J., Barron, K. D., & Rodichok, L. D. (1982). Biofeedback and relaxation training with three kinds of headache: Treatment effects and their prediction. *Journal of Consulting and Clinical Psychology, 50,* 562–575.

Blanchard, E. B., Appelbaum, K. A., Radniz, C. L., Michultka, D., Morrill, B., Kirsch, C., Hillhouse, J., Evans, D. D., Guarnieri, P., Attanasio, V., Andrasik, F., Jaccard, J., & Dentinger, M. P. (1990a). Placebo-controlled evaluation of abbreviated progressive muscle relaxation and of relaxation combined with cognitive therapy in the treatment of tension headache. *Journal of Consulting and Clinical Psychology, 58,* 210–215.

Blanchard, E. B., Appelbaum, K. A., Radniz, C. L., Morrill, B., Michultka, D., Kirsch, C., Guarnieri, P., Hillhouse, J., Evans, D. D., Jaccard, J., & Barron, K. D. (1990b). A controlled evaluation of thermal biofeedback and thermal biofeedback combined with cognitive therapy in the treatment of vascular headache. *Journal of Consulting and Clinical Psychology, 58,* 216–224.

Blanchard, E. B., & Epstein, L. H. (1977). The clinical usefulness of biofeedback. In M. Hersen, R. M. Eisler, & P. M. Miller (Eds.), *Progress in behavior modification* (Vol. 4, pp. 163–249). New York: Academic Press.

Blankenhorn, D. H., Johnson, R. L., Mack, W. J., Zein, H. A., & Vailas, L. I. (1990). The influence of diet on the appearance of new lesions in human coronary arteries. *Journal of the American Medical Association, 263,* 1646–1652.

Blevins, D. R. (1979). An overview. In D. R. Blevins (Ed.), *The diabetic and nursing care* (pp. 1–9). New York: McGraw-Hill.

Bloemburg, B. P., Kromhout, D., Goddjin, H. E., Jansen, A., & Obermann-de Boer, G. L. (1991). The impact of the guidelines for a healthy diet of the Netherlands Nutrition Council on total and high density lipoprotein cholesterol in hypercholesterolemic free-living men. *American Journal of Epidemiology, 134,* 39–49.

Bloom, C., Kogel, L., & Zaphiropoulos, L. (1994). Beginning the eating and body work: Stance and tools. In C. Bloom, A. Gitter, S. Gutwill, L. Kogel, & L. Zaphiropoulos (Eds.), *Eating problems: A feminist psychoanalytic treatment model* (pp. 67–82). New York: Basic Books.

Blose, J. O., & Holder, H. D. (1991). Injury-related medical care utilization in a problem drinking population. *American Journal of Public Health, 81,* 1571–1575.

Blum, E. M. (1966). Psychoanalytic views of alcoholism: A review. *Quarterly Journal of Studies on Alcohol, 27,* 259–299.

Blume, S. B. (1985). Psychodrama and the treatment of alcoholism. In S. Zimberg, J. Wallace, & S. B. Blume (Eds.), *Practical approaches to alcoholism psychotherapy* (2nd ed.). New York: Plenum.

Blumstein, P., & Schwartz, P. (1983). *American couples.* New York: Pocket Books.

Bly, J. L., Jones, R. C., & Richardson, J. E. (1986). Impact of worksite health promotion on health care costs and utilization: Evaluation of Johnson & Johnson's Live for Life program. *Journal of the American Medical Association, 256,* 3235–3240.

Bodnar, J. C., & Kiecolt-Glaser, J. K. (1994). Caregiver depression after bereavement: Chronic stress isn't over when it's over. *Psychology and Aging, 9,* 372–380.

Bohman, M., Sigvardsson, S., & Cloninger, C. R. (1981). Maternal inheritance of alcohol abuse. *Archives of General Psychiatry, 38,* 965–969.

Bolinder, G., Alfredsson, L., England, A., & de Faire, U. (1994). Smokeless tobacco use and increased cardiovascular mortality among Swedish construction workers. *American Journal of Public Health, 84,* 399–404.

Boll, T. J. (1987). Predoctoral education and training in health psychology. In G. C. Stone, S. M. Weiss, J. D. Matarazzo, N. E. Miller, J. Rodin, C. D. Belar, M. J. Follick, & J. E. Singer (Eds.), *Health psychology: A discipline and a profession* (pp. 335–349). Chicago: University of Chicago Press.

Bond, G. G., Aiken, L. S., & Somerville, S. C. (1992). The health belief model and adolescents with insulin-dependent diabetes mellitus. *Health Psychology, 11,* 190–198.

Boney McCoy, S., Gibbons, F. X., Reis, T. J., Gerrard, M., Luus, C. A. E., & Von Wald Sufka, A. (1992). Perceptions of smoking risk as a function of smoking status. *Journal of Behavior Medicine, 15,* 469–488.

Bonica, J. J. (1980). Cancer pain. In J. J. Bonica (Ed.), *Pain.* New York: Raven.

Bonica, J. J. (1990a). Definitions and taxonomy of pain. In J. J. Bonica (Ed.), *The management of pain* (2nd ed., pp. 18–27). Malvern, PA: Lea & Febiger.

Bonica, J. J. (1990b). General considerations of chronic pain. In J. J. Bonica (Ed.), *The management of pain* (2nd ed., pp. 180–196). Malvern, PA: Lea & Febiger.

Bonica, J. J., Ventafridda, V., & Twycross, R. G. (1990). Cancer pain. In J. J. Bonica (Ed.), *The management of pain* (2nd ed., pp. 400–460). Malvern, PA: Lea & Febiger.

Bonneau, R., Sheridan, J. F., Feng, N., & Glaser, R. (1991). Stress-induced suppression of herpes simplex virus (HSV)-specific sytotoxic T lymphocyte and natural killer cell activity and enhancement of acute pathogenesis following local HSV infection. *Brain, Behavior, and Immunity, 5,* 170–192.

Borkan, G. A., Sparrow, D., Wisniewski, C., & Vokonas, P. S. (1986). Body weight and coronary disease risk: Patterns of risk factor change associated with long-term weight change. The Normative Aging Study. *American Journal of Epidemiology, 124,* 410–419.

Borrelli, B., & Mermelstein, R. (1994). Goal setting and behavior change in a smoking cessation program. *Cognitive Therapy and Research, 18,* 69–82.

Boskind-White, M., & White, W. C., Jr. (1983). *Bulimarexia: The binge/purge cycle.* New York: Norton.

Bosscher, R. J. (1993). Running and mixed physical exercises with depressed psychiatric patients. Special Issue: Exercise and psychological well-being. *International Journal of Sport Psychology, 24,* 170–184.

Botvin, G. J., Baker, E., Dusenburg, L., Botvin, E. M., & Diaz, T. (1995). Long-term follow-up results of a randomized drug abuse prevention trial in a White middle class population. *Journal of the American Medical Association, 273,* 1106–1112.

Bouchard, C., Tremblay, A., Després, J-P., Nadeau, A., Lupien, P. J., Thériault, G., Dussault, J., Moorjani, S., Pinault, S., & Fournier, G. (1990). The response to long-term overfeeding in identical twins. *New England Journal of Medicine, 322,* 1477–1482.

Bovbjerg, V. E., McCann, B. S., Brief, D. J., Follette, W. C., Retzlaff, B. M., Dowdy, A. A., Walden, C. E., & Knopp, R. H. (1995). Spouse support and long-term adherence to lipid-lowering diets. *American Journal of Epidemiology, 141,* 451–460.

Boyd, J. R., Covington, T. R., Stanaszek, W. F., & Coussons, R. T. (1974). Drug-defaulting II: Analysis of noncompliance patterns. *American Journal of Hospital Pharmacy, 31,* 485–491.

Bradley, L. A. (1993). Pain measurement in arthritis. *Arthritis Care and Research, 6,* 178–186.

Bradley, L. A., Prokop, C. K., Gentry, W. D., Van der Heide, L. H., & Prieto, E. J. (1981). Assessment of chronic pain. In C. K. Prokop & L. A. Bradley (Eds.), *Medical psychology: Contributions to behavioral medicine.* New York: Academic Press.

Bradley, L. A., Prokop, C. K., Margolis, R., & Gentry, W. D. (1978). Multivariate analysis of the MMPI profiles of low back pain patients. *Journal of Behavioral Medicine, 1,* 253–272.

Bradley, L. A., & Van der Heide, L. H. (1984). Pain-related correlates of MMPI profile subgroups among back pain patients. *Health Psychology, 3,* 157–174.

Brandsma, J. M., Maultsby, M. C., & Welsh, R. J. (1980). *The outpatient treatment of alcoholism: A review and comparative study.* Baltimore: University Park Press.

Brannon, L., & Papadimitriou, M. (1985, October). *Smokers vs. nonsmokers: Perception of risks.* Paper presented at convention of the Louisiana Psychological Association, Lake Charles, LA.

Braun, A. C. (1977). *The story of cancer.* Reading, MA: Addison-Wesley.

Bray, G. A. (1992). Pathophysiology of obesity. *American Journal of Clinical Nutrition, 55,* 488S–494S.

Brecher, E. M. (1972). *Licit and illicit drugs.* Boston: Little, Brown.

Brehm, J. W. (1966). *A theory of psychological reactance.* New York: Academic Press.

Breuer, J., & Freud, S. (1955). Studies on hysteria. In J. Strachey (Ed. and Trans.), *The standard edition of the complete pyschological works of Sigmund Freud* (Vol. 2). London: Hogarth Press. (Original work published 1895)

Brewer, B. W., & Karoly, P. (1992). Recurrent pain in college students. *Journal of American College Health, 41,* 67–69.

Brewer, R. D., Morris, P. D., Cole, T. B., Watkins, S., Patetta, M. J., & Popkin, C. (1994). The risk of dying in alcohol-related automobile crashes among habitual drunk drivers. *New England Journal of Medicine, 331,* 513–517.

Brock, D. W., & Wartman, S. A. (1990). When competent patients make irrational choices. *New England Journal of Medicine, 322,* 1595–1599.

Broman, C. L. (1993). Social relationships and health-related behavior. *Journal of Behavioral Medicine, 16,* 335–350.

Brown, B. (1970). Recognition of aspects of consciousness through association with EEG alpha activity represented by a light signal. *Psychophysics, 6,* 442–446.

Brown, D. (1988, October 25). The beat goes on: Framingham Heart Study at 40. *Health, Science, and Society,* pp. 12–16.

Brown, D. (1994, June 2). Baby boomers have greater cancer risk, researchers report. *The Houston Chronicle,* p. 2A.

Brown, G. W., Bhrolcháin, M. N., & Harris, T. O. (1975). Social class and psychiatric disturbance among women in an urban population. *Sociology, 9,* 225–254.

Brown, G. W., & Harris, T. O. (1989). *Life events and illness.* New York: Guilford Press.

Brown, J. D. (1991). Staying fit and staying well: Physical fitness as a moderator of life stress. *Journal of Personality and Social Psychology, 60,* 555–561.

Brown, J. D., & Lawton, M. (1986). Stress and well-being in adolescence: The moderating role of physical exercise. *Journal of Human Stress, 12,* 125–131.

Brown, J. D., & McGill, K. L. (1989). The cost of good fortune: When positive life events produce negative health consequences. *Journal of Personality and Social Psychology, 57,* 1103–1110.

Brown, J. D., & Siegel, J. M. (1988). Exercise as a buffer of life stress: A prospective study of adolescent health. *Health Psychology, 7,* 341–353.

Brownell, K. D. (1982). The addictive disorders. In C. M. Franks, G. T. Wilson, P. C. Kendall, & K. D. Brownell, *Annual review of behavior therapy: Theory and practice* (Vol. 8, pp. 208–272). New York: Guilford Press.

Brownell, K. D. (1984a). The addictive disorders. In G. T. Wilson, C. M. Franks, K. D. Brownell, & P. C. Kendall. *Annual review of behavior therapy: Theory and practice* (Vol. 9, pp. 211–258). New York: Guilford Press.

Brownell, K. D. (1984b). Behavioral medicine. In G. T. Wilson, C. M. Franks, K. D. Brownell, & P. C. Kendall, *Annual review of behavior therapy: Theory and practice* (Vol. 9). New York: Guilford Press.

Brownell, K. D. (1991). Personal responsibility and control over our bodies: When expectation exceeds reality. *Health Psychology, 10,* 303–310.

Brownell, K. D. (1993). Whether obesity should be treated. *Health Psychology, 12,* 339–341.

Brownell, K. D., & Rodin, J. (1994a). The dieting maelstrom: Is it possible and advisable to lose weight? *American Psychologist, 49,* 781–791.

Brownell, K. D., & Rodin, J. (1994b). Medical, metabolic, and psychological effects of weight cycling. *Archives of Internal Medicine, 154,* 1325–1330.

Brownell, K. D., & Stein, L. J. (1989). Metabolic and behavioral effects of weight loss and regain: A review of the animal and human literature. In A. J. Stunkard & A. Baum (Eds.), *Perspectives in behavioral medicine: Eating, sleeping, and sex* (pp. 39–52). Hillsdale, NJ: Erlbaum.

Browning, C. H., & Miller, S. I. (1968). Anorexia nervosa: A study in prognosis and management. *American Journal of Psychiatry, 124,* 1128–1132.

Brownlee-Duffeck, M., Peterson, L., Simonds, J. F., Goldstein, D., Kilo, C., & Hoette, S. (1987). The role of health beliefs in the regimen adherence and metabolic control of adolescents and adults with diabetes mellitus. *Journal of Consulting and Clinical Psychology, 55,* 139–144.

Brownson, R. C., Alavanja, M. C. R., Hock, E. T., & Loy, T. S. (1992). Passive smoking and lung cancer in nonsmoking women. *American Journal of Public Health, 82,* 1525–1530.

Brownson, R. C., Jackson-Thompson, J., Wilkerson, J. C., Davis, J. R., Owens, N. W., & Fisher, E. B., Jr. (1992). Demographic and socioeconomic differences in beliefs about the health effects of smoking. *American Journal of Public Health, 82,* 99–103,

Bru, E., Mykletun, R. J., Berge, W. T., & Svebak, S. (1994). Effects of different psychological interventions on neck, shoulder and low back pain in female hospital staff. *Psychology and Health, 9,* 371–382.

Bruch, H. (1973). *Eating disorders: Obesity, anorexia nervosa and the person within.* New York: Basic Books.

Bruch, H. (1978). *The golden cage: The enigma of anorexia nervosa.* Cambridge, MA: Harvard University Press.

Bruch, H. (1982). Anorexia nervosa: Therapy and theory. *American Journal of Psychiatry, 139,* 1531–1538.

Brunnquell, D., & Hall, M. D. (1984). Issues in the psychological care of pediatric oncology patients. In R. H. Moos (Ed.), *Coping with physical illness 2: New perspectives* (pp. 195–207). New York: Plenum Press.

Bryant, R. A. (1993). Beliefs about hypnosis: A survey of acute and chronic pain therapists. *Contemporary Hypnosis, 10,* 89–98.

Bryson, Y. J., Pang, S., Wei, L. S., Dickover, A. D., & Chen, I. S. Y. (1995). Clearance of HIV infection in a perinatally infected infant. *New England Journal of Medicine, 332,* 833–838.

Bucholz, K. K. (1992). Alcohol abuse and dependence from a psychiatric epidemiologic perspective. *Alcohol Health and Research World, 16,* 197–208.

Buckley, W. E., Yesalis, C. E., III, Friedl, K. E., Anderson, W. A., Streit, A. L., & Wright, J. E. (1988). Estimated prevalence of anabolic steroid use among male high school seniors. *Journal of the American Medical Association, 260,* 3441–3445.

Buffone, G. W. (1980). Exercise as therapy: A closer look. *Journal of Counseling and Psychotherapy, 3,* 101–115.

Bullock, K. M., Reed, R. J., & Grant, I. (1992). Reduced mortality risk in alcoholics who achieve long-term abstinence. *Journal of the American Medical Association, 262,* 668–672.

Bulman, R. J., & Wortman, C. B. (1977). Attribution of blame and coping in the "real world": Severe accident victims react to their lot. *Journal of Personality and Social Psychology, 35,* 351–363.

Burbach, D. J., & Peterson, L. (1986). Children's concepts of physical illness: A review and critique of the cognitive-developmental literature. *Health Psychology, 5,* 307–325.

Burish, T. G., Meyerowitz, B. E., Carey, M. P., & Morrow, G. R. (1987). The stressful effects of cancer in adults. In A. Baum & J. E. Singer (Eds.), *Handbook of psychology and health: Vol. 5. Stress* (pp. 137–173). Hillsdale, NJ: Erlbaum.

Burns, J. W., & Katkin, E. S., (1993). Psychological, situational, and gender predictors of cardiovascular reactivity to stress: A multivariate approach. *Journal of Behavioral Medicine, 16,* 445–465.

Burns, T., & Crisp, A. H. (1990). Outcome of anorexia nervosa in males. In A. E. Andersen (Ed.), *Males with eating disorders* (pp. 163–186). New York: Brunner/Mazel.

Burros, M. (1996, January 3). In an about-face, U.S. says alcohol has health benefits. *New York Times,* pp. A1, C2.

Bush, C., Ditto, B., & Feuerstein, M. (1985). A controlled evaluation of paraspinal EMG biofeedback in the treatment of chronic low back pain. *Health Psychology, 4,* 307–321.

Bush, J. P., Melamed, B. G., Sheras, P. L., & Greenbaum, P. E. (1986). Mother-child patterns of coping with anticipatory medical stress. *Health Psychology, 5,* 137–157.

Buss, A. H., & Durkee, A. (1957). An inventory for assessing different kinds of hostility. *Journal of Consulting Psychology, 21,* 343–349.

Byers, T. E., Graham, S., Haughey, B. P., Marshall, J. R., & Swanson, M. K. (1987). Diet and lung cancer risk: Findings from the Western New York Diet Study. *American Journal of Epidemiology, 125,* 351–363.

Byrne, J., Fears, T. R., Steinhorn, S. C., Mulvihill, J. J., Connelly, R. R., Austin, D. F., Holmes, G. F., Holmes, F. F., Latourette, H. B., Teta, J., Strong, L. C., & Myers, M. H. (1989). Marriage and divorce after childhood and adolescent cancer. *Journal of the American Medical Association, 262,* 2693–2699.

Caddy, G. R., Addington, H. J., & Perkins, D. (1978). Individualized behavior therapy for alcoholics: A third year indepen-

dent double-blind follow-up. *Behavior Research and Therapy, 16,* 345–362.

Caetano, R. (1994). Drinking and alcohol-related problems among minority women. *Alcohol Health and Research World, 18,* 233–241.

Caggiula, A. W., Christakis, G., Farrand, M., Hulley, S. B., Johnson, R., Lasser, N. L., Stamler, J., & Widdowson, G. (1981). The Multiple Risk Factor Intervention Trial (MRFIT): IV. Intervention on blood lipids. *Preventive Medicine, 10,* 443–475.

Caldwell, J. R., Cobb, S., Dowling, M. D., & DeJongh, D. (1970). The dropout problem in antihypertensive therapy. *Journal of Chronic Diseases, 22,* 579–592.

Calermajer, D. S., Adams, M. R., Clarkson, P., Robinson, J., McCredie, R., Donald, A., & Deanfield, J. E. (1996). Passive smoking and impaired endothelium-dependent arterial dilation in healthy young adults. *New England Journal of Medicine, 334,* 150–154.

Calhoun, J. B. (1956). A comparative study of the social behavior of two inbred strains of house mice. *Ecological Monogram, 26,* 81.

Calhoun, J. B. (1962, February). Population density and social pathology. *Scientific American, 206,* 139–148.

Calhoun, J. B. (1971). Space and the strategy of life. In A. H. Esser (Ed.), *Behavior and environment: The use of space by animals and men.* New York: Plenum.

Calle, E. E., Miracle-McMahill, H. L., Thun, M. J., & Heath, C. W., Jr. (1994). Cigarette smoking and risk of fatal breast cancer. *American Journal of Epidemiology, 139,* 1001–1007.

Camacho, T. C., Roberts, R. E., Lazarus, N. B., Kaplan, G. A., & Cohen, R. D. (1991). Physical activity and depression: Evidence from the Alameda County Study. *American Journal of Epidemiology, 134,* 220–231.

Camacho, T. C., & Wiley, J. A. (1983). Health practices, social networks, and change in physical health. In L. F. Berkman & L. Breslow (Eds.), *Health and ways of living: The Alameda County Study.* New York: Oxford University Press.

Cameron, E., Pauling, L., & Leibowitz, B. (1979). Ascorbic acid and cancer: A review. *Cancer Research, 39,* 663–681.

Cameron, L., Leventhal, E. A., & Leventhal, H. (1993). Symptom representations and affect as determinants of care seeking in a community-dwelling, adult sample population. *Health Psychology, 12,* 171–179.

Cameron, L., Leventhal, E. A., & Leventhal, H. (1995). Seeking medical care in response to symptoms and life stress. *Psychosomatic Medicine, 57,* 37–47.

Campfield, L. A., Smith, F. J., Guisez, Y., Devos, R., & Burn, P. (1995). Recombinant mouse OB protein: Evidence for a peripheral signal linking adiposity and central neural networks. *Science, 269,* 546–549.

Cannon, W. (1932). *The wisdom of the body.* New York: Norton.

Caragata, W. (1995, April 3). Medicare wars: Canada's health care cuts. *Maclean's, 108,* 14–15.

Carden, A. D. (1994). Wife abuse and the wife abuser: Review and recommendations. *Counseling Psychologist, 22,* 539–582.

Carmach, M. A., & Martens, R. (1979). Measuring commitment to running: A survey of runners' attitudes and mental state. *Journal of Sports Psychology, 1,* 25–42.

Carmelli, D., Dame, A., & Swan, G. E. (1992). Age-related changes in behavioral components in relation to changes in global Type A behavior. *Journal of Behavioral Medicine, 15,* 143–154.

Carmelli, D., Dame, A., Swan, G., & Rosenman, R. (1991). Long-term changes in Type A behavior: A 27-year follow-up of the Western Collaborative Group Study. *Journal of Behavioral Medicine, 14,* 593–606.

Caron, H. S., & Roth, H. P. (1968). Patients' cooperation with a medical regimen: Difficulties in identifying the noncooperator. *Journal of the American Medical Association, 203,* 922–926.

Carron, H. (1984). Management of low back pain. In C. Benedetti, C. R. Chapman, & G. Moricca (Eds.), *Advances in pain research and therapy: Vol. 7. Recent advances in the management of pain.* New York: Raven.

Carruthers, M. (1983). Instrumental stress tests. In H. Selye (Ed.), *Selye's guide to stress research* (Vol. 2). New York: Scientific and Academic Editions.

Carson, B. S. (1987). Neurologic and neurosurgical approaches to cancer pain. In D. B. McGuire & C. H. Yarbro (Eds.), *Cancer pain management* (pp. 223–243). Philadelphia: Saunders.

Case, R. B., Moss, A. J., Case, N., McDermott, M., & Eberly, S. (1992). Living alone after myocardial infarction. *Journal of the American Medical Association, 267,* 515–519.

Caspersen, C. J., Bloemberg, B. P. M., Saris, W. H. M., Merritt, R. K., & Kromhout, D. (1991). The prevalence of selected physical activities and their relation with coronary heart disease risk factors in elderly men: The Zutphen Study, 1985. *American Journal of Epidemiology, 133,* 1078–1092.

Cassel, J. (1976). The contribution of the social environment to host resistance. *American Journal of Epidemiology, 104,* 107–123.

Cassileth, B. R., Lusk, E. J., Miller, D. S., Brown, L. L., & Miller, C. (1985). Psychosocial correlates of survival in advanced malignant diseases? *New England Journal of Medicine, 312,* 1551–1555.

Catalano, R. B. (1987). Pharmacologic management in the treatment of cancer pain. In D. B. McGuire & C. H. Yarbro (Eds.), *Cancer pain management* (pp. 151–201). Philadelphia: Saunders.

Caudill, B. D., & Marlatt, G. A. (1975). Modeling influences in social drinking: An experimental analogue. *Journal of Consulting and Clinical Psychology, 143,* 405–415.

Cauwells, J. M. (1983). *Bulimia: The binge-purge compulsion.* Garden City, NY: Doubleday.

Cavaliere, F. (1995, July). APA and CDC join forces to combat illness. *APA Monitor, 26*(7), 1, 13.

Centers for Disease Control and Prevention (CDC). (1992). 1993 revised classification system for HIV infection and expanded surveillance case definition for AIDS among adolescents and adults. *Morbidity and Mortality Weekly Report, 41,* No. RR-17.

Centers for Disease Control and Prevention (CDC). (1993). Cigarette smoking—attributable mortality and years of potential life lost—United States, 1990. *Morbidity and Mortality Weekly Report, 42,* 645–649.

Centers for Disease Control and Prevention (CDC). (1994a). Mortality patterns—United States, 1992. *Morbidity and Mortality Weekly Report, 43,* 916–920.

Centers for Disease Control and Prevention (CDC). (1994b). Prevalence of selected risk factors for chronic disease by education level in racial/ethnic populations—United States, 1991–1992. *Morbidity and Mortality Weekly Report, 43,* 894–899.

Centers for Disease Control and Prevention (CDC). (1994c). Preventing tobacco use among young people: A report of the Surgeon General. *Morbidity and Mortality Weekly Report, 43,* No. RR-4.

Centers for Disease Control and Prevention (CDC). (1994d). Reasons for tobacco use and symptoms of nicotine withdrawal among adolescent and young adult tobacco users—United States, 1993. *Morbidity and Mortality Weekly Report, 43,* 745–750.

Centers for Disease Control and Prevention (CDC). (1994e). Recommendations of the U.S. Public Health Service Task Force on the use of zidovudine to reduce perinatal transmission of human immunodeficiency virus. *Morbidity and Mortality Weekly Report, 43,* No. RR-11.

Centers for Disease Control and Prevention (CDC). (1994f). Revised classification system for human immunodeficiency virus infection in children less than 13 years of age. *Morbidity and Mortality Weekly Report, 43,* No. RR-12.

Centers for Disease Control and Prevention (CDC). (1994g). Trends in AIDS diagnoses and reporting under the expanded surveillance definition for adolescents and adults—United States, 1993. *Morbidity and Mortality Weekly Report, 43,* 826–831.

Centers for Disease Control and Prevention (CDC). (1994h). Update: Alcohol-related traffic fatalities—United States, 1982–1993. *Morbidity and Mortality Weekly Report, 43,* 861–863.

Centers for Disease Control and Prevention (CDC). (1995a). Sociodemographic and behavioral characteristics associated with alcohol consumption during pregnancy—United States, 1988. *Morbidity and Mortality Weekly Report, 44,* 261–264.

Centers for Disease Control and Prevention (CDC). (1995b). Update: Acquired immunodeficiency syndrome—United States, 1994. *Morbidity and Mortality Weekly Report, 44,* 64–67.

Centers for Disease Control and Prevention (CDC). (1995c). Update: AIDS among women—United States, 1994. *Morbidity and Mortality Weekly Report, 44,* 81–84.

Centers for Disease Control and Prevention (CDC). (1995d). Update: Trends in fetal alcohol syndrome—United States, 1979–1993. *Morbidity and Mortality Weekly Report, 44,* 249–251.

Centerwall, B. S. (1984). Race, socioeconomic status, and domestic homicide, Atlanta, 1971–72. *American Journal of Public Health, 74,* 813–815.

Centerwall, B. S. (1995). Race, socioeconomic status, and domestic homicide. *Journal of the American Medical Association, 273,* 1755–1768.

Champion, V. L. (1994). Strategies to increase mammography utilization. *Medical Care, 32,* 118–129.

Chapman, C. R., & Gunn, C. C. (1990). Acupuncture. In J. J. Bonica (Ed.), *The management of pain* (2nd ed., pp. 1805–1821). Malvern, PA: Lea & Febiger.

Chapman, C. R., & Syrjala, K. L. (1990). Measurement of pain. In J. J. Bonica (Ed.), *The management of pain* (2nd ed., pp. 580–594). Malvern, PA: Lea & Febiger

Chapman, S., Wong, W. L., & Smith, W. (1993). Self-exempting beliefs about smoking and health: Differences between smokers and ex-smokers. *American Journal of Public Health, 83,* 215–219.

Chaves, J. F., & Brown, J. M. (1987). Spontaneous cognitive strategies for the control of clinical pain and stress. *Journal of Behavioral Medicine, 10,* 263–276.

Cheadle, A., Pearson, D., Wagner, E., Psaty, B. M., Diehr, P., & Koepsell, T. (1994). Relationship between socioeconomic status, health status, and lifestyle practices of American Indians: Evidence from a Plains reservation population. *Public Health Reports, 109,* 405–413.

Chen, K., & Kandel, D. B. (1995). The natural history of drug use from adolescence to the mid-thirties in a general population sample. *American Journal of Public Health, 85,* 41–47.

Chen, Y., Horne, S. L., & Dosman, J. A. (1993). The influence of smoking cessation on body weight may be temporary. *American Journal of Public Health, 83,* 1330–1332.

Chesney, M. A. (1993). Health psychology in the 21st century: Acquired immunodeficiency syndrome as a harbinger of things to come. *Health Psychology, 12,* 259–268.

Chesney, M. A., Hecker, M. H., & Black, G. W. (1988). Coronary-prone components of Type A behavior in the WCGS: A new methodology. In B. K. Houston & G. R. Snyder (Eds.), *Type A behavior pattern: Research, theory, and intervention.* New York; Wiley.

Chesney, M. A., & Shelton, J. L. (1976). A comparison of muscle relaxation and electromyogram biofeedback treatments for muscle contraction headache. *Journal of Behavior Therapy and Experimental Psychiatry, 7,* 221–225.

Chilcoat, H. D., Deshion, T. J., & Anthony, J. C. (1995). Parent monitoring and the incidence of drug sampling in urban elementary school children. *American Journal of Epidemiology, 141,* 25–31.

Chi-Lum, B. I. (1995). Putting prevention into medical training. *Journal of the American Medical Association, 273,* 1402–1403.

Chimonczyk, B. A., Salmun, L. M., Megathlin, F. N., Neveux, L. M., Palomadi, G. E., Knight, G. J., Pulkkinen, A. J., & Haddow, J. E. (1993). Association between exposure to environmental tobacco smoke and exacerbations of asthma in children. *New England Journal of Medicine, 328,* 1665–1669.

Ching, P. L. Y. H., Willett, W. C., Rimm, E. B., Colditz, G. A., Gortmaker, S. L., & Stampfer, M. J. (1996). Activity level and risk of overweight in male health professionals. *American Journal of Public Health, 86,* 25–30.

Christ, G. H., Siegel, K., Freund, B., Langosch, D., Hendersen, S., Sperber, D., & Weinstein, L. (1993). Impact of parental terminal cancer on latency-age children. *American Journal of Orthopsychiatry, 63,* 417–425.

Christensen, A. J., Smith, T. W., Turner, C. W., Holman, J. M., Gregory, M. C., & Rich, M. A. (1992). Family support, physical impairment, and adherence in hemodialysis: An investigation of main and buffering effects. *Journal of Behavioral Medicine, 15,* 313–325.

Chrombie, I. (1979). Variation of melanoma incidence with latitude in North America and Europe. *British Journal of Cancer, 40,* 774–781.

Chu, S. Y., Lee, N. C., Wingo, P. A., & Webster, L. A. (1988). Alcohol consumption and the risk of breast cancer. *American Journal of Epidemiology, 130,* 867–877.

Cinciripini, P. M., Lapitsky, L., Seay, S., Wallfisch, A., Kitchens, K., & Van Vunakis, H. (1995). The effects of smoking schedules on cessation outcome: Can we improve on common methods of gradual and abrupt nicotine withdrawal? *Journal of Consulting and Clinical Psychology, 63,* 388–399.

Clark, W. B., & Cahalan, D. (1976). Changes in problem drinking over a four-year span. *Addictive Behaviors, 1,* 251–259.

Clarke, J. C. (with Saunders, J. B.). (1988). *Alcoholism and problem drinking: Theories and treatment* (pp. 1–39). Sydney, Australia: Pergamon Press.

Cloninger, C. R., Bohman, M., & Sigvardsson, S. (1981). Inheritance of alcohol abuse. *Archives of Psychiatry, 38,* 861–868.

Coambs, R. B., Li, S., & Kozlowski, L. T. (1992). Age interacts with heaviness of smoking in predicting success in cessation of smoking. *American Journal of Epidemiology, 135,* 240–246.

Coate, D. (1993). Moderate drinking and coronary heart disease mortality: Evidence from NHANES I and the NHANES I follow-up. *American Journal of Public Health, 83,* 888–890.

Coates, R. J., & Li, V. C. (1983). Does smoking cessation lead to weight gain? The experience of asbestos-exposed shipyard workers. *American Journal of Public Health, 11,* 1303–1304.

Cochran, S. D. (1984). Preventing medical noncompliance in the outpatient treatment of bipolar affective disorders. *Journal of Consulting and Clinical Psychology, 52,* 873–878.

Cochran, S. D., & Mays, V. M. (1993). Applying social psychological models to predicting HIV-related sexual risk behaviors among African-Americans. Special Issue: Psychosocial aspects of AIDS prevention among African Americans. *Journal of Black Psychology, 19,* 142–154.

Cohen, R. Y., Stunkard, A. J., & Felix, M. R. J. (1987). Comparison of three worksite weight-loss competitions. *Journal of Behavioral Medicine, 10,* 467–479.

Cohen, S. (1980). Aftereffects of stress on human performance and social behavior: A review of research and theory. *Psychological Bulletin, 88,* 82–108.

Cohen, S. (1988). Psychosocial models of the role of social support in the etiology of physical disease. *Health Psychology, 7,* 269–297.

Cohen, S., Doyle, W. J., Skoner, D. P., Fireman, P., Gwatney, J. M., Jr., & Newson, J. T. (1995). State and trait negative affect as predictors of objective and subjective symptoms of respiratory viral infections. *Journal of Personality and Social Psychology, 68,* 159–169.

Cohen, S., Glass, D. C., & Phillips, S. (1977). Environment and health. In H. E. Freeman, S. Levine, & L. G. Reeder (Eds.), *Handbook of medical sociology.* Englewood Cliffs, NJ: Prentice-Hall.

Cohen, S., Kamarck, T., & Mermelstein, R. (1983). A global measure of perceived stress. *Journal of Health and Social Behavior, 24,* 385–396.

Cohen, S., Krantz, D. S., Evans, G. W., & Stokols, D. (1982). Community noise, behavior, and health: The Los Angeles Noise Project. In A. Baum & J. E. Singer (Eds.), *Advances in environmental psychology: Vol. 4. Environment and health* (pp. 295–317). Hillsdale, NJ: Erlbaum.

Cohen, S., Lichtenstein, E., Prochaska, J. O., Rossi, J. S., Gritz, E. R., Carr, C. R., Orleans, C. T., Schoenbach, V. J., Beiner, L., Abrams, D., DiClemente, C., Curry, S., Marlatt, G. A., Cummings, K. M., Emont, S. L., Giovino, G. & Ossip-Klein, D. (1989). Debunking myths about self-quitting: Evidence from 10 prospective studies of persons who attempt to quit smoking by themselves. *American Psychologists, 44,* 1355–1365.

Cohen, S., & McKay, G. (1984). Social support, stress and the buffering hypothesis: A theoretical analysis. In A. Baum, S. E. Taylor, & J. E. Singer (Eds.), *Handbook of psychology and health: Vol. 4. Social psychology and health* (pp. 253–267). Hillsdale, NJ: Erlbaum.

Cohen, S., Tyrrell, D. A. J., Russell, M. A. H., Jarvis, M. J., & Smith, A. P. (1993). Smoking, alcohol consumption, and susceptibility to the common cold. *American Journal of Public Health, 83,* 1277–1283.

Cohen, S., Tyrrell, D. A. J., & Smith, A. P. (1991). Psychological stress and susceptibility to the common cold. *New England Journal of Medicine, 325,* 606–612.

Cohen, S., Tyrrell, D. A. J., & Smith, A. P. (1993). Negative life events, perceived stress, negative affect, and susceptibility to the common cold. *Journal of Personality and Social Psychology, 64,* 131–140.

Cohler, B. J., Groves, L., Borden, W., & Lazarus, L. (1989). Caring for family members with Alzheimer's disease. In E. Light & B. D. Lebowitz (Eds.), *Alzheimer's disease treatment and family stress: Direction for research* (pp. 50–105). (DHHS Publication No. ADM 89-1569). Washington, DC: U.S. Government Printing Office.

Colditz, G. A., Bonita, R., Stampfer, M. J., Willett, W. C., Rosner, B., Speizer, F. E., & Hennekens, C. H. (1988). Cigarette smoking and risk of stroke in middle-aged women. *New England Journal of Medicine, 318,* 937–941.

Colditz, G. A., Willett, W. C., Hunter, D. J., Stampfer, M. J., Manson, J. E., Hennekens, C. H., Rosner, B. A., & Speizer, F. E. (1993). Family history, age, and risk of breast cancer. *Journal of the American Medical Association, 270,* 338–343.

Coles, C. D., Smith, I. E., Lancaster, J. S., & Falek, A. (1987). Persistence over the first month of neurobehavioral alternations in infants exposed to alcohol prenatally. *Infant Behavior and Development, 10,* 23–37.

Colligan, R. C., & Offord, K. P. (1988). The risky use of the MMPI Hostility Scale in assessing risk for coronary heart disease. *Psychosomatics, 29,* 188–196.

Colon, I. (1992). Race, belief in destiny, and seat belt usage: A pilot study. *American Journal of Public Health, 82,* 875–877.

Colt, E. W. D., Dunner, D. L., Hall, K., & Fieve, R. R. (1981). A high prevalence of affective disorder in runners. In M. H. Sacks & M. L. Sachs (Eds.), *Psychology of running.* Champaign, IL: Human Kinetics Publishers.

COMMIT Research Group. (1995a). Community intervention trial for smoking cessation (COMMIT): I. Cohort results from a four-year community intervention. *American Journal of Public Health, 85,* 183–192.

COMMIT Research Group. (1995b). Community intervention trial for smoking cessation (COMMIT): II. Changes in adult cigarette smoking prevalence. *American Journal of Public Health, 85,* 193–200.

Conboy, J. K. (1994). The effects of exercise withdrawal and mood states in runners. *Journal of Sport Psychology, 17,* 188–203.

Condiotte, M. M., & Lichtenstein, E. (1982). Self-efficacy and relapse in smoking cessation programs. *Journal of Consulting and Clinical Psychology, 49,* 648–658.

Conger, J. (1956). Reinforcement theory and the dynamics of alcoholism. *Quarterly Journal of Studies on Alcohol, 17,* 296–305.

Conn, J. M., Chorba, T. L., Peterson, T. D., Rhodes, P., & Annest, J. L. (1993). Effectiveness of safety-belt use: A study using hospital-based data for nonfatal motor-vehicle crashes. *Journal of Safety Research, 24,* 223–232.

Connell, C. M., & D'Augelli, A. R. (1990). The contribution of personality characteristics to the relationship between social support and perceived physical health. *Health Psychology, 9,* 192–207.

Connor, W. E. (1990). Dietary fiber—Nostrum or critical nutrient? *New England Journal of Medicine, 322,* 193–195.

Consumers Union. (1992a, August). Wasted health care dollars. *Consumer Reports, 57,* 435–448.

Consumers Union. (1992b, September). Health care in crisis: The search for solutions. *Consumer Reports, 57,* 579–592.

Contrada, R. J. (1989). Type A behavior, personality hardiness, and cardiovascular response to stress. *Journal of Personality and Social Psychology, 57,* 895–903.

Cook, W., & Medley, D. (1954). Proposed hostility and pharisaic-virtue scales for the MMPI. *Journal of Applied Psychology, 38,* 414–418.

Cooper, C. L., & Faragher, E. B. (1993). Psychosocial stress and breast cancer: The inter-relationship between stress events, coping strategies and personality. *Psychological Medicine, 23,* 653–662.

Cooper, K. H. (1968). *Aerobics.* New York: Evans.

Cooper, K. H. (1970). *The new aerobics.* New York: Evans.

Cooper, K. H. (1982). *The aerobics program for total well-being.* New York: Evans.

Cooper, K. H. (1985). *Running without fear: How to reduce the risks of heart attack and sudden death during aerobic exercise.* New York: Evans.

Cooper, K. H. (1988). *Controlling cholesterol.* Toronto: Bantam.

Cooper, K. H. (1994). *Dr. Kenneth H. Cooper's antioxidant revolution.* Nashville, TN: Nelson.

Cooper, K. H., & Cooper, M. (1972). *Aerobics for women.* New York: Evans.

Coppotelli, H. C., & Orleans, C. T. (1985). Partner support and other determinants of smoking cessation and maintenance among women. *Journal of Consulting and Clinical Psychology, 53,* 455–460.

Corbitt, G., Bailey, A., & Williams, G. (1990). HIV infection in Manchester, 1959. *Lancet, 336,* 51.

Corcoran, K. J. (1994, August). *Party on? Age, gender, and drinking at a college festival.* Presented at the 102nd convention of the American Psychological Association, Los Angeles, CA.

Corcoran, K. J., & Kisler, V. (1994, August). *Perception of seriousness of binging and drinking in young women.* Presented at the 102nd convention of the American Psychological Association, Los Angeles, CA.

Cornelius, L. J. (1991). Health habits of school-age children. *Journal of Health Care for the Poor and Underserved, 2,* 374–395.

Corti, M. C., Guralnik, J. M., Salive, M. D., Harris, T., Field, T. S., Wallace, R. B., Berkman, L. F., Seeman, T. W., Glynn, R. J., Hennekens, C. H., & Havlik, R. J. (1995). HDL cholesterol predicts coronary heart disease mortality in older persons. *Journal of the American Medical Association, 274,* 539–544.

Cotanch, P. H. (1984). Health promotion in hospitals. In J. D. Matarazzo, S. M. Weiss, J. A. Herd, N. E. Miller, & S. M. Weiss (Eds.), *Behavioral health: A handbook of health enhancement and disease prevention* (pp. 1125–1136). New York: Wiley.

Cotten, N. U., Resnick, J., Browne, D. C., Martin, S. L., McCarraher, D. R., & Woods, J. (1994). Aggression and fighting behavior among African-American adolescents: Individual and family factors. *American Journal of Public Health, 84,* 618–622.

Cottington, E. M., & House, J. S. (1987). Occupational stress and health: A multivariate relationship. In A. Baum & J. E. Singer (Eds.), *Handbook of psychology and health: Vol. 5. Stress* (pp. 41–62). Hillsdale, NJ: Erlbaum.

Cotton, D. H. G. (1990). *Stress management: An integrated approach to therapy.* New York: Brunner/Mazel.

Cotton, P. (1994). Alzheimer's/apo E link grows stronger. *Journal of the American Medical Association, 272,* 1483.

Cousins, N. (1983). *The healing heart: Antidote to panic and helplessness.* New York: Norton.

Cover, H., & Irwin, M. (1994). Immunity and depression: Insomnia, retardation, and reduction of natural killer cell activity. *Journal of Behavioral Medicine, 17,* 217–223.

Cowley, G., King, P., Hager, M., & Rosenberg, D. (1995, June 26). Going mainstream. *Newsweek, 125,* 56–57.

Cox, D. J., Freundlich, A., & Meyer, R. G. (1975). Differential effectiveness of electromyographic feedback, verbal relaxation instructions and medication placebo with tension headaches. *Journal of Consulting and Clinical Psychology, 43,* 892–898.

Cox, D. J., & Gonder-Frederick, L. A. (1991). The role of stress in diabetes mellitus. In P. M. McCabe, N. Schniederman, T. M. Field, & J. S. Skyler (Eds.), *Stress, coping and disease* (pp. 119–134). Hillsdale, NJ: Erlbaum.

Cox, D. J., & Gonder-Frederick, L. (1992). Major developments in behavioral diabetes research. *Journal of Consulting and Clinical Psychology, 60,* 628–638.

Cox, T., & Mackay, C. (1982). Psychosocial factors and psychophysiological mechanisms in the aetiology and development of cancer. *Social Science and Medicine, 16*, 381–396.

Coyne, J. C., & DeLongis, A. (1986). Going beyond social support: The role of social relationships in adaptation. *Journal of Consulting and Clinical Psychology, 54*, 454–460.

Cramer, J. A., Mattson, R. H., Prevey, M. L., Scheyer, R. D., & Ouellette, V. L. (1989). How often is medication taken as prescribed? *Journal of the American Medical Association, 261*, 3273–3277.

Crandall, C. S. (1988). Social contagion of binge eating. *Journal of Personality and Social Psychology, 55*, 588–598.

Crandall, C. S., Preisler, J. J., & Aussprung, J. (1992). Measuring life event stress in the lives of college students: The Undergraduate Stress Questionnaire (USQ). *Journal of Behavioral Medicine, 15*, 627–662.

Crandall, J. E., & Lehman, R. E. (1977). Relationship of stressful life events to social interest, locus of control, and psychological adjustment. *Journal of Consulting and Clinical Psychology, 45*, 1208.

Crawford, S. L., McGraw, S. A., Smith, K. W., McKinlay, J. B., & Pierson, J. E. (1994). Do blacks and whites differ in their use of health care for symptoms of coronary heart disease? *American Journal of Public Health, 84*, 957–964.

Creager, J. G. (1983). *Human anatomy and physiology.* Belmont, CA: Wadsworth.

Creer, T. L., & Bender, B. G. (1993). Asthma. In R. J. Gatchel & E. B. Blanchard (Eds.), *Psychophysiological disorders: Research and clinical applications* (pp. 151–203). Washington, DC: American Psychological Association.

Crisp, A. H., & Burns, T. (1990). Primary anorexia nervosa in the male and female: A comparison of clinical features and prognosis. In A. E. Andersen (Ed.), *Males with eating disorders* (pp. 77–99). New York: Brunner/Mazel.

Crisp, A. H., Palmer, R. L., & Kalucy, R. S. (1976). How common is anorexia nervosa? A prevalence study. *British Journal of Psychiatry, 128*, 549–554.

Critchlow, B. (1986). The powers of John Barleycorn: Beliefs about the effects of alcohol on social behavior. *American Psychologist, 41*, 751–764.

Cullen, K. J., Knuiman, M. W., & Ward, N. J. (1993). Alcohol and mortality in Busselton, Western Australia. *American Journal of Epidemiology, 137*, 242–248.

Cummings, K. M., Hellmann, R., & Emont, S. L. (1988). Correlates of participation in a worksite stop-smoking contest. *Journal of Behavioral Medicine, 11*, 267–277.

Cummings, K. M., Sciandra, R., & Markello, S. (1987). Impact of a newspaper mediated quit smoking program. *American Journal of Public Health, 77*, 1452–1453.

Cummings, P., & Psaty, B. M. (1994). The association between cholesterol and death from injury. *Annals of Internal Medicine, 120*, 848–855.

Cunningham, A. J. (1981). Mind, body, and immune response. In R. Ader (Ed.), *Psychoneuroimmunology* (pp. 609–617). New York: Academic Press.

Curfman, G. D. (1993a). The health benefits of exercise: A critical reapprasial. *New England Journal of Medicine, 328*, 574–575.

Curfman, G. D. (1993b). Is exercise beneficial—or hazardous—to your heart? *New England Journal of Medicine, 329*, 1730–1731.

Curry, S. J., Marlatt, G. A., & Gordon, J. R. (1987). Abstinence violation effect: Validation of an attributional construct with smoking cessation. *Journal of Consulting and Clinical Psychology, 55*, 145–149.

Cushman, R., James, W., & Waclawik, H. (1991). Physicians promoting bicycle helmets for children: A randomized trial. *American Journal of Public Health, 81*, 1044–1046.

Czeisler, C. A., Johnson, M. P., Duffy, J. F., Brown, E. N., Ronda, J. M., & Kronauer, R. E. (1990). Exposure to bright light and darkness to treat physiologic maladaptation to night work. *New England Journal of Medicine, 322*, 1253–1259.

D'Agostino, R. B., Belanger, A. J., Kannel, W. B., & Higgins, M. (1995). Role of smoking in the U-shaped relation of cholesterol to mortality in men: The Framingham Study. *American Journal of Epidemiology, 141*, 822–827.

Dahlquist, L. N., Gil, K. M., Armstrong, D., DeLawyer, D. D., Green, P., & Wvori, D. (1986). Preparing children for medical examinations: The importance of previous medical experience. *Health Psychology, 5*, 249–259.

Daling, J. R., Weiss, N. S., Hislop, T. G., Maden, C., Coates, R. J., Sherman, K. J., Ashley, R. L., Beagrie, M., Ryan, J. A., & Corey, L. (1987). Sexual practices, sexually transmitted diseases, and the incidence of anal cancer. *New England Journal of Medicine, 317*, 973–977.

Daling, J. R., Weiss, N. S., Klopfenstein, L. L., Cochran, L. E., Chow, W. H., & Daifuku, R. (1982). Correlates of homosexual behavior and the incidence of anal cancer. *Journal of the American Medical Association, 247*, 1988–1990.

Damkot, D. K., Kirk, R. S., & Huntley, M. S., Jr. (1983). Influences of alcohol, monetary incentive and visual interruption upon control use during automobile driving. *Alcohol and Alcoholism, 18*, 81–88.

Damon, A. (1973). Smoking attitudes and practices in seven preliterate societies. In W. L. Dunn, Jr. (Ed.), *Smoking behavior: Motives and incentives* (pp. 219–230). Washington, DC: Winston.

Daniell, H. W. (1971). Smokers' wrinkles. *Annals of Internal Medicine, 75*, 873–880.

Danneberg, A. L., Gielen, A. C., Beilenson, P. L., Wilson, D. H., & Joffe, A. (1993). Bicycle helmet laws and educational campaigns: An evaluation of strategies to increase children's helmet use. *American Journal of Public Health, 83*, 667–674.

Darby, P. L., Garfinkel, P. E., Garner, D. M., & Coscina, D. V. (Eds.). (1983). *Anorexia nervosa: Recent developments in research.* New York: Liss.

Dattore, P. J., Shontz, F. C., & Coyne, L. (1980). Premorbid personality differentiation of cancer and noncancer groups: A list of the hypotheses of cancer proneness. *Journal of Consulting and Clinical Psychology, 48*, 388–394.

Davenport, D. (1995, May). Fiscal fitness. *World Traveler, 27*, 20, 22, 24–25.

Davidson, L. L., Durkin, M. S., Kuhn, L., O'Connor, P., Barlow, B., & Heagarity, M. C. (1994). The impact of the Safe Kids/Healthy Neighborhoods Injury Prevention Program in Harlem, 1988–1991. *American Journal of Public Health, 84*, 580–586.

Davidson, P. O., & Schrag, A. R. (1969). Factors affecting the outcome of child psychiatric consultations. *American Journal of Orthopsychiatry, 39*, 774–778.

Davies, D. L. (1962). Normal drinking in recovered alcohol addicts. *Quarterly Journal of Studies on Alcohol, 24*, 321–332.

Davis, C., Brewer, H., & Ratusny, D. (1993). Behavioral frequency and psychological commitment: Necessary concepts in the study of excessive exercising. *Journal of Behavioral Medicine, 16*, 611–628.

Davis, C., Kennedy, S. H., Ravelski, E., & Dionne, M. (1994). The role of physical activity in the development and maintenance of eating disorders. *Psychological Medicine, 24*, 957–964.

Davis, D. L., Dinse, G. E., & Hoel, D. G. (1994). Decreasing cardiovascular disease and increasing cancer among whites in the United States from 1973 through 1987: Good news and bad news. *Journal of the American Medical Association, 271,* 431–437.

Davis, G. P., & Park, E. (1981). *The heart: The living pump.* Washington, DC: U.S. News Books.

Davis, K. L., Thal, L. J., Gamzer, E. R., Davis, C. S., Woolson, R. F., Gracon, S. I., Dranchman, D. A., Schneider, L. S., Whitehouse, P. J., Hoover, T. M., Morris, J. C., Kawas, C. H., Knopman, D. S., Earl, N. L., Kumar, V., & Doody, R. S. (1992). A double-blind, placebo-controlled multicenter study of tacrine for Alzheimer's disease. *New England Journal of Medicine, 327,* 1253–1259.

Davis, M. F., & Iverson D. C. (1984). An overview and analysis of the Health Style campaign. *Health Education Quarterly, 11,* 253–272.

Davis, M. S. (1966). Variation in patients' compliance with doctors' orders: Analysis of congruence between survey responses and results of empirical investigations. *Journal of Medical Education, 41,* 1039–1048.

Davis, M. S. (1968). Physiologic, psychological and demographic factors in patient compliance with doctors' orders. *Medical Care, 6,* 115–122.

Davis, R. M. (1988). Health education on the six-o'clock news: Motivating television coverage of news in medicine. *Journal of the American Medical Association, 259,* 1036–1038.

Davison, G. C., Williams, M. E., Nezami. E., Bice, T. L., & DeQuattro, V. L. (1991). Relaxation, reduction in angry articulated thoughts, and improvements in borderline hypertension and heart rate. *Journal of Behavioral Medicine, 14,* 453–468.

Dawber, T. R. (1980). *The Framingham study: The epidemiology of atherosclerotic disease.* Cambridge, MA: Harvard University Press.

de Benedittis, G., & Lorenzetti, A. (1992). The role of stressful life events in the persistence of primary headache: Major events vs. daily hassles. *Pain, 51,* 35-42.

Deffenbacher, J. L. (1994). Anger reduction: Issues, assessment, and intervention strategies. In A. W. Siegman & T. W. Smith (Eds.), *Anger, hostility, and the heart* (pp. 239–269). Hillsdale, NJ: Erlbaum.

Deffenbacher, J. L., & Stark, R. S. (1992). Relaxation and cognitive-relaxation treatments of general anger. *Journal of Counseling Psychology, 39,* 158–167.

Deitrich, R. A., & Spuhler, K. (1984). Genetics of alcoholism and alcohol actions. In R. G. Smart, H. D. Cappell, F. B. Glasser, Y. Israel, H. Kalant, R. E. Popham, W. Schmidt, & E. M. Sellers (Eds.), *Research advances in alcohol and drug problems* (Vol. 8). New York: Plenum.

De Leo, D., Carollo, G., & Dello Bueno, M. (1995). Lower suicide rates associated with a Tele-Help/Tele-Check service for the elderly at home. *American Journal of Psychiatry, 152,* 632–634.

DeJong, W., & Wallack, L. (1992). The role of designated driver programs in the prevention of alcohol-impaired driving: A critical reassessment. *Health Education Quarterly, 19,* 429–442.

DeLong, R. D. (1971). Individual differences in patterns of anxiety arousal, stress-relevant information, and recovery from surgery (Doctoral dissertation, University of California, Los Angeles, 1970). *Dissertation Abstracts International, 32,* 554B.

Dembroski, T. M., & Costa, P. T, Jr. (1987). Coronary-prone behavior: Components of the Type A pattern and hostility. *Journal of Personality, 55,* 211–236.

Dembroski, T. M., & MacDougall, J. M. (1985). Beyond global Type A: Relationships of paralinguistic attributes, hostility, and anger-in to coronary heart disease. In T. Field, P. McCabe,

& N. Scheiderman (Eds.), *Stress and coping* (pp. 223–241). Hillsdale, NJ: Erlbaum.

Dembroski, T. M., MacDougall, J. M., Costa, P. T., Jr., & Grandits, G. A. (1989). Components of hostility as predictors of sudden death and myocardial infarction in the Multiple Risk Factor Intervention Trial. *Psychosomatic Medicine, 51,* 514–522.

Dembroski, T. M., MacDougall, J. M., Williams, R. B., Haney, T. L., & Blumenthal, J. A. (1985). Components of Type A, hostility, and anger-in: Relationship to angiographic findings. *Psychosomatic Medicine, 47,* 219–233.

Dembroski, T. M., & Williams, R. B., Jr. (1989). Definition and assessment of coronary-prone behavior. In N. Schneiderman, S. M. Weiss, & P. G. Kaufman (Eds.), *Handbook of research methods in cardiovascular behavioral medicine* (pp. 553–569). New York: Plenum.

DeNitto, E. (1993, September 29). 100 leaders monopolize pain relievers. *Advertising Age, 64,* 2.

Derogatis, L. R., Abeloff, M. D., & Melisaratos, N. (1979). Psychological coping mechanisms and survival time in metastatic breast cancer. *Journal of the American Medical Association, 242,* 1504–1508.

Derogatis, L. R., Morrow, G. R., Fetting, J., Penman, D., Piasetsky, S., Schmale, A. M., Henrichs, M., & Carnicke, C. L. M. (1983). The prevalence of psychiatric disorders among cancer patients. *Journal of the American Medical Association, 249,* 751–757.

Des Jarlais, D. C. (1995). Editorial: Harm reduction—A framework for incorporating science into drug policy. *American Journal of Public Health, 85,* 10–12.

de Vincenzi, I. (1994). A longitudinal study of human immunodeficiency virus transmission by heterosexual partners. *New England Journal of Medicine, 331,* 341–346.

Devins, G. M., Mandin, H., Hons, R. B., Burgess, E. D., Klassen, J., Taub, K., Schorr, S., Letourneau, P. K., & Buckle, S. (1990). Illness intrusiveness and quality of life in end-stage renal disease: Comparison and stability across treatment modalities. *Health Psychology, 9,* 117–142.

Dew, M. A., Bromet, E. J., Brent, D., & Greenhouse, J. B. (1987). A quantitative literature review of the effectiveness of suicide prevention centers. *Journal of Consulting and Clinical Psychology, 55,* 239–244.

DiClemente, C. C. (1981). Self-efficacy and smoking cessation maintenance: A preliminary report. *Cognitive Therapy and Research, 5,* 175–187.

DiMatteo, M. R. (1994). Enhancing patient adherence to medical recommendations. *Journal of the American Medical Association, 271,* 79, 83.

DiMatteo, M. R., & DiNicola, D. D. (1982). *Achieving patient compliance: The psychology of the medical practitioner's role.* New York: Pergamon Press.

Dinges, D. F., Douglas, S. D., Zaugg, L., Campbell, D. E., McMann, J. M., Whitehouse, W. G., Orme, E. C., Kapoor, S. C., Icaza, E., & Orne, M. T. (1994). Leukocytosis and natural killer cell function parallel neurobehavioral fatigue induced by 64 hours of sleep deprivation. *Journal of Clinical Investigation, 93,* 1930–1939.

Dinh, K. T., Sarason, I. G., Peterson, A. V., & Onstad, L. E. (1995). Children's perceptions of smokers and nonsmokers: A longitudinal study. *Health Psychology, 14,* 32–40.

DiNicola, D. D., & DiMatteo, M. R. (1984). Practitioners, patients, and compliance with medical regimens: A social psychological perspective. In A. Baum, S. E. Taylor, & J. E. Singer (Eds.), *Handbook of psychology and health: Vol. 4. Social psychological aspects of health* (pp. 55–84). Hillsdale, NJ: Erlbaum.

Dishman, R. K. (1982). Compliance/adherence in health-related exercise. *Health Psychology, 1,* 237–267.

Doherty, W. J., Schrott, H. G., Metcalf, L., & Iasiello-Vailas, L. (1983). Effects of spouse support and health beliefs on medication adherence. *Journal of Family Practice, 17,* 837–841.

Dohrenwend, B. P. (1979). Stressful life events and psychopathology: Some issues of theory and method. In J. E. Barrett, R. M. Rose, & G. L. Klerman (Eds.), *Stress and mental disorder* (pp. 1–15). New York: Raven.

Dohrenwend, B. S., Dohrenwend, B. P., Dodson, M., & Shrout, P. E. (1984). Symptoms, hassles, social supports and life events: Problem of confounded measures. *Journal of Abnormal Psychology, 93,* 222–230.

Dohrenwend, B. S., Krasnoff, L., Askenasy, A. R., & Dohrenwend, B. P. (1978). Exemplification of a method for scaling life events: The PERI Life Event Scale. *Journal of Health and Social Behavior, 19,* 205–229.

Dohrenwend, B. S., Krasnoff, L., Askenasy, A. R., & Dohrenwend, B. P. (1982). The Psychiatric Epidemiology Research Interview Life Events Scale. In L. Goldberger & S. Breznitz (Eds.), *Handbook of stress: Theoretical and clinical aspects* (pp. 332–363). New York: Free Press.

Dolan, B. (1991). Cross-cultural aspects of anorexia nervosa and bulimia: A review. *International Journal of Eating Disorders, 10,* 67–79.

Dolan, C. A., Sherwood, A., & Light, K. C. (1992). Cognitive coping strategies and blood pressure responses to real-life stress in healthy young men. *Health Psychology, 11,* 233–240.

Dolecek, T. A., Milas, N. C., Van Horn, L. V., Farrand, M. E., Gorder, D. D., Duchene, A. G., Dyer, J. R., Stone, P. A., & Randall, B. L. (1986). A long-term nutrition experience: Lipid responses and dietary adherence patterns in the Multiple Risk Factor Intervention Trial. *Journal of the American Dietetic Association, 86,* 752–758.

Doll, J., & Ajzen, I. (1992). Accessibility and stability of predictors in the theory of planned behavior. *Journal of Personality and Social Psychology, 63,* 754–765.

Doll, R. (1991). Progress against cancer: An epidemiologic assessment: The 1991 John C. Cassel Memorial lecture. *American Journal of Epidemiology, 134,* 675–688.

Doll, R., & Hill, A. B. (1950). Smoking and carcinoma of the lung, *British Medical Journal,* 739–748.

Doll, R., & Hill, A. B. (1956). Lung cancer and other causes of death in relation to smoking: A second report on the mortality of British doctors. *British Medical Journal,* 1071–1081.

Doll, R., & Peto, R. (1981). *The causes of cancer.* New York: Oxford University Press.

Dollinger, M., Rosenbaum, E. H., & Cable, G. (1991). *Everyone's guide to cancer therapy.* Kansas City: Somerville.

Donaldson, C. S., Stanger, L. M., Donaldson, M. W., Cram, J., & Skubick, D. L. (1993). A randomized crossover investigation of a back pain and disability prevention program: Possible mechanisms of change. *Journal of Occupational Rehabilitation, 3,* 83–94.

Donaldson, S. I., Graham, J. W., Piccinin, A. M., & Hansen, W. B. (1995). Resistance-skills training and onset of alcohol use: Evidence for beneficial and potentially harmful effects in public schools and in private Catholic schools. *Health Psychology, 14,* 291–300.

Donovan, J. E., Jessor, R., & Costa, F. M. (1993). Structure of health-enhancing behavior in adolescence: A latent-variable approach. *Journal of Health and Social Behavior, 34,* 346–362.

Donovan, M. I. (1989). Relieving pain: The current basis for practice. In S. G. Funk, E. M. Tornquist, M. T. Champagne, L. A. Copp, & R. A. Wiese (Eds.), *Key aspects of comfort: Management of pain, fatigue, and nausea* (pp. 25–31). New York: Springer.

Dorgan, J. F., Brown, C., Barrett, M., Splansky, G. L., Kreger, B. E., D'Agostino, R. B., Albanes, D., & Schatzkin, A. (1994). Physical activity and risk of breast cancer in the Framingham Heart Study. *American Journal of Epidemiology, 139,* 662–669.

Doyne, E. J., Ossip-Klein, D. J., Bowman, E. D., Osborn, K. M., McDougall-Wilson, I. B., & Neimeyer, R. A. (1987). Running versus weight lifting in the treatment of depression. *Journal of Consulting and Clinical Psychology, 55,* 748–754.

Dreon, D. M., Vranizan, K. M., Krauss, R. M., Austin, M. A., & Wood, P. D. (1990). The effects of polyunsaturated fat vs. monounsaturated fat on plasma lipoproteins. *Journal of the American Medical Association, 263,* 2462–2466.

Drewnowski, A., Hopkins, S. A., & Kessler, R. C. (1988). The prevalence of bulimia nervosa in the U. S. college student population. *American Journal of Public Health, 78,* 1322–1325.

Driver, H. E., & Swann, P. F. (1987). Alcohol and human cancer [review]. *Anticancer Research, 7,* 309–320.

Dubuisson, D., & Melzack, R. (1976). Classification of clinical pain descriptions by multiple group discriminant analysis. *Experimental Neurology, 51,* 480–487.

Dudgeon, D., Raubertas, R. F., & Rosenthal, S. M. (1993). The Short-Form McGill Pain Questionnaire in chronic cancer pain. *Journal of Pain and Symptom Management, 8,* 191–195.

Dunbar, H. F. (1943). *Psychosomatic diagnosis.* New York: Hoeber.

Dunbar, J. (1979). Issues in assessment. In S. J. Cohen (Ed.), *New directions in patient compliance* (pp. 41–57). Lexington, MA: Lexington Books.

Duncan, J. J., Gordon, N. F., & Scott, C. B. (1991). Women walking for health and fitness: How much is enough? *Journal of the American Medical Association, 266,* 3295–3299.

Duncan, T. E., & McAuley, E. (1993). Social support and efficacy cognitions in exercise adherence: A latent growth curve analysis. *Journal of Behavioral Medicine, 16,* 199–218.

Dunkel-Schetter, C. (1984). Social support and cancer: Findings based on patient interviews and their implications. *Journal of Social Issues, 40*(4), 77-98.

Dunkel-Schetter, C., Feinstein, L. G., Taylor, S. E., & Falke, R. L. (1992). Patterns of coping with cancer. *Health Psychology, 11,* 79–87.

Dunkel-Schetter, C., & Wortman, C. B. (1982). The interpersonal dynamics of cancer: Problems in social relationships and their impact on the patient. In H. S. Friedman & M. R. DiMatteo (Eds.), *Interpersonal issues in health care.* New York: Academic Press.

Dwyer, J. H. (1995). Genes, blood pressure, and African heritage. *Lancet, 346,* 392.

Dwyer, J. T., Feldman, J. J., & Mayer, J. (1967). Adolescent dieters: Who are they? *Journal of Clinical Nutrition, 20,* 1045–1056.

Eaker, E. D., Pinsky, J., & Castelli, W. P. (1992). Myocardial infarction and coronary death among women: Psychosocial predictors from a 20-year follow-up of women in the Framingham Study. *American Journal of Epidemiology, 135,* 854–864.

Eckardt, M. J., Harford, T. C., Kaelber, C. T., Parker, E. S., Rosenthal, L. S., Ryback, R. S., Salmoiraghi, G. C., Vanderveen, E., & Warren, K. R. (1981). Health hazards associated with alcohol consumption. *Journal of the American Medical Association, 246,* 648–666.

Eckert, E. D. (1983). Behavior modification in anorexia nervosa: A comparison of two reinforcement schedules. In P. L. Darby, P. E. Garfinkel, D. M. Garner, & D. V. Coscina (Eds.), *Anorexia nervosa: Recent developments in research.* New York: Liss.

Eckert, E. D., Goldberg. S. C., Halmi, K. A., Casper, R. C., & Davis, J. M. (1979). Behavior therapy in anorexia nervosa. *British Journal of Psychiatry, 134,* 55–59.

Eckholm, E. (1977). *The picture of health: Environmental sources of disease.* New York: Norton.

Eckholm, E., & Tierney, J. (1990, September 16). AIDS in Africa: A killer rages on. *The New York Times,* pp. A1, A10.

Edlin, B. R., Irwin, K., Faruque, S., McCoy, C. B., Word, C., Serrano, Y., Inciardi, J. A., Bowser, B. P., Schilling, R. F., & Holmberg, S. D. (1994). Intersecting epidemics: Crack cocaine use and HIV infection among inner-city young adults. *New England Journal of Medicine, 331,* 1422–1427.

Edwards, G. (1977). The alcohol dependence syndrome: Usefulness of an idea. In G. Edwards & M. Grant (Eds.), *Alcoholism: New knowledge and new responses.* London: Croom Helm.

Edwards, G., & Gross, M. M. (1976). Alcohol dependence: Provisional description of a clinical syndrome. *British Medical Journal, 1,* 1058–1061.

Edwards, G., Gross, M. M., Keller, M., Moser, J., & Room, R. (1977). *Alcohol-related disabilities* (WHO Offset Pub. No. 32). Geneva, Switzerland: World Health Organization.

Eisenberg, D. M., Kessler, R. C., Foster, C., Norlock, F. E., Calkins, D. R., & Delbanco, T. L. (1993). Unconventional medicine in the United States: Prevalence, costs, and patterns of use. *New England Journal of Medicine, 328,* 246–252.

Eisinger, R. A. (1972). Psychosocial predictors of smoking behavior change. *Journal of Health and Social Behavior, 13,* 137–144.

Ekstrand, M. L., Coates, T. J., Guydish, J. R., Hauck, W. W., Collette, L., & Hulley, S. B. (1994). Are bisexually identified men in San Francisco a common vector for spreading HIV infection to women? *American Journal of Public Health, 84,* 915–919.

Elder, J. P., Sallis, J. F., Woodruff, S. I., & Wildey, M. D. (1993). Tobacco-refusal skills and tobacco use among high-risk adolescents. *Journal of Behavioral Medicine, 16,* 629–642.

Elder, J. P., Wildey, M., de Moor, C., Sallis, J. F., Jr., Eckhardt, L., Edwards, C., Erickson, A., Golbeck, A., Hovell, M., Johnston, D., Levitz, M. D., Molgaard, C., Young, R., Vito, D., & Woodruff, S. I. (1993). The long-term prevention of tobacco use among junior high school students: Classroom and telephone interventions. *American Journal of Public Health, 83,* 1239–1244.

El-Faizy, M., & Reinsch, S. (1994). Home safety intervention for the prevention of falls. *Physical and Occupational Therapy in Geriatrics, 12,* 33–49.

Elkins, P. D., & Roberts, M. C. (1983). Psychological preparation for pediatric hospitalization. *Clinical Psychology Review, 3,* 275–295.

Ellestad, M. H. (1986). *Stress testing* (3rd ed.). Philadelphia: Davis.

Elliott, G. R., & Eisdorfer, C. (Eds.). (1982). *Stress and human health: Analysis and implications of research.* New York: Springer.

Elliott, T. E., & Elliott, B. A. (1992). Physician attitudes and beliefs about use of morphine for cancer pain. *Journal of Pain and Symptom Management, 7,* 141–148.

Ellis, A. (1962). *Reason and emotion in psychotherapy.* New York: Stuart.

Ellis, A. (1986, Summer). Thoughts on supervising counselors and therapists. *Association for Counselor Education and Supervision Newsletter,* pp. 3–5.

Elton, D. (1993). Combined use of hypnosis and EMG biofeedback in the treatment of stress-induced conditions. *Stress Medicine, 9,* 25–35.

Emery, C. F., Hauck, E. R., Blumenthal, J. A. (1992). Exercise adherence or maintenance among older adults: 1-year follow-up study. *Psychology and Aging, 7,* 466–470.

Emrick, C. D., & Hansen, J. (1983). Assertions regarding effectiveness of treatment for alcoholism: Fact or fantasy? *American Psychologist, 38,* 1078–1088.

Engel, G. L. (1977). The need for a new medical model: A challenge for biomedicine. *Science, 196,* 129–136.

Engelberg, H. (1992). Low serum cholesterol and sucide. *Lancet, 339,* 727–729.

Ennett, S. T., Tobler, N. S., Ringwalt, C. L., & Flewelling, R. L. (1994). How effective is drug abuse resistance education? A meta-analysis of Project DARE outcome evaluations. *American Journal of Public Health, 84,* 1394–1401.

Epstein, L. H., & Perkins, K. A. (1988). Smoking, stress, and coronary heart disease. *Journal of Consulting and Clinical Psychology, 56,* 342–349.

Epstein, L. H., Valoski, A. M., Vara, L. S., McCurley, J., Wisniewski, L., Kalarchian, M. A., Klein, K. R., & Shrager, L. R. (1995). Effects of decreasing sedentary behavior and increasing activity on weight change in obese children. *Health Psychology, 14,* 109–115.

Epstein, L. H., Valoski, A., Wing, R. R., & McCurley, J. (1994). Ten-year outcomes of behavioral family-based treatment for childhood obesity. *Health Psychology, 13,* 373–383.

Epstein, L. H., & Wing, R. R. (1980). Aerobic exercise and weight. *Addictive Behaviors, 5,* 371–388.

Epstein, L. H., & Wing, R. R. (1987). Behavioral treatment of childhood obesity. *Psychological Bulletin, 101,* 331–342.

Epstein, Y. M. (1982). Crowding stress and human behavior. In G. W. Evans (Ed.), *Environmental stress* (pp. 133–148). Cambridge, England: Cambridge University Press.

Ernster, V. L., Grady, D. G., Greene, J. C., Walsh, M., Robertson, P., Daniels, T. E., Benowitz, N., Siegel, D., Gerbert, B., & Hauck, W. W. (1990). Smokeless tobacco use and health effects among baseball players. *Journal of the American Medical Association, 264,* 218–224.

Ernster, V. L., Grady, D., Müke, R., Black, D., Selby, J., & Kerlikowske, K. (1995). Facial wrinkling in men and women by smoking status. *American Journal of Public Health, 85,* 78–82.

Esterling, B. A., Kiecolt-Glaser, J. K., Bodnar, J. C., & Glaser, R. (1994). Chronic stress, social support, and persistent alterations in the natural killer cell response to cytokines in older adults. *Health Psychology, 13,* 291–298.

Evans, D. A., Funkenstein, H., Albert, M. S., Scherr, P. A., Cook, N. R., Chown, M. J., Hebert, L. E., Hennekens, C. H., & Taylor, J. O. (1989). Prevalence of Alzheimer's disease in a community population of older persons: Higher than previously reported. *Journal of the American Medical Association, 262,* 2551–2556.

Evans, F. J. (1985). Expectancy, therapeutic instructions, and the placebo response. In L. White, B. Tursky, & G. E. Schwartz (Eds.), *Placebo: Theory, research, and mechanisms* (pp. 215–228). New York: Guilford Press.

Evans, F. J. (1988). Hypnosis and pain control. *Advances, 5,* 31–39.

Evans, G. W., Palsane, M. N., Lepore, S. J., & Martin, J. (1989). Residental density and psychological health: The mediating effects of social support. *Journal of Personality and Social Psychology, 57,* 994–999.

Evans, L. (1987). Fatality risk reduction from safety belt use. *Journal of Trauma, 27,* 746–749.

Evans, R. I. (1976). Smoking in children: Developing a social psychological strategy of deterrence. *Preventive Medicine, 5,* 122–127.

Evans, R. I., Rozelle, R. M., Maxwell, S. E., Raines, B. E., Dill, C. A., Guthrie, T. J., Henderson, A. H., & Hill, D. C. (1981). Social modeling films to deter smoking in adolescents: Results of a three year field investigation. *Journal of Applied Psychology, 66,* 399–414.

Evans, R. I., Rozelle, R. M., Mittlemark, M. B., Hansen, W. B., Bane, A. L., & Havis, J. (1978). Determining the onset of smoking in children: Knowledge of immediate physiological effects and coping with peer pressure, media pressure and parent modeling. *Journal of Applied Social Psychology, 8*, 126–135.

Evans, R. I., Smith, C. K., & Raines, B. E. (1984). Deterring cigarette smoking in adolescents: A psychosocial-behavioral analysis of an intervention strategy. In A. Baum, S. E. Taylor, & J. E. Singer (Eds.), *Handbook of psychology and health: Vol. 4. Social psychological aspects of health* (pp. 301–318). Hillsdale, NJ: Erlbaum.

Evans, W. N., Neville, D., Graham, J. D. (1991). General deterrence of drunk driving: Evaluation of recent American policies. *Risk Analysis, 11*, 278–289.

Everhart, J., & Wright, D. (1995). Diabetes mellitus as a risk factor for pancreatic cancer: A meta analysis. *Journal of the American Medical Association, 273*, 1605–1609.

Eysenck, H. J. (1984). Lung cancer and the stress-personality inventory. In C. L. Cooper (Ed.), *Psychosocial stress and cancer*. Chichester, England: Wiley.

Eysenck, H. J. (1987, November). *Personality, stress and cancer: Prediction and prophylaxis*. Paper presented at the meeting of the Louisiana Psychological Association, New Orleans.

Eysenck, H. J. (1988, December). Health's character. *Psychology Today, 22*, 28–35.

Eysenck, H. J. (1991a). Personality, stress, and disease: An interactionist perspective. *Psychological Inquiry, 2*, 221–232.

Eysenck, H. J. (1991b). *Smoking, personality and stress: Psychosocial factors in the prevention of cancer and coronary heart disease*. New York: Springer-Verlag.

Eysenck, H. J. (1991c). Were we really wrong? *American Journal of Epidemiology, 133*, 429–433.

Eysenck, H. J. (1993). Prediction of cancer and coronary heart disease: Mortality by means of a personality inventory: Results of a 15-year follow-up study. *Psychological Reports, 72*, 499–516.

Faberow, N. L. (1986). Noncompliance as indirect self-destructive behavior. In K. E. Gerber & A. M. Nehemkis (Eds.), *Compliance: The dilemma of the chronically ill*. New York: Springer.

Faden, R. R. (1987). Ethical issues in government sponsored public health campaigns. *Health Education Quarterly, 14*, 27–37.

Fairburn, C. G., Hay, P. J., & Welch, S. L. (1993). Binge eating and bulimia nervosa: Distribution and determinants. In C. G Fairburn & G. T. Wilson (Eds.), *Binge eating: Nature, assessment, and treatment* (pp. 123–143). New York: Guilford Press.

Falk, A., Hanson, B. S., Issacsson, S., & Ostergren, P. (1992). Job strain and mortality in elderly men: Social network, support, and influence as buffers. *American Journal of Public Health, 82*, 1136–1139.

Farley, C., Haddad, S., & Brown, B. (1996). The effects of a 4-year program promoting bicycle helmet use among children in Quebec. *American Journal of Public Health, 86*, 46–51.

Farquhar, J. W., Fortmann, S. P., Flora, J. A., Taylor, C. B., Haskell, W. L., Williams, P. T., Maccoby, N., & Wood, P. D. (1990). Effects of communitywide education on cardiovascular disease risk factors: The Stanford Five-City Project. *Journal of the American Medical Association, 264*, 359–365.

Farquhar, J. W., Fortmann, S. P., Maccoby, N., Wood, P. D., Haskell, W. L., Taylor, C. B., Flora, J. A., Solomon, D. S., Rogers, T., Adler, E., Breitrose, P., & Weiner, L. (1984). The Stanford Five City Project: An overview. In J. D. Matarazzo, S. M. Weiss, J. A. Herd, N. E. Miller, & S. M. Weiss (Eds.), *Behavioral health: A handbook of health enhancement and disease prevention* (pp. 1154–1165). New York: Wiley.

Fawzy, F. I., Fawzy, N. W., Hyun, C. S., Elashoff, R., Guthrie, D., Fahley, J. L., & Morton, D. L. (1993). Malignant melanoma: Effects of an early structures psychiatric intervention, coping, and affective state on recurrence and survival 6 years later. *Archives of General Psychiatry, 50*, 681–689.

Feinstein, A. R. (1988). Scientific standards in epidemiologic studies of the menace of daily life. *Science, 242*, 1257–1263.

Feist, G. J., Bodner, T. E., Jacobs, J. F., Miles, M., & Tan, V. (1995). Integrating top-down and bottom-up structural models of subjective well-being: A longitudinal investigation. *Journal of Personality and Social Psychology, 68*, 138–150.

Feist, J. (1994). *Theories of personality* (3rd ed.). Fort Worth: Harcourt Brace.

Feldman, J. (1966). *The dissemination of health information*. Chicago: Aldine.

Feldman, R. H. L. (1984). Evaluating health promotion in the workplace. In J. D. Matarazzo, S. M. Weiss, J. A. Herd, N. E. Miller, & S. M. Weiss (Eds.), *Behavioral health: A handbook of health enhancement and disease prevention* (pp. 1087–1093). New York: Wiley.

Feletti, G., Firman, D., & Sanson-Fisher, R. (1986). Patient satisfaction and primary-care consultations. *Journal of Behavioral Medicine, 9*, 389–399.

Felson, D. T., Zhang, Y., Hannan, M. T., Kannel, W. B., & Kiel, D. P. (1995). Alcohol intake and bone mineral density in elderly men and women: The Framingham Study. *American Journal of Epidemiology, 142*, 485–492.

Ferraro, D. P. (1980). Acute effects of marijuana on human memory and cognition. In R. C. Peterson (Ed.), *Marijuana research findings*. National Institute on Drug Abuse. Washington, DC: U.S. Government Printing Office.

Fichten, C. S., Creti, L., Amsel, R., Brender, W., Weinstein, N., & Libman, E. (1995). Poor sleepers who do not complain of insomnia: Myths and realities about psychological and lifestyle characteristics of older good and poor sleepers. *Journal of Behavioral Medicine, 18*, 189–223.

Fielding, J. E. (1985). Smoking: Health effects and control. *New England Journal of Medicine, 313*, 491–498.

Fielding, J. E., & Piserchia, P. V. (1989). Frequency of worksite health promotion activities. *American Journal of Public Health, 79*, 16–20.

Fife, B. L. (1994). The conceptualization of meaning in illness. *Social Science in Medicine, 38*, 309–316.

Fife, B. L., Irick, N., & Painter, J. D. (1993). A comparative study of the attitudes of physicians and nurses toward the management of cancer pain. *Journal of Pain Symptom Management, 8*, 132–139.

Fillmore, K. M. (1987a). Prevalence, incidence and chronicity of drinking patterns and problems among men as a function of age: A longitudinal and cohort analysis. *British Journal of Addiction, 82*, 77–83.

Fillmore, K. M. (1987b). Women's drinking across the adult life course as compared to men's. *British Journal of Addiction, 82*, 801–811.

Fincham, J. E., & Wertheimer, A. I. (1986). Initial drug noncompliance in the elderly. *Journal of Geriatric Drug Therapy, 1*, 19–29.

Finkelhor, D., Asdigian, N., & Dziuba-Leatherman, J. (1995). Victimization prevention programs for children: A follow-up. *American Journal of Public Health, 85*, 1684–1689.

Fiore, M. C., Jorenby, D. E., Baker, T. B., & Kenford, S. L. (1992). Tobacco dependence and the nicotine patch. *Journal of the American Medical Association, 268*, 2687–2694.

Fiore, M. C., Smith, S. S., Jorenby, D. E., & Baker, T. B. (1994). The effectiveness of the nicotine patch for smoking cessation:

A meta-analysis. *Journal of the American Medical Association, 271,* 1940–1947.

Fischer, P. M., Richards, J. W., Jr., Berman, E. J., & Krugman, D. M. (1989). Recall and eye tracking study of adolescents viewing tobacco advertisements. *Journal of the American Medical Association, 261,* 84–89.

Fishbein, M., & Ajzen, I. (1975). *Belief, attitude, intention, and behavior: An introduction to theory and research.* Reading, MA: Addison-Wesley.

Fisher, M. J. (1995, April 3). Health coverage lacking among minority-Americans. *National Underwriter Property & Casualty-Risk & Benefits Management, 14,* 3.

Fisher, R. C. (1992). Patient education and compliance: A pharmacist's perspective. *Patient Education and Counseling, 19,* 261–271.

Fitzgerald, T. E., Tennen, H., Afflect, G., & Pransky, G. S. (1993). The relative importance of dispositional optimism and control appraisals in quality of life after coronary artery bypass surgery. *Journal of Behavioral Medicine, 16,* 25–43.

Fixx, J. F. (1977). *The complete book of running.* New York: Random House.

Fixx, J. F. (1980). *Jim Fixx's second book of running.* New York: Random House.

Flanders, W. D., & Rothman, K. J. (1982). Interaction of alcohol and tobacco in laryngeal cancer. *American Journal of Epidemiology, 115,* 371–379.

Flaxman, J. (1978). Quitting smoking now or later: Gradual, abrupt, immediate, and delayed quitting. *Behavior Therapy, 9,* 260–270.

Flay, B. R., Koepke, D., Thomson, S. J., Santi, S., Best, A., & Brown, S. (1989). Six-year follow-up of the first Waterloo school smoking prevention trial. *American Journal of Public Health, 79,* 1371–1376.

Flegal, K. M., Troiano, R. P., Pamuk, E. R., Kuczmarski, R. J., & Campbell, S. M. (1995). The influence of smoking cessation on the prevalence of overweight in the United States. *New England Journal of Medicine, 333,* 1165–1170.

Fleishman, J. A., & Fogel, B. (1994). Coping and depressive symptoms among people with AIDS. *Health Psychology, 13,* 156–169.

Fleshner, M., Laudenslager, M. L., Simons, L., & Maier, S. F. (1989). Reduced serum antibodies associated with social defeat in rats. *Physiological Behavior, 45,* 1183–1187.

Fleury, J. (1992). The application of motivational theory to cardiovascular risk reduction. *Image: Journal of Nursing Scholarship, 24,* 229–239.

Flor, H., & Birbaumer, N. (1993). Comparison of the efficacy of electromyographic biofeedback, cognitive-behavioral therapy, and conservative medical interventions in the treatment of chronic musculoskeletal pain. *Journal of Consulting and Clinical Psychology, 61,* 653–658.

Flynn, B. S., Worden, J. K., Secker-Walker, R. H., Badger, G. J., Geller, B. M., & Costanza, M. C. (1992). Prevention of cigarette smoking through mass media intervention and school programs. *American Journal of Public Health, 82,* 827–834.

Flynn, B. S., Worden, J. K., Secker-Walker, R. H., Pirie, P. L., Badger, G. J., Carpenter, J. H., & Geller, B. M. (1994). Mass media and school interventions for cigarette smoking prevention: Effects 2 years after completion. *American Journal of Public Health, 84,* 1148–1150.

Foley, K. M. (1989). The "decriminalization" of cancer pain. In C. S. Hill, Jr., & W. S. Fields (Eds.), *Advances in pain research and therapy: Vol. 11. Drug treatment of cancer pain in a drug-oriented society* (pp. 5–18). New York: Raven.

Folkman, S. (1993). Psychosocial effects of HIV infection. In L. Goldberger & S. Breznitz (Eds.), *Handbook of stress: Theo-*

retical and clinical aspects (2nd ed., pp. 658–681). New York: Free Press.

Follick, M. J., Ahern, D. K., & Aberger, E. W. (1985). Development of an audiovisual taxonomy of pain behavior: Reliability and discriminant validity. *Health Psychology, 4,* 555–568.

Folsom, A. R., Kaye, S. A., Sellers, T. A., Hong, C.-P., Cerhan, J. D., Potter, J. D., & Prineas, R. J. (1993). Body fat distribution and 5-year risk of death in older women. *Journal of the American Medical Association, 269,* 483–487.

Fontana, A. F., Kerns, R. D., Rosenberg, R. L., & Colonese, K. L. (1989). Support, stress, and recovery from coronary heart disease: A longitudinal causal model. *Health Psychology, 8,* 175–193.

Fontham, E. T. H., Correa, P., Reynolds, P., Wu-Williams, A., Buffler, P. A., Greenberg, R. S., Chen, V. W., Alterman, T., Boyd, P., Austin, D. F., & Liff, J. (1994). Environmental tobacco smoke and lung cancer in nonsmoking women: A multicenter study. *Journal of the American Medical Association, 271,* 1952–1759.

Forbes, G. B. (1992). Exercise and lean weight: The influence of body weight. *Nutrition Reviews, 50,* 147–161.

Forde, D. R. (1993). Perceived crime, fear of crime, and walking alone at night. *Psychological Reports, 73,* 403–407.

Fordyce, W. E. (1974). Pain viewed as learned behavior. In J. J. Bonica (Ed.), *Advances in neurology* (Vol. 4). New York: Raven.

Fordyce, W. E. (1976). *Behavioral methods for chronic pain and illness.* St. Louis: Mosby.

Fordyce, W. E. (1990a). Contingency management. In J. J. Bonica (Ed.), *The management of pain* (2nd ed., pp. 1702–1710). Malvern, PA: Lea & Febiger.

Fordyce, W. E. (1990b). Learned pain: Pain as behavior. In J. J. Bonica (Ed.), *The management of pain* (2nd ed., pp. 291–299). Malvern, PA: Lea & Febiger.

Fordyce, W. E., Brockway, J. A., Bergman, J. A., & Spengler, D. (1986). Acute back pain: A control-group comparison of behavioral vs. traditional management methods. *Journal of Behavioral Medicine, 9,* 127–140.

Fordyce, W. E., Fowler, R., Lehmann, J., DeLateur, B., Sand, P., & Treischmann, R. (1973). Operant conditioning in the treatment of chronic pain. *Archives of Physical Medicine and Rehabilitation, 54,* 399–408.

Fordyce, W. E., Shelton, J. L., & Dundore, D. E. (1982). The modification of avoidance learning pain behavior. *Journal of Behavioral Medicine, 5,* 405–414.

Fortmann, S. P., & Killen, J. D. (1994). Who shall quit? Comparisons of volunteer and population-based recruitment in two minimal-contact smoking cessation studies. *American Journal of Epidemiology, 140,* 39–51.

Fortmann, S. P., Taylor, C. B., Flora, J. A., & Jatulis, D. E. (1993). Changes in adult cigarette smoking prevalence after 5 years of community health education: The Stanford Five-City Project. *American Journal of Epidemiology, 137,* 82–96.

Fortmann, S. P., Taylor, C. B., Flora, J. A., & Winkleby, M. A. (1993). Effect of community health education on plasma cholesterol levels and diet: The Stanford Five-City Project. *American Journal of Epidemiology, 137,* 1039–1055.

Fowkes, F. G. R., Leng, G. C., Donnan, P. T., Deary, I. J., Riemersma, R. A., & Housley, E. (1992). Serum cholesterol, triglycerides, and aggression in the general population. *Lancet, 340,* 995–998.

Francis, M. E., & Pennebaker, J. W. (1992). Putting stress into words: The impact of writing on physiological, absentee, and self-reported emotional well-being measures. *Americal Journal of Health Promotion, 6,* 280–287.

Frank, E., Winkleby, M. A., Altman, D. G., Rockhill, B., & Fortmann, S. P. (1991). Predictors of physicians' smoking cessation advice. *Journal of the American Medical Association, 266,* 3139–3144.

Frank, R. G., Bouman, D. E., Cain, K., & Watts, C. (1992). A preliminary study of a traumatic injury program. *Psychology and Health, 8,* 129–140.

Franz, I. D. (1913). On psychology and medical education. *Science, 38,* 555–566.

Fraser, D. W. (1987). Epidemiology as a liberal art. *New England Journal of Medicine, 316,* 309–314.

Fraser, G. E., Beeson, W. L., & Phillips, R. L. (1991). Diet and lung cancer in California Seventh-day Adventists. *American Journal of Epidemiology, 133,* 683–693.

Frasure-Smith, N., Lespérance, F., & Talajic, M. (1995). The impact of negative emotions on prognosis following myocardial infarction: Is it more than depression? *Health Psychology, 14,* 388–398.

Freedman, D. S., Byers, T., Barrett, D. H., Stroup, N. E., & Monroe-Blum, H. (1995). Plasma lipid levels and psychologic characteristics in men. *American Journal of Epidemiology, 141,* 507–517.

Freedman, D. S., Williamson, D. F., Croft, J. B., Ballew, C., & Byers, T. (1995). Relationship of body fat distribution to ischemic heart disease: The National Health and Nutrition Examination Survey I (NHANES I): Epidemiologic Follow-up Study. *American Journal of Epidemiology, 142,* 53–63.

Freeman, R. C., Rodriguez, G. M., & French, J. F. (1994). A comparison of male and female intravenous drug users' risk behaviors for HIV infection. *American Journal of Drug and Alcohol Abuse, 20,* 129–157.

Freimuth, V. S., Hammond, S. L., & Stein, J. A. (1988). Health advertising: Prevention for profit. *American Journal of Public Health, 78,* 557–561.

French, S. A., Perry, C. L., Leon, G. R., & Fulkerson, J. A. (1994). Weight concerns, dieting behavior and smoking initiation among adolescents: A prospective study. *American Journal of Public Health, 84,* 1818–1820.

French, S. A., Story, M., Downes, B., Resnick, M. D., & Blum, R. W. (1995). Frequent dieting among adolescents: Psychosocial and health behavior correlates. *American Journal of Public Health, 85,* 695–701.

Freund, K. M., D'Agostino, R. B., Belanger, A. J., Kannel, W. B., & Stokes, J. III. (1992). Predictors of smoking cessation: The Framingham Study. *American Journal of Epidemiology, 135,* 957–964.

Frezza, M., di Padova, C., Pozzato, G., Terpin, M., Baraona, E., & Lieber, C. S. (1990). High blood alcohol levels in women: The role of decreased gastric alcohol dehydrogenase activity and first-pass metabolism. *New England Journal of Medicine, 322,* 95–99.

Fricton, J. R. (1982). Medical evaluation of patients with chronic pain. In J. Barber & C. Adrian (Eds.), *Psychological approaches to the management of pain.* New York: Brunner/Mazel.

Friedländer, L. (1968). *Roman life and manners under the early empire.* New York: Barnes & Noble.

Friedman, Emily. (1993). Changing the system: Implications for physicians. *Journal of the American Medical Association, 269,* 2437–2440.

Friedman, Edward S., Clark, D. B., & Gershon, S. (1992). Stress, anxiety, and depression: Review of biological, diagnostic, and nosologic issues. *Journal of Anxiety Disorders, 6,* 337–363.

Friedman, H. S. (1987). Postdoctoral training for research. In G. C. Stone, S. M. Weiss, J. D. Matarazzo, N. E. Miller, J. Rodin, C. D. Belar, M. J. Follick, & J. E. Singer (Eds.), *Health psychology: A discipline and a profession* (pp. 361–369). Chicago: University of Chicago Press.

Friedman, H. S. (Ed.). (1990). *Personality and disease.* New York: Wiley.

Friedman, H. S. (1991). *The self-healing personality: Why some people achieve health and others succumb to illness.* New York: Holt.

Friedman, H. S., & Booth-Kewley, S. (1987). The "disease-prone personality": A meta-analytic view of the construct. *American Psychologist, 42,* 539–555.

Friedman, H. S., Tucker, J. S., Schwartz, J. E., Martin, L. R., Tomlinson-Keasey, C., Wingard, D. L., & Criqui, M. H. (1995). Childhood conscientiousness and longevity: Health behaviors and cause of death. *Journal of Personality and Social Psychology, 68,* 696–703.

Friedman, H. S., Tucker, J. S., Schwartz, J. E., Tomlinson-Keasey, C., Martin, L. R., Wingard, D. L., & Criqui, M. H. (1995). Psychosocial and behavioral predictors of longevity: The aging and death of the "Termites." *American Psychologist, 50,* 69–78.

Friedman, H. S., Tucker, J. S., Tomlinson-Keasey, C., Schwartz, J. E., Wingard, D. L., & Criqui, M. H. (1993). Does childhood personality predict longevity? *Journal of Personality and Social Psychology, 65,* 176–185.

Friedman, L. A., & Kimball, A. W. (1986). Coronary heart disease mortality and alcohol consumption in Framingham. *American Journal of Epidemiology, 124,* 481–489.

Friedman, M., & Rosenman, R. H. (1974). *Type A behavior and your heart.* New York: Knopf.

Friedman, M., Thoresen, C. E., Gill, J. J., Powell, L. H., Ulmer, D., Thompson, L., Price, V. A., Rabin, D. D., Breall, W. S., Dixon, T., Levy, R., & Bourg, E. (1984). Alteration of Type A behavior and reduction in cardiac recurrences in post-myocardial infarction patients. *American Heart Journal, 108,* 237–248.

Friedman, M., & Ulmer, D. (1984). *Treating Type A behavior and your heart.* New York: Knopf.

Frisch, R. E., Wyshak, G., Albright, N. L., Albright, T. E., Schiff, I., Witschi, J., & Marguglio, M. (1985). Lower prevalence of breast cancer and cancers of the reproductive system among former college athletes compared to non-athletes. *British Journal of Cancer, 53,* 885–891.

Froland, S. S., Jenum, P., Lendboe, C. F., Wefring, K. W., Linnestad, P. J., & Bohmer, T. (1988). HIV-1 infection in a Norwegian family before 1970. *Lancet, i,* 1344–1345.

Fuchs, C. S., Stampfer, M. J., Colditz, G. A., Giovannucci, E. L., Manson, J. E., Kawachi, I., Hunter, D. J., Hankinson, S. E., Hennekens, C. H., Rosner, B., Speizer, F. E., & Willett, W. C. (1995). Alcohol consumption and mortality among women. *New England Journal of Medicine 332,* 1245–1250.

Fuchs, V. R. (1993). Dear President Clinton. *Journal of the American Medical Association, 269,* 1678–1679.

Fuller, R. K., Branchey, L., Brightwell, D. R., Derman, R. M., Emrick, C. D., Iber, F. L., James, K. E., Lacoursiere, R. B., Lee, K. K., Lowenstam, I., Maany, I., Neiderhiser, D., Nocks, J. J., & Shaw, S. (1986). Disulfiram treatment of alcoholism: A Veterans Administration cooperative study. *Journal of the American Medical Association, 256,* 1449–1455.

Fullilove, M. T., Wiley, J., Fullilove, R. E., Golden, E., Catania, J., Peterson, J., Garrett, K., Siegel, D., Marin, B., Kegeles, S., Coates, T., & Hulley, S. (1992). Risk for AIDS in multi-ethnic neighborhoods in San Francisco, California. The population-based AMEN study. *The Western Journal of Medicine, 157,* 32–40.

Funk, S. C. (1992). Hardiness: A review of theory and research. *Health Psychology, 11,* 335–345.

Funk, S. C., & Houston, B. K. (1987). A critical analysis of the hardiness scale's validity and utility. *Journal of Personality and Social Psychology, 53,* 572–578.

Furnham, A., & Kramers, M. (1989). Eating-problem patients' conceptions of normality. *Journal of Genetic Psychology, 150,* 147–153.

Futterman, A. D., Kemeny, M. E., Shapiro, D., & Fahey, J. L. (1994). Immunological and physiological changes associated with induced positive and negative mood. *Psychosomatic Medicine, 56,* 499–511.

Gallagher, D., Wrabetz, A., Lovett, S., Del Maestro, S., & Rose, J. (1989). Depression and other negative affects in family caregivers. In E. Light & B. D. Lebowitz (Eds.), *Alzheimer's disease treatment and family stress: Direction for research* (pp. 218–244). (DHHS Publication No. ADM 89-1569). Washington, DC: U.S. Government Printing Office.

Gallagher, E. B. (1988). Chronic illness management: A focus for future research applications. In D. S. Gochman (Ed.), *Health behavior: Emerging research perspectives* (pp. 397407). New York: Plenum.

Gallagher, E. J., Viscoli, C. M., & Horwitz, R. I. (1993). The relationship of treatment adherence to the risk of death after myocardial infarction in women. *Journal of the American Medical Association, 270,* 742–743.

Galton, F. (1879). Psychometric experiments. *Brain, 2,* 149–162.

Galton, F. (1883). *Inquiries into human faculty and its development.* London: Macmillan.

Ganellen, R. J., & Blaney, P. H. (1984). Hardiness and social support as moderators of the effects of life stress. *Journal of Personality and Social Psychology, 47,* 156–163.

Garfinkel, P. E., & Garner, D. M. (1982). *Anorexia nervosa: A multidimensional perspective.* New York: Brunner/Mazel.

Garfinkel, P. E., & Garner, D. M. (1984). Bulimia in anorexia nervosa. In R. C. Hawkins, II, W. J. Fremouw, & P. F. Clement (Eds.), *The binge-purge syndrome: Diagnosis, treatment and research.* New York: Springer.

Garfinkel, P. E., Moldofsky, H., & Garner, D. M. (1977). The outcome of anorexia nervosa: Significance of clinical features, body image, and behavior modification. In R. A. Vigersky (Ed.), *Anorexia nervosa* (pp. 315–329). New York: Raven.

Garland, A. F., & Zigler, E. F. (1994). Psychological correlates of help-seeking attitudes among children and adolescents. *American Journal of Orthopsychiatry, 64,* 586–593.

Garner, D. M., Fairburn, C. G., & Davis, R. (1987). Cognitive-behavioral treatment of bulimia nervosa: A critical appraisal. *Behavior Modification, 11,* 398–431.

Garner, D. M., & Garfinkel, P. E. (1980). Social-cultural factors in the development of anorexia nervosa. *Psychological Medicine, 10,* 647–656.

Garner, D. M., Garfinkel, P. E., & Bemis, K. M. (1982). A multidimensional psychotherapy for anorexia nervosa. *International Journal of Eating Disorders, 1,* 3–46.

Garner, D. M., Garfinkel, P. E., Schwartz, D., & Thompson, M. (1980). Cultural expectations of thinness in women. *Psychological Reports, 47,* 483–491.

Garrison, W. T., & McQuiston, S. (1989). *Chronic illness during childhood and adolescence: Psychological aspects.* Newbury Park, CA: Sage.

Gastorf, J. W., & Galanos, A. N. (1983). Patient compliance and physicians' attitude. *Family Practice Research Journal, 2,* 190–198.

Gatchel, R. J. (1993). Psychophysiological disorders: Past and present perspectives. In R. J. Gatchel & E. B. Blanchard (Eds.), *Psychophysiological disorders: Research and clinical applications* (pp. 1–21). Washington, DC: American Psychological Association.

Gatz, M., Pearson, C., & Weicker, W. (1987). Older persons and health psychology. In G. C. Stone, S. M. Weiss, J. D. Matarazzo, N. E. Miller, J. Rodin, C. D. Belar, M. J. Follick, & J. E. Singer (Eds.), *Health psychology: A discipline and a profession* (pp. 303–319). Chicago: University of Chicago Press.

Gaziano, J. M., Buring, J. E., Breslow, J. L., Goldhaber, S. Z., Rosner, B., VanDenburgh, M., Willett, W., & Hennekens, C. H. (1993). Moderate alcohol intake, increased levels of high-density lipoprotein and its subfractions, and decreased risk of myocardial infarction. *New England Journal of Medicine, 329,* 1829–1834.

Gebhardt, D. L., & Crump, C. E. (1990). Employee fitness and wellness programs in the workplace. *American Psychologist, 43,* 262–272.

Gibbons, A. (1991). Does war on cancer equal war on poverty? *Science, 253,* 260.

Gibbons, F. X., McGovern, P. G., & Lando, H. A. (1991). Relapse and risk perception among members of a smoking cessation clinic. *Health Psychology, 10,* 42–45.

Gilbar, O. (1989). Who refuses chemotherapy: A profile. *Psychological Reports, 64,* 1291–1297.

Gilbert, D. G. (1995). *Smoking: Individual differences, psychopathology, and emotion.* Washington DC: Taylor & Francis.

Ginsburg, K. R., Slap, G. B., Chaan, A., Forke, C. M., Balsley, C. M., & Rouselle, D. M. (1995). Adolescents' perception of factors affecting their decisions to seek health care. *Journal of the American Medical Association, 273,* 1913–1918.

Ginzberg, E. (1991). Access to health care for Hispanics. *Journal of the American Medical Association, 265,* 238–241.

Givovino, G. A., Schooley, M. W., Zhu, B., Chrismon, J. H., Tomar, S. L., Peddicord, J. P., Merritt, R. K., Housten, C. G., & Eriksen, M. P. (1994). Surveillance for selected tobacco-use behaviors—United States, 1990–1994. *Morbidity and Mortality Weekly Report, 43,* No. SS-3.

Glantz, S. A., & Parmley, W. W. (1995). Passive smoking and heart disease: Mechanisms and risk. *Journal of the American Medical Association, 273,* 1047–1053.

Glanz, K., Patterson, R. E., Kristal, A. R., DiClemente, C. C., Heimendinger, J., Linnan, L., & McLerran, D. F. (1994). Stages of change in adopting healthy diets: Fat, fiber, and correlates of nutrient intake. *Health Education Quarterly, 21,* 499–519.

Glascoff, M. A., Knight, S. M., & Jenkins, L. K. (1994). Designated driver programs: College students' experiences and opinions. *Journal of American College Health, 43,* 65–70.

Glasgow, R. E., McCaul, K. D., & Fisher, K. J. (1993). Participation in worksite health promotion: A critique of the literature and recommendations for future practice. *Health Education Quarterly, 20,* 391–408.

Glasgow, R. E., Toobert, D. J., Riddle, M., Donnelly, J., Mitchell, D. L., & Calder, D. (1989). Diabetes-specific social learning variables and self-care behaviors among persons with Type II diabetes. *Health Psychology, 8,* 285–303.

Glasner, P. D., & Kaslow, R. A. (1990). The epidemiology of human immunodeficiency virus infection. *Journal of Consulting and Clinical Psychology, 58,* 13–21.

Glass, D. C., & Singer, J. E. (1972). *Urban stress: Experiments on noise and social stressors.* New York: Academic Press.

Glasser, R. J. (1976). *The body is the hero.* New York: Random House.

Glasser, W. (1976). *Positive addiction.* New York: Harper & Row.

Glynn, C. J., Lloyd, J. W., & Folkard, S. (1981). Ventilatory responses to chronic pain. *Pain, 11,* 201–212.

Goedert, M., Strittmatter, W. J., & Roses, A. D. (1994). Risky apolipoprotein in brain. *Nature, 372,* 45.

Goffman, E. (1961). *Asylums.* Garden City, NY: Doubleday.

Goldman, L. S., & Kimball, C. P. (1985). Cardiac surgery: Enhancing postoperative outcomes. In A. M. Razin (Ed.), *Helping cardiac patients: Biobehavioral and psychotherapeutic approaches* (pp. 113–155). San Francisco: Jossey-Bass.

Goldman, S. L., Whitney-Saltiel, D., Granger, J., & Rodin, J. (1991). Children's representations of "everyday" aspects of health and illness. *Journal of Pediatric Psychology, 16,* 747–766.

Goldner, E. M., & Birmingham, C. L. (1994). Anorexia nervosa: methods of treatment. In L. Alexander-Mott & D. B. Lumsden (Eds.), *Understanding eating disorders: Anorexia nervosa, bulimia nervosa, and obesity* (pp. 135–157). Washington, DC: Taylor & Francis.

Goldstein, A. (1976). Opoid peptides (endorphins) in pituitary and brain. *Science, 193,* 1081–1086.

Goldstein, I. B. (1972). Electromyography: A measure of skeletal muscle response. In N. S. Greenfield & R. A. Sternbach (Eds.), *Handbook of psychophysiology.* New York: Holt, Rinehart and Winston.

Goldston, D. B., Kovacs, M., Obrosky, D. S., & Iyengar, S. (1995). A longitudinal study of life events and metabolic control among youths with insulin-dependent diabetes mellitus. *Health Psychology, 14,* 409–414.

Goleman, D. (1982, March). Staying up: The rebellion against sleep's gentle tyranny. *Psychology Today, 16,* 24–35.

Gomberg, E. S. L. (1989). Suicide risk among women with alcohol problems. *American Journal of Public Health, 79,* 1363–1365.

Gonder-Frederick, L. A., Carter, W. R., Cox, D. J., & Clarke, W. L. (1990). Environmental stress and blood glucose change in insulin-dependent diabetes mellitus. *Health Psychology, 9,* 503–515.

Gonder-Frederick, L. A., Cox, D. J., Bobbitt, S. A., & Pennebaker, J. W. (1986). Blood glucose symptom beliefs of diabetic patients: Accuracy and implications. *Health Psychology, 5,* 327–341.

Gonder-Frederick, L. A., Julian, D. M., Cox, D. J., Clarke, W. L., & Carter, W. (1988). Self-measurement of blood glucose: Accuracy of self reported data and adherence to recommended regimen. *Diabetes Care, 11,* 579–585.

Goodall, T. A., & Halford, W. K. (1991). Self-management of diabetes mellitus: A critical review. *Health Psychology, 10,* 1–8.

Goodwin, D. G. (1976). *Is alcoholism hereditary?* New York: Oxford University Press.

Goodwin, D. W., Schulsinger, F., Hermansen, L., Guze, S. B., & Winokur, G. (1973). Alcohol problems in adoptees raised apart from alcoholic biological parents. *Archives of General Psychiatry, 28,* 238–243.

Goodwin, J. S., Hunt, W. C., Key, C. R., & Samet, J. M. (1987). The effect of marital status on stage, treatment, and survival of cancer patients. *Journal of the American Medical Association, 258,* 3125–3130.

Gordon, D., & Rifkind, B. (1989). Treating high blood cholesterol in the older patient. *American Journal of Caardiology, 63* (Suppl.), 48H–52H.

Gordon, T., & Doyle, J. T. (1987). Drinking and mortality: The Albany Study. *American Journal of Epidemiology, 125,* 263–270.

Gordon, T., Castelli, W. P., Hjortland, M. C., Kannel, W. B., & Dawber, T. R. (1977). High density lipoprotein as a protective factor against coronary heart disease. The Framingham study. *American Journal of Medicine, 62,* 707–714.

Gordon, T., & Kannel, W. B. (1984). Drinking and mortality: The Framingham Study. *American Journal of Epidemiology, 120,* 97–107.

Gore, J. M., & Fallon, J. T. (1994). Case records of the Massachusetts General Hospital: A 25-year-old man with the recent onset of diabetes mellitus and congestive heart failure. *New England Journal of Medicine, 331,* 460–466.

Gorman, C. (1991, September 16). Why do Blacks die young? *Time, 138,* 50–52.

Gottlieb, A. M., Killen, J. D., Marlatt, G. A., & Taylor, C. B. (1987). Pyschological and pharmacological influences in cigarette smoking withdrawal: Effects of nicotine gum and expectancy on smoking withdrawal symptoms and relapse. *Journal of Consulting and Clinical Psychology, 55,* 606–608.

Gottman, J. M. (1991). Predicting the longitudinal course of marriages. *Journal of Marital and Family Therapy, 17,* 3–7.

Grady, D., & Ernster, V. (1992). Does cigarette smoking make you ugly and old? *American Journal of Epidemiology, 135,* 839–842.

Graham, D. Y. (1993). Treatment of peptic ulcers caused by Helicobacter pylori. *New England Journal of Medicine, 328,* 349–350.

Graham, R. B. (1990). *Physiological psychology.* Belmont, CA: Wadsworth.

Graham, S. (1983). Toward a dietary prevention of cancer. *Epidemiologic Reviews, 5,* 38–50.

Graham, S., Zielezny, M., Marshall, J., Priore, R., Freudenheim, J., Brasure, J., Haughey, B., Nasco, P., & Zdeb, M. (1992). Diet in the epidemiology of postmenopausal breast cancer in the New York cohort. *American Journal of Epidemiology, 136,* 1327–1337.

Graig, E. (1993). Stress as a consequence of the urban physical environment. In L. Goldberger & S. Breznitz (Eds.), *Handbook of stress: Theoretical and clinical aspects* (2nd ed., pp. 316–332). New York: Free Press

Green, B. L. (1986). On the confounding of "hassles" stress and outcome. *American Psychologist, 41,* 714–715.

Green, L. W. (1984). Health education models. In J. D. Matarazzo, S. M. Weiss, J. A. Herd, N. E. Miller, & S. M. Weiss (Eds.), *Behavioral health: A handbook of health enhancement and disease prevention* (pp. 181–198). New York: Wiley.

Greenberg, M. R., & Schneider, D. (1994). Violence in American cities: Young Black males is the answer, but what was the question? *Social Science and Medicine, 39,* 179–187.

Greenberger, E., & O'Neil, R. (1993). Spouse, parent, worker: Role commitments and role-related experiences in the construction of adults' well-being. *Developmental Psychology, 29,* 181–197.

Greendale, G. A., Barrett-Connor, E., Edelstein, S., Ingles, S., & Halle, R. (1995). Lifetime leisure exercise and osteoporosis: The Rancho Bernardo Study. *American Journal of Epidemiology, 141,* 951–959.

Greenley, J. R., & Davidson, R. E. (1988). Organizational influences on patient health behavior. In D. S. Gochman (Ed.), *Health behavior: Emerging research perspectives* (pp. 215–229). New York: Plenum.

Greenwood, J., Love, E. R., & Pratt, O. E. (1983). The effects of alcohol or of thiamine deficiency upon reproduction in the female rat and fetal development. *Alcohol and Alcoholism, 18,* 45–51.

Greer, S., & Morris, T. (1975). Psychological attributes of women who develop breast cancer: A controlled study. *Journal of Psychosomatic Research, 19,* 147–153.

Greer, S., & Morris, T. (1978). The study of psychological factors in breast cancer: Problems of method. *Social Science and Medicine, 12,* 129–134.

Greist, J. H. (1984). Exercise in the treatment of depression. *Coping with mental stress: The potential and limits of exercise intervention.* Washington, DC: National Institute of Mental Health.

Greist, J. H., Eischens, R. R., Klein, M. H., & Linn, D. (1981). Addendum to "Running through your mind." In M. H. Sacks & M. L. Sachs (Eds.), *Psychology of running.* Champaign, IL: Human Kinetics Publishers.

Greist, J. H., & Greist, T. H. (1979). *Antidepressant treatment: The essentials.* Baltimore: Williams & Wilkins.

Greist, J. H., Klein, M. H., Eischens, R. R., Faris, J., Gurman, A. S., & Morgan, W. P. (1978). Running through your mind. *Journal of Psychosomatic Research, 22,* 259–294.

Greist, J. H., Klein, M. H., Eischens, R. R., Faris, J., Gurman, A. S., & Morgan, W. P. (1979). Running as treatment of depression. *Comprehensive Psychiatry, 20,* 41–54.

Grinspoon, L., & Bakalar, J. B. (1976). *Cocaine: A drug and its social evolution.* New York: Basic Books.

Grinspoon, L., & Bakalar, J. B. (1995). Marihuana as medicine: A plea for reconsideration. *Journal of the American Medical Association, 273,* 1875–1876.

Grønbaek, M., Deis, A., Sørense, T. I. A., Becker, U., Schnohr, P., & Jensen, G. (1995). Mortality associated with moderate intakes of wine, beer, or spirits. *British Medical Journal, 310,* 1165–1169.

Gross, L. (1983). *How much is too much? The effects of social drinking.* New York: Random House.

Gross, N. J. (1994). Lung health study: Disappointment and triumph. *Journal of the American Medical Association, 272,* 1539.

Grossarth-Maticek, R., & Eysenck, H. J. (1989). Length of survival and lymphocyte percentage in women with mammary cancer as a function of psychotherapy. *Psychological Reports, 65,* 315–321.

Grossarth-Maticek, R., Eysenck, H. J., Vetter, H., & Frentzel-Beyme, R. (1986). The Heidelberg Prospective Intervention Study. In W. J. Eylenbasch, A. M. Depoorter, & N. van Larbeke (Eds.), *Primary prevention of cancer* (pp. 199–212). New York: Raven.

Grossarth-Maticek, R., Vetter, H., Frentzel-Beyme, R., & Heller, W. D. (1988). Precursor lesions of the GI tract and psychosocial risk factors for prediction and prevention of gastric cancer. *Cancer Detection and Prevention, 13,* 23–29.

Grossman, D. C., Krieger, J. W., Sugarman, J. R., & Forquera, R. A. (1994). Health status of urban American Indians and Alaska Natives: A population-based study. *Journal of the American Medical Association, 271,* 845–850.

Grover, S. A., Gray-Donald, K., Joseph, L., Abrahamowicz, M., & Coupal, L. (1994). Life expectancy following dietary modification or smoking cessation. *Archives of Internal Medicine, 154,* 1697–1704.

Groves, P. M., & Rebec, G. V. (1988). *Introduction to biological psychology* (3rd ed.). Dubuque, IA: Brown.

Grunau, R. V. E., & Craig, K. D. (1988). Pain. In W. Linden (Ed.), *Biological barriers in behavioral medicine* (pp. 257–279). New York: Plenum.

Guerci, A. D., & Ross, R. R. (1989). TIMI II and the role of angioplasty in acute myocardial infarction. *New England Journal of Medicine, 320,* 663–665.

Guerra, N. G. (1994). Violence prevention. Symposium: Disease prevention research at NIH: An agenda for all (1993, Bethesda, Maryland). *Preventive Medicine, 23,* 661–664

Gugler, R., Rohner, H-G., Kratochvil, P., Branditätter, G., & Schmitz, H. (1982). Effects of smoking on duodenal ulcer healing with cimetidine and ormetidine. *Gut, 23,* 866–871.

Gull, W. W. (1874). Anorexia nervosa (apepsia hysterica, anorexia hysterica). *Transactions of the Clinical Society of London, 7,* 22–28. (Reprinted in R. M. Kaufman & M. Heiman [Eds.], *Evolution of psychosomatic concepts: Anorexia nervosa, a paradigm.* New York: International University Press, 1964.)

Gwinup, G. (1975). Effect of exercise alone on the weight of obese women. *Archives of Internal Medicine, 135,* 676–680.

Gwinup, G., Chelvam, R., & Steinberg, T. (1971). Thickness of subcutaneous fat and activity of underlying muscles. *Annals of Internal Medicine, 74,* 408–411.

Haddon, W. H., Jr. (1970). On the escape of tigers: An ecologic note. *Technology Reviews, 72,* 3–7.

Haddon, W. H., Jr. (1972). A logical framework for categorizing highway safety phenomena and activity. *Journal of Trauma, 12,* 193–207.

Haddon, W. H., Jr. (1980, September–October). The basic strategies for reducing damage from hazards of all kinds. *Hazard Prevention, 6,* 16–22.

Haddon, W. H., Jr., & Baker, S. P. (1987). Injury control. In D. W. Clark & B. MacMahon (Eds.). *Preventive and community medicine* (2nd ed., pp. 109–140). Boston: Little, Brown.

Haglund, B., & Cnattingius, S. (1990). Cigarette smoking as a risk factor for sudden infant death syndrome: A population-based study. *American Journal of Public Health, 80,* 29–32.

Hains, A. A., & Ellmann, S. W. (1994). Stress inoculation training as a preventive intervention for high school youths. *Journal of Cognitive Psychotherapy, 8,* 219–232.

Halaas, J. L., Gajiwala, K. S., Maffei, M., Cohen, S. L., Chait, B. T., Rabinowitz, D., Lallone, R. L., Burley, S. K., & Friedman, J. M. (1995). Weight-reducing effects of the plasma protein encoded by the *obese* gene. *Science, 269,* 543–546.

Hall, G. R. (1994). Caring for people with Alzheimer's disease using the conceptual model of Progressively Lowered Stress Threshold in the clinical setting. *Nursing Clinics of North America, 27,* 129–141.

Hall, J. A., Irish, J. T., Roter, D. L., Ehrlich, C. M., & Miller, L. H. (1994). Gender in medical encounters: An analysis of physician and patient communication in a primary care setting. *Health Psychology, 13,* 384–392.

Hall, N. R., & Goldstein, A. L. (1981). Neurotransmitters and the immune system. In R. Ader (Ed.), *Psychoneuroimminology* (pp. 521–543). New York: Academic Press.

Hall, R. C., Tice, L., Beresford, T. P., Wooley, B., & Hall, A. K. (1989). Sexual abuse in patients with anorexia nervosa and bulimia. *Psychosomatics, 30,* 73–79.

Hall, S. M., Havassy, B. E., & Wasserman, D. A. (1990). Commitment to abstinence and acute stress in relapse to alcohol, opiates, and nicotine. *Journal of Consulting and Clinical Psychology, 58,* 175–181.

Hall, S. M., Tunstall, C. D., Ginsberg, D., Benowitz, N. L., & Jones, R. T. (1987). Nicotine gum and behavioral treatment: A placebo controlled trial. *Journal of Consulting and Clinical Psychology, 55,* 603–605.

Halmi, K. A. (1982). Cyproheptadine for anorexia nervosa. *Lancet, i,* 1357–1358.

Halmi, K. A., Falk, J. R., & Schwartz, E. (1981). Binge-eating and vomiting: A survey of a college population. *Psychological Medicine, 11,* 697–706.

Hammel, R. W., & Williams, P. O. (1964). Do patients receive prescribed medication? *American Pharmacy Association Journal, 4,* 331–334.

Hansen, W. B., Graham, J. W., Sobel, J. L., Shelton, D. R., Flay, B. R., & Johnson, C. A. (1987). The consistency of peer and parent influences on tobacco, alcohol, and marijuana use among young adolescents. *Journal of Behavioral Medicine, 10,* 559–579.

Hansen, W. B., Raynor, A. E., & Wolkenstein, B. H. (1991). Perceived personal immunity to the consequences of drinking alcohol: The relationship between behavior and perception. *Journal of Behavioral Medicine, 14,* 205–224.

Hanvik, L. J. (1951). MMPI profiles in patients with low back pain. *Journal of Consulting and Clinical Psychology, 15,* 350–353.

Hardy, J. D., & Smith, T. W. (1988). Cynical hostility and vulnerability to disease: Social support, life stress, and physiological response to conflict. *Health Psychology, 7,* 447–459.

Harris, M. B. (1981). Runners' perceptions of the benefits of running. *Perceptual and Motor Skills, 52,* 153–154.

Harris, R. E., & Wynder, E. L. (1988). Breast cancer and alcohol consumption: A study in weak associations. *Journal of the American Medical Association, 259,* 2867–2871.

Harris, S. S., Caspersen, C. J., DeFriese, G. H., & Estes, H. (1989). Physical activity counseling for healthy adults as a primary preventive intervention in the clinical setting: Report for the US Preventive Services Task Force. *Journal of the American Medical Association, 261,* 3590–3598.

Harris, T. B., Ballard-Barbasch, R., Madans, J., Makuc, D. M., & Feldman, J. J. (1993). Overweight, weight loss and risk of coronary heart disease in older women: The NHANES I Epidemiologic Follow-up Study. *American Journal of Epidemiology, 137,* 1318–1327.

Hartz, A. J., Rupley, D. C., & Rimm, A. A. (1984). The association of girth measurements with disease in 32,856 women. *American Journal of Epidemiology, 119,* 71–80.

Hatch, J. P. (1993). Headache. In R. J. Gatchel & E. B. Blanchard (Eds.), *Psychophysiological disorders: Research and clinical applications* (pp. 111–149). Washington, DC: American Psychological Association.

Haug, M. R. (1988). Power, authority, and health behavior. In D. S. Gochman (Ed.), *Health behavior: Emerging research perspectives* (pp. 325–336). New York: Plenum.

Hawkins, W. E. (1992). Problem behaviors and health-enhancing practices of adolescents: A multivariate analysis. *Health Values: The Journal of Health Behavior, Education and Promotion, 16,* 46–54.

Hayashida, M., Alterman, A. I., McLellan, A. T., O'Brien, C. P., Purtill, J. J., Volpicelli, J. R., Raphaelson, A. H., & Hall, C. P. (1989). Comparative effectiveness and costs of inpatient and outpatient detoxification of patients with mild-to-moderate alcohol withdrawal syndrome. *New England Journal of Medicine, 320,* 358–365.

Haynes, R. B. (1976a). A critical review of the "determinants" of patient compliance with therapeutic regimens. In D. L. Sackett & R. B. Haynes (Eds.), *Compliance with therapeutic regimens* (pp. 26–39). Baltimore: Johns Hopkins University Press.

Haynes, R. B. (1976b). Strategies for improving compliance: A methodologic analysis and review. In D. L. Sackett & R. B. Haynes (Eds.), *Compliance with therapeutic regimens* (pp. 69–82). Baltimore: Johns Hopkins University Press.

Haynes, R. B. (1979a). Determinants of compliance: The disease and the mechanics of treatment. In R. B. Haynes, D. W. Taylor, & D. L. Sackett (Eds.), *Compliance in health care* (pp. 49–62). Baltimore: Johns Hopkins University Press.

Haynes, R. B. (1979b). Introduction. In R. B. Haynes, D. W. Taylor, & D. L. Sackett (Eds.), *Compliance in health care* (pp. 1–7). Baltimore: Johns Hopkins University Press.

Haynes, R. B. (1979c). Strategies to improve compliance with referrals, appointments, and prescribed medical regimens. In R. B. Haynes, D. W. Taylor, & D. L. Sackett (Eds.), *Compliance in health care* (pp. 121–143). Baltimore: Johns Hopkins University Press.

Haynes, R. B., Wang, E., & da Mota Gomes, M. (1987). A critical review of interventions to improve compliance with prescribed medications. *Patient Education and Counseling, 10,* 155–166.

Haynes, S. G. (1989, August). *Women, work, and coronary heart disease.* Paper presented at the convention of the American Psychological Association, New Orleans, LA.

Haynes, S. G., Feinleib, M., & Kannel, W. B. (1980). The relationship of psychosocial factors to coronary heart disease in the Framingham study: III. Eight-year incidence of coronary heart disease. *American Journal of Epidemiology, 111,* 37–58.

Haynes, S. N., Griffin, P., Mooney, D., & Parise, M. (1975). Electromyographic feedback and relaxation instructions in the treatment of muscle contraction headaches. *Behavior Therapy, 6,* 672–678.

Hays, R. D., Kravitz, R. L., Mazel, R. M., Sherbourne, C. D., DiMatteo, M. R., Rogers, W. H., & Greenfield, S. (1994). The impact of patient adherence on health outcomes for patients with chronic disease in the Medical Outcomes Study. *Journal of Behavioral Medicine, 17,* 347–360.

Haythornthwaite, J. S. (1992-93). Behavioral stress, sodium intake, and blood pressure. *Homeostasis in Health and Disease, 34,* 302–312.

Hazuda, H. P. (1994). A critical evaluation of U.S. epidemiological evidence and ethnic variation. In S. A. Shumaker & S. M. Czajkowski (Eds.), *Social support and cardiovascular disease* (pp. 119–142). New York: Plenum.

Hearn, M. D., Murray, D. M., & Luepker, R. V. (1989). Hostility, coronary heart disease, and total mortality: A 33-year follow-up study of university students. *Journal of Behavioral Medicine, 12,* 105–121.

Hearn, W. L., Flynn, D. D., Hime, G. W., Rose, S., Cofino, J. C., Mantero-Atienza, E., Wetli, C. V., & Mash, D. C. (1991). Cocaethylene: A unique cocaine metabolite displays high affinity for the dopamine transporter. *Journal of Neurochemistry, 56,* 698–701.

Heather, N., & Robertson, I. (1983). *Controlled drinking* (rev. ed.). London: Methuen.

Heather, N., & Robertson, I. (1990). *Problem drinking* (2nd ed.). Oxford, England: Oxford University Press.

Heatherton, T. F., Polivy, J., & Herman, C. D. (1989). Restraint and internal responsiveness: Effects of placebo manipulations of hunger state on eating. *Journal of Abnormal Psychology, 98,* 89–92.

Hebert, L. E., Scheer, P. A., Becett, L. A., Albert, M. S., Pilgrim, D. M., Chown, M. J., Feenkenstein, H., & Evans, D. A. (1995). Age-specific incidence of Alzheimer's disease in a community population. *Journal of the American Medical Association, 273,* 1354–1359.

Hegel, M. T., Ayllon, T., Thiel, G., & Oulton, B. (1992). Improving adherence to fluid restrictions in male hemodialysis patients: A comparison of cognitive and behavioral approaches. *Health Psychology, 11,* 324–330.

Heinrich, R. L., Cohen, M. J., Naliboff, B. D., Collins, G. A., & Bonebakker, A. D. (1985). Comparing physical and behavioral therapy for chronic low back pain on physical abilities, psychological distress, and patients' perceptions. *Journal of Behavioral Medicine, 8,* 61–78.

Heitzmann, C. A., & Kaplan, R. M. (1988). Assessment of methods for measuring social support. *Health Psychology, 7,* 75–109.

Helby, E. M., Gafarian, C. T., & McCann, S. C. (1989). Situational and behavioral correlates of compliance to a diabetic regimen. *Journal of Compliance in Health Care, 4,* 101–116.

Helgeson, V. S. (1993). The onset of chronic illness: Its effect on the patient-spouse relationship. *Journal of Social and Clinical Psychology, 12,* 406–428.

Hellmich, N. (1995, May 25). Wake-up call for the sleep deprived. *USA Today,* pp. D1, D2.

Helmer, D. C., Ragland, D. R., & Syme, S. L. (1991). Hostility and coronary artery disease. *American Journal of Epidemiology, 133,* 112–122.

Helmers, K. F., Posluszny D. M., & Krantz, D. S. (1994). Associations of hostility and coronary artery disease: A review of studies. In A. W. Siegman & T. W. Smith (Eds.), *Anger, hostility, and the heart* (pp. 67–96). Hillsdale, NJ: Erlbaum.

Helmrich, S. P., Ragland, D. R., Leung, R. W., & Paffenbarger, R. S., Jr. (1991). Physical activity and reduced occurrence of non-insulin-dependent diabetes mellitus. *New England Journal of Medicine, 325,* 147–152.

Helsing, K. J., Sandler, D. P., Comstock, G. W., & Chee, E. (1988). Heart disease mortality in nonsmokers living with smokers. *American Journal of Epidemiology, 127,* 915–922.

Helsing, K. J., Szklo, M., & Comstock, G. W. (1981). Factors associated with mortality after widowhood. *American Journal of Public Health, 71,* 802–809.

Helzer, J. E., Robins, L. N., & McEvoy, L. (1987). Post-traumatic stress disorder in the general population: Findings of the Epidemiologic Catchment Area survey. *New England Journal of Medicine, 317,* 1630–1634.

Helzer, J. E., Robins, L. N., Taylor, J. R., Carey, K., Miller, R. H., Combs-Orme, T., & Farmer, A. (1985). The extent of long-term moderate drinking among alcoholics discharged from medical and psychiatric treatment facilities. *New England Journal of Medicine, 312,* 1678–1682.

Hepler, R. S., & Frank, I. M. (1971). Marijuana smoking and intraocular pressure. *Journal of the American Medical Association, 217,* 1392.

Herbert, T. B., & Cohen, S. (1993a). Depression and immunity: A meta-analytic review. *Psychological Bulletin, 113,* 472–486.

Herbert, T. B., & Cohen, S. (1993b). Stress and immunity in humans: A meta-analytic review. *Psychosomatic Medicine, 55,* 364–379.

Herbert, T. B., & Cohen, S. (1994). Stress and illness. In V. S. Ramachandran (Ed.), *Encyclopedia of human behavior, Vol. 4* (pp. 325–332). San Diego, CA: Academic Press.

Herity, B. (1984). Role of alcohol, tobacco, and socio-economic factors. In B. A. Stoll (Ed.), *Risk factors and multiple cancer* (pp. 83–102). Chichester, England: Wiley.

Herning, R. I., Jones, R. T., Bachman, J., & Mines, A. H. (1981). Puff volume increases when low-nicotine cigarettes are smoked. *British Medical Journal, 283,* 187–189.

Hersey, J. C., Klibanoff, L. S., Lam, D. J., & Taylor, R. L. (1984). Promoting social support: The impact of California's "Friends Can Be Good Medicine" campaign. *Health Education Quarterly, 11,* 293–311.

Heston, L. L., & White, J. A. (1991). *The vanishing mind: A practical guide to Alzheimer's disease and other dementias* (2nd ed.). New York: Freeman.

Heszen-Klemens, I. (1987). Patients' noncompliance and how doctors manage this. *Social Science and Medicine, 24,* 409–416.

Heuch, I., Kvale, G., Jacobsen, B. K., & Bjelke, E. (1983). Use of alcohol, tobacco and coffee, and risk of pancreatic cancer. *British Journal of Cancer, 48,* 637–643.

Hewitt, P. L., Flett, G. L., & Mosher, S. W. (1992). The Perceived Stress Scale: Factor structure and relation to depression symptoms in a psychiatric sample. *Journal of Psychopathology and Behavioral Assessment, 14,* 247–257.

Higgins, M. W., Kjelsberg, M., & Metzner, H. (1967). Characteristics of smokers and nonsmokers in Tecumseh, Michigan. I: The distribution of smoking habits in persons and families and their relationship to social characteristics. *American Journal of Epidemiology, 86,* 45–59.

Higgins, R. L., & Marlatt, G. A. (1973). Effects of anxiety arousal on the consumption of alcohol by alcoholics and social drinkers. *Journal of Consulting and Clinical Psychology, 41,* 426–433.

Higgins, R. L., & Marlatt, G. A. (1975). Fear of interpersonal evaluation as a determinant of alcohol consumption in male social drinkers. *Journal of Abnormal Psychology, 84,* 644–651.

Hilgard, E. R. (1975). The alleviation of pain by hypnosis. *Pain, 1,* 213–231.

Hilgard, E. R. (1978). Hypnosis and pain. In R. A. Sternbach (Ed.), *The psychology of pain.* New York: Raven.

Hilgard, E. R. (1979). Divided consciousness in hypnosis: The implications of the hidden observer. In E. Fromm & R. E. Shor (Eds.), *Hypnosis: Development in research and new perspectives* (pp. 45–79). Chicago: Aldine.

Hilgard, E. R., & Hilgard, J. R. (1975). *Hypnosis in the relief of pain.* Los Altos, CA: Kaufmann.

Hill, C. S., Jr. (1995). When will adequate pain treatment be the norm? *Journal of the American Medical Association, 274,* 1881–1882.

Hill, J. O., Drougas, H. J., & Peters, J. C. (1994). Physical activity, fitness, and moderate obesity. In C. Bouchard, R. J. Shephard, & T. Stephens (Eds.), *Physical activity, fitness, and health: International proceedings and consensus statement* (pp. 684–695). Champaign, IL: Human Kinetics.

Hillbrand, M., Spitz, R. T., & Foster, H. G. (1995). Serum cholesterol and aggression in hospitalized male forensic patients. *Journal of Behavioral Medicine, 18,* 33–43.

Hinds, M. W., Kolonel, L. N., Hankin, J. H., & Lee, J. (1984). Dietary vitamin A, carotene, vitamin C and risk of lung cancer in Hawaii. *American Journal of Epidemiology, 119,* 227–237.

Hingson, R. W., Strunin, L., Berlin, B. M., & Heeren, T. (1990). Beliefs about AIDS, use of alcohol and drugs, and unprotected sex among Massachusetts adolescents. *American Journal of Public Health, 80,* 295–299.

Hinkle, J. S. (1992). Aerobic running behavior and psychotherapeutics: Implications for sports counseling and psychology. *Journal of Sport Behavior, 15,* 263–277.

Hobfoll, S. E., & Vaux, A. (1993). Social support: Resources and context. In L. Goldberger & S. Breznitz (Eds.), *Handbook of stress: Theoretical and clinical aspects* (2nd ed., pp. 685–705). New York: Free Press.

Hochbaum, G. (1958). *Public participation in medical screening programs* (DHEW Publication No. 572, Public Health Service). Washington, DC: U. S. Government Printing Office.

Hochschild, A. (with Machung, A.). (1989). *The second shift: Working parents and the revolution at home.* New York: Viking.

Hoek, H. W. (1993). Review of the epidemiological studies of eating disorders. *International Review of Psychiatry, 5,* 61–74.

Hogan, J. (1989). Personality correlates of physical fitness. *Journal of Personality and Social Psychology, 56,* 284–288.

Holahan, C. J., & Moos, R. H. (1985). Life stress and health: Personality, coping and family support in stress resistance. *Journal of Personality and Social Psychology, 49,* 739–747.

Holahan, C. J., Moos, R. H., Holahan, C. K., & Brennan, P. L. (1995). Social support, coping, and depressive symptoms in a late-middle-aged sample of patients reporting cardiac illness. *Health Psychology, 14,* 152–163.

Holderness, C. C., Brooks-Gunn, J., & Warren, M. P. (1994). Comorbidity of eating disorders and substance abuse: Review of the literature. *International Journal of Eating Disorders, 16,* 1–34.

Holland, J. C., & Lewis, S. (1993). Emotions and cancer: Who do we really know? In D. Goleman & J. Gurin (Eds.), *Mind/body medicine: How to use your mind for better health* (pp. 85–109). Yonkers, NY: Consumer Reports Books.

Hollis, J. F., Connett, J. E., Stevens, V. J., & Greenlick, M. R. (1990). Stressful life events, Type A behavior, and the prediction of cardiovascular and total mortality over six years. *Journal of Behavioral Medicine, 13,* 263–280.

Holme, I. (1990). An analysis of randomized trials evaluating the effect of cholesterol reduction on total mortality and coronary heart disease incidence. *Circulation, 82,* 1916–1924.

Holmes, T. H., & Masuda, M. (1974). Life change and illness susceptibility. In B. S. Dohrenwend & B. P. Dohrenwend (Eds.), *Stressful life events: Their nature and effects* (pp. 45–72). New York: Wiley.

Holmes, T. H., & Rahe, R. H. (1967). The Social Readjustment Rating Scale. *Journal of Psychosomatic Research, 11,* 213–218.

Holroyd, K. A., Appel, M. A., & Andrasik, F. (1983). A cognitive-behavioral approach to psychophysiological disorders. In D. Meichenbaum & M. E. Jaremko (Eds.), *Stress reduction and prevention* (pp. 219–259). New York: Plenum.

Holt, N. L., Daling, J. R., McKnight, B., Moore, D. E., Stergachis, A., & Weiss, N. S. (1994). Cigarette smoking and functional ovarian cysts. *American Journal of Epidemiology, 139,* 781–786.

Holt, R R. (1993). Occupational stress. In L. Goldberger & S. Breznitz (Eds.), *Handbook of stress: Theoretical and clinical aspects* (2nd ed., pp. 333–367). New York: Free Press.

Honkanen, R. (1993). Alcohol in home and leisure injuries. International Symposium on Alcohol-related Accidents and Injuries (1991, Yverdon-les-Bains, Switzerland). *Addiction, 88,* 939–944.

Hopper, J. L., & Seeman E. (1994). The bone density of female twins discordant for tobacco use. *New England Journal of Medicine, 330,* 387–392.

Horan, J. L. (1973). "In vivo" emotive imagery: A technique for reducing childbirth anxiety and discomfort. *Psychological Reports, 32,* 1328.

Horan, J. J., & Dellinger, J. K. (1974). "In vivo" emotive imagery: A preliminary test. *Perceptual and Motor Skills, 39,* 359–362.

Horan, J. J., Layng, F. C., & Pursell, C. H. (1976). Preliminary study of effects of "in vivo" emotive imagery on dental discomfort. *Perceptual and Motor Skills, 42,* 105–106.

Hornbrook, M. C., Stevens, V. J., Wingfield, D. J., Hollis, J. F., Greenlick, M. R., & Ory, M. G. (1994). Preventing falls among community-dwelling older persons: Results from a randomized trial. *Gerontologist, 34,* 16–23.

Horne, J. (1988). *Why we sleep: The functions of sleep in humans and other mammals.* Oxford, England: Oxford University Press.

Horne, R. L., & Picard, R. S. (1979). Psychosocial risk factors for lung cancer. *Psychosomatic Medicine, 41,* 503–514.

Horwitz, R. I., Viscoli, C. M., Berkman, L., Donaldson, R. M., Horwitz, S. M., Murray, C. J., Ransohoff, D. F., & Sindelar, J. (1990). Treatment adherence and risk of death after myocardial infarction. *Lancet, 336,* 542–545.

House, J. S., Robbins, C., & Metzner, H. L. (1982). The association of social relationships and activities with mortality: Prospective evidence from the Tecumseh Community Health Study. *American Journal of Epidemiology, 116,* 123–140.

Houston, B. K. (1986). Psychological variables and cardiovascular and neuroendocrine reactivity. In K. A. Matthews, S. M. Weiss, T. Detre, T. M. Dembroski, B. Falkner, S. B. Manuck, & R. B. Williams, Jr. (Eds.), *Handbook of stress, reactivity, and cardiovascular disease* (pp. 207–209). New York: Wiley-Interscience.

Houston, B. K. (1988). Division 38 survey: Synopsis of results. *The Health Psychologist, 10,* 2–3.

Houston, B. K., & Vavak, C. R. (1991). Cynical hostility: Developmental factors, psychosocial correlates, and health behaviors. *Health Psychology, 10,* 9–17.

Hsu, J. S. J., & Williams, S. D. (1991). Injury prevention awareness in an urban Native American population. *American Journal of Public Health, 81,* 1466–1468.

Hsu, L. K. G. (1990). *Eating disorders.* New York: Guilford Press.

Hudgens, R. W. (1974). Personal catastrophe and depression. In B. S. Dohrenwend & B. P. Dohrenwend (Eds.), *Stressful life events: Their nature and effects.* New York: Wiley.

Hughes, J. (1975). Isolation of an endogenous compound from the brain with pharmacological properties similar to morphine. *Brain Research, 88,* 295–308.

Hughes, J. R., Gulliver, S. B., Fenwick, J. W., Valliere, W. A., Cruser, K., Pepper, S., Shea, P., Solomon, L. J., & Flynn, B. S. (1992). Smoking cessation among self-quitters. *Health Psychology, 11,* 331–334.

Hughes, J. R., Gust, S. W., Keenan, R. M., Fenwick, J. W., & Healey, M. L. (1989). Nicotine vs. placebo gum in general medical practice. *Journal of the American Medical Association, 261,* 1300–1305.

Hull, J. G. (1981). A self-awareness model of the causes and effects of alcohol consumption. *Journal of Abnormal Psychology, 90,* 586–600.

Hull, J. G. (1987). Self-awareness model. In H. T. Blane & K. E. Leonard (Eds.), *Psychological theories of drinking and alcoholism* (pp. 272–304). New York: Guilford Press.

Hull, J. G., & Bond, C. F. (1986). Social and behavioral consequences of alcohol consumption and expectancy: A meta-analysis. *Psychological Bulletin, 99,* 347–360.

Hull, J. G., Van Treuren, R. R., & Virnelli, S. (1987). Hardiness and health: A critique and alternative approach. *Journal of Personality and Social Psychology, 53,* 518–530.

Humble, C., Croft, J., Gerber, A., Casper, M., Hames, C. G., & Tyroler, H. A. (1990). Passive smoking and 20-year cardiovascular disease mortality among nonsmoking wives, Evans County, Georgia. *American Journal of Public Health, 80,* 599–601.

Hunt, L. M., Jordan, B., Irwin, S., & Browner, C. H. (1989). Compliance and the patient's perspective: Controlling symptoms in everyday life. *Culture, Medicine, and Psychiatry, 13,* 315–334.

Hunt, W. A., Barnett, L. W., & Branch, L. G. (1971). Relapse rates in addiction programs. *Journal of Clinical Psychology, 27,* 455–456.

Hunter, C., Jr. (1982). Freestanding alcohol treatment centers—A new approach to an old problem. *Psychiatric Annals, 12,* 396–408.

Hunter, D. J., Manson, J. E., Colditz, G. A., Stampfer, M. J., Rosner, B., Hennekens, C. H., Speizer, F. E., & Willett, W. C. (1993). A prospective study of the intake of vitamins C, E, and A and the risk of breast cancer. *New England Journal of Medicine, 329,* 234–240.

Hunter, M., & Philips, C. (1981). The experience of headache: An assessment of the qualities of tension headache pain. *Pain, 10,* 209–219.

Huon, G. F., Brown, L., & Morris, S. (1988). Lay beliefs about disordered eating. *International Journal of Eating Disorders, 7,* 239–252.

Hurley, B. F., Seals, D. R., Hagberg, J. M., Goldberg, A. C., Ostrove, S. M., Holloszy, J. O., Wiest, W. G., & Goldberg, A. P. (1984). High-density lipoprotein cholesterol in body-builders vs. powerlifters: Negative effects of androgen use. *Journal of the American Medical Association, 252,* 507–513.

Hurt, R. D., Dale, L. C., Fredrickson, P. A., Caldwell, C. C., Lee, G. A., Offord, K. P., Lauger, G. G., Marušic, Z., Neese, L. W., & Lunberg, T. G. (1994). Nicotine patch therapy for smoking cessation combined with physician advice and nurse follow-up: One-year outcome and percentage of nicotine replacement. *Journal of the American Medical Association, 271,* 595–600.

Hyman, R. B., Baker, S., Ephraim, R., Moadel, A., & Philip, J. (1994). Health Belief Model variables as predictors of screening mammography utilization. *Journal of Behavior Medicine, 17,* 391–406.

Hypertension Detection and Follow-up Program Cooperative Group. (1979). Five-year findings of the Hypertension Detection and Follow-up Program. *Journal of the American Medical Association, 242,* 2562–2577.

Ickovics, J. R., & Rodin, J. (1992). Women and AIDS in the United States: Epidemiology, natural history, and mediating mechanisms. *Health Psychology, 11,* 1–16.

Ikard, F. F., Green, D., & Horn, D. A. (1969). A scale to differentiate between types of smoking as related to the management of affect. *International Journal of Addictions, 4,* 649–659.

Ikegami, N. (1992). The economics of health care in Japan. *Science, 258,* 614–618.

Ilacqua, G. E. (1994). Migraine headaches: Coping efficacy of guided imagery training. *Headache, 34,* 99–102.

Imber, S., Schultz, E., Funderburk, F., Allen, R., & Flanner, R. (1976). The fate of the untreated alcoholic: Toward a natural history of the disorder. *Journal of Nervous and Mental Disorders, 162,* 238–247.

Ingraham, J., & Ingraham, C. (1995). *Introduction to Mirobiology* (1st ed.). Belmont, CA: Wadsworth.

International Association for the Study of Pain (IASP), Subcommittee on Taxonomy. (1979). Pain terms: A list with definitions and notes on usage. *Pain, 6,* 249–252.

International Society of Sport Psychology. (1992). Physical activity and psychological benefits: A position statement from the International Society of Sport Psychology. *Journal of Applied Sport Psychology, 4,* 94–98.

Irwin, M., Mascovich, M., Gillin, C., Willoughby, R., Pike, J., & Smith, T. L. (1994). Partial sleep deprivation reduces natural killer cell activity in humans. *Psychosomatic Medicine, 56,* 493–498.

Ismail, A. I., Burt, B. A., & Eklund, S. A. (1983). Epidemiologic patterns of smoking and peridontal disease in the United States. *Journal of the American Dental Association, 106,* 617–621.

Iso, H., Jacobs, D. R., Jr., Wentworth, P., Neaton, J. D., & Cohen, J. D. (1989). Serum cholesterol levels and six-year mortality from stroke in 350,977 men screened for the Multiple Risk Factor Intervention Trial. *New England Journal of Medicine, 320,* 904–910.

Istvan, J., & Hatton, D. C. (1987). Curricula of graduate training programs in health psychology. In G. C. Stone, S. M. Weiss, J. D. Matarazzo, N. E. Miller, J. Rodin, C. D. Belar, M. J. Follick, & J. E. Singer (Eds.), *Health psychology: A discipline and a profession* (pp. 425–448). Chicago: University of Chicago Press.

Jablon, S., Hrubec, Z., & Boise, J. D. (1991). Cancer in populations living near nuclear facilities. *Journal of the American Medical Association, 265,* 1403–1408.

Jackson, R., Scragg, R., & Beaglehole, R. (1992). Does recent alcohol consumption reduce the risk of acute myocardial infarction and coronary death in regular drinkers? *American Journal of Epidemiology, 136,* 819–824.

Jacobs, A. L., Kurtz, R. M., & Strube, M. J. (1995). Hypnotic analgesia, expectancy effects, and choice of a design: A reexamination. *International Journal of Clinical and Experimental Hypnosis, 43,* 55–68.

Jacobs, D., Blackburn, H., Higgins, M., Reed, D., Iso, H., McMillian, G., Neaton, J., Nelson, J., Potter, J., Rifkind, B., Jossouw, J., Shekelle, R., & Yusuf, S. (1992). Report of the conference on low blood cholesterol: Mortality associations. *Circulation, 86,* 1046–1060.

Jacobs, D. R., Jr., Muldoon, M. F., & Råstam, L. (1995). Invited Commentary: Low blood cholesterol, nonillness mortality, and other nonatherosclerotic disease mortality: A search for causes and confounders. *American Journal of Epidemiology, 141,* 518–522.

Jacobs, M. (1972). The addictive personality: Prediction of success in a smoking withdrawal program. *Psychosomatic Medicine, 34,* 30–38.

Jacobson, E. (1934). *You must relax.* New York: McGraw-Hill.

Jacobson, E. (1938). *Progressive relaxation: A physiological and clinical investigation of muscle states and their significance in psychology and medical practice* (2nd ed.). Chicago: University of Chicago Press.

Jagal, S. B., Kreiger, N., & Darlington, G. (1993). Past and recent physical activity and risk of hip fracture. *American Journal of Epidemiology, 138,* 107–118.

Jamison, K. R., & Akiskal, H. (1983). Medication compliance in patients with bipolar disorder. *Psychiatric Clinics of North America, 6,* 175–192.

Jamison, R. N., Burish, T. G., & Wallston, K. A. (1987). Psychogenic factors in predicting survival of breast cancer patients. *Journal of Clinical Oncology, 5,* 768–772.

Janis, I. L. (1958). *Psychological stress.* New York: Wiley.

Janis, I. L. (1983). The role of social support in adherence to stressful decisions. *American Psychologist, 38,* 143–160.

Janis, I. L. (1984). Improving adherence to medical recommendations: Prescriptive hypotheses derived from recent research in social psychology. In A. Baum, S. E. Taylor, & J. E. Singer (Eds.), *Handbook of psychology and health: Vol. 4. Social psychological aspects of health* (pp. 113–148). Hillsdale, NJ: Erlbaum.

Janis, I. L., & Feshbach, S. (1953). Effects of fear-arousing communications. *Journal of Abnormal and Social Psychology, 48,* 78–92.

Janis, I. L., & Rodin, J. (1979). Attribution, control, and decision making: Social psychology and health care. In G. C. Stone, F. Cohen, & N. E. Adler (Eds.), *Health psychology — A handbook* (pp. 487–521). San Francisco: Jossey-Bass.

Japsen, B. (1994). Indians seek supplemental fundings. *Modern Healthcare, 24,* 78.

Jarvik, M. (1977). Biological factors underlying the smoking habit. In M. Jarvik, J. Cullen, E. Gritz, T. Vogt, & L. West (Eds.), *Research on smoking and behavior* (NIDA Publication No. ADM 78-581). Rockville, MD: National Institute on Drug Abuse.

Jarvik, M., Killen, J. D., Varady, A., & Fortmann, S. P. (1993). The favorite cigarette of the day. *Journal of Behavioral Medicine, 16,* 413–422

Jason, L. A., Jayaraj, S., Blitz, C. C., Michaels, M. H., & Klett, L. E. (1990). Incentives and competition in a worksite smoking cessation intervention. *American Journal of Public Health, 80,* 205–206.

Jay, S. M., Elliott, C. H., Katy, E., & Siegel, S. E. (1987). Cognitive-behavioral and pharmacological interventions for children's distress during painful medical procedures. *Journal of Consulting and Clinical Psychology, 55,* 860–865.

Jay, S. M., Elliott, C. H., Woody, P. D., & Siegel, S. (1991). An investigation of cognitive-behavior therapy combined with oral valium for children undergoing painful medical procedures. *Health Psychology, 10,* 317–322.

Jellinek, E. M. (1960). *The disease concept of alcoholism.* New Haven, CT: College and University Press.

Jemmott, J. B., III, Borysenko, J. Z., Borysenko, M., McClelland, D. C., Chapman, R., Meyer, D., & Benson, H. (1983). Academic stress, power motivation, and decrease in secretion rate of salivary secretory immunoglobulin A. *Lancet, i,* 1400–1402.

Jemmott, J. B., III, Croyle, R. T., & Ditto, P. H. (1988). Common-sense epidemiology: Self-based judgments from laypersons and physicians. *Health Psychology, 7,* 55–73.

Jemmott, J. B., III, Hellman, C., McClelland, D. C., Locke, S. E., Kraus, L., Williams, R. M., & Valeri, C. R. (1990). Motivational syndromes associated with natural killer cell activity. *Journal of Behavioral Medicine, 13,* 53-73.

Jemmott, J. B., III, & Locke, S. E. (1984). Psychosocial factors, immunologic mediation, and human susceptibility to infectious diseases: How much do we know? *Psychological Bulletin, 95,* 78-108.

Jemmott, J. B., III, & Magloire, K. (1988). Academic stress, social support, and secretory immunoglobulin A. *Journal of Personality and Social Psychology, 55,* 803-810.

Jenkins, C. D., Rosenman, R. H., & Zyzanski, S. J. (1965). *The Jenkins Activity Survey for health prediction.* Chapel Hill, NC: Author.

Jenkins, C. D., Zyzanski, S. J., & Rosenman, R. H. (1979). *Jenkins Activity Survey.* New York: Psychological Corporation.

Jenner, J. L., Ordovas, J. M., Lamon-Fava, S., Schaefer, M. M., Wilson, W. F., Castelli, W. P., & Schaefer, E. J. (1993). Effects of age, sex, and menopausal states on plasma lipoprotein(a) levels: The Framingham Offspring Study. *Circulation, 87,* 1135-1141.

Job, R. F. S. (1988). Effective and ineffective use of fear in health promotion campaigns. *American Journal of Public Health, 78,* 163-167.

Joesting, J. (1981). Running and depression. *Perceptual and Motor Skills, 52,* 442.

John, E. M., Savitz, D. A., & Sandler, D. P. (1991). Prenatal exposure to parents' smoking and childhood cancer. *American Journal of Epidemiology, 133,* 123-132.

Johnson, J. V., & Hall, E. M. (1988). Job strain, work place social support, and cardiovascular disease: A cross-sectional study of a random sample of the Swedish working population. *American Journal of Public Health, 78,* 1336-1342.

Johnson, M., & Vögele, C. (1993). Benefits of psychological preparation for surgery: A meta-analysis. *Annals of Behavioral Medicine, 15,* 245-256.

Johnson, S. B., Freund, A., Silverstein, J., Hansen, C. A., & Malone, J. (1990). Adherence-health status relationships in childhood diabetes. *Health Psychology, 9,* 606-631.

Johnson, S. B., Tomer, A., Cunningham, W. R., & Henretta, J. C. (1990). Adherence in childhood diabetes: Results of a confirmatory factor analysis. *Health Psychology, 9,* 493-501.

Johnston, L. D., O'Malley, P. M., & Bachman, J. G. (1989). *Drug use, drinking, and smoking: National survey results from high school, college, and young adult populations, 1975-1988.* (DHHS Publication No. ADM 89-1638). Washington, DC: U.S. Government Printing Office.

Johnston, L. D., O'Malley, P. M., & Bachman, J. G. (1994a). *National survey results on drug use from the Monitoring the Future study, 1975-1993, Vol. I: Secondary school students.* NIH Publication No. 94-3809. Rockville, MD: National Institute on Drug Abuse.

Johnston, L. D., O'Malley, P. M., & Bachman, J. G. (1994b). *National survey results on drug use from the Monitoring the Future study, 1975-1993, Vol. II: College students and young adults.* NIH Publication No. 94-3810. Rockville, MD: National Institute on Drug Abuse.

Jones, J. A., Eckhardt, L. E., Mayer, J. A., Bartholomew, S., Malcarne, V. L., Hovell, M. F., & Elder, J. P. (1993). The effects of an instructional audiotape on breast self-examination proficiency. *Journal of Behavioral Medicine, 16,* 225-235.

Jones, N. L. (1988). *Clinical exercise testing.* Philadelphia: Saunders.

Jones, R. B., & Moberg, D. P. (1988). Correlates of smokeless tobacco use in a male adolescent population. *American Journal of Public Health, 78,* 61-63.

Jousilahti, P., Vartiainen, E., Toumilehto, J., Pekkanen, J., & Puska, P. (1995). Effect of risk factors and changes in risk factors on coronary mortality in three cohorts of middle-aged people in Eastern Finland. *American Journal of Epidemiology, 141,* 50-60.

Julien, R. M. (1978). *A primer of drug action* (2nd ed.). San Francisco: Freeman.

Kabat, G. C., Stellman, S. D., & Wynder, E. L. (1995). Relation between exposure to environmental tobacco smoke and lung cancer in lifetime nonsmokers. *American Journal of Epidemiology, 142,* 141-148.

Kabat-Zinn, J. (1991). *Full catastrophe living: Using the wisdom of your body and mind to face stress, pain and illness.* New York: Delacorte.

Kabat-Zinn, J. (1993). Mindfulness meditation: Health benefits of an ancient Buddhist practice. In D. Goleman & J. Gurin (Eds.), *Mind/body medicine: How to use your mind for better health* (pp. 259-275). Yonkers, NY: Consumer Reports Books.

Kabat-Zinn, J., & Chapman-Waldrop, A. (1988). Compliance with an outpatient stress reduction program: Rates and predictors of program completion. *Journal of Behavioral Medicine, 11,* 333-352.

Kabat-Zinn, J., Lipworth, L., & Burney, R. (1985). The clinical use of mindfulness meditation for the self-regulation of chronic pain. *Journal of Behavioral Medicine, 8,* 163-190.

Kabat-Zinn, J., Massion, A. O., Kristeller, J., Peterson, L. G., Fletcher, K. E., Pbert, L., Lenderking, W. R., & Santorelli, S. F. (1992). Effectiveness of a meditation-based stress reduction program in the treatment of anxiety disorders. *American Journal of Psychiatry, 149,* 936-943.

Kahn, H. A. (1963). The relationship of reported coronary heart disease mortality to physical activity of work. *American Journal of Public Health, 53,* 1058-1067.

Kalafat, J., & Elias, M. (1994). An evaluation of a school-based suicide awareness intervention. *Suicide and Life Threatening Behavior, 24,* 224-233.

Kamarck, T. W., Jennings, R., Pogue-Geile, M., & Manuck, S. B. (1994). A multidimensional measurement model for cardiovascular reactivity: Stability and cross-validation in two adult samples. *Health Psychology, 13,* 471-478.

Kaminski, P. L., & McNamara, K. (1996). A treatment for college women at risk for bulimia: A controlled evaluation. *Journal of Counseling & Development, 74,* 288-294.

Kamiya, J. (1969). Operant control of the EEG alpha rhythm and some of its reported effects on consciousness. In C. Tart (Ed.), *Altered states of consciousness.* New York: Wiley.

Kaniasty, K., & Norris, F. H. (1993). How general is the cost of good fortune? Attempting to replicate Brown and McGill (1989). Special Issue: Replication research in the social sciences. *Journal of Social Behavior and Personality, 8,* 31-49.

Kann, L., Warren, C. W., Harris, W. A., Collins, J. L., Douglas, K. A., Collins, M. E., Williams, B. I., Ross, J. G., & Kolbe, L. J. (1995). Youth Risk Behavior Surveillance—United States, 1993. *Morbidity and Mortality Weekly Report, 44,* No. SS-1.

Kannel, W. B., & Cupples, L. A. (1989). Cardiovascular and noncardiovascular consequences of obesity. In A. J. Stunkard & A. Baum (Eds.), *Perspectives in behavioral medicine: Eating, sleeping, and sex* (pp. 109-129). Hillsdale, NJ: Erlbaum.

Kanner, A. D., Coyne, J. C., Schaefer, C., & Lazarus, R. S. (1981). Comparison of two modes of stress measurement: Daily hassles and uplifts versus major life events. *Journal of Behavioral Medicine, 4,* 1-39.

Kaplan, B. H. (1992). Social health and the forgiving heart: The Type B story. *Journal of Behavioral Medicine, 15,* 3-14.

Kaplan, B. H., Cassel, J. C., & Gore, S. (1977). Social support and health. *Medical Care, 15,* 47–58.

Kaplan, G. A., & Reynolds, P. (1988). Depression and cancer mortality and morbidity: Prospective evidence from the Alameda County study. *Journal of Behavioral Medicine, 11,* 1–13.

Kaplan, G. A., Salonen, J. T., Cohen, R. D., Brand, R. J., Syme, S. L., & Puska, P. (1988). Social connections and mortality from all causes and from cardiovascular disease: Prospective evidence from eastern Finland. *American Journal of Epidemiology, 128,* 370–380.

Kaplan, H. I. (1985). Psychological factors affecting physical conditions (psychosomatic disorders). In H. I. Kaplan & B. J. Saddock (Eds.), *Comprehensive textbook of psychiatry IV* (pp. 1106–1113). Baltimore: Williams & Wilkins.

Kaplan, H. I., & Kaplan, H. S. (1957). The psychosomatic concept of obesity. *Journal of Nervous and Mental Disorders, 125,* 181–189.

Kaplan, J. R., Manuck, S. B., & Shively, C. A. (1991). The effects of fat and cholesterol on social behavior in monkeys. *Psychomatic Medicine, 53,* 634–642.

Kaplan, J. R., Shively, C. A., Fontenot, M. B., Morgan, T. M., Howell, S. M., Manuck, S. B., Muldoon, M. F., & Mann, J. J. (1994). Demonstration of an association among dietary cholesterol, central serotonergic activity, and social behavior in monkeys. *Psychosomatic Medicine, 56,* 479–484.

Kaplan, R. M. (1984). The connection between clinical health promotion and health status. *American Psychologist, 39,* 755–765.

Kaplan, R. M. (1990). Behavior as the central outcome in health care. *American Psychologist, 45,* 1211–1220.

Kaplan, R. M. (1994). Measures of health outcome in social support research. In S. A. Shumaker & S. M. Czajkowski (Eds.), *Social support and cardiovascular disease* (pp. 65–94). New York: Plenum.

Kaplan, R. M., & Anderson, J. P. (1988). The Quality of Well-Being Scale: Rationale for a single quality of life index. In S. R. Walker & R. M. Rosner (Eds.), *Quality of life: Assessment and application* (pp. 51–77). Lancaster, Great Britain: MTP Press.

Kaplan, R. M., & Bush, J. W. (1982). Health-related quality of life measurement for evaluation research and policy analysis. *Health Psychology, 1,* 61–80.

Karasek, R. A., Theorell, T., Schwartz, J. E., Schnall, P. L., Pieper, C. F., & Michela, J. L. (1988). Job characteristics in relation to the prevalence of myocardial infarction in the U. S. Health Examination Survey (HES) and the Health and Nutrition Examination Survey (HANES). *American Journal of Public Health, 78,* 910–918.

Kasl, S. V., & Cobb, S. (1966a). Health behavior, illness behavior, and sick role behavior I. Health and illness behavior. *Archives of Environmental Health, 12,* 246–266.

Kasl, S. V., & Cobb, S. (1966b). Health behavior, illness behavior, and sick role behavior II. Sick role behavior. *Archives of Environmental Health, 12,* 531–541.

Katz, D. (1985). Cable television and health promotion: A feasibility study with arthritis patients. *Health Education Quarterly, 12,* 379–389.

Kavanagh, T., & Shepard, R. J. (1973). The immediate antecedents of myocardial infarction in active men. *Canadian Medical Association Journal, 109,* 19–22.

Kawachi, I., Colditz, G. A., Ascherio, A., Rimm, E. B., Giovannucci, E., Stampfer, M. J., & Willett, W. C. (1994). Prospective study of phobic anxiety and risk of coronary heart disease in men. *Circulation, 89,* 1992–1997.

Kawachi, I., Colditz, G. A., Stampfer, M. J., Willett, W. C., Manson, J. E., Rosner, B., Speizer, F. E., & Hennekens, C. H. (1993).

Smoking cessation and decreased risk of stroke in women. *Journal of the American Medical Association, 269,* 232–236.

Kawachi, I., Sparrow, D., Vokonas, P. S., & Weiss, S. T. (1994). Symptoms of anxiety and risk of coronary heart disease: The Normative Aging Study. *Circulation, 90,* 2225–2229.

Keefe, F. J. (1982). Behavioral assessment and treatment of chronic pain: Current status and future directions. *Journal of Consulting and Clinical Psychology, 50,* 896–911.

Keefe, F. J., & Block, A. R. (1982). Development of an observation method for assessing pain behavior in chronic low back pain patients. *Behavior Therapy, 13,* 363–375.

Keefe, F. J., Brown, G. K., Wallston, K. A., & Caldwell, D. S. (1989). Coping with rheumatoid arthritis pain: Catastrophizing as a maladaptive strategy. *Pain, 37,* 51–56.

Keefe, F. J., & Van Horn, Y. (1993). Cognitive-behavioral treatment of rheumatoid arthritis pain: Maintaining treatment gains. Special Issue: The challenges of pain in arthritis. *Arthritis Care and Research, 6,* 213–222.

Keefe, F. J., & Williams, D. A. (1992). Assessment of pain behaviors. In D. C. Turk & R. Melzack (Eds.), *Handbook of pain assessment* (pp. 277–292). New York: Guilford Press.

Keesey, R. E. (1980). A set-point analysis of the regulation of body weight. In A. J. Stunkard (Ed.), *Obesity* (pp. 144–165). Philadelphia: Saunders.

Keil, J. E., Sutherland, S. E., Knapp, R. G., & Tyroler, H. A. (1992). Does equal socioeconomic status in Black and White men mean equal rates of mortality? *American Journal of Public Health, 82,* 1133–1136.

Kelly, J. A., St. Lawrence, J. S., Brasfield, T. L., Lemke, A., Amideé, T., Roffman, R. E., Hood, H. V., Smith, J. E., Kilgore, H., & McNeill, C., Jr. (1990). Psychological factors that predict AIDS high-risk versus AIDS precautionary behavior. *Journal of Consulting and Clinical Psychology, 58,* 117–120.

Keltikangas-Järvinen, L., & Räikkönen, K. (1990a). Developmental trends in Type A behavior as predictors for the development of somatic coronary heart disease risk factors. *Psychotherapy and Psychosomatics, 51,* 210–215..

Keltikangas-Järvinen, L., & Räikkönen, K. (1990b). Type A factors as predictors of somatic risk factors of coronary heart disease in young Finns: A six-year follow-up study. *Journal of Psychomatic Research, 34,* 89–97.

Kelly, G. A. (1955). *The psychology of personal constructs* (Vols. 1 and 2). New York: Norton.

Kelly, M. A., McKinty, H. R., & Carr, R. (1988). Utilization of hypnosis to promote compliance with routine dental flossing. *American Journal of Clinical Hypnosis, 31,* 57–60.

Kendall, P. C., & Watson, D. (1981). Psychological preparation for stressful medical procedures. In C. K. Prokop & L. A. Bradley (Eds.), *Medical psychology: Contributions to behavioral medicine* (pp. 197–221). New York: Academic Press.

Kenford, S. L., Fiore, M. C., Jorenby, D. E., Smith, S. S., Wetter, D., & Baker, T. B. (1994). Predicting smoking cessation: Who will quit with and without the nicotine patch. *Journal of the American Medical Association, 271,* 589–604.

Kerner, J. F., & Alexander, J. (1981). Activities of daily living: Reliability and validity of gross vs. specific ratings. *Archives of Physical Medicine and Rehabilitation, 62,* 161–166.

Kerns, R. D., Haythornthwaite, J., Rosenberg, R., Southwick, S., Giller, E. L., & Jacob, M. C. (1991). The Pain Behavior Check List (PBCL): Factor structure and psychometric properties. *Journal of Behavioral Medicine, 14,* 155–167.

Kerns, R. D., Turk, D. C., & Rudy, T. E. (1985). The West Haven-Yale Multidimensional Pain Inventory. *Pain, 23,* 345–356.

Keyes, J. B., & Dean, S. F. (1988). Stress inoculation training for direct contact staff working with mentally retarded persons. *Behavioral Residential Treatment, 3,* 315–323.

Keys, A. (1980). *Seven countries: A multivariate analysis of death and coronary heart disease.* Cambridge, MA: Harvard University Press.

Keys, A., Brozek, J., Henschel, A., Mickelsen, O., & Taylor, H. L. (1950). *The biology of human starvation.* 2 vols. Minneapolis: University of Minnesota Press.

Khantzian, E. J. (1980). The ego, the self, and opiate addiction: Theoretical and treatment considerations. *International Review of Psychoanalysis, 5,* 189–198.

Kiecolt-Glaser, J. K., Dura, J. R., Speicher, C. E., Trask, J., & Glaser, R. (1991). Spousal caregivers of dementia victims: Longitudinal changes in immunity and health. *Psychosomatic Medicine, 53,* 345–362.

Kiecolt-Glaser, J. K., Dyer, C. S., & Shuttleworth, E. C. (1988). Upsetting social interactions and distress among Alzheimer's disease family care-givers: A replication and extension. *American Journal of Community Psychology, 16,* 825–837.

Kiecolt-Glaser, J. K., Fisher, L., Ogrocki, P., Stout, J. C., Speicher, C. E., & Glaser, R. (1987). Marital quality, marital disruption, and immune function. *Psychosomatic Medicine, 49,* 13–35.

Kiecolt-Glaser, J. K., & Glaser, R. (1988). Psychological influences on immunity: Making sense of the relationship between stressful life events and health. In G. P. Chrousos, D. L. Loriaux, & P. W. Gold (Eds.), *Mechanisms of physical and emotional stress* (pp. 237–247). New York: Plenum.

Kiecolt-Glaser, J. K., & Glaser, R. (1989). Psychoneuroimmunology: Past, present, and future. *Health Psychology, 8,* 677–682.

Kiecolt-Glaser, J. K., & Glaser, R. (1993). Mind and immunity. In D. Goleman & J. Gurin (Eds.), *Mind/body medicine: How to use your mind for better health* (pp. 39–61). Yonkers, NY: Consumer Reports Books.

Kiecolt-Glaser, J. K., Glaser, R., Dyer, C., Shuttleworth, E. C., Ogrocki, P., & Speicher, C. E. (1987). Chronic stress and immune function in family caregivers of Alzheimer's disease victims. *Psychosomatic Medicine, 49,* 523–535.

Kiecolt-Glaser, J. K., Glaser, R., Williger, D., Stout, J., Messick, G., Sheppard, S., Ricker, D., Romisher, S. C., Briner, W., Bonnell, G., & Donnerberg, R. (1985). Psychosocial enhancement of immunocompetence in a geriatric population. *Health Psychology, 4,* 25–41.

Kiecolt-Glaser, J. K., Marucha, P. T., Malarkey, W. B., Mercado, A. M., & Glaser, R. (1995). Slowing of wound healing by psychological stress. *Lancet, 346,* 1194–1196.

Kiecolt-Glaser, J. K., Speicher, C. E., Holliday, J. E., & Glaser, R. (1984). Stress and the transformation of lymphocytes in Epstein-Barr virus. *Journal of Behavioral Medicine, 7,* 1–12.

Kiely, D. K., Wolf, P. A., Cupples, L. A., Beiser, A. S., & Kannel, W. B. (1994). Physical activity and stroke risk: The Framingham Study. *American Journal of Epidemiology, 140,* 608–620.

Kiernan, M., Rodin, J., Brownell, K. D., Wilmore, J. H., & Crandall, C. (1992). Relation of level of exercise, age, and weight-cycling history to weight and eating concerns in male and female runners. *Health Psychology, 11,* 418–421.

Killen, J. D., Taylor, B., Telch, M. J., Robinson, T. N., Maron, D. J., & Saylor, K. E. (1987). Depressive symptoms and substance use among adolescent binge eaters and purgers: A defined population study. *American Journal of Public Health, 77,* 1539–1541.

Kimball, C. P. (1981). *The biopsychosocial approach to the patient.* Baltimore: Williams & Wilkins.

King, A. C., Taylor, C. B., Haskell, W. L., & DeBusk, R. F. (1989). Influence of regular aerobic exercise on psychological health: A randomized, controlled trial of healthy, middle-aged adults. *Health Psychology, 8,* 305–324.

Kinney, R. D., Gatchel, R. J., Polatin, P. B., Fogarty, W. T., & Mayer, T. G. (1993). Prevalence of psychopathology in acute and chronic low back pain patients. *Journal of Occupational Rehabilitation, 3,* 95–103.

Kinosian, B. P., & Eisenberg, J. M. (1988). Cutting into cholesterol: Cost effective alternatives for treating hypercholesterolemia. *Journal of the American Medical Association, 259,* 2249–2254.

Kirby, R. W., Anderson, J. W., Sieling, B., Rees, E. D., Chen, W. J., Miller, R. E., & Kay, R. M. (1981). Oat bran intake selectively lowers serum low-density lipoprotein cholesterol concentrates in hypercholesterolemic men. *American Journal of Clinical Nutrition, 34,* 824–829.

Kirscht, J. P., & Rosenstock, I. M. (1977). Patient adherence to antihypertensive medical regimens. *Journal of Community Health, 3,* 115–124.

Kiselica, M, S., Baker, S. B., Thomas, R, N., & Reedy, S. (1994). Effects of stress inoculation training on anxiety, stress, and academic performance among adolescents. *Journal of Counseling Psychology, 41,* 335–342.

Kiyak, H. A., Vitalinao, P. P., & Crinean, J. (1988). Patients' expectations as predictors of orthognathic surgery outcomes. *Health Psychology, 7,* 251–268.

Kizer, W. M. (1987). *The healthy workplace: A blueprint for corporate action.* New York: Wiley.

Klag, M. J., Ford, D. E., Mead, L. A., He, J., Whelton, P. K., Liang, K., & Levine, D. M. (1993). Serum cholesterol in young men and subsequent cardiovascular disease. *New England Journal of Medicine, 328,* 313–318.

Klatsky, A. L. (1987). The cardiovascular effects of alcohol. *Alcohol and Alcoholism, 22,* 117–124.

Klatsky, A. L., & Armstrong, M. A. (1992). Alcohol, smoking, coffee, and cirrhosis. *American Journal of Epidemiology, 136,* 1248–1257.

Klatsky, A. L., Friedman, G. D., & Siegelaub, A. B. (1981). Alcohol and mortality: A ten-year Kaiser-Permanente experience. *Annals of Internal Medicine, 95,* 139–145.

Klein, D. N., & Rubovits, D. R. (1987). The reliability of subjects' reports of stressful life events inventories: A longitudinal study. *Journal of Behavioral Medicine, 10,* 501–512.

Klohn, L. S., & Rogers, R. W. (1991). Dimensions of the severity of a health threat: The persuasive effects of visibility, time of onset, and rate of onset on young women's intentions to prevent osteoporosis. *Health Psychology, 10,* 323–329.

Klonoff, E. A., Annechild, A., & Landrine, H. (1994). Predicting exercise adherence in women: The role of psychological and physiological factors. *Preventive Medicine: An International Journal Devoted to Practice and Theory, 23,* 257–262.

Klonoff, E. A., & Landrine, H. (1993). Cognitive representations of bodily parts and products: Implications for health behavior. *Journal of Behavioral Medicine, 16,* 497–508.

Klonoff, E. A., & Landrine, H. (1994). Culture and gender diversity in commonsense beliefs about the causes of six illnesses. *Journal of Behavioral Medicine, 17,* 407–418.

Knowles, J. H. (1977). The responsibility of the individual. In J. H. Knowles (Ed.), *Doing better and feeling worse: Health in the United States* (pp. 57–80). New York: Norton.

Kobasa, S. C. O. (1979). Stressful life events, personality, and health: An inquiry into hardiness. *Journal of Personality and Social Psychology, 37,* 1–11.

Kobasa, S. C. O., & Maddi, S. R. (1977). Existential personality theory. In R. Corsini (Ed.), *Current personality theories* (pp. 242–276). Itasca, IL: Peacock.

Kobasa, S. C. O., Maddi, S. R., & Courington, S. (1981). Personality and constitution as mediators in the stress-illness relationship. *Journal of Health and Social Behavior, 22,* 368–378

Kobasa, S. C. O., Maddi, S. R., & Kahn, S. (1982). Hardiness and health: A prospective study. *Journal of Personality and Social Psychology, 42,* 168–177.

Kobernick, S. D., & Niwayana, G. (1960). Physical activity in experimental cholesterol atherosclerosis in rabbits. *American Journal of Pathology, 36,* 393–409.

Kofoed, L. L. (1987). Chemical monitoring of disulfiram compliance: A study of alcoholic outpatients. *Alcoholism, 11,* 481–485.

Kog, E., & Vandereycken, W. (1985). Family characteristics of anorexia nervosa and bulimia: A review of the research literature. *Clinical Psychology Review, 5,* 159–180.

Kohn, P. M. (1991). Reactivity and anxiety in the laboratory and beyond. In J. Strelau & A. Angleitner (Eds.), *Explorations in temperament: International perspectives on theory and measurement* (pp. 273–286). New York: Plenum.

Kohn, P. M., & Gurevich, M. (1993). The adequacy of the indirect method of measuring the primary appraisal of hassles-based stress. *Personality and Individual Differences, 14,* 679–684.

Kohn, P. M., Lafreniere, K., & Gurevich, M. (1990). The Inventory of College Students' Recent Life Experiences: A decontaminated hassles scale for a special population. *Journal of Behavioral Medicine, 13,* 619–630.

Kohn, P. M., Lafreniere, K., & Gurevich, M. (1991). Hassles, health, and personality. *Journal of Personality and Social Psychology, 61,* 478–482.

Kohn, P. M., & Macdonald, J. E. (1992). The Survey of Recent Life Experiences: A decontaminated hassles scale for adults. *Journal of Behavioral Medicine, 15,* 221–236.

Kolata, G. (1983). Some bypass surgery unnecessary. *Science, 222,* 605.

Koniak-Griffin, D. (1994). Aerobic exercise, psychological well-being, and physical discomforts during adolescent pregnancy. *Research in Nursing and Health, 17,* 253–268.

Koop, C. E. (1989). A parting shot at tobacco. *Journal of the American Medical Association, 262,* 2894–2895.

Koplan, J. P., Powell, K. E., Sikes, R. K., Shirley, R. W., & Campbell, C. C. (1982). An epidemiologic study of the benefits and risks of running. *Journal of the American Medical Association, 248,* 3118–3121.

Kotler, P., & Wingard, D. L. (1989). The effect of occupational, marital and parental roles on mortality: The Alameda County study. *American Journal of Public Health, 79,* 607–612.

Kottke, T. W., Battista, R. N., DeFriese, G. H., & Brekke, M. L. (1988). Attributes of successful smoking cessation interventions in medical practice: A meta-analysis of 39 controlled trials. *Journal of the American Medical Association, 259,* 2882–2889.

Kottke, T. E., Puska, P., Salonen, J. T., Tuomilehto, J., & Nissinen, A. (1985). Projected effects of high risk versus population-based prevention strategies in coronary heart disease. *American Journal of Epidemiology, 121,* 697–704.

Kovacs, J. A., Baseler, M., Dewar, R. J., Vogel, S., Davey, R. T., Jr., Fallon, J., Polis, M. A., Walker, R. E., Stevens, R., Salzan, N. P., Metcalf, J. A., Masur, H., & Lane, H. C. (1995). Increases in CD4 T lymphocytes with intermittent courses of interleukin-2 in patients with human immunodeficiency virus infection. *New England Journal of Medicine, 332,* 567–575.

Kovacs, M., Iyengar, S., Goldston, D., Obrosky, D. S., Stewart, J., & Marsh, J. (1990). Psychological functioning among mothers of children with insulin-dependent diabetes mellitus: A longitudinal study. *Journal of Consulting and Clinical Psychology, 58,* 189–195.

Kozlowski, L. T., Wilkinson, A., Skinner, W., Kent, C., Franklin, T., & Pope, M. (1989). Comparing tobacco cigarette dependence with other drug dependences. *Journal of the American Medical Association, 261,* 898–901.

Kral, J. G. (1992). Overview of surgical techniques for treating obesity. *American Journal of Clinical Nutrition, 55,* 552S–555S.

Kramer, A. M. (1995). Health care for elderly persons—myths and realities. *New England Journal of Medicine, 332,* 1027–1029.

Kramsch, D. M., Aspen, A. J., Abramowitz, B. M., Kreimendahl, T., & Hood, W. B., Jr. (1981). Reduction of coronary atherosclerosis by moderate conditioning exercise in monkeys on an atherogenic diet. *New England Journal of Medicine, 305,* 1483–1489.

Krantz, D. S., Contrada, R. J., Hill, D. R., & Friedler, E. (1988). Environmental stress and biobehavioral antecedents of coronary heart disease. *Journal of Consulting and Clinical Psychology, 56,* 333–341.

Krause, N. (1991). Stress and isolation from close ties in later life. *Journals of Gerontology, 46,* S183–S184.

Kremer, E. F., Atkinson, J. H., Jr., & Ignelzi, R. J. (1981). Measurement of pain: Patient preference does not confound pain measurement. *Pain, 10,* 241–248.

Kremer, E. F., Atkinson, J. H., Jr., & Ignelzi, R. J. (1981). Pain measurement: The affective dimensional measure of the McGill Pain Questionnaire with a cancer pain population. *Pain, 12,* 153–163.

Krokosky, N. J., & Reardon, R. C. (1989). The accuracy of nurses' and doctors' perception of patient pain. In S. G. Funk, E. M. Tornquist, M. T. Champagne, L. A. Copp, & R. A. Wiese (Eds.), *Key aspects of comfort: Management of pain, fatigue, and nausea* (pp. 127–140). New York: Springer.

Kronmal, R. A., Cain, K. C., Ye, Z. S., & Omenn, G. (1993). Total serum cholesterol levels and mortality risk as a function of age: A report based on the Framingham data. *Archives of Internal Medicine, 153,* 1065–1073.

Krumholz, H. M., Seeman, T. E., Merrill, S. S., Mendes de Leon, C. F., Vaccarino, V., Silverman, D. I., Tsukahara, R., Ostfeld, A. M., & Berkman, L. F., (1994). Lack of association between cholesterol and coronary heart disease mortality and morbidity and all-cause mortality in persons older than 70 years. *Journal of the American Medical Association, 272,* 1335–1340.

Kubik, A. (1984). The influence of smoking and other etiopathogenetic factors on the incidence of bronchogenic carcinoma and chronic nonspecific respiratory disease. *Czechoslovakian Medicine, 7,* 25–34.

Kuczmarski, R. J. (1992). Prevalence of overweight and weight gain in the United States. *American Journal of Clinical Nutrition, 55,* 495S–502S.

Kuder, G. F., & Richardson, M. W. (1937). The theory of estimation of test reliability. *Psychometrika, 2,* 151–160.

Kuhn, C. M. (1989). Adrenocortical and gonadal steroids in behavioral cardiovascular medicine. In N. Scheiderman, S. M. Weiss, & P. G. Kaufmann (Eds.), *Handbook of research methods in cardiovascular behavioral medicine* (pp. 185–204). New York: Plenum.

Kulich, R., Follick, M. J., & Conger, R. (1983, November). *Development of a pain behavior classification system: Importance of multiple data sources.* Paper presented at the annual meeting of the American Pain Society, Chicago.

Kulik, J. A., & Carlino, P. (1987). The effect of verbal commitment and treatment choice on medication compliance in a pediatric setting. *Journal of Behavioral Medicine, 10,* 367–376.

Kulik, J. A., & Mahler, H. I. M. (1987). Effects of preoperative roommate assignments on preoperative anxiety and recovery from coronary-bypass surgery. *Health Psychology, 6,* 525–543.

Kulik, J. A., & Mahler, H. I. M. (1989). Social support and recovery from surgery. *Health Psychology, 8,* 221–238.

Kulik, J. A., & Mahler, H. I. M. (1993). Emotional support as a moderator of adjustment and compliance after coronary artery bypass surgery: A longitudinal study. *Journal of Behavioral Medicine, 16,* 48–63.

Kuntzleman, C. T. (1978). *Rating the exercises.* New York: Morrow.

Laabs, J. J. (1994). Companies kick the smoking habit. *Personnel Journal,* 38–48.

LaCroix, A. Z., & Haynes, S. G. (1987). Gender differences in the health effects of work place roles. In R. C. Barnett, L. B. Biener, & G. K. Baruch (Eds.), *Gender and stress* (pp. 96–121). New York: Free Press.

Laforge, R. G., Greene, G. W., & Prochaska, J. O. (1994). Psychosocial factors influencing low fruit and vegetable consumption. *Journal of Behavioral Medicine, 17,* 361–374.

Lahad, A., Malter, A. D., Berg, A. O., & Deyo, R. A. (1994). The effectiveness of four interventions for the prevention of low back pain. *Journal of the American Medical Association, 272,* 1286–1291.

Lakka, T. A., & Salonen, J. T. (1992). Physical activity and serum lipids: A cross-sectional population study in Eastern Finnish men. *American Journal of Epidemiology, 136,* 806–816.

Lakka, T. A., Venäläinen, J. M., Rauramaa, R., Salonen, R., Tuomilehto, J., & Salonen, J. T. (1994). Relations of leisure-time physical activity and cardiorespiratory fitness to the risk of acute myocardial infarction in men. *New England Journal of Medicine, 330,* 1549–1554.

Lando, H. A., Pechacek, T. F., Pirie, P. L., Murray, D. M., Mittlemark, M. B., Lichtenstein, E., Nothwehr, F., & Gray, C. (1995). Changes in adult cigarette smoking in the Minnesota Heart Health Program. *American Journal of Public Health, 85,* 201–208.

Landrine, H., & Klonoff, E. A. (1994). Cultural diversity in causal attributions for illness: The role of the supernatural. *Journal of Behavioral Medicine, 17,* 181–193.

Lang, A., & Marlatt, G. A. (1982). Problem drinking: A social learning perspective. In R. J. Gatchel, A. Baum, & J. E. Singer (Eds.), *Handbook of psychology and health: Vol. 1. Clinical psychology and behavioral medicine: Overlapping disciplines.* Hillsdale, NJ: Erlbaum.

Lange, L. G., & Kinnumen, P. M. (1987). Cardiovascular effects of alcohol. *Advances in Alcohol and Substance Abuse, 6,* 47–52.

Langer, E. J., & Rodin, J. (1976). The effects of choice and enhanced personal responsibility for the aged: A field experiment in an institutional setting. *Journal of Personality and Social Psychology, 34,* 191–198.

Langford, H. G., Blaufox, D., Oberman, A., Hawkins, M., Curb, J. D., Cutter, G. R., Wassertheil-Smoller, S., Pressel, S., Babcock, C., Abernethy, J. D., Hotchkiss, J., & Tyler, M. (1985). Dietary therapy slows the return of hypertension after stopping prolonged medication. *Journal of the American Medical Association, 253,* 657–664.

Langlie, J. K. (1977). Social networks, health beliefs and preventive behavior. *Journal of Health and Social Behavior, 18,* 244–260.

Laporte, R., Brenes, G., & Dearwarter, S. (1983). HDL-cholesterol across a spectrum of physical activity from quadriplegia to marathon running. *Lancet, I,* 1212–1213.

LaRosa, J. H. (1990). Executive women and health: Perceptions and practices. *American Journal of Public Health, 80,* 1450–1454.

Larroque, B., Kaminski, M., Dehaene, P., Subtil, D., Delfosse, M-J., & Querleu, D. (1995) Moderate prenatal alcohol exposure and psychomotor development at preschool age. *American Journal of Public Health, 85,* 1654–1661.

Lasater, T., Abrams, D., Artz., L., Beaudin, P., Cabrera, L., Elder, J., Ferreira, A., Knisley, P., Peterson, G., Rodrigues, A., Rosenberg, P., Snow, R., & Carleton, R. (1984). Lay volunteer delivery of a community-based cardiovascular risk factor change program: The Pawtuckett experiment. In J. D. Matarazzo, S. M. Weiss, J. A. Herd, N. E. Miller, & S. M. Weiss (Eds.), *Behavioral health: A handbook of health enhancement and disease prevention* (pp. 1166–1170). New York: Wiley.

Lau, R. R. (1988). Beliefs about control and health behavior. In D. S. Gochman (Ed.), *Health behavior: Emerging research perspectives* (pp. 43–63). New York: Plenum.

Lau, R. R., Bernard, T. M., & Hartman, K. A. (1989). Further explorations of common-sense representations of common illnesses. *Health Psychology, 8,* 195–219.

Lau, R. R., & Hartman, K. A. (1983). Common sense representations of common illnesses. *Health Psychology, 2,* 167–185.

Laudenslager, M. L., Ryan, S. M., Drugan, R. C., Hyson, R. L., & Maier, S. F. (1983). Coping and immunosuppression: Inescapable but not escapable shock suppresses lymphocyte proliferation. *Science, 221,* 568–570.

Lautch, H. (1971). Dental phobia. *British Journal of Psychiatry, 119,* 151–158.

Lavey, R. S., & Taylor, C. B. (1985). The nature of relaxation therapy. In S. R. Burchfield (Ed.), *Stress: Psychological and physiological interactions.* Washington, DC: Hemisphere.

Law, A., Logan, H., & Baron, R. S. (1994). Desire for control, felt control, and stress intervention training during dental treatment. *Journal of Personality and Social Psychology, 67,* 926–936.

Lazarus, R. S. (1984a). Puzzles in the study of daily hassles. *Journal of Behavioral Medicine, 7,* 375–389.

Lazarus, R. S. (1984b). The trivialization of distress. In B. L. Hammonds & C. J. Scheirer (Eds.), *Psychology and health: The Master Lecture Series* (pp. 125–144). Washington, DC: American Psychological Association.

Lazarus, R. S. (1993). From psychological stress to the emotions: A history of changing outlooks. *Annual Review of Psychology, 44,* 1–21.

Lazarus, R. S., & DeLongis, A. (1983). Psychological stress and coping in aging. *American Psychologist, 38,* 245–254.

Lazarus, R. S., DeLongis, A., Folkman, S., & Gruen, R. (1985). Stress and adaptational outcomes. *American Psychologist, 40,* 770–779.

Lazarus, R. S., & Folkman, S. (1984). *Stress, appraisal, and coping.* New York: Springer.

Lecky, P. (1945). *Self-consistency.* New York: Island Press.

Lee, I-M. (1994). Physical activity, fitness, and cancer. In C. Bouchard, R. J. Shephard, & T. Stephens (Eds.), *Physical activity, fitness, and health: International proceedings and consensus statement* (pp. 814–831). Champaign, IL: Human Kinetics.

Lee, I-M., Hsieh, C-c., & Paffenbarger, R. S., Jr. (1995). Exercise intensity and longevity in men. *Journal of the American Medical Association, 273,* 1179–1184.

Lee, I-M., & Paffenbarger, R. S., Jr. (1992). Change in body weight and longevity. *Journal of the American Medical Association, 268,* 2045–2049.

Lee, I-M., Paffenbarger, R. S., Jr., & Hsieh, C-c. (1992). Physical activity and risk of prostatic cancer among college alumni. *American Journal of Epidemiology, 135,* 169–179.

Leevy, C. M., Gellene, R., & Ning, M. (1964). Primary liver cancer in cirrhosis of the alcoholic. *Annals of the New York Academy of Science, 114,* 1026–1040.

Lefebvre, R. C., & Flora, J. A. (1988). Social marketing and public health intervention. *Health Education Quarterly, 15,* 299–315.

Lehman, A. K., & Rodin, J. (1989). Styles of self-nurturance and disordered eating. *Journal of Consulting and Clinical Psychology, 57,* 117–122.

Lehrer, P. M., Carr, R., Sargunaraj, D., & Woolfolk, R. L. (1994). Stress management techniques: Are they all equivalent, or do they have specific effects? *Biofeedback and Self-Regulation, 19,* 353–401.

Leibel, R. L., Rosenbaum, M., & Hirsch, J. (1995). Changes in energy expenditure resulting from altered body weight. *New England Journal of Medicine, 332,* 621–629.

Leiss, J. K., & Savitz, D. A. (1995). Home pesticide use and childhood cancer: A case-control study. *American Journal of Public Health, 85,* 249–252.

Leitenberg, H., Rosen, J. C., Gross, J., Nudelman, S., & Vara, L. S. (1988). Exposure plus response-prevention treatment of bulimia nervosa. *Journal of Consulting and Clinical Psychology, 56,* 535–541.

Le Marchand, L., Kolonel, L. N., & Yoshizawa, C. N. (1991). Lifetime occupational physical activity and prostate cancer risk. *American Journal of Epidemiology, 133,* 103–111.

Lemp, G. F., Hirozawa, A. M., Givertz, D., Nieri, G. N., Anderson, L., Lindegren, M. L., Janssen, R. S., & Katz, M. (1994). Seroprevalence of HIV and risk behaviors among young homosexual and bisexual men: The San Francisco/Berkeley Young Men's Survey. *Journal of the American Medical Association, 272,* 449–454.

Lenderking, W. R., Gelber, R. D., Cotton, D. J., Cole, B. F., Goldhirsch, A., Volberding, P. A., & Testa, M. A. (1994). Evaluation of the quality of life associated with zidovudine treatment in asymptomatic human immunodeficiency virus infection. *New England Journal of Medicine, 330,* 738–743.

Leon, A. S., Connett, J., Jacobs, D. R., Jr., & Rauramaa, R. (1987). Leisure-time physical activity levels and risk of coronary heart disease and death: The Multiple Risk Factor Intervention Trial. *Journal of the American Medical Association, 258,* 2388–2395.

LeResche, L. (1982). Facial expression of pain: A study of candid photographs. *Journal of Non-verbal Behavior, 7,* 46–56.

Lerman, C., Trock, B., Rimer, B. K., Jepson, C., Brody, D., & Boyce, A. (1991). Psychological side effects of breast cancer screening. *Health Psychology, 10,* 259–267.

Lerner, M. J., & Simmons, C. (1966). Observer's reaction to the 'innocent victim': Compassion or rejection? *Journal of Personality and Social Psychology, 4,* 203–210.

Lerner, W. D., & Fallon, H. J. (1985). The alcohol withdrawal syndrome. *New England Journal of Medicine, 313,* 951–952.

LeRoy, P. L., & Filasky, R. (1990). Thermography. In J. J. Bonica (Ed.), *The management of pain* (2nd ed., pp. 610–621). Malvern, PA: Lea & Febiger.

Lester, D. (1994). Are there unique features of suicide in adults of different ages and developmental stages? *Omega Journal of Death and Dying, 29,* 337–348.

Leutwyler, K. (1995, April). The price of prevention. *Scientific American, 272,* 124–129.

Levenson, R. L., & Mellins, C. A. (1992). Pediatric HIV disease: What psychologists need to know. *Professional Psychology Research and Practice, 23,* 410–415.

Levenson, R. W., Sher, K. J., Grossman, L. M., Newman, J., & Newlin, D. B. (1980). Alcohol and stress response dampening: Pharmacological effects, expectancy, and tension reduction. *Journal of Abnormal Psychology, 89,* 528–538.

Leventhal, H. (1970). Findings and theory in the study of fear communications. *Advances in Experimental Social Psychology, 5,* 119–186.

Leventhal, H. (1971). Fear appeals and persuasion: The differentiation of a motivational construct. *American Journal of Public Health, 61,* 120–124.

Leventhal, H., & Avis, N. (1976). Pleasure, addiction, and habit: Factors in verbal report or factors in smoking behavior? *Journal of Abnormal Psychology, 85,* 478–488.

Leventhal, H., & Cleary, P. D. (1980). The smoking problem: A review of the research and theory in behavioral risk modification. *Psychological Bulletin, 88,* 370–405.

Leventhal, H., & Diefenbach, M. (1991). The active side of illness cogntion. In J. A. Skelton & R. T. Croyle (Eds.), *Mental representation in health and illness* (pp. 247–272). New York: Springer-Verlag.

Leventhal, H., Diefenbach, M., & Leventhal, E. A. (1992). Illness cognition: Using common sense to understand treatment adherence and affect cognition interactions. *Cognitive Therapy and Research, 16,* 143–163.

Leventhal, H., Meyer, D., & Nerenz, D. (1980). The common-sense representation of illness danger. In S. Rachman (Ed.), *Medical psychology* (Vol. 2). New York: Pergamon Press.

Leventhal, H., Nerenz, D. R., & Steele, D. J. (1984). Illness representations and coping with health threats. In A. Baum, S. E. Taylor, & J. E. Singer (Eds.), *Handbook of psychology and health: Vol. 4. Social psychological aspects of health* (pp. 219–252). Hillsdale, NJ: Erlbaum.

Levi, L. (1974). Psychosocial stress and disease: A conceptual model. In E. K. E. Gunderson & R. H. Rahe (Eds.), *Life stress and illness* (pp. 8–33). Springfield, IL: Thomas.

Levine, H. G. (1980). Temperance and women in 19th century United States. In O. J. Kalant (Ed.), *Alcohol and drug problems in women: Research advances in alcohol and drug problems* (pp. 25–66). New York: Plenum.

Levine, J. D., Gordon, N. C., & Fields, H. L. (1978). The mechanism of placebo analgesia. *Lancet, ii,* 654–657.

Levy, A. S., & Heaton, A. W. (1993). Weight control practices of U.S. adults trying to lose weight. *Annals of Internal Medicine, 119,* 661–666.

Levy, S. M. (1985). *Behavior and cancer: Life-style and psychosocial factors in the initiation and progression of cancer.* San Francisco: Jossey-Bass.

Levy, S. M. (1989, August). *The psychological response to terminal illness: Hope, autonomy, and the right to die.* Paper presented at the American Psychological Association Convention, New Orleans.

Levy, S. M., Herberman, R. B., Simons, A. Whiteside, T., Lee, J., McDonald, R., & Beadle, M. C. (1989). Persistently low natural killer cell activity in normal adults: Immunological, hormonal and mood correlates. *Natural Immunity and Cell Growth Regulation, 8,* 173–186.

Ley, P., & Spelman, M. S. (1967). *Communication with the patient.* London: Staples Press.

Li, G., & Baker, S. P. (1994). Alcohol in fatally injured bicyclists. 37th Annual Meeting of the Association for Advancement of Automotive Medicine (1993, San Antonio, Texas). *Accident Analysis and Prevention, 26,* 543–548.

Li, G., Smith, G. S., & Baker, S. P. (1994). Drinking behavior in relation to cause of death among US adults. *American Journal of Public Health, 84,* 1402–1406.

Liddell, A. (1990). Personality characteristics versus medical and dental experiences of dentally anxious children. *Journal of Behavioral Medicine, 13,* 183–194.

Lied, E. R., & Marlatt, G. A. (1979). Modeling as a determinant of alcohol consumption: Effect of subject sex and prior drinking history. *Addictive Behaviors, 4,* 47–54.

Lierman, L. M., Kasprzyk, D., Benoliel, J. Q. (1991). Understanding adherence to breast self-examination in older women. *Western Journal of Nursing Research, 13*, 46–66.

Light, K. C., Kopke, J. P., Obrist, P. A., & Willis, P. W. (1983). Psychological stress induces sodium fluid retention in men at high risk for hypertension. *Science, 220*, 429–431.

Light, K. C., Turner, J. R., Hinderliter, A. L., & Sherwood, A. (1993a). Race and gender comparisons: I. Hemodynamic responses to a series of stressors. *Health Psychology, 12*, 354–365.

Light, K. C., Turner, J. R., Hinderliter, A. L., & Sherwood, A. (1993b). Race and gender comparisons: II. Predictions of work blood pressure from laboratory baseline and cardiovascular reactivity measures. *Health Psychology, 12*, 366–375.

Lilienfeld, A. M., & Lilienfeld, D. E. (1980). *Foundations of epidemiology* (2nd ed.). New York: Oxford University Press.

Linden, W. (1988). Biopsychological barriers to the behavioral treatment of hypertension. In W. Linden (Ed.), *Biological barriers in behavioral medicine* (pp. 163–191). New York: Plenum.

Lindman, R. E., Sjöholm, B. A., & Lang, A. R. (1994, August). *Cross-cultural comparison of global positive alcohol expectancies*. Presented at the 102nd convention of the American Psychological Association, Los Angeles, CA.

Lingswiler, V. M., Crowther, J. H., & Stephens, M. A. P. (1987). Emotional reactivity and eating in binge eating and obesity. *Journal of Behavioral Medicine, 10*, 287–299.

Link, R. P., Pedersoli, W. M., & Safanie, A. H. (1972). Effect of exercise on development of atherosclerosis in swine. *Atherosclerosis, 15*, 107–122.

Linn, R. (1976). *The last chance diet*. New York: Bantam.

Linn, S., Carroll, M., Johnson, C., Fulwood, R., Kalsbeek, W., & Briefel, R. (1993). High-density lipoprotein cholesterol and alcohol consumption in US White and Black adults: Data from NHANES II. *American Journal of Public Health, 83*, 811–816.

Lipid Research Clinics Program. (1984). The Lipid Research Clinics coronary primary prevention trial results II. The relationship of reduction in the incidence of coronary heart disease to cholesterol lowering. *Journal of the American Medical Association, 253*, 365–374.

Lipton, R. I. (1994). The effects of moderate alcohol use on the relationship between stress and depression. *American Journal of Public Health, 84*, 1913–1917.

Liska, A. E., & Baccaglini, W. (1990). Feeling safe by comparison: Crime in the newspapers. *Social Problems, 37*, 360–374.

Lissner, L., Bengtsson, C., Björkelund, C., & Wedel, H. (1996). Physical activity levels and changes in relation to longevity. *American Journal of Epidemiology, 143*, 54–62.

Lissner, L., Odell, P. M., D'Agostino, R. B., Stokes, J., III, Kreger, B. E., Belanger, A. J., & Brownell, K. D. (1991). Variability of body weight and health outcomes in the Framingham population. *New England Journal of Medicine, 324*, 1839–1844.

Lloyd, C. (1980a). Life events and depressive disorder reviewed. II: Events as precipitating factors. *Archives of General Psychiatry, 37*, 541–548.

Lloyd, C. (1980b). Life events and depressive disorder reviewed. I: Events as predisposing factors. *Archives of General Psychiatry, 37*, 529–535.

Lobel, M., Dunkel-Schetter, C., & Scrimshaw, S. C. M. (1992). Prenatal maternal stress and prematurity: A prospective study of socioeconomically disadvantaged women. *Health Psychology, 11*, 32–40.

Loeser, J. D. (1980). Low back pain. In J. J. Bonica (Ed.), *Pain*. New York: Raven.

Loeser, J. D. (1990). Pain after amputation: Phantom limb and stump pain. In J. J. Bonica (Ed.), *The management of pain* (2nd ed., pp. 244–256). Malvern, PA: Lea & Febiger.

Loeser, J. D. (1989). Chronic pain. In F. C. Seitz, J. E. Carr, & M. Covey (Eds.), *Issues in behavioral medicine* (pp. 16–20). Bozeman, MT: Clinical Management Consultants.

Loimer, H., & Guarnieri, M. (1996). Accidents and acts of God: A history of the terms. *American Journal of Public Health, 86*, 101–107.

Long, C. J. (1981). The relationship between surgical outcome and MMPI profiles in chronic back patients. *Journal of Clinical Psychology, 37*, 744–749.

Long, R. T., & Cope, O. (1961). Emotional problems of burned children. *New England Journal of Medicine, 264*, 1121–1127.

Lopez, M. A., & Silber, S. (1991). Stress management for the elderly: A preventive approach. *Clinical Gerontologist, 10*, 73–76.

Lorber, J. (1975). Good patients and problem patients: Conformity and deviance in a general hospital. *Journal of Health and Social Behavior, 16*, 213–225.

Lovastatin Study Group III. (1988). A multicenter comparison of lovastatin and cholestyramine therapy for severe hypercholesterolemia. *Journal of the American Medical Association, 260*, 359–366.

Lovibond, S. H., & Caddy, G. R. (1970). Discriminated aversive control in the moderation of alcoholics' drinking behavior. *Behavior Therapy, 1*, 437–441.

Lowenfels, A. B., & Zevola, S. A. (1989). Alcoholism and breast cancer: An overview. *Alcoholism, 13*, 109–111.

Lowry, R., Holtzman, D., Truman, B. I., Kann, L., Collins, J. L., & Kolbe, L. J. (1994). Substance use and HIV-related sexual behaviors among US high school students: Are they related? *American Journal of Public Health, 84*, 1116–1120.

Loxley, W. M., & Hawks, D. V. (1994). AIDS and injecting drug use: Very risky behaviour in a Perth sample of injecting drug users. *Drug and Alcohol Review, 13*, 21–30.

Lubin, J. H., Blot, W. J., Berrino, F., Flamant, R., Gillis, C. R., Kunzer, M., Schmahl, D., & Visco, G. (1984). Patterns of lung cancer according to type of cigarette smokers. *International Journal of Cancer, 33*, 569–576.

Lubin, J. H., Richter, B. S., & Blot, W. J. (1984). Lung cancer risk with cigar and pipe use. *Journal of the National Cancer Institute, 73*, 377–381.

Lucas, A. R., Beard, C. M., O'Fallon, W. M., & Kurland, L. T. (1991). 50-year trends in the incidence of anorexia nervosa in Rochester, Minn.: A population-based study. *American Journal of Psychiatry, 7*, 917–922.

Lucas, F., & Sclafani, A. (1990). Hyperphagia in rats produced by a mixture of fats and sugar. *Physiology and Behavior, 47*, 51–55.

Lucchesi, B. R., Schuster, C. R., & Emley, G. S. (1967). The role of nicotine as a determinant of cigarette smoking frequency in man with observations of certain cardiovascular effects associated with the tobacco alkaloid. *Clinical Pharmacology and Therapeutics, 8*, 791.

Ludel, J. (1978). *Introduction to sensory processes*. San Francisco: Freeman.

Lukaski, H. C. (1987). Methods for the assessment of human body composition: Traditional and new. *American Journal of Clinical Nutrition, 46*, 537–556.

Lundgren, J. D., Melbye, M., Pedersen, C., Rosenberg, P. S., & Gerstoft, J. (1995). Changing patterns of Kaposi's sarcoma in Danish acquired immunodeficiency syndrome patients with complete follow-up. *American Journal of Epidemiology, 141*, 652–658.

Lutz, R. W., Silbret, M., & Olshan, W. (1983). Treatment outcome and compliance with therapeutic regimens: Long-term follow-up of a multidisciplinary pain program. *Pain, 17,* 301–308.

Lux, K. M., & Petosa, R. (1994). Using the health belief model to predict safer sex intentions of incarcerated youth. *Health Education Quarterly, 21,* 487–497.

Lyles, J. N., Burish, T. G., Krozely, M. G., & Oldham, R. K. (1982). Efficacy of relaxation training and guided imagery in reducing the aversiveness of cancer chemotherapy. *Journal of Consulting and Clinical Psychology, 50,* 509–524.

Lynch, D. J., Birk, T. J., Weaver, M. T., Gohara, A. F., Leighton, R. F., Repka, F. J., & Walsh, M. E. (1992). Adherence to exercise interventions in the treatment of hypercholesterolemia. *Journal of Behavior Medicine, 15,* 365–377.

Macarthur, C., Saunders, N., & Feldman, W. (1995). *Helicobacter pylori,* gastroduodenal disease, and recurrent abdominal pain in children. *Journal of the American Medical Association, 273,* 729–734.

Maccoby, N., & Alexander, J. (1980). Use of media in lifestyle programs. In P. O. Davidson & S. M. Davidson (Eds.), *Behavioral medicine: Changing health lifestyles* (pp. 351–370). New York: Brunner/Mazel.

MacCoun, R. J. (1993). Drugs and the law: A psychological analysis of drug prohibition. *Psychological Bulletin, 113,* 497–512.

MacDougal, J. M., Dembroski, T. M., Dimsdale, J. E., & Hackett, T. P. (1985). Components of Type A, hostility, and anger-in: Further relationships to angiographic findings. *Health Psychology, 4,* 137–142.

Mace, N. L., & Rabins, P. V. (1981). *The 36-hour day: A family guide to caring for persons with Alzheimer's disease, related dementing illnesses, and memory loss in later life.* Baltimore: Johns Hopkins University Press.

Macharia, W. M., Leon, G., Rowe, B. H., Stephenson, B. J., & Haynes, R. B. (1992). An overview of interventions to improve compliance with appointment keeping for medical services. *Journal of the American Medical Association, 267,* 1813–1817.

MacLean, D., & Reichlin, S. (1981). Neuroendocrinology and the immune process. In R. Ader (Ed.), *Psychoneuroimmunology* (pp. 475–520). New York: Academic Press.

Madden, T. J., Ellen, P. S., & Ajzen, I. (1992). A comparison of the theory of planned behavior and the theory of reasoned action. *Personality and Social Psychology Bulletin, 18,* 3–9.

Mahboubi, E. (1977). The epidemiology of oral cavity, pharyngeal and oesophageal cancer outside of North American and Western Europe. *Cancer, 40,* 1879–1886.

Maier, S. F., Watkins, L. R., & Fleshner, M. (1994). Psychoneuroimmunology: The interface between behavior, brain, and immunity. *American Psychologist, 49,* 1004–1017.

Malarkey, W. B., Kiecolt-Glaser, J. K., Pearl, D., & Glaser, R. (1994). Hostile behavior during marital conflict alters pituitary and adrenal hormones. *Psychosomatic Medicine, 56,* 41–51.

Malley, P. B., Kush, F., & Bogo, R. J. (1994). School-based adolescent suicide prevention and intervention programs: A survey. *School Counselor, 42,* 130–136.

Malmivaara, A., Hakkinen, U., Aro, T., Heinrichs, M., Koskenniemi, L., Klosma, E., Lappi, S., Paloheimo, R., Servo, C., Vaaranen, V., & Hernberg, S. (1995). The treatment of acute low back pain—bed rest, exercise, or ordinary activity. *New England Journal of Medicine, 332,* 351–355.

Mancuso, R. A., & Pennebaker, J. W. (1994). *Resolving vs. dredging up past traumas: The effects of writing.* Paper presented at the convention of the American Psychological Association, Los Angeles, CA.

Manley, R. S., & Boland, F. J. (1983). Side-effects and weight gain following a smoking cessation program. *Addictive Behaviors, 8,* 375–380.

Manne, S. L., Bakeman, R., Jacobsen, P. B., Gorfinkle, K., Bernstein, D., & Redd, W. H. (1992). Adult-child interaction during invasive medical procedures. *Health Psychology, 11,* 241–249.

Mannino, D. M., Klevens, R. M., & Flanders, W. D. (1994). Cigarette smoking: An independent risk factor for impotence? *American Journal of Epidemiology, 140,* 1003–1008.

Manolio, T. A., Pearson, T. A., Wenger, N. K., Barrett-Connor, E., Payne, G. H., & Harlan, W. R. (1992). Cholesterol and heart disease in older persons and women: Review of an NHBLI workshop. *Annals of Epidemiology, 2,* 161–176.

Manson, J. E., Nathan, D. M., Krolewski, A. S., Stampfer, M. J., Willett, W. C., & Hennekens, C. H. (1992). A prospective study of exercise and incidence of diabetes among US male physicians. *Journal of the American Medical Association, 268,* 63–67.

Manson, J. E., Willett, W. C., Stampfer, M. J., Colditz, G. A., Hunter, D. J., Hankinson, S. E., Hennekens, C. H., & Speizer, F. E. (1995). Body weight and mortality among women. *New England Journal of Medicine, 333,* 677–685.

Manyande, A., Berg, S., Getting, D., Stanford, S. C., Mazhero, S., Marks, D. F., & Salmon, P. (1995). Preoperative rehearsal of active coping imagery influences subjective and hormonal responses to abdominal surgery. *Psychosomatic Medicine, 57,* 177–182.

Markovitz, J. H., Matthews, K. A., Kannel, W. B., Cobb, J. L., & D'Agostino, R. B. (1993). Psychological predictors of hypertension in the Framingham study: Is there tension in hypertension? *Journal of the American Medical Association, 270,* 2439–2443.

Marlatt, G. A. (1983). The controlled-drinking controversy: A commentary. *American Psychologist, 38,* 1097–1110.

Marlatt, G. A. (1987). Alcohol, the magic elixir: Stress, expectancy, and the transformation of emotional states. In E. Gottheil, K. A. Druly, S. Pashko, & S. P. Weinstein (Eds.), *Stress and addiction* (pp. 302–322). New York: Brunner/ Mazel.

Marlatt, G. A., Demming, B., & Reid, J. (1973). Loss of control drinking in alcoholics: An experimental analogue. *Journal of Abnormal Psychology, 81,* 233–241.

Marlatt, G. A., & Gordon, J. R. (1980). Determinants of relapse: Implication for the maintenance of behavior change. In P. O. Davidson & S. M. Davidson (Eds.), *Behavioral medicine: Changing health lifestyles* (pp. 410–452). New York: Brunner/ Mazel.

Marlatt, G. A., & Rohsenow, D. J. (1980). Cognitive processes in alcohol use: Expectancy and the balanced placebo design. In N. Mello (Ed.), *Advances in substance abuse: Behavioral and biological research.* Greenwich, CT: JAI Press.

Maron, D. J., & Fortmann, S. P. (1987). Nicotine yield and measures of cigarette smoke exposure in a large population: Are lower-yield cigarettes safer? *American Journal of Public Health, 77,* 546–549.

Marshall, B. J. (1995). Helicobacter pylori: The etiologic agent for peptic ulcers. *Journal of the American Medical Association, 274,* 1064–1066.

Marston, A. R., & Bettencourt, B. A. (1988). An evaluation of the American Lung Association's home video smoking cessation program. *American Journal of Public Health, 78,* 1226–1227.

Martin, J. E., & Dubbert, P. M. (1985). Adherence to exercise. In R. L. Terjung (Ed.), *Exercise and sport sciences reviews* (Vol. 13). New York: Macmillan.

Martin, P. R., Adinoff, B., Weingarter, H., Mukherjee, A. B., & Eckardt, M. J. (1986). Alcoholic organic brain disease: Nosology and pathophysiologic mechanisms. *Progress in Neuropsychopharmacology and Biological Psychiatry, 10,* 147–164.

Martin, T. R., & Bracken, M. B. (1986). Association of low birth weight with passive smoke exposure in pregnancy. *American Journal of Epidemiology, 124,* 633–642.

Marwick, C. (1991). Hispanic HANES takes long look at Latino health. *Journal of the American Medical Association, 265,* 177, 181.

Marwick, C. (1995). Administration attacks increasing use of marijuana. *Journal of the American Medical Association, 274,* 598–596.

Marx, J. (1992). Familial Alzheimer's linked to chrosome 14 gene. *Science, 258,* 550.

Maslach, C. (1976). Burned-out. *Human Behavior, 5,* 16–22.

Mason, J. W. (1971). A reevaluation of the concept of "nonspecificity" in stress theory. *Journal of Psychiatric Research, 8,* 323–333.

Mason, J. W. (1975). A historical view of the stress field. Pt. 2. *Journal of Human Stress, 1,* 22–36.

Masur, F. T., III. (1981). Adherence to health care regimens. In C. K. Prokop & L. A. Bradley (Eds.), *Medical psychology: Contributions to behavioral medicine.* New York: Academic Press.

Matanoski, G., Kanchanaraksa, S., Lantry, D., & Chang, Y. (1995). Characteristics of nonsmoking women in NHANES I and NHANES I Epidemiologic Follow-up Study with exposure to spouses who smoke. *American Journal of Epidemiology, 142,* 149–157.

Matarazzo, J. D. (1980). Behavioral health and behavioral medicine: Frontiers for a new health psychology. *American Psychologist, 35,* 807–817.

Matarazzo, J. D. (1982). Behavioral health's challenge to academic, scientific, and professional psychology. *American Psychologist, 37,* 1–14.

Matarazzo, J. D. (1984a). Behavioral health: A 1990 challenge for the health sciences professions. In J. D. Matarazzo, S. M. Weiss, J. A. Herd, N. E. Miller, & S. M. Weiss (Eds.), *Behavioral health: A handbook of health enhancement and disease prevention* (pp. 3–40). New York: Wiley.

Matarazzo, J. D. (1984b). Behavioral immunogens and pathogens in health and illness. In B. L. Hammonds & C. J. Scheirer (Eds.), *Psychology and health: The Master Lecture Series, Vol. 3* (pp. 9–43). Washington, DC: American Psychological Association.

Matarazzo, J. D. (1987a). Postdoctoral education and training of service providers in health psychology. In G. C. Stone, S. M. Weiss, J. D. Matarazzo, N. E. Miller, J. Rodin, C. D. Belar, M. J. Follick, & J. E. Singer (Eds.), *Health psychology: A discipline and a profession* (pp. 371–388). Chicago: University of Chicago Press.

Matarazzo, J. D. (1987b). Relationships of health psychology to other segments of psychology. In G. C. Stone, S. M. Weiss, J. D. Matarazzo, N. E. Miller, J. Rodin, C. D. Belar, M. J. Follick, & J. E. Singer (Eds.), *Health psychology: A discipline and a profession* (pp. 41–59). Chicago: University of Chicago Press.

Matarazzo, J. D. (1994). Health and behavior: The coming together of science and practice in psychology and medicine after a century of benign neglect. *Journal of Clinical Psychology in Medical Settings, 1,* 7–39.

Materi, M. (1977). Assertiveness training: A catalyst for behavior change. *Alcohol Health and Research World, 1,* 23–26.

Maton, K. I. (1988). Social support, organizational characteristics, psychological well-being, and group appraisal in three self-help group populations. *American Journal of Community Psychology, 16,* 53–77.

Matthews, K. A. (1986a). Preface. In K. A. Matthews, S. M. Weiss, T. Detre, T. M. Dembroski, B. Falkner, S. B. Manuch, & R. B. Williams, Jr. (Eds.), *Handbook of stress, reactivity, and cardiovascular disease* (pp. xi–xii). New York: Wiley-Interscience.

Matthews, K. A. (1986b). Summary, conclusions, and implications. In K. A. Matthews, S. M. Weiss, T. Detre, T. M. Dembroski, B. Falkner, S. B. Manuch, & R. B. Williams, Jr. (Eds.), *Handbook of stress, reactivity, and cardiovascular disease.* New York: Wiley-Interscience.

Matthews, K. A. (1989). Interactive effects of behavior and reproductive hormones on sex differences in risk for coronary heart disease. *Health Psychology, 8,* 373–387.

Matthews, K. A., Woodall, K. L., Kenyon, K., & Jacob, T. (1996). Negative family environment as a predictor of boys' future status on measures of hostile attitudes, interview behavior, and anger expression. *Health Psychology, 15,* 30–37.

Mayeux, R., & Schupf, N. (1995). Apolipoprotein E and Alzheimer's disease: The implications of progress in molecular medicine. *American Journal of Public Health, 85,* 1280–1284.

Mayfield, D. (1976). Alcoholism, alcohol intoxication, and assaultive behavior. *Diseases of the Nervous System, 37,* 228–291.

Mazze, R. S., Shamoon, H., Pasmantier, R., Lucido, D., Murphy, J., Hartmann, K., Kuykendall, V., & Lopatin, W. (1984). Reliability of blood glucose monitoring by patients with diabetes mellitus. *American Journal of Medicine, 77,* 211–217.

McAuley, E. (1992). The role of efficacy cognitions in the prediction of exercise behavior in middle-aged adults. *Journal of Behavioral Medicine, 15,* 65–88

McAuley, E. (1993). Self-efficacy and the maintenance of exercise participation in older adults. *Journal of Behavioral Medicine, 16,* 103–113.

McAuley, E. (1994). Physical activity and psychosocial outcomes. In C. Bouchard, R. J. Shephard, & T. Stephens (Eds.), *Physical activity, fitness, and health: International proceedings and consensus statement* (pp. 551–568). Champaign, IL: Human Kinetics.

McCaffery, M. (1979). *Nursing management of the patient with pain* (2nd ed.). Philadelphia: Lippincott.

McCaul, K. D., Monson, N., & Maki, R. H. (1992). Does distraction reduce pain-produced distress among college students? *Health Psychology, 11,* 210–217.

McCaul, K. D., Sandgren, A. K., O'Neill, H. K., & Hinsz, V. B. (1993). The value of the theory of planned behavior, perceived control, and self-efficacy for predicting health-protective behaviors. *Basic and Applied Social Psychology, 14,* 231–252.

McClintic, J. R. (1978). *Physiology of the human body* (2nd ed.). New York: Wiley.

McClure, M. O., Bieniasz, P. D., Weber, J. N., Tedder, R. S., O'Shea, S., Banatvala, J. E., Tudor-Williams, G., Simmonds, P., Holmes, E. C., Bryson, Y., & Chen, I. S. Y. (1995). HIV clearance in an infant? *Nature, 375,* 637–638.

McCracken, L. M., Zayfert, C., & Gross, R. T. (1992). The Pain Anxiety Symptoms Scale: Development and validation of a scale to measure fear of pain. *Pain, 50,* 67–73.

McCracken, L. M., Zayfert, C., & Gross, R. T. (1993). The Pain Anxiety Symptoms Scale (PASS): A multimodal measure of pain-specific anxiety symptoms. *Behavior Therapy, 16,* 183–184.

McCranie, E. W., Watkins, L. O., Brandsma, J. M., & Sisson, B. D. (1986). Hostility, coronary heart disease (CHD) incidence, and total mortality: Lack of association in a 25-year follow-up study of 478 physicians. *Journal of Behavioral Medicine, 9,* 119–125.

McCutchan, J. A. (1990). Virology, immunology, and clinical course of HIV infection. *Journal of Consulting and Clinical Psychology, 58,* 5–12.

McDowell, J., & Mondi, L. (1995, April 10). A tiny win against AIDS? *Time, 145,* 62.

McGill, J. C., Lawlis, G. F., Selby, D., Mooney, V., & McCoy, C. E. (1983). The relationship of Minnesota Multiphasic Personality Inventory (MMPI) profile clusters to pain behaviors. *Journal of Behavioral Medicine, 6,* 77–92.

McGinnis, J. M., & Foege, W. H. (1993). Actual causes of death in the United States. *Journal of the American Medical Association, 270,* 2207–2212.

McGlashan, T. H., Evans, F. J., & Orne, M. T. (1969). The nature of hypnotic analgesia and the placebo response to experimental pain. *Psychosomatic Medicine, 31,* 227–246.

McGrady, A., Wauquier, A., McNeil, A., & Gerard, G. (1994). Effect of biofeedback-assisted relaxation on migraine headache and changes in cerebral blood flow velocity in the middle cerebral artery. *Headache, 34,* 424–428.

McHugh, S., & Vallis, M. (1986). Illness behavior: Operationalization of the biopsychosocial model. In S. McHugh & J. M. Vallis (Eds.), *Illness behavior: A multidisciplinary model* (pp. 1–31). New York: Plenum.

McKinnon, W., Weisse, C. S., Reynolds, C. P., Bowles, C. A., & Baum, A. (1989). Chronic stress, leucocyte subpopulations, and humoral response to latent viruses. *Health Psychology, 8,* 389–402.

McLean, S., Skirboll, L. R., & Pert, C. B. (1985). Comparison of substance P and enkephalin distribution in rat brain: An overview using radioimmunocytochemistry. *Neuroscience, 14,* 837–852.

McLellan, A. T., Arndt, I. O., Metzger, D. S., Woody, G. E., & O'Brien, C. P. (1993). The effects of psychosocial services in substance abuse treatment. *Journal of the American Medical Association, 269,* 1953–1959.

McMurran, M. (1994). *The psychology of addiction.* London: Taylor & Francis.

McMurray, R. G., Sheps, D. S., & Guinan, D. M. (1984). Effects of naloxone on maximal stress testing in females. *Journal of Applied Physiology, 56,* 436–440.

Mechanic, D. (1978). *Medical sociology* (2nd ed.). New York: Free Press.

Medical Essay (1993, June). Cholesterol. In Supplement to *Mayo Clinic Health Letter,* pp. 1–8. Also reprinted in R. Yarian (Ed.), *Health: Annual editions 95/96* (pp. 177–180). Guilford, CT: Dushkin.

Meichenbaum, D. (1977). *Cognitive behavior modification: An integrative approach.* New York: Plenum.

Meichenbaum, D., & Cameron, R. (1983). Stress inoculation training: Toward a general paradigm for training coping skills. In D. Meichenbaum & M. E. Jaremko (Ed.), *Stress reduction and prevention* (pp. 115–154). New York: Plenum.

Meichenbaum, D., & Jaremko, M. E. (Eds.). (1982). *Stress prevention and management: A cognitive-behavioral approach.* New York: Plenum.

Meichenbaum, D., & Jaremko, M. E. (Eds.). (1983). *Stress reduction and prevention.* New York: Plenum.

Meichenbaum, D., & Turk, D. C. (1976). The cognitive-behavioral management of anxiety, anger and pain. In P. O. Davidson (Ed.), *The behavioral management of anxiety, depression, and pain.* New York: Brunner/Mazel.

Melamed, B. G. (1984). Health intervention: Collaboration for health and science. In B. L. Hammonds & C. J. Scheirer (Eds.), *Psychology and health: The Master Lecture Series*

Vol. 3 (pp. 49–119). Washington, DC: American Psychological Association.

Meltzer, A. A., & Everhart, J. E. (1995). Unintentional weight loss in the United States. *American Journal of Epidemiology, 142,* 1039–1046.

Melzack, R. (1973). *The puzzle of pain.* New York: Basic Books.

Melzack, R. (1975a). How acupuncture can block pain. In M. Weisenberg (Ed.), *Pain: Clinical and experimental perspectives* (pp. 251–257). St. Louis: Mosby.

Melzack, R. (1975b). The McGill Pain Questionnaire: Major properties and scoring methods. *Pain, 1,* 277–299.

Melzack, R. (1987). The short-form McGill Pain Questionnaire. *Pain, 30,* 191–197.

Melzack, R. (1992, April). Phantom limbs. *Scientific American, 266,* 120–126.

Melzack, R. (1993). Pain: Past, present and future. *Canadian Journal of Experimental Psychology, 47,* 615–629.

Melzack, R., & Torgerson, W. S. (1971). On the language of pain. *Anesthesiology, 34,* 50–59.

Melzack, R., & Wall, P. D. (1965). Pain mechanisms: A new theory. *Science, 150,* 971–979.

Melzack, R., & Wall, P. D. (1982). *The challenge of pain.* New York: Basic Books.

Melzack, R., & Wall, P. D. (1988). *The challenge of pain* (rev. ed.). London: Penguin.

Mendes de Leon, C. F. (1992). Anger and impatience/irritability in patients of low socioeconomic status with acute coronary heart disease. *Journal of Behavioral Medicine, 15,* 273–284.

Mensink, R. P., & Katan, M. B. (1989). Effects of a diet enriched with monounsaturated or polyunsaturated fatty acids on levels of low-density and high-density lipoprotein cholesterol in healthy men and women. *New England Journal of Medicine, 321,* 436–441.

Mermelstein, R., Cohen, S., Lichtenstein, E., Baer, J. S., & Kamarck, T. (1986). Social support and smoking cessation and maintenance. *Journal of Consulting and Clinical Psychology, 54,* 447–453.

Metropolitan Life Insurance Company. (1959). New weight standards for men and women. *Statistical Bulletin, 40,* 1.

Meyer, D., Leventhal, H., & Gutman, M. (1985). Common-sense models of illness: The example of hypertension. *Health Psychology, 4,* 115–135.

Meyer, T. J., & Mark, M. M. (1995). Effects of psychosocial interventions with adult cancer patients: A meta-analysis of randomized experiments. *Health Psychology, 14,* 101–108.

Michela, J. L. (1987). Interpersonal and individual impacts of a husband's heart attack. In A. Baum & J. E. Singer (Eds.), *Handbook of psychology and health: Vol. 5. Stress* (pp. 255–301). Hillsdale, NJ: Erlbaum.

Michie, S., Marteau, T. M., & Kidd, J. (1992). Predicting antenatal class attendance: Attitudes of self and others. *Psychology and Health, 7,* 225–234.

Midanik, L. T., & Clark, W. B. (1994). The demographic distribution of US drinking patterns in 1990: Description and trends from 1984. *American Journal of Public Health, 84,* 1218–1222.

Mikail, S. F., DuBreuil, S. C., & D'Eon, J. L. (1993). A comparative analysis of measures used in the assessment of chronic pain patients. *Psychological Assessment, 5,* 117–120.

Millar, M. G., & Millar, K. (1995). Negative affective consequences of thinking about disease detection behaviors. *Health Psychology, 14,* 141–146.

Millar, W. J. (1983). Sex differentials in mortality by income level in urban Canada. *Canadian Journal of Public Health, 74,* 329–334.

Millard, R. W., Waranch, H. R., & McEntee, M. (1992). Compliance to nicotine gum recommendations in a multicomponent group smoking cessation program: An exploratory study. *Addictive Behaviors, 17,* 201–207.

Miller, A. B. (1994). How do we interpret the "bad news" about cancer? *Journal of the American Medical Association, 271,* 468.

Miller, A. L. (1993, March). *The U. S. smoking-material fire problem through 1990: The role of lighted tobacco products in fire.* Paper presented at the meeting of the National Fire Protection Association, Quincy, MA.

Miller, F. T., Bentz, W. K., Aponte, J. F., & Brogan, D. R. (1974). Perception of life crises events: A comparative study of rural and urban samples. In B. S. Dohrenwend & B. P. Dohrenwend (Eds.), *Stressful life events: Their nature and effects.* New York: Wiley.

Miller, J. D., & Cisin, I. H. (1983). *Highlights from the National Survey on Drug Abuse: 1982.* (DHHS Publication No. ADM 83-1277). Washington, DC: U.S. Government Printing Office.

Miller, M. F., Barabasz, A. F., & Barabasz, M. (1991). Effects of active alert and relaxation hypnotic inductions on cold pressor pain. *Journal of Abnormal Psychology, 100,* 223–226.

Miller, N. E. (1969). Learning of visceral and glandular responses. *Science, 163,* 434–445.

Miller, P., Wikoff, R., & Hiatt, A. (1992). Fishbein's model of reasoned action and compliance behavior of hypertensive patients. *Nursing Research, 41,* 104–109.

Miller, W. R. (1983). Controlled drinking: A history and a critical review. *Journal of Studies on Alcohol, 44,* 68–83.

Miller, W. R., & Hester, R. K. (1980). Treating the problem drinker: Modern approaches. In W. R. Miller (Ed.), *The addictive behaviors* (pp. 11–141). Oxford, England: Pergamon Press.

Mills, P. K., Annegers, J. F., & Phillips, R. L. (1988). Animal product consumption and subsequent fatal breast cancer risk among Seventh-day Adventists. *American Journal of Epidemiology, 127,* 440–453.

Millstein, S. G., & Irwin, C. E. (1987). Concepts of health and illness: Different constructs or variations on a theme? *Health Psychology, 6,* 515–524.

Minuchin, S., Rosman, B. L., & Baker, L. (1978). *Psychosomatic families: Anorexia nervosa in context.* Cambridge, MA: Harvard University Press.

Mitchell, J. E., & de Zwaan, M. (1993). Pharmacological treatments of binge eating. In C. G. Fairburn & G. T. Wilson (Eds.), *Binge eating: Nature, assessment, and treatment* (pp. 250–269). New York: Guilford Press.

Mittelmark, M. B., Luepker, R. V., Grimm, R., Jr., Kottke, T. E., & Blackburn, H. (1988). The role of physicians in a community-wide program for prevention of cardiovascular disease: The Minnesota Heart Health Program. *Public Health Reports, 103,* 360–365.

Mittelmark, M. B., Murray, D. M., Luepker, R. V., Pechacek, T. F., Pirie, P. L., & Pallonen, U. E. (1987). Predicting experimentation with cigarettes: The Childhood Antecedents of Smoking Study (CASS). *American Journal of Public Health, 77,* 206–208.

Mittleman, H. A., Maclure, M., Tofler, G. H., Sherwood, J. B., Goldberg, R. J., & Muller, J. E. (1993). Triggering of acute myocardial infarction by heavy physical exertion: Protection against triggering by regular exertion. *New England Journal of Medicine, 329,* 1677–1683.

Mobily, P. R., Herr, K. A., Clark, M. K., & Wallace, R. B. (1994). An epidemiologic analysis of pain in the elderly: The Iowa 65+ Rural Health Study. *Journal of Aging and Health, 6,* 139–154.

Modesti, D. G., & Tryon, W. W. (1994, August). *Emotional strain on adult children of a parent with Alzheimer's disease.* Paper presented at the American Psychological Association convention, Los Angeles, CA.

Moffatt, R. J., Wallace, M. B., & Sady, S. P. (1990). Effects of anabolic steroids on lipoprotein profiles of female weight lifters. *The Physician and Sportsmedicine, 18*(9), 106–115.

Mohide, E. A. (1993). Informal care of community-dwelling patients with Alzheimer's disease: Focus on the family caregiver. *Neurology, 43* (Suppl 4), S16–S19.

Moldofsky, H., Lue, F. A., Eisen, J., Keystone, E., & Gorczynski, R. M. (1986). The relationship of interleukin-1 and immune function to sleep in humans. *Psychosomatic Medicine, 48,* 309–318.

Monroe, S. M. (1982). The assessment of life events: Event-symptom associations and the cause of disorder. *Journal of Abnormal Psychology, 91,* 14–24.

Monson, R. R., & Lyon, J. L. (1975). Proportional mortality among alcoholics. *Cancer, 36,* 1077–1079.

Montano, D. E., & Taplin, S. H. (1991). A test of an expanded theory of reasoned action to predict mammography participation. *Social Science and Medicine, 32,* 733–741.

Moolgavkar, S. H. (1983). A model for human carcinogenesis: Hereditary cancers and premalignant lesions. In R. G. Crispen (Ed.), *Cancer: Etiology and prevention* (pp. 71–77). New York: Elsevier Biomedical.

Moore, J. E., Armentrout, D. P., Parker, J. C., & Kivlahan, D. R. (1986). Empirically derived pain-patient MMPI subgroups: Prediction of treatment outcome. *Journal of Behavioral Medicine, 9,* 51–63.

Moos, R. H. (1984). The crisis of illness: Chronic conditions. In R. H. Moos (Ed.), *Coping with physical illness 2: New perspectives* (pp. 139–143). New York: Plenum.

Moos, R. H., & Schaefer, J. A. (1984). The crisis of physical illness: An overview and conceptual analysis. In R. H. Moos (Ed.), *Coping with physical illness 2: New perspectives* (pp. 3–25). New York: Plenum.

Moret, V., Forster, A., Laverriere, M. C., Lambert, H., Gaillard, R. C., Bourgeois, P., Haynal, A., Gemperle, M., & Buchser, E. (1991). Mechanism of analgesia induced by hypnosis and acupuncture: Is there a difference? *Pain, 45,* 135–140.

Morgan, R. E., Palinkas, L. A., Barrett-Connor, E. L., & Wingard, D. L. (1993). Plasma cholesterol and depressive symptoms in older men. *Lancet, 341,* 75–79.

Morgan, W. P. (1973). Influence of acute physical activity on state anxiety. In *Proceedings of the College Physical Education Association,* Pittsburgh, PA.

Morgan, W. P. (1979, February). Negative addiction in runners. *The Physician and Sportsmedicine,* pp. 56–63, 67–70.

Morgan, W. P. (1981). Psychological benefits of physical activity. In F. J. Nagle & H. J. Montoye (Eds.), *Exercise in health and disease.* Springfield, IL: Thomas.

Morris, D. B. (1994, Autumn). Pain's dominion: What we make of pain. *Wilson Quarterly,* pp. 8–33.

Morris, D. L., Kritchevsky, S. B., & Davis, C. E. (1994). Serum carotenoids and coronary heart disease: The Lipid Research Clinics Coronary Primary Prevention Trial and Follow-up Study. *Journal of the American Medical Association, 272,* 1439–1441.

Morris, J. N., Heady, J. A., Raffle, P. A. B., Roberts, C. G., & Parks, J. W. (1953). Coronary heart-disease and physical activity of work. *Lancet, ii,* 1053–1057, 1111–1120.

Mosbach, P., & Leventhal, H. (1988). Peer group identification and smoking: Implications for intervention. *Journal of Abnormal Psychology, 97,* 238–245.

Moser, R., McCance, K. L., & Smith, K. R. (1991). Results of a national survey of physicians' knowledge and application of prevention capabilities. *American Journal of Preventive Medicine, 7,* 384–390.

Moss, M., Bucher, B., Moore, F. A., Moore, E. E., & Parsons, P. E. (1996). The role of chronic alcohol abuse in the development of Acute Respiratory Distress Syndrome. *Journal of the American Medical Association, 275,* 50–54.

Moy, C. S., Songer, T. J., LaPorte, R. E., Dorman, J. S., Kriska, A. M., Orchard, T. J., Becker, D. J., & Drash, A. L. (1993). Insulindependent diabetes mellitus, physical activity, and death. *American Journal of Epidemiology, 137,* 74–81.

Moyer, M. A. (1989). Use of patient-controlled analgesia for burn pain. In S. C. Funk, E. M. Tornquist, M. T. Champagne, L. A. Copp, & R. A. Wiese (Eds.), *Key aspects of comfort: Management of pain, fatigue, and nausea* (pp. 135–140). New York: Springer.

Muldoon, M. F., Kaplan, J. R., Manuck, S. B., & Mann, J. J. (1992). Effects of a low-fat diet on brain serontonergic responsivity in cynomolgus monkeys. *Biological Psychiatry, 31,* 739–742.

Muldoon, M. F., Manuck, S. B., & Matthews, K. A. (1992). Lowering cholesterol concentrations and mortality: A quantitative review of primary prevention trials. *British Medical Journal, 301,* 309–314.

Multiple Risk Factor Intervention Trial Research Group. (1977). Statistical design considerations in the NHLI Multiple Risk Factor Intervention Trial. *Journal of Chronic Diseases, 30,* 261–275.

Multiple Risk Factor Intervention Trial Research Group. (1982). Risk factor changes and mortality. *Journal of the American Medical Association, 248,* 1465–1477.

Multiple Risk Factor Intervention Trial Research Group. (1990). Mortality rates after 10.5 years for participants in the Multiple Risk Factor Intervention Trial. *Journal of the American Medical Association, 263,* 1795–1801.

Murphy, J. K., Stoney, C. M., Alpert, B. S., & Walker, S. S. (1995). Gender and ethnicity in children's cardiovascular reactivity: 7 years of study. *Health Psychology, 14,* 48–55.

Murphy, K. R., & Davidshofer, C. O. (1994). *Psychological testing: Principles and applications* (3rd ed.). Englewood Cliffs, NJ: Prentice-Hall.

Murray, D. M., Davis-Hearn, M., Goldman, A. I., Pirie, P., & Luepker, R. V. (1988). Four- and five-year follow-up results from four seventh-grade smoking prevention strategies. *Journal of Behavioral Medicine, 11,* 395–405.

Murray, D. M., Richards, P. S., Luepker, R. V., & Johnson, C. A. (1987). The prevention of cigarette smoking in children: Two- and three-year follow-up comparisons of four prevention strategies. *Journal of Behavioral Medicine, 10,* 595–611.

Murray, D. M., Pirie, P., Luepker, R. V., & Pallonen, U. (1989). Five- and six-year follow-up results from four seventh-grade smoking prevention strategies. *Journal of Behavioral Medicine, 12,* 207–218.

Mushlin, A. I., & Appel, F. A. (1977). Diagnosing patient noncompliance. *Archives of Internal Medicine, 137,* 318–321.

Mustard, T. R., & Harris, A. V. E. (1989). Problems in understanding prescription labels. *Perceptual and Motor Skills, 69,* 291–299.

Myasnikov, A. L. (1958). Influence of some factors on development of experimental cholesterol atherosclerosis. *Circulation, 17,* 99–113.

Myers, L., Coughlin, S. S., Webber, L. S., Srinivasan, S. R., Berenson, G. S. (1995). Prediction of adult cardiovascular multifactorial risk status from childhood risk factor levels: The Bogalusa Heart Study. *American Journal of Epidemiology, 142,* 918–924.

Naditch, M. P. (1984). The Staywell program. In J. D. Matarazzo, S. M. Weiss, J. A. Herd, N. E. Miller, & S. M. Weiss (Eds.), *Behavioral health: A handbook of health enhancement and disease prevention* (pp. 1071–1078). New York: Wiley.

Nathan, P. E. (1984a). Johnson & Johnson's Live for Life: A comprehensive positive lifestyle change program. In J. D. Matarazzo, S. M. Weiss, J. A. Herd, N. E. Miller, & S. M. Weiss (Eds.), *Behavioral health: A handbook of health enhancement and disease prevention* (pp. 1064–1070). New York: Wiley.

Nathan, P. E. (1984b). The worksite as a setting for health promotion and positive lifestyle change. In J. D. Matarazzo, S. M. Weiss, J. A. Herd, N. E. Miller, & S. M. Weiss (Eds.), *Behavioral health: A handbook of health enhancement and disease prevention* (pp. 1061–1063). New York: Wiley.

National Center for Health Statistics. (1994). *Health, United States, 1993.* (DHHS, Publication No. PHS 94-1232). Hyattsville, MD: U.S. Government Printing Office.

National Center for Health Statistics. (1995). *Health, United States.* Hyattsville, MD: U.S. Government Printing Office.

National Institute of Alcohol Abuse and Alcoholism (NIAAA). (1983). *Fifth special report to the U.S. Congress on alcohol and health.* (DHHS Publication No. ADM 84-1291). Washington, DC: U.S. Government Printing Office.

National Institute on Alcohol Abuse and Alcoholism (NIAAA). (1988). Alcohol and aging. *Alcohol Alert, 2,* 1–4.

National Institute of Alcohol Abuse and Alcoholism (NIAAA). (1983). *Seventh special report to the U.S. Congress on alcohol and health.* (DHHS Publication No. ADM 90-1656). Washington, DC: U.S. Government Printing Office.

National Task Force on the Prevention and Treatment of Obesity. (1993). Very low-calorie diets. *Journal of the American Medical Association, 270,* 967–974.

Navarro, V. (1990). Race or class versus race and class: Mortality differentials in the United States. *Lancet, 336,* 1238–1240.

Neimark, J., Conway, C., & Doskoch, P. (1994, September–October). Back from the drink. *Psychology Today, 27,* 46–49.

Nelson, D. E., Giovino, G. A., Shepland, D. R., Mowery, P. D., Mills, S. L., & Eridsen, M. P. (1995). Trends in cigarette smoking among US adolescents, 1974 through 1991. *American Journal of Public Health, 85,* 34–40.

Nelson, H. D., Nevitt, M. C., Scott, J. C., Stone, K. L., & Cummings, S. R. (1994). Smoking, alcohol, and neuromuscular and physical functioning of older women. *Journal of the American Medical Association, 272,* 1825–1831.

Nelson, M. E., Fiatarone, M. A., Marganti, C. M., Trice, I., Greenberg, R. A., & Evans, W. J. (1994). Effects of high-intensity strength training on multiple risk factors for osteoporatic fractures. *Journal of the American Medical Association, 272,* 1909–1914.

Nelson, T. S., & Planchock, N. Y. (1989). The effects of transcutaneous electrical nerve stimulation (TENS) on postoperative patients' pain and narcotic use. In S. G. Funk, E. M. Tornquist, M. T. Champagne, L. A. Copp, & R. A. Wiese (Eds.), *Key aspects of comfort: Management of pain, fatigue, and nausea* (pp. 134–145). New York: Springer.

Nemeroff, C. J. (1995). Magical thinking about illness virulence: Conceptions of germs from "safe" versus "dangerous" others. *Health Psychology, 14,* 147–151.

Nethercut, G., & Piccione, A. (1984). The physician perspective of health psychologists in medical settings. *Health Psychology, 3,* 175–184.

Neugebauer, R. (1984). The reliability of life-event reports. In B. S. Dohrenwend & B. P. Dohrenwend (Eds.), *Stressful life events & their contexts* (pp. 85–107). New Brunswick, NJ: Rutgers University Press.

Neuman, P. A., & Halvorson, P. A. (1983). *Anorexia nervosa and bulimia*. New York: Van Nostrand Reinhold.

Newacheck, P. W., & Taylor, W. R. (1992). Childhood chronic illness: Prevalence, severity, and impact. *American Journal of Public Health, 82,* 364–371.

Newberne, P. M., & Suphakarn, V. (1983). Nutrition and cancer: A review, with emphasis on the role of vitamins C and E and selenium. *Nutrition and Cancer, 5,* 107–119.

Newell, M. L., Dunn, D., De Maria, A., Ferrazin, A., De Rossi, A., Giaquinto, C., Levy, J., Alimenti, A., Ehrnst, A., Bohlin, A. B., Ljung, R., Peckham, C. (1996). Detection of virus in vertically exposed HIV-antibody-negative children. *Lancet, 347,* 213–215.

Newschaffer, C. J., Bush, T. L., & Hale, W. E. (1992). Aging and total cholesterol levels: Cohort, period, and survivorship effects. *American Journal of Epidemiology, 136,* 23–34.

Nicholson, N. L., & Blanchard, E. B. (1993). A controlled evaluation of behavioral treatment of chronic headache in the elderly. *Behavior Therapy, 24,* 395–408.

Nides, M., Rand, C., Dolce, J., Murray, R., O'Hara, P., Voelker, H., & Connett, J. (1994). Weight gain as a function of smoking cessation and 2-mg nicotine gum use among middle-aged smokers with mild lung impairment in the first 2 years of the Lung Health Study. *Health Psychology, 13,* 354–361

Nigl, A. J. (1984). *Biofeedback and behavioral strategies in pain treatment*. New York: Medical and Scientific Books.

NIH Technology Assessment Conference Panel. (1993). Methods for voluntary weight loss and control. *Annals of Internal Medicine, 119,* 764–770.

Nisbett, R. E. (1972). Hunger, obesity, and the ventromedial hypothalamus. *Psychological Review, 79,* 433–453.

Nivision, M. E., & Endresen, I. M. (1993). An analysis of relationships among environmental noise, annoyance and sensitivity to noise, and the consequences for health and sleep. *Journal of Behavior Medicine, 16,* 257–276.

Nolen-Hoeksema, S. (1994, August). *Rumination in response to depression*. Presented at the American Psychological Association convention, Los Angeles, CA.

Norman, P., & Conner, M. (1993). The role of social cognition models in predicting attendance at health checks. *Psychology and Health, 8,* 447–462.

Norvell, N., & Belles, D. (1993). Psychological and physical benefits of circuit weight training in law enforcement personnel. *Journal of Consulting and Clinical Psychology, 61,* 520–527.

Oken, D. (1987). Coping and psychosomatic illness. In A. Baum & J. E. Singer (Eds.), *Handbook of psychology and health: Vol. 5. Stress* (pp. 109–136). Hillsdale, NJ: Erlbaum.

Oldridge, N. B., & Steiner, D. (1990). The health belief model: Predicting compliance and dropout in cardiac rehabilitation. *Medicine and Science in Sports and Exercise, 22,* 678–683.

Oldridge, N. B., Guyatt, G. H., Fischer, M. E., & Rimm, A. A. (1988). Cardiac rehabilitation after myocardial infarction. *Journal of the American Medical Association, 260,* 945–950.

O'Leary, A. (1990). Stress, emotion, and human immune function. *Psychological Bulletin, 108,* 363–382.

Olkkonen, S., & Honkanen, R. (1990). The role of alcohol in nonfatal bicycle injuries. *Accident Analysis and Prevention, 22,* 89–96.

Olness, K. (1993). Hypnosis: The power of attention. In D. Goleman & J. Gurin (Eds.), *Mind/body medicine: How to use your mind for better health* (pp. 277–290). Yonkers, NY: Consumer Reports Books.

Olshansky, S. J., Carnes, B. A., & Cassel, C. K. (1993, April). The aging of the human species. *Scientific American, 268,* 46–52.

Orme, C. M., & Binik, Y. M. (1987). Recidivism and self-cure of obesity: A test of Schachter's hypothesis in diabetic patients. *Health Psychology, 6,* 467–475.

Orme, C. M., & Binik, Y. M. (1989). Consistency of adherence across regimen demands. *Health Psychology, 8,* 27–43.

Orme, M. T. (1976). Mechanisms of hypnotic pain control. In J. J. Bonica & D. Abel-Fessard (Eds.), *Advances in pain research and therapy* (Vol. 1). New York: Raven.

Orme, M. T. (1980). Hypnotic control of pain: Toward a clarification of the different psychological processes involved. In J. J. Bonica (Ed.), *Pain* (pp. 155–172). New York: Raven.

Ornish, D. (1993). *Eat more, weigh less*. New York: Harper Collins.

Ornish, D. (1995, May). *Reversing heart disease*. Presented by St. Patrick's Hospital, Lake Charles, LA.

Ornish, D., Brown, S. E., Scherwitz, L. W., Billings, J. H., Armstrong, W. T., Ports, T., McLanahan, S. M., Kirkeeide, R. L., Brand, R. J., & Gould, K. L. (1990). Can lifestyle changes reverse coronary heart disease? The Lifestyle Heart Trial. *Lancet, 336,* 129–133.

Ornstein, R., & Sobel, D. (1987). *The healing brain*. New York: Simon & Schuster.

Orr, E., & Westman, M. (1990). Does hardiness moderate stress, and how? A review. In M. Rosenbaum (Ed.), *Learned resourcefulness: On coping skills, self-control, and adaptive behavior* (pp. 64–94). New York: Springer.

Osman, A., Barrios, F. X., Osman, J. R., Schneekloth, R., & Troutman, J. A. (1994). The Pain Anxiety Symptoms Scale: Psychometric properties in a community sample. *Journal of Behavioral Medicine, 17,* 511–522.

Ott, P. J., & Levy, S. M. (1994). Cancer in women. In V. J. Adesso, D. M. Reddy, & R. Fleming (Eds.), *Psychological perspectives on women's health* (pp. 83–98). Washington, DC: Taylor & Francis.

Ouellette, E. M., Rosett, H. L., Rosman, N. P., & Weinen, L. (1977). Adverse effects in offspring of maternal alcohol abuse during pregnancy. *New England Journal of Medicine, 297,* 528–530.

Ouellette, S. C. (1993). Inquiries into hardiness. In L. Goldberger & S. Breznitz (Eds.), *Handbook of stress: Theoretical and clinical aspects* (2nd ed., pp. 77–100). New York: Free Press

Oxman, T. E., Berkman, L. F., Kasl, S., Freeman, D. H., Jr., & Barrett, J. (1992). Social support and depressive symptoms in the elderly. *American Journal of Epidemiology, 135,* 356–368.

Padian, N. S., Shiboski, S. C., & Jewell, N. P. (1991). Female-to-male transmission of human immunodeficiency virus. *Journal of the American Medical Association, 266,* 1664–1667.

Paffenbarger, R. S., Jr. (1972). Factors predisposing to fatal stroke in longshoremen. *Preventive Medicine, 1,* 522–527.

Paffenbarger, R. S., Jr., Gima, A. S., Laughlin, M. E., & Black, R. A. (1971). Characteristics of longshoremen related to fatal coronary heart disease and stroke. *American Journal of Public Health, 61,* 1362–1370.

Paffenbarger, R. S., Jr., & Hale, W. E. (1975). Work activity and coronary heart mortality. *New England Journal of Medicine, 292,* 545–550.

Paffenbarger, R. S., Jr., Hyde, R. T., & Wing, A. L. (1987). Physical activity and incidence of cancer in diverse populations: A preliminary report. *American Journal of Clinical Nutrition, 45,* 312–315.

Paffenbarger, R. S., Jr., Hyde, R. T., Wing, A. L., & Hsieh, C-c. (1986). Physical activity, all-cause mortality, and longevity of college alumni. *New England Journal of Medicine, 314,* 605–613.

Paffenbarger, R. S., Jr., Hyde, R. T., Wing, A. L., Lee, I-M., Jung, D., & Klampert, J. B. (1993). The association of changes in physical activity level and other lifestyle characteristics with mortality among men. *New England Journal of Medicine, 328,* 538.

Paffenbarger, R. S., Jr., Hyde, R. T., Wing, A. L., & Steinmetz, C. H. (1984). A natural history of athleticism and cardiovascular health. *Journal of the American Medical Association, 252,* 491–495.

Paffenbarger, R. S., Jr., Laughlin, M. E., Gima, A. S., & Black, R. A. (1970). Work activity of longshoremen as related to death from coronary heart disease and stroke. *New England Journal of Medicine, 282, 1109–1114.*

Paffenbarger, R. S., Jr., Wing, A. L., & Hyde, R. T. (1978). Physical activity as an index of heart attack risk in college alumni. *American Journal of Epidemiology, 108,* 161–175.

Palazzoli, M. S. (1974). *Self-starvation.* London: Chaucer.

Palmblad, J., Petrini, B., Wasserman, J., & Åkerstedt, T. (1979). Lymphocyte and granulocyte reactions during sleep deprivation. *Psychosomatic Medicine, 41,* 273–278.

Palmer, S. E., Canzona, L., & Wai, L. (1984). Helping families respond effectively to chronic illness: Home dialysis as a case example. In R. H. Moos (Ed.), *Coping with physical illness 2: New perspectives* (pp. 283–294). New York: Plenum.

Pamuk, E. R., Williamson, D. F., Madans, J., Serdula, M. K., Kleinman, J. C., & Byers, T. E. (1992). Weight loss and mortality in a national cohort of adults, 1971–1987. *American Journal of Epidemiology, 136,* 668–697.

Pamuk, E. R., Williamson, D. F., Serdula, M. K., Madans, J., & Byers, T. E. (1993). Weight loss and subsequent death in a cohort of U.S. adults. *Annals of Internal Medicine, 119,* 744–748.

Pappas, G. (1994). Elucidating the relationships between race, socioeconomic status, and health. *American Journal of Public Health, 84,* 892–893.

Parkes, C. M. (1964). The effects of bereavement on physical and mental health—A study of the medical records of widows. *British Medical Journal,* 274–279.

Parsons, T. (1951). *The social system.* New York: Free Press.

Parsons, T. (1978). *Action theory and the human condition.* New York: Free Press.

Pate, R. R., & Macera, C. A. (1994). Risks of exercising: Musculoskeletal injuries. In C. Bouchard, R. J. Shephard, & T. Stephens (Eds.), *Physical activity, fitness, and health: International proceedings and consensus statement* (pp. 1008–1018). Champaign, IL: Human Kinetics.

Pate, R. R., Pratt, M., Blair, S. N., Haskell, W. L., Macera, C. A., Bouchard, C., Buchner, D., Ettinger, W., Heath, G. W., King, A. C., Kriska, A., Leon, A. S., Marcus, B. H., Morris, J., Paffenbarger, R. S., Jr., Patrick, K., Pollock, M. L., Rippe, J. M., Sallis, J., & Wilmore, J. H. (1995). Physical activity and public health: A recommendation from the Centers for Disease Control and Prevention and the American College of Sports Medicine. *Journal of the American Medical Association, 273,* 402–407.

Pattishall, E. G. (1989). The development of behavioral medicine: Historical models. *Annals of Behavioral Medicine, 11,* 43–48.

Pattison, E. M., Sobell, M. B., & Sobell, L. C. (Eds.). (1977). *Emerging concepts of alcohol dependence.* New York: Springer.

Paul, C. L., Sanson-Fisher, R. W., Redman, S., & Carter, S. (1994). Preventing accidental injury to young children in the home using volunteers. *Health Promotion International, 9,* 241–249.

Pauling, L. (1980). Vitamin C therapy of advanced cancer. *New England Journal of Medicine, 302,* 694–698.

Paulus, P. B., McCain, G., & Cox, V. C. (1978). Death rates, psychiatric commitments, blood pressure, and perceived crowding as a function of institutional crowding. *Environmental Psychology and Nonverbal Behavior, 3,* 107–116.

Paykel, E. S., Brayne, C., Huppert, F. A., Gill, C., Barley, C., Gehlhaar, E., Beardsall, L., Girling, D. M., Pollitt, P., & O'Connor, D. (1994). Incidence of dementia in a population older than 75 years in the United Kingdom. *Archives of General Psychiatry, 51,* 324–332.

Paykel, E. S., Prusoff, B. A., & Uhlenhuth, E. H. (1971). Scaling of life events. *Archives of General Psychiatry, 25,* 340–347.

Pbert, L., Doerfler, L. A., & DeCosimo, D. (1992). An evaluation of the Perceived Stress Scale in two clinical populations. *Journal of Psychopathology and Behavioral Assessment, 14,* 363–375.

Pearce, J. M. S. (1994). Headache. *Journal of Neurology, Neurosurgery and Psychiatry, 57,* 134–143.

Pearl, R. (1938). Tobacco and longevity. *Science, 87,* 216–217.

Pearlin, L. I., Turner, H., & Semple, S. (1989). Coping and the mediation of caregiver stress. In E. Light & B. D. Lebowitz (Eds.), *Alzheimer's disease treatment and family stess: Directions for research* (pp. 198–217). (DHHS Publication No. ADM 89-1569). Washington, DC: U.S. Government Printing Office.

Peele, S. (1984). The cultural context of psychological approaches to alcoholism: Can we control the effects of alcohol? *American Psychologist, 39,* 1337–1351.

Peele, S. (1993). The conflict between public health goals and the temperance mentality. *American Journal of Public Health, 83,* 805–810.

Pekkanen, J., Linn, S., Heiss, G., Suchindran, C. M., Leon, A., Rifkind, B. M., & Tyroler, H. A. (1990). Ten-year mortality from cardiovascular disease in relation to cholesterol level among men with and without preexisting cardiovascular disease. *New England Journal of Medicine, 322,* 1700–1707.

Pell, S., & Fayerweather, W. E. (1985). Trends in the incidence of myocardial infarction and in associated mortality and morbidity in a large employed population, 1957–1983. *New England Journal of Medicine, 312,* 1005–1011.

Pelletier, K. R. (1984). *Healthy people in unhealthy places: Stress and fitness at work.* New York: Merloyd Lawrence.

Pelleymounter, M. A., Cullen, M. J., Baker, M. B., Hecht, R., Winters, D., Boone, T., & Collins, F. (1995). Effects of *obese* gene production body weight regulation in *ob/ob* mice. *Science, 269,* 540–543.

Pendery, M. L., Maltzman, I. M., & West, L. J. (1982). Controlled drinking by alcoholics? New findings and a reevaluation of a major affirmative study. *Science, 217,* 169–175.

Penkower, L., Dew, M. A., Kingsley, L., Becker, J. T., Satz, P., Schaerf, F. W., & Sheridan, K. (1991). Behavioral, health and psychosocial factors and risk for HIV infection among sexually active homosexual men: The Multicenter AIDS Cohort Study. *American Journal of Public Health, 81,* 194–196.

Pennebaker, J. W. (1982). *The psychology of physical symptoms.* New York: Springer-Verlag.

Pennebaker, J. W. (1993). Putting stress into words: Health, linguistic, and therapeutic implications. *Behavior Research and Therapy, 31,* 539–548.

Pennebaker, J. W., Barger, S. D., & Tiebout, J. (1989). Disclosure of traumas and health among Holocaust survivors. *Psychosomatic Medicine, 51,* 577–589.

Pennebaker, J. W., Colder, M., & Sharp, L. K. (1990). Accelerating the coping process. *Journal of Personality and Social Psychology, 58,* 528–537.

Pennebaker, J. W., Kiecolt-Glaser, J. K., & Glaser, R. (1988). Disclosure of trauma and immune function: Health implications for psychotherapy. *Journal of Consulting and Clinical Psychology, 56,* 239–245.

Penty, M. A., MacKinnon, D. P., Flay, B. R., Hansen, W. B., Johnson, C. A., & Dwyer, J. H. (1989). Primary prevention of chronic diseases in adolescence: Effects of the Midwestern

Prevention Project on tobacco use. *American Journal of Epidemiology, 130,* 713–724.

Pérez-Stable, E. J., Sabogal, F., Otero-Sabogal, R., Hiatt, R. A., & McPhee, S. J. (1992). Misconceptions about cancer among Latinos and Anglos. *Journal of the American Medical Association, 288,* 3219–3223.

Perkins, K. A., Dubbert, P. M., Martin, J. E., Faulstich, M. E., & Harris, J. K. (1986). Cardiovascular reactivity to psychological stress in aerobically trained versus untrained mild hypertensives and normotensives. *Health Psychology, 5,* 407–421.

Perkins, K. A., Epstein, L. H., Marks, B. L., Stiller, R. L., & Jacob, R. G. (1989). The effect of nicotine on energy expenditure during light physical activity. *New England Journal of Medicine, 320,* 898–903.

Perri, M. G., McAllister, D. A., Gange, J. J., Jordan, R. C., McAdoo, W. G., & Nezu, A. M. (1988). Effects of four maintenance programs on the long-term managment of obesity. *Journal of Consulting and Clinical Psychology, 56,* 529–534.

Persky, V. W., Kempthrone-Rawson, J., & Shekelle, R. B. (1987). Personality and risk of cancer: 20-year followup of the Western Electric Study. *Psychosomatic Medicine, 49,* 435–439.

Persons, J. B., & Rao, P. A. (1985). Longitudinal study of cognitions, life events, and depression in psychiatric inpatients. *Journal of Abnormal Psychology, 94,* 51–63.

Pert, C. B., & Snyder, S. H. (1973). Opiate receptor: Demonstration in nervous tissue. *Science, 179,* 1011–1014.

Pertschuk, M. J. (1977). Behavior therapy: Extended follow-up. In R. A. Vigersky (Ed.), *Anorexia nervosa.* New York: Raven.

Peters, R. K., & Mack, T. M. (1983). Pattern of anal carcinoma by gender and marital status in Los Angeles County. *British Journal of Cancer, 48,* 629–636.

Peterson, L., & Brown, D. (1994). Integrating child injury and abuse-neglect research: Common histories, etiologies, and solutions. *Psychological Bulletin, 116,* 293–315.

Peterson, L., Gillies, R., Cook, S. C., Schick, B. & Little, T. (1994). Developmental patterns of expected consequences for simulated bicycle injury events. *Health Psychology, 13,* 218–223.

Peterson, L., & Schick, B. (1993). Empirically derived injury prevention rules. Special Section: Behavioral pediatrics. *Journal of Applied Behavior Analysis, 26,* 451–460.

Peto, R., Doll, R., Buckley, J. D., & Spron, M. B. (1981). Can dietary beta-carotene materially reduce human cancer rates? *Nature, 290,* 201–208.

Pettingale, K. W., Morris, T., Greer, S., & Haybittle, J. L. (1985). Mental attitudes to cancer: An additional prognostic factor. *Lancet, i,* 750.

Pfohl, B., Barrash, J., True, B., & Alexander, B. (1989). Failure of two Axis II measures to predict medication noncompliance among hypertensive outpatients. *Journal of Personality Disorders, 3,* 45–52.

Philips, H. C., & Hunter, M. (1982). A laboratory technique for the assessment of pain behavior. *Journal of Behavioral Medicine, 5,* 283–294.

Pierce, E. F., Eastman, N. W., Tripathi, H. L., Olson, K. G., & Dewey, W. L. (1993). b-Endorphin response to endurance exercise: Relationship to exercise dependence. *Perceptual and Motor Skills, 77,* 767–770.

Pierce, E. F., & Pate, D. W. (1994). Mood alterations in older adults following acute exercise. *Perceptual and Motor Skills, 79,* 191–194.

Pierce, J. P., Lee, L., & Gilpin, E. A. (1994). Smoking initiation by adolescent girls, 1944 through 1988: An association with targeted advertising. *Journal of the American Medical Association, 271,* 608–611

Pietschmann, R. J. (1984, November). Probing death on the run. *Runner's World,* pp. 38–44, 90–94.

Pike, J. L., Smith, T. L., Hauger, R. L., Nicassio, P. M., & Irwin, M. R. (1994, August). *Immunologic effects of acute stress: Chronic life stress as a moderator.* Presented at the American Psychological Association convention, Los Angeles, CA.

Pike, K. M., & Rodin, J. (1991). Mothers, daughters, and disordered eating. *Journal of Abnormal Psychology, 100,* 198–204.

Pinkney, D. S. (1994). Barriers to Medicare remain, especially for blacks. *American Medical News, 37*(44), 20.

Pinto, R. P., & Hollandsworth, J. G., Jr. (1989). Using videotape modeling to prepare children psychologically for surgery: Influence of parents and costs versus benefits of providing preparation services. *Health Psychology, 8,* 79–95.

Pipes, T. V., & Wilmore, J. H. (1975). Isokinetic vs. isotonic strength training in adult men. *Medical Science Sports, 7,* 262–274.

Pirie, P. L., McBride, C. M., Hollerstedt, W., Jeffery, R. W., Hatsukami, D., Allen, S., & Lando, H. (1992). Smoking cessation in women concerned about weight gain. *American Journal of Public Health, 82,* 1238–1243.

Pirie, P. L., Murray, D. M., & Luepker, R. V. (1991). Gender differences in cigarette smoking and quitting in a cohort of young adults. *American Journal of Public Health, 81,* 324–327.

Pi-Sunyer, X. (1993). Medical hazards of obesity. *Annals of Internal Medicine, 119,* 655–660.

Plaut, S. M., & Friedman, S. B. (1981). Psychosocial factors in infectious disease. In R. Ader (Ed.), *Psychoneuroimmunology* (pp. 3–30). New York: Academic Press.

Po-Huang, C., Nomura, A. M. Y., & Stemmermann, G. N. (1992). A prospective study of the attributable risk of cancer due to cigarette smoking. *American Journal of Public Health, 82,* 37–40.

Polich, J. M., Armor, D. J., & Braiker, H. B. (1980). *The course of alcoholism: Four years after treatment.* Santa Monica, CA: Rand.

Polivy, J., Heatherton, T. F., & Herman, C. P. (1988). Self-esteem, restraint, and eating behavior. *Journal of Abnormal Psychology, 97,* 354–356.

Polivy, J., & Herman, C. P. (1983). *Breaking the diet habit: The natural weight alternative.* New York: Basic Books.

Pollock, M. L., Wilmore, J. H., & Fox, S. M., III. (1978). *Health and fitness through physical activity.* New York: Wiley.

Pomerleau, O. F. (1980). Why people smoke: Current psychobiological models. In P. O. Davidson & S. M. Davidson (Eds.), *Behavioral medicine: Changing health lifestyles* (pp. 94–115). New York: Brunner/Mazel.

Pomerleau, O. F. (1982). A discourse on behavioral medicine: Current status and future trends. *Journal of Consulting and Clinical Psychology, 50,* 1030–1039.

Pomerleau, O. F., Fertig, J. B., Seyler, E. L., & Jaffe, J. (1983). Neuroendocrine reactivity to nicotine in smokers. *Psychopharmacology, 81,* 61–67.

Pope, H. G., Jr., & Hudson, J. I. (1984). *New hope for binge eaters: Advances in the understanding and treatment of bulimia.* New York: Harper & Row.

Pope, H. G., Jr., Hudson, J. I., Jonas, J. M., & Yurgelun-Todd, D. (1983). Bulimia treated with imipramine: A placebo-controlled double-blind study. *American Journal of Psychiatry, 140,* 554–558.

Pope, H. G., Jr., Hudson, J. I., & Yurgelun-Todd, D. (1984). Anorexia nervosa and bulimia among 300 suburban women shoppers. *American Journal of Psychiatry, 141,* 292–293.

Popham, R. E. (1978). The social history of the tavern. In Y. Israel, F. B. Glaser, H. Kalant, R. E. Popham, W. Schmidt, & R. G. Smart (Eds.), *Research advances in alcohol and drug problems* (Vol. 2, pp. 225–302). New York: Plenum.

Popham, R. E., Schmidt, W., & Israelstam, S. (1984). Heavy alcohol consumption and physical health problems: A review of the epidemiologic evidence. In R. G. Smart, H. D. Cappell, F. B. Glaser, Y. Israel, H. Kalant, R. E. Popham, W. Schmidt, & E. M. Sellers (Eds.), *Research advances in alcohol and drug problems* (Vol. 8). New York: Plenum.

Porter, J., & Jick, H. (1980). Addiction rate in patients treated with narcotics. *New England Journal of Medicine, 302,* 123.

Pratt, O. E. (1980). The fetal alcohol syndrome: Transport of nutrients and transfer of alcohol and acetaldehyde from mother to fetus. In M. Sandler (Ed.), *Psychopharmacology of alcohol.* New York: Raven.

Pratt, O. E. (1982). Alcohol and the developing fetus. *British Medical Bulletin, 38,* 48–52.

Price, J. H., Desmond, S. M., & Losh, D. P. (1991). Patients' expectations of the family physician in health promotion. *American Journal of Preventive Medicine, 7,* 33–39.

Prochaska, J. O. (1994). Strong and weak principles for progressing from precontemplation to action on the basis of twelve problem behaviors. *Health Psychology, 13,* 47–51.

Prochaska, J. O., & DiClemente, C. C. (1983). Stages and processes of self-change of smoking: Toward an integrative model of change. *Journal of Consulting and Clinical Psychology, 51,* 390–395.

Prochaska, J. O., DiClemente, C. C., & Norcross, J. C. (1992). In search of how people change: Applications to addictive behaviors. *American Psychologist, 47,* 1102–1114.

Prochaska, J. O., Redding, C. A., Harlow, L. L., Rossi, J. S., & Velicer, W. F. (1994). The transtheoretical model of change and HIV prevention: A review. *Health Education Quarterly, 21,* 471–486.

Prochaska, J. O., Velicer, W. F., Rossi, J. S., Goldstein, M. G., Marcus, B. H., Rakowski, W., Flore, C., Harlow, L. L., Redding, C. A., Rosenbloom, D., & Rossi, S. R. (1994). Stages of change and decisional balance for 12 problem behaviors. *Health Psychology, 13,* 39–46.

Prohaska, T. R., Keller, U. L., Leventhal, E. A., & Leventhal, H. (1987). Impact of symptoms and aging attribution on emotions and coping. *Health Psychology, 6,* 495–514.

Prokop, C. K., Bradley, L. A., Margolis, R., & Gentry, W. D. (1980). Multivariate analysis of the MMPI profiles of multiple pain patients. *Journal of Personality Assessment, 44,* 246–252.

Ptacek, J. T., Smith, R. E., & Zanas, J. (1992). Gender, appraisal, and coping: A longitudinal analysis. *Journal of Personality, 60,* 747–770.

Public Health Service. (1981). Surgeon General's advisory on alcohol and pregnancy. *FDA Drug Bulletin, 11*(2), 9–10.

Pukish, M. M., & Tucker, J. A. (1994, August). *Natural recovery from alcoholism: Contexts surrounding abstinent and moderation outcomes.* Paper presented at the 102nd convention of the American Psychological Association, Los Angeles, CA.

Puska, P. (1984). Community-based prevention of cardiovascular disease: The North Karelia Project. In J. D. Matarazzo, S. M. Weiss, J. A. Herd, N. E. Miller, & S. M. Weiss (Eds.), *Behavioral health: A handbook of health enhancement and disease prevention* (pp. 1140–1147). New York: Wiley.

Puska, P., & Mustaniemi, H. (1975). Incidence and presentation of myocardial infarction in North Karelia, Finland. *Acta Medicus Scandinavia, 197,* 211–216.

Pyle, R. L., Mitchell, J. E., & Eckert, E. D. (1981). Bulimia: A report of 34 cases. *Journal of Clinical Psychiatry, 42,* 60–64.

Pyle, R. L., Mitchell, J. E., Eckert, E. D., Halvorson, P. A., Neuman, P. A., & Goff, G. M. (1983). The incidence of bulimia in freshman college students. *International Journal of Eating Disorders, 2,* 75–85.

Rabins, P. V. (1989). Behavior problems in the demented. In E. Light & B. D. Lebowitz (Eds.), *Alzheimer's disease treatment and family stress: Directions for research* (pp. 322–339). (DHHS Publication No. ADM 89-1569). Washington, DC: U.S. Government Printing Office.

Rabkin, J. G. (1993). Stress and psychiatric disorders. In L. Goldberger & S. Breznitz (Eds.), *Handbook of stress: Theoretical and clinical aspects* (2nd ed., pp. 477–495). New York: Free Press

Rabkin, J. G., & Struening, E. L. (1976). Life events, stress, and illness. *Science, 194,* 1013–1020.

Radford, E. P., & Renard, K. G. S. C. (1984). Lung cancer in Swedish iron miners exposed to low doses of radon daughters. *New England Journal of Medicine, 310,* 1485–1494.

Ragland, D. R., & Brand, R. J. (1988a). Coronary heart disease mortality in the Western Collaborative Group Study: Follow-up experience of 22 years. *American Journal of Epidemiology, 127,* 462–475.

Ragland, D. R., & Brand, R. J. (1988b). Type A behavior and mortality from coronary heart disease. *New England Journal of Medicine, 318,* 65–69.

Rahe, R. H. (1984). Developments in life change measurement: Subjective life change unit scaling. In B. S. Dohrenwend & B. R. Dohrenwend (Eds.), *Stressful life events and their contexts.* New Brunswick, NJ: Rutgers University Press.

Rahe, R. H., Romo, M., Bennett, L., & Siltanen, P. (1974). Recent life changes, myocardial infarction, and abrupt coronary death. *Archives of Internal Medicine, 133,* 221–228.

Raitakari, O. T., Porkka, V. K., Taimela, S., Telama, R., Räsänen, L. & Vükai, J. S. A. (1994). Effects of persistent physical activity and inactivity on coronary risk factors in children and young adults: The Cardiovascular Risk in Young Finns study. *American Journal of Epidemiology, 140,* 195–205.

Ramirez, S. (1995). Key elements for quality health promotion programs. *Wellness Management: Newsletter of the National Wellness Association, 11*(2), 1, 4.

Rand, C. S. W., & Stunkard, A. J. (1983). Obesity and psychoanalysis: Treatment and four-year follow-up. *American Journal of Psychiatry, 140,* 1140–1144.

Rankin, R. (1969). Air pollution control and public apathy. *Journal of the Air Pollution Control Association, 19,* 565–569.

Raphael, K. G., Cloitre, M., & Dohrenwend, B. P. (1991). Problems of recall and misclassification with checklist methods of measuring stressful life events. *Health Psychology, 10,* 62–74.

Rasmussen, B. K. (1993). Migraine and tension-type headache in a general population: Precipitating factors, female hormones, sleep patttern and relation to lifestyle. *Pain, 53,* 65–72.

Ratliff-Crain, J., Temoshok, L., Kiecolt-Glaser, J. K., & Tamarkin, L. (1989). Issues in psychoneuroimmunology. *Health Psychology, 8,* 747–752.

Ratner, H., Gross, L., Casas, J., & Castells, S. (1990). A hypnotherapeutic approach to improvement of compliance in adolescent diabetics. *American Journal of Clinical Hypnosis, 32,* 154–159.

Reed, D. M., LaCroix, A. Z., Karasek, R. A., Miller, D., & MacLean, C. A. (1989). Occupational strain and the incidence of coronary heart disease. *American Journal of Epidemiology, 129,* 495–502.

Reed, D. M., MacLean, C. J., & Hayash, T. (1987). Predictors of atherosclerosis in the Honolulu Heart Program: Biologic, dietary, and lifestyle characteristics. *American Journal of Epidemiology, 126,* 214–225.

Reifler, B. V., & Larson, E. (1989). Excess disability in dementia of the Alzheimer's type. In E. Light & B. D. Lebowitz (Eds.), *Alzheimer's disease treatment and family stess: Directions for research* (pp. 363–382). (DHHS Publication No. ADM 89-1569). Washington, DC: U.S. Government Printing Office.

Reis, H. T., Wheeler, L., Kernis, M. H., Spiegel, N., & Nezlek, J. (1985). On specificity in the impact of social participation on physical and psychological health. *Journal of Personality and Social Psychology, 48,* 456–471.

Rejeski, W. J., Brubaker, P. H., Herb, R. A., Kaplan, J. R., & Koritnik, D. (1988). Anabolic steroids and aggressive behavior in Cynomolgus monkeys. *Journal of Behavioral Medicine, 11,* 95–105.

Rejeski, W. J., Thompson, A., Brubaker, P. H., & Miller, H. S. (1992). Acute exercise: Buffering psychosocial stress responses in women. *Health Psychology, 11,* 355–362.

Remington, P. L., Forman, M. R., Gentry, E. M., Marks, J. S., Hogelin, G. S., & Trowbridge, F. L. (1985). Current smoking trends in the United States. The 1981–1983 Behavioral Risk Factor Surveys. *Journal of the American Medical Association, 253,* 2975–2978.

Repetti, R. L. (1993a). The effects of workload and the social environment at work on health. In L. Goldberger & S. Breznitz (Eds.), *Handbook of stress: Theoretical and clinical aspects* (2nd ed., pp. 368–385). New York: Free Press.

Repetti, R. L. (1993b). Short-term effects of occupational stressors on daily mood and health complaints. *Health Psychology, 12,* 125–131.

Reppucci, J. D., Revenson, T. A., Aber, M., & Reppucci, N. D. (1991). Unrealistic optimism among adolescent smokers and nonsmokers. *Journal of Primary Prevention, 11,* 227–236.

Resnick, H. S., Kilpatrick, D. G., Best, C. L., & Kramer, T. L. (1992). Vulnerability-stress factors in development of post-traumatic stress disorder. *Journal of Nervous and Mental Disease, 180,* 424–430.

Revicki, D. A., & May, H. J. (1985). Occupational stress, social support, and depression. *Health Psychology, 4,* 61–77.

Reynolds, P., & Kaplan, G. A. (1990). Social connections and risk for cancer: Prospective evidence from the Alameda County Study. *Behavioral Medicine, 16,* 101–110.

Richardson, J. L., Zarnegar, Z., Bisno, B., & Levine, A. (1990). Psychosocial status at initiation of cancer treatment and survival. *Journal of Psychosomatic Research, 34,* 189–201.

Ridker, P. M., Hennekens, C. H., & Stampfer, M. J. (1993). A prospective study of lipoprotein(a) and the risk of myocardial infarction. *Journal of the American Medical Association, 270,* 2195–2199.

Ridker, P. M., Vaughan, D. E., Stampfer, M. J., Glynn, R. J., & Hennekens, C. H. (1994). Association of moderate alcohol consumption and plasma concentration of endogenous tissue-type plasminogen activator. *Journal of the American Medical Association, 272,* 929–933.

Riger, S. (1985). Crime as an environmental stressor. *Journal of Community Psychology, 13,* 270–280.

Rimberg, H. M., & Lewis, R. J. (1994). Older adolescents and AIDS: Correlates of self-reported safer sex practices. *Journal of Research on Adolescence, 4,* 453–464.

Rimer, B., & Glassman, B. (1984). How do persuasive health messages work: A health education field study. *Health Education Quarterly, 11,* 313–321.

Rimm, E. B., Stampfer, M. J., Ascherio, A., Giovannucci, E., Colditz, G. A., & Willett, W. C. (1993). Vitamin E consumption and risk of coronary heart disease in men. *New England Journal of Medicine, 328,* 1450–1456.

Rimm, E. B., Stampfer, M. J., Giovannucci, E., Ascherio, A., Spiegelman, D., Colditz, G. A., & Willett, W. C. (1995). Body size and fat distribution as predictors of coronary heart disease among middle-age and older US men. *American Journal of Epidemiology, 141,* 1117–1127.

Risch, H. A., Howe, G. R., Jain, M., Burch, J. D., Holoway, E. J., & Miller, A. G. (1993). Are female smokers at higher risk for lung cancer than male smokers? *American Journal of Epidemiology, 138,* 281–293.

Ritchie, K., & Kildea, D. (1995). Is senile dementia "age-related" or "ageing-related"? — Evidence from meta-analysis of dementia prevalence in the oldest old. *Lancet, 346,* 931–934.

Roberts, T. G., Fournet, G. P., & Penland, E. (1995). A comparison of the attitudes toward alcohol and drug use and school support by grade level, gender, and ethnicity. *Journal of Alcohol and Drug Education, 40,* 112–127.

Robertson, I. H., & Heather, N. (1982). A survey of controlled drinking treatment in Britain. *British Journal on Alcohol and Alcoholism, 17,* 102–105.

Robertson, L. S. (1984). Behavior and injury prevention: Whose behavior? In J. D. Matarazzo, S. M. Weiss, J. A. Herd, N. E. Miller, & S. M. Weiss (Eds.), *Behavioral health: A handbook of health enhancement and disease prevention* (pp. 980–989). New York: Wiley.

Robertson, L. S. (1996). Reducing death on the road: The effects of minimum safety standards, publicized crash tests, seat belts, and alcohol. *American Journal of Public Health, 86,* 31–34.

Robine, J-M., & Ritchie, K. (1991). Healthy life expectancy: Evaluation of global indicator of change in population health. *British Medical Journal, 302,* 457–460.

Robins, L. N. (1995). Editorial: The natural history of substance use as a guide to setting drug policy. *American Journal of Public Health, 85,* 12–13.

Rodin, J. (1992). *Body traps.* New York: William Morrow.

Rodin, J., & Baum, A. (1978). Crowding and helplessness: Potential consequences of density and loss of control. In A. Baum & Y. M. Epstein (Eds.), *Human response to crowding* (pp. 389–401). Hillsdale, NJ: Erlbaum.

Rodin, J., & Langer, E. J. (1977). Long-term effects of a control-relevant intervention with the institutionalized aged. *Journal of Personality and Social Psychology, 35,* 897–902.

Rodin, J., & Salovey, P. (1989). Health psychology. *Annual Review of Psychology, 40,* 533–579.

Rodin, J., & Stone, G. C. (1987). Historical highlights in the emergence of the field. In G. C. Stone, S. M. Weiss, J. D. Matarazzo, N. E. Miller, J. Rodin, C. D. Belar, M. J. Follick, & J. E. Singer (Eds.), *Health psychology: A discipline and a profession* (pp. 15–26). Chicago: University of Chicago Press.

Rogers, R. G. (1992). Living and dying in the U.S.A.: Sociodemographic determinants of death among blacks and whites. *Demography, 29,* 287–303.

Rohsenow, D. J. (1982). Social anxiety, daily moods, and alcohol use over time among heavy social drinking men. *Addictive Behaviors, 7,* 311–315.

Ronis, D. L., & Kaiser, M. K. (1989). Correlates of breast self-examination in a sample of college women: Analyses of linear structural relations. *Journal of Applied Social Psychology, 19,* 1068–1084.

Room, R. (1972). Comments on Robinson, D. "The alcohologist's addiction." *Quarterly Journal of Studies on Alcohol, 33,* 1049–1059.

Room, R., & Day, N. (1974). Alcohol and mortality. In M. Keller (Ed.), *Second special report to the U.S. Congress: Alcohol and health.* Washington, DC: U.S. Government Printing Office.

Room, R., & Greenfield, T. (1993). Alcoholics Anonymous, other 12-step movements and psychotherapy in the US population, 1990. *Addiction, 88,* 555–562.

Rorabaugh, W. C. (1979). *The alcoholic republic: An American tradition.* New York: Oxford University Press.

Rorer, B., Tucker, C. M., & Blake, H. (1988). Long-term nurse-patient interactions: Factors in patient compliance or noncompliance to the dietary regimen. *Health Psychology, 7,* 35–46.

Rosen, G. (1958). *A history of public health.* New York: MD Publications.

Rosen, J. C., & Gross, J. (1987). Prevalence of weight reducing and weight gaining in adolescent girls and boys. *Health Psychology, 6,* 131–147.

Rosen, M., Nystrom, L., & Wall, S. (1988). Diet and cancer mortality in the counties of Sweden. *American Journal of Epidemiology, 127,* 42–49.

Rosenbaum, M. (1988). Learned resourcefulness, stress, and self-regulation. In S. Fisher & J. Reason (Eds.), *Handbook of life stress, cognition, and health* (pp. 483–496). Chichester, UK: Wiley.

Rosenbaum, M. (1990). The role of learned resourcefulness in the self-control of health behavior. In M. Rosenbaum (Ed.), *Learned resourcefulness: On coping skills, self-control, and adaptive behavior* (pp. 3–30). New York: Springer.

Rosenberg, H. (1993). Prediction of controlled drinking by alcoholics and problem drinkers. *Psychological Bulletin, 113,* 129–139.

Rosenberg, M. L., & Fenley, M. A. (1992). The federal role in injury control. *American Psychologist, 47,* 1931–1935.

Rosenberg, L., Palmer, J. R., Miller, D. R., Clarke, E. A., & Shapiro, S. (1990). A case-control study of alcoholic beverage consumption and breast cancer. *American Journal of Epdemiology, 131,* 6–14.

Rosenberg, L., Palmer, J. R., & Shapiro, S. (1990). Decline in the risk of myocardial infarction among women who stop smoking. *New England Journal of Medicine, 322,* 213–217.

Rosenfield, S. (1992). The costs of sharing: Wives' employment and husbands' mental health. *Journal of Health and Social Behavior, 33,* 213–225.

Rosengren, A., Tibblin, G., & Wilhelmsen, L. (1991). Self-perceived psychological stress and incidence of coronary artery disease in middle-aged men. *American Journal of Cardiology, 68,* 1171–1175.

Rosenman, R. H. (1993). Relationships of the Type A Behavior Pattern with Coronary Heart Disease. In L. Goldberger & S. Breznitz (Eds.), *Handbook of stress: Theoretical and clinical aspects* (2nd ed., pp. 449–476). New York: Free Press.

Rosenman, R. H., Brand, R. J., Jenkins, C. D., Friedman, M., Straus, R., & Wurm, M. (1975). Coronary heart disease in the Western Collaborative Group Study: Final follow-up of 8½ years. *Journal of the American Medical Association, 233,* 872–877.

Rosenstock, I. M. (1990). The health belief model: Explaining health behavior through expectancies. In K. Glanz, F. M. Lewis, & B. K. Rimer (Eds.), *Health behavior and health education: Theory, research, and practice* (pp. 39–62). San Francisco: Jossey-Bass.

Rosenstock, I., M., Strecher, V. J., & Becker, M. H. (1988). Social learning theory and the Health Belief Model. *Health Education Quarterly, 15,* 175–183.

Rosenstock, I. M., & Kirscht, J. P. (1979). Why people seek health care. In G. C. Stone, F. Cohen, & N. E. Adler (Eds.), *Health psychology—A handbook* (pp. 161–188). San Francisco: Jossey-Bass.

Rosenthal, D. (1970). *Genetic theory and abnormal behavior.* New York: McGraw-Hill.

Roskies, E., Seraganian, P., Oseasohn, R., Hanley, J. A., Collu, R., Martin, N., & Smilga, C. (1986). The Montreal Type A Intervention Project: Major findings. *Health Psychology, 5,* 45–69.

Ross, C. E. (1993). Fear of victimization and health. *Journal of Quantitative Criminology, 9,* 159–175.

Ross, C. E., & Hayes, D. (1988). Exercise and psychologic well-being in the community. *American Journal of Epidemiology, 127,* 762–771.

Rost, K., Carter, W., & Innui, T. (1989). Introduction of information during the initial medical visit: Consequences for patient follow-through with physician recommendations for medication. *Social Science and Medicine, 28,* 315–321.

Roter, D. L. (1988). Reciprocity in the medical encounter. In D. S. Gochman (Ed.), *Health behavior: Emerging research perspectives* (pp. 293–303). New York: Plenum.

Roth, D. L., & Holmes, D. S. (1985). Influence of physical fitness in deterring the impact of stressful events on physical and psychologic health. *Psychosomatic Medicine, 47,* 164–173.

Roth, H. P. (1987). Measurement of compliance. *Patient Education and Counseling, 10,* 107–116.

Roth, H. P., & Caron, H. S. (1978). Accuracy of doctors' estimates and patients' statements on adherence to a drug regimen. *Clinical Pharmacology and Therapeutics, 23,* 361–370.

Rotter, J. B. (1966). Generalized expectancies for internal versus external control of reinforcement. *Psychological Monographs, 80* (Whole No. 609).

Rotter, J. B. (1982). *The development and applications of social learning theory: Selected papers.* New York: Praeger.

Rotton, J., Yoshikawa, J., & Kaplan, F. (1979). *Perceived control, malodorous air pollution and behavioral aftereffects.* Paper presented at the annual meeting of the Southeastern Psychological Association, New Orleans.

Routh, D. K., & Sanfilippo, M. D. (1991). Helping children cope with painful medical procedures. In J. P. Bush & S. W. Harkins (Eds.), *Children in pain: Clinical and research issues from a developmental perspective* (pp. 397–424). New York: Springer-Verlag.

Ruch-Ross, H. S., & O'Connor, K. G. (1993). Bicycle helmet counseling by pediatricians: A random national survey. *American Journal of Public Health, 83,* 728–730.

Rudy, T. E., Turk, D. C., Zaki, H. S., & Curtin, H. D. (1989). An empirical taxometric alternative to traditional classification of temporomandibular disorders. *Pain, 36,* 311–320.

Rueter, M. A., & Harris, D. V. (1980, August). *The effects of running on individuals who are clinically depressed.* Paper presented at the annual meeting of the American Psychological Association, Montreal.

Ruiz, P., & Ruiz, P. P. (1983). Treatment compliance among Hispanics. *Journal of Operational Psychiatry, 14,* 112–114.

Runyon, C. W., & Runyon, D. K. (1991). How can physicians get kids to wear bicycle helmets? A prototypic challenge in injury prevention. *American Journal of Public Health, 81,* 972–973.

Russell, L. B. (1986). *Is prevention better than cure?* Washington, DC: Brookings Institution.

Russell, L. B. (1987). *Evaluating preventive care.* Washington, DC: Brookings Institution.

Russell, N K., & Roter, D. L. (1993). Health promotion counseling of chronic-disease patients during primary care visits. *American Journal of Public Health, 83,* 979–982.

Ruuskanen, J. M., & Parkatti, T. (1994). Physical activity and related factors among nursing home residents. *Journal of the American Geriatrics Society, 42,* 987–991.

Ryan, W. (1971). *Blaming the victim.* New York: Pantheon.

Rybstein-Blinchik, E. (1979). Effects of different cognitive strategies on chronic pain experience. *Journal of Behavioral Medicine, 2,* 93–101.

Rzewnicki, R., & Forgays, D. G. (1987). Recidivism and self-cure of smoking and obesity: An attempt to replicate. *American Psychologist, 42,* 97–100.

Saah, A. J., Hoover, D. R., Peng, Y., Phair, J. P., Visscher, B., Kingsley, L. A., & Schrager, L. K. (1995). Predictors for failure of *Pneumocystis carinii* pneumonia prophylaxis. *Journal of the American Medical Association, 273,* 1197–1202.

Sachs, M. L. (1981). Running addiction. In M. H. Sacks (Ed.), *Psychology of running* (pp. 116–126). Champaign, IL: Human Kinetics Publishers.

Sachs, M. L. (1982). Compliance and addiction to exercise. In R. C. Cantu (Ed.), *The exercising adult* (pp. 19–27). Lexington, MA: Collamore Press.

Sachs, M. L., & Pargman, D. (1979). Running addiction: A depth interview examination. *Journal of Sport Behavior, 2,* 143–155.

Sackett, D. L. (1976). The magnitude of compliance and non-compliance. In D. L. Sackett & R. B. Haynes (Eds.), *Compliance with therapeutic regimen* (pp. 9–25). Baltimore: Johns Hopkins University Press.

Sackett, D. L., & Haynes, R. B. (Eds.). (1976). *Compliance with therapeutic regimen.* Baltimore: Johns Hopkins University Press.

Sackett, D. L., & Snow, J. C. (1979). The magnitude of compliance and noncompliance. In R. B. Haynes, D. W. Taylor, & D. L. Sackett (Eds.), *Compliance in health care* (pp. 11–22). Baltimore: Johns Hopkins University Press.

Sacks, F. M., Donner, A., Castelli, W. P., Gronemeyer, J., Pletka, P., Margolius, H. S., Landsberg, L., & Kass, E. H. (1981). Effect of ingestion of meat on plasma cholesterol of vegetarians. *Journal of the American Medical Association, 246,* 640–644.

Sacks, J. J., Holingreen, P., Smith, S. M., & Sosin, D. M. (1991). Bicycle-associated head injuries and deaths in the United States from 1984 through 1988. *Journal of the American Medical Association, 266,* 3016–3018.

Sacks, J. J., & Nelson, D. E. (1994). Smoking and injuries: An overview. *Preventive Medicine, 23,* 515–520.

Sacks, M. H. (1993). Exercise for stress control. In D. Goleman & J. Gurin (Eds.), *Mind/body medicine: How to use your mind for better health* (pp. 316–327). Yonkers, NY: Consumer Reports Books.

Sallan, S. E., Zinberg, N. E., & Frei, E., III. (1975). Antiemetic effect of delta-9-tetrahydrocannabinol in patients receiving cancer chemotherapy. *New England Journal of Medicine, 293,* 795–797.

Salonen, J. T., Alfthan, G., Huttunen, J. K., & Puska, P. (1984). Association between serum selenium and the risk of cancer. *American Journal of Epidemiology, 120,* 342–349.

Sanchez-Craig, M., Wilkinson, A., & Davila, R. (1995). Empirically based guidelines for moderate drinking: 1-year results from three studies with problem drinkers. *American Journal of Public Health, 85,* 823–828.

Sanders, M. R., Shepherd, R. W., Cleghorn, G., & Woolford, H. (1994). The treatment of recurrent abdominal pain in children: A controlled comparison of cognitive-behavioral family intervention and standard pediatric care. *Journal of Consulting and Clinical Psychology, 62,* 306–314.

Sandivk, L., Eridssen, J., Thaulow, E., Erikssen, G., Mundal, R., & Rodahl, K. (1993). Physical fitness as a predictor of mortality among healthy, middle-aged Norwegian men. *New England Journal of Medicine, 328,* 533–537.

Sandler, D. P., Comstock, G. W., Helsing, K. J., & Shore, D. L. (1989). Deaths from all causes in non-smokers who lived with smokers. *American Journal of Public Health, 79,* 163–167.

Sarason, B. R., & Sarason, I. G. (1994). Assessment of social support. In S. A. Shumaker & S. M. Czajkowski (Eds.), *Social support and cardiovascular disease* (pp. 41–63). New York: Plenum.

Sarason, I. G., Sarason, B. R., & Johnson, J. H. (1985). Stressful life events: Measurement, moderators, and adaptation. In S. R. Burchfield (Ed.), *Stress: Psychological and physiological interactions.* Washington, DC: Hemisphere.

Sargent, J., Solbach, P., Coyne, L., Spohn, H., & Segerson, J. (1986). Results of a controlled, experimental outcome study of nondrug treatments for the control of migraine headaches. *Journal of Behavioral Medicine, 9,* 291–323.

Satariano, W. A., & Syme, S. L. (1981). Life changes and disease in elderly populations: Coping with change. In J. L. McGaugh & S. B. Kiesler (Eds.), *Aging: Biology and behavior* (pp. 311–327). New York: Academic Press.

Schachter, S. (1980). Urinary pH and the psychology of nicotine addiction. In P. O. Davidson & S. M. Davidson (Eds.), *Behavioral medicine: Changing health lifestyles* (pp. 70–93). New York: Brunner/Mazel.

Schachter, S. (1982). Recidivism and self-cure of smoking and obesity. *American Psychologist, 37,* 436–444.

Schachter, S., Goldman, R., & Gordon, A. (1968). Effects of fear, food deprivation, and obesity on eating. *Journal of Personality and Social Psychology, 10,* 107–116.

Schachter, S., & Singer, J. E. (1962). Cognitive, social, and physiological determinants of emotional state. *Psychological Review, 69,* 379–399.

Schaefer, E. J., Lamon-Fava, S., Jenner, J. L., McNamara, J. R., Ordovas, J. M., Davis, C. E., Abolafia, J. M., Lippel, K., & Levy, R. I. (1994). Lipoprotein(a) levels and risk of coronary heart disease in men: The Lipid Research Clinics Coronary Primary Prevention Trial. *Journal of the American Medical Association, 271,* 999–1003.

Schaeffer, M., Street, S., Singer, J., & Baum, A. (1988). Effects of control on the stress reaction of commuters. *Journal of Applied Social Psychology, 18,* 944–957.

Scharff, L., & Marcus, D. A. (1994). Interdisciplinary outpatient group treatment of intractable headache. *Headache, 34,* 73–78.

Schatzkin, A., Jones, D. Y., Hoover, R. N., Taylor, P. R., Brinton, L. A., Ziegler, R. G., Harvey, E. B., Carter, C. L., Licitra, L. M., Dufour, M. C., & Larson, D. B. (1987). Alcohol consumption and breast cancer in the epidemiologic follow-up study of the first National Health and Nutrition Examination Survey. *New England Journal of Medicine, 316,* 1169–1173.

Scheier, M. F., Matthews, K. A., Owens, J. F., Magovern, G. J., Sr., Lefebvre, R. C., Abbott, R. A., & Carver, C. S. (1989). Dispositional optimism and recovery from coronary artery bypass surgery: The beneficial effects on physical and psychological well-being. *Journal of Personality and Social Psychology, 57,* 1024–1040.

Scherr, P. A., LaCroix, A. Z., Wallace, R. B., Berkman, L., Curb, J. D., Cornoni-Huntley, J., Evans, D. A., & Hennekens, C. H. (1992). Light to moderate alcohol consumption and mortality in the elderly. *Journal of the American Geriatrics Society, 40,* 651–657.

Scherwitz, L., Perkins, L., Chesney, M., & Hughes, G. (1991). Cook-Medley Hostility Scale and subsets: Relationship to demographic and psychosocial characteristics in young adults in the CARDIA study. *Psychomatic Medicine, 53,* 36–49.

Scherwitz, L. W., Perkins, L. L., Chesney, M. A., Hughes, G. H., Sidney, S., & Manollo, T. A. (1992). Hostility and health behaviors in young adults: The CARDIA Study. *American Journal of Epidemiology, 136,* 136–145.

Schiffman, S. S. (1983). Taste and smell in disease (Second of two parts). *New England Journal of Medicine, 308,* 1337–1342.

Schiffman, S. S., Musante, G., & Conger, J. (1978). Application of multidimensional scaling to ratings of foods for obese and normal weight individuals. *Physiology and Behavior, 21,* 417–422.

Schindler, L. W. (1992). *Understanding the immune system.* NIH Publication No. 92-529. Washington, DC: U.S. Department of Health and Human Services.

Schinke, S. P. (1994). Prevention science and practice: An agenda for action. *Journal of Primary Prevention, 15,* 45–57.

Schleifer, S. J., Keller, S. E., Camerino, M., Thorton, J. C., & Stein, M. (1983). Suppression of lymphocyte stimulation following bereavement. *Journal of the American Medical Association, 250,* 374–377.

Schmelkin, L. P., Wachtel, A. B., Schneiderman, B. E., & Hecht, D. (1988). The dimensional structure of medical students' perception of diseases. *Journal of Behavioral Medicine, 11,* 171–183.

Schmied, L. A., & Lawler, K. A. (1986). Hardiness, Type A behavior, and the stress-illness relation in working women. *Journal of Personality and Social Psychology, 51,* 1218–1223.

Schmitz, A. (1991, November). Food news blues. *Health,* 40-47. Also in R. Yarian (Ed.), *Health 95/96* (pp. 237–240). Guilford, CT: Dushkin Publishing Group.

Schnall, P. L., Pieper, C., Schwartz, J. E., Karasek, R. A., Schlussel, Y., Devereaux, R. B., Ganau, A., Alderman, M., Warren, K., & Pickering, T. G. (1990). The relationship between "job-strain" workplace diastolic blood pressure, and left ventricular mass index. *Journal of the American Medical Association, 263,* 1929–1935.

Schneider, W. J., & Nevid, J. S. (1993). Overcoming math anxiety: A comparison of stress inoculation training and systemic desensitization. *Journal of College Student Development, 34,* 283–288.

Schoenbach, V. J., Kaplan, B. H., Fredman, L., & Kleinbaum, D. G. (1986). Social ties and mortality in Evans County, Georgia. *American Journal of Epidemiology, 123,* 577–591.

Schoenberg, J. B., Wilcox, H. B., Mason, T. J., Bill, J., & Sternhagen, A. (1989). Variation in smoking-related lung cancer risk among New Jersey women. *American Journal of Epidemiology, 130,* 688–695.

Schofield, W. (1969). The role of psychology in the delivery of health services. *American Psychologist, 24,* 568–584.

Schotte, D. E., & Stunkard, A. J. (1987). Bulimia vs. bulimic behaviors on a college campus. *Journal of the American Medical Association, 258,* 1213–1215.

Schradle, S. B., & Dougher, M. J. (1985). Social support as a mediator of stress: Theoretical and empirical issues. *Clinical Psychology Review, 5,* 641–661.

Schuman, M. (1982). Biofeedback in the management of chronic pain. In J. Barber & C. Adrian (Eds.), *Psychological approaches to the management of pain* (pp. 150–167). New York: Brunner/Mazel.

Schürmann, K. (1975). Surgical treatment: Fundamental principles of the surgical treatment of pain. In M. Weisenberg (Ed.), *Pain: Clinical and experimental perspectives* (pp. 261–274). St. Louis: Mosby.

Schwartz, D. M., & Thompson, M. G. (1981). Do anorectics get well? Current research and future needs. *American Journal of Psychiatry, 138,* 319–323.

Schwartz, G. E., & Weiss, S. M. (1978). Behavioral medicine revisited: An amended definition. *Journal of Behavioral Medicine, 1,* 249–251.

Schwartz, J. L. (1987). *Review and evaluation of smoking cessation methods, the United States and Canada, 1978–1985.* (NIH Publication No. 87-2940). Washington, DC: U.S. Government Printing Office.

Schwarz, D. F., Grisso, J. A., Miles, C., Holmes, J. H., & Sutton, R. L. (1993). An injury prevention program in an urban African-American community. *American Journal of Public Health, 83,* 675–680.

Schwarzer, R., & Leppin, A. (1989). Social support and health: A meta-analysis. *Psychology and Health, 3,* 1–15.

Schwarzer, R., & Leppin, A. (1992). Possible impact of social ties and support on morbidity and mortality. In H. O. E. Veiel & U. Baumann (Eds.), *The meaning and measurement of social support* (pp. 65–83). New York: Hemisphere.

Sclafani, A., & Springer, D. (1976). Dietary obesity in adult rats: Similarities to hypothalamic and human obesity. *Physiology and Behavior, 17,* 461–471.

Scragg, R., Stewart, A., Jackson, R., & Beaglehole, R. (1987). Alcohol and exercise in myocardial infarction and sudden coronary death in men and women. *American Journal of Epidemiology, 126,* 77–85.

Sechrest, L. (1987). Postdoctoral training in health policy studies. In G. C. Stone, S. M. Weiss, J. D. Matarazzo, N. E. Miller, J. Rodin, C. D. Belar, M. J. Follick, & J. E. Singer (Eds.), *Health psychology: A discipline and a profession* (pp. 389–402). Chicago: University of Chicago Press.

Secretary's Task Force on Alzheimer's Disease. (1984). *Alzheimer's disease.* (DHHS Publication No. ADM 84-1323). Washington, DC: U.S. Government Printing Office.

Self, C. A., & Rogers, R. W. (1990). Coping with threats to health: Effects of persuasive appeals on depressed, normal, and antisocial personalities. *Journal of Behavioral Medicine, 13,* 343–357.

Seligman, M. E. P. (1975). *Helplessness.* San Francisco: Freeman.

Selik, R. M., Chu, S. Y., & Buehler, J. W. (1993). HIV infection as leading cause of death among young adults in US cities and states. *Journal of the American Medical Association, 269,* 2991–2994.

Sellwood, W., & Tarrier, N. (1994). Demographic factors associated with extreme non-compliance in schizophrenia. *Social Psychiatry and Psychiatric Epidemiology, 29,* 172–177.

Selye, H. (1956). *The stress of life.* New York: McGraw-Hill.

Selye, H. (1976). *Stress in health and disease.* Reading, MA: Butterworths.

Selye, H. (1982). History and present status of the stress concept. In L. Goldberger & S. Breznitz (Eds.), *Handbook of stress: Theoretical and clinical aspects* (pp. 7–17). New York: Free Press.

Serdula, M. K., Collins, M. E., Williamson, D. F., Anda, R. F., Pamuk, E., & Byers, T. E. (1993). Weight control practices of U.S. adolescents and adults. *Annals of Internal Medicine, 119,* 667–671.

Shaffer, J. W., Graves, P. L., Swank, R. T., & Pearson, T. A. (1987). Clustering of personality traits in youth and the subsequent development of cancer among physicians. *Journal of Behavioral Medicine, 10,* 441–447.

Shapiro, A. K. (1970). Placebo effects in psychotherapy and psychoanalysis. *Journal of Clinical Pharmacology, 10,* 73–78.

Shapiro, D. H. (1985). Meditation and behavioral medicine: Application of a self-regulation strategy to the clinical management of stress. In S. R. Burchfield (Ed.), *Stress: Psychological and physiological interactions.* Washington, DC: Hemisphere.

Shapiro, S. (1994). Meta-analysis/shmeta-analysis. *American Journal of Epidemiology, 140,* 771–778

Shaw, C. R. (1981). What is cancer and how much is caused by occupational exposure? In C. R. Shaw (Ed.), *Prevention of occupational cancer.* Boca Raton, FL: CRC Press.

Sheidler, V. R. (1987). New methods in analgesic delivery. In D. B. McGuire & C. H. Yarbro (Eds.), *Cancer pain management* (pp. 203–222). Philadelphia: Saunders.

Shekelle, R. B., Hulley, S. B., Neaton, J. D., Billings, J. H., Borhani, N. O., Gerace, T. A., Jacobs, D. R., Lasser, N. L., Mittlemark, M. B., & Stamler, J. (1985). The MRFIT behavior pattern study: II. Type A behavior and incidence of coronary heart disease. *American Journal of Epidemiology, 122,* 559–570.

Shekelle, R. B., Raynar, W. J., Ostfield, A. M., Garron, D. C., Bieliauskas, L. A., Liu, S. C., Maliza, C., & Paul, O. (1981). Psychological depression and 17-year risk of death from cancer. *Psychosomatic Medicine, 43,* 117–125.

Shekelle, R. B., Rossof, A. H., & Stamler, J. (1991). Dietary cholesterol and incidence of lung cancer: The Western Electric study. *American Journal of Epidemiology, 134,* 480–484.

Sher, K. J. (1987). Stress response dampening. In H. T. Blane & K. E. Leonard (Eds.), *Psychological theories of drinking and alcoholism* (pp. 227–271). New York: Guilford Press.

Sher, K. J., & Levenson, R. W. (1982). Risk for alcoholism and individual differences in the stress-response-dampening effect of alcohol. *Journal of Abnormal Psychology, 91,* 350–367.

Sherbourne, C. D., Hays, R. D., Ordway, L., DiMatteo, M. R., & Kravitz, R. L. (1992). Antecedents of adherence to medical recommendations: Results from the Medical Outcomes Study. *Journal of Behavioral Medicine, 15,* 447–468.

Sheridan, E. P., Matarazzo, J. D., Boll, T. J., Perry, N. W., Jr., Weiss, S. M., & Belar, C. D. (1988). Postdoctoral education and training for clinical service providers in health psychology. *Health Psychology, 7,* 1–17.

Sherman, J. E., & Liebeskind, J. C. (1980). An endorphinergic centrifugal substrate of pain modulation: Recent findings, current concepts, and complexities. In J. J. Bonica (Ed.), *Pain.* New York: Raven.

Sherwood, R. J. (1983). Compliance behavior of hemodialysis patients and the role of the family. *Family Systems Medicine, 1,* 60–72.

Shiffman, S. (1989). Trans-situational consistency in smoking relapse. *Health Psychology, 8,* 471–481.

Shipley, R. H., Butt, J. H., Horwitz, B., & Farbry, J. E. (1978). Preparation for a stressful medical procedure: Effects of amount of stimulus preexposure and coping style. *Journal of Consulting and Clinical Psychology, 46,* 499–507.

Shilts, R. (1987). *And the band played on.* New York: St. Martin's Press.

Shore, E. R., Gregory, T., & Tatlock, L. (1991). College students' reactions to a designated driver program: An exploratory study. *Journal of Alcohol and Drug Education, 37,* 1–6.

Shroyer, J. A. (1990). Getting tough on anabolic steroids: Can we win the battle? *The Physician and Sportsmedicine, 18* (2), 106–118.

Sibthorpe, B., & Lear, B. (1994). Circumstances surrounding needle use and transitions among injection drug users: Implications for HIV intervention. *International Journal of the Addictions, 29,* 1245–1257.

Sidney, S., Friedman, G. D., & Siegelaub, A. B. (1987). Thinness and mortality. *American Journal of Public Health, 77,* 317–322.

Siegel, J. M. (1984). Anger and cardiovascular risk in adolescents. *Health Psychology, 3,* 293–313.

Siegel, M. (1993a). Involuntary smoking in the restaurant workplace: A review of employee exposure and health effects. *Journal of the American Medical Association, 270,* 490–493.

Siegel, M. (1993b). Smoking and leukemia: Evaluation of a causal hypothesis. *American Journal of Epidemiology, 138,* 1–9.

Siegel, P. Z., Brackbill, R. M., & Heath, G. W. (1995). The epidemiology of walking for exercise: Implications for promoting activity among sedentary groups. *American Journal of Public Health, 85,* 706–710.

Siegler, I. C., Peterson, B. L., Barefoot, J. C., & Williams, R. B. (1992). Hostility during late adolescence predicts coronary risk factors at mid-life. *American Journal of Epidemiology, 136,* 146–154.

Siegman, A. W. (1993a). Cardiovascular consequences of expressing, experiencing, and repressing anger. *Journal of Behavioral Medicine, 16,* 539–569.

Siegman, A. W. (1993b). Paraverbal correlates stress: Implications for stress identification and management. In L. Goldberger & S. Breznitz (Eds.), *Handbook of stress: Theoretical and clinical aspects* (2nd ed., pp. 274–299). New York: Free Press

Siegman, A. W. (1994). From Type A to hostility to anger: Reflections on the history of coronary-prone behavior. In A. W. Siegman & T. W. Smith (Eds.), *Anger, hostility, and the heart* (pp. 1–21). Hillsdale, NJ: Erlbaum.

Siegman, A. W., Dembroski, T. M., & Ringel, N. (1987). Components of hostility and the severity of coronary artery disease. *Psychosomatic Medicine, 49,* 127–135.

Siegman, A. W., Anderson, R., Herbst, J., Boyle, S., & Wilkinson, J. (1992). Dimensions of anger-hostility and cardiovascular reactivity in provoked and angered men. *Journal of Behavioral Medicine, 15,* 257–272.

Silverberg, I. J. (1991). Kaposi's sarcoma and AIDS-related lymphosarcoma. In M. Dollinger, E. H. Rosenbaum, & G. Cable (Eds.), *Everyone's guide to cancer therapy* (pp. 366–374). Kansas City: Somerville.

Silverstein, B., Feld, S., & Kozlowski, L. T. (1980). The availability of low-nicotine cigarettes as a cause of cigarette smoking in teenage females. *Journal of Health and Social Behavior, 21,* 383–388.

Simone, C. B. (1983). *Cancer and nutrition.* New York: McGraw-Hill.

Simons, A. D., McGowan, C. R., Epstein, L. H., Kupfer, D. J., & Robertson, R. J. (1985). Exercise as a treatment for depression: An update. *Clinical Psychology Review, 5,* 553–568.

Simonton, O. C., & Simonton, S. S. (1975). Belief systems and management of emotional aspects of malignancy. *Journal of Transpersonal Psychology, 7,* 29–47.

Sims, E. A. H. (1974). Studies in human hyperphagia. In G. Bray & J. Bethune (Eds.), *Treatment and management of obesity.* New York: Harper & Row.

Sims, E. A. H. (1976). Experimental obesity, dietary-induced thermogenesis, and their clinical implications. *Clinics in Endocrinology and Metabolism, 5,* 377–395.

Sims, E. A. H., Danforth, E., Jr., Horton, E. S., Bray, G. A., Glennon, J. A., & Salans, L. B. (1973). Endocrine and metabolic effects of experimental obesity in man. *Recent Progress in Hormonal Research, 29,* 457–496.

Sims, E. A. H., & Horton, E. S. (1968). Endocrine and metabolic adaptation to obesity and starvation. *American Journal of Clinical Nutrition, 21,* 1455–1470.

Sinyor, D., Golden, M., Steinert, Y., & Seraganian, P. (1986). Experimental manipulation of aerobic fitness and the response to psychosocial stress: Heart rate and self-report measures. *Psychosomatic Medicine, 48,* 324–337.

Siscovick, D. S., Weiss, N. S., Fletcher, R. H., & Lasky, T. (1984). The incidence of primary cardiac arrest during vigorous exercise. *New England Journal of Medicine, 311,* 874–877.

Siscovick, D. S., Weiss, N. S., Hallstrom, A. P., Inui, T. S., & Peterson, D. R. (1982). Physical activity and primary cardiac arrest. *Journal of the American Medical Association, 248,* 3113–3117.

Sjöström, L. V. (1992a). Morbidity of severely obese subjects. *American Journal of Clinical Nutrition, 55,* 508S–515S.

Sjöström, L. V. (1992b). Mortality of severely obese subjects. *American Journal of Clinical Nutrition, 55,* 516S–523S.

Skelton, J. A. (1991). Laypersons' judgments of patient credibility and the study of illness representations. In J. A. Skelton & R. T. Croyle (Eds.), *Mental representation in health and illness* (pp. 108–131). New York: Springer-Verlag.

Skinner, B. F. (1938). *The behavior of organisms.* Englewood Cliffs, NJ: Prentice-Hall.

Skinner, B. F. (1953). *Science and human behavior.* New York: Macmillan.

Skinner, B. F. (1987). *Upon further reflection.* Englewood Cliffs, NJ: Prentice-Hall.

Slater, J., & Depue, R. A. (1981). The contribution of environmental events and social support to serious suicide attempts in primary depressive disorder. *Journal of Abnormal Psychology, 90,* 275–285.

Slattery, M. L., & Kerber, R. A. (1993). A comprehensive evaluation of family history and breast cancer risk. *Journal of the American Medical Association, 270,* 1563–1568.

Slattery, M. L., Schumacher, M. C., Smith, K. R., West, D. W., & Abd-Elghany, N. (1990). Physical activity, diet, and risk of colon cancer in Utah. *American Journal of Epidemiology, 128,* 989–999.

Slattery, M. L., Sorenson, A. W., Mahoney, A. W., French, T. K., Kritchevsky, D., & Street, J. C. (1988). Diet and colon cancer: Assessment of risk by fiber type and food source. *Journal of the National Cancer Institute, 80,* 474–480.

Sloan, R. P., & Gruman, J. C. (1988). Participation in workplace health promotion programs: The contribution of health and organizational factors. *Health Education Quarterly, 15,* 269–288.

Slochower, J. A. (1983). *Excessive eating: The role of emotions and environment.* New York: Human Sciences Press.

Slyper, A. H. (1994). Low-density lipoprotein density and atherosclerosis: Unraveling the connection. *Journal of the American Medical Association, 272,* 305–308.

Smart, R. G. (1976). Spontaneous recovery in alcoholics: A review and analysis of the available research. *Drug and Alcohol Dependence, 1,* 277–285.

Smith, E. M., Sowers, M. F., & Burns, T. (1984). Effects of smoking on the development of female reproductive cancers. *Journal of the National Cancer Institute, 73,* 371–376.

Smith, M., Colligan, M., Horning, R. W., & Hurrel, J. (1978). *Occupational comparison of stress-related disease incidence.* Cincinnati: National Institute for Occupational Safety and Health.

Smith, T. W. (1994). Concepts and methods in the study of anger, hostility, and health. In A. W. Siegman & T. W. Smith (Eds.), *Anger, hostility, and the heart* (pp. 23–42). Hillsdale, NJ: Erlbaum.

Smith, T. W., & Allred, K. D. (1989). Blood-pressure responses during social interaction in high- and low-cynically hostile males. *Journal of Behavioral Medicine, 12,* 135–143.

Smith, T. W., & Brown, P. C. (1991). Cynical hostility, attempts to exert social control, and cardiovascular reactivity in married couples. *Journal of Behavioral Medicine, 14,* 581–592.

Smith, T. W., Sanders, J. D., & Alexander, J. F. (1990). What does the Cook and Medley Hostility Scale measure? Affect, behavior, and attributions in the marital context. *Journal of Personality and Social Psychology, 58,* 699–708.

Snyder, S. H. (1977, March). Opiate receptors and internal opiates. *Scientific American, 236,* 44–56.

Sobel, D. S. (1995). Rethinking medicine: Improving health outcomes with cost-effective psychosocial interventions. *Psychosomatic Medicine, 57,* 234–244.

Sobell, M. B. (1978). Alternatives to abstinence: Evidence, issues and some proposals. In P. E. Nathan, G. A. Marlatt, & T. Loberg (Eds.), *Alcoholism: New directions in behavioral research and treatment.* New York: Plenum.

Sobell, M. B., & Sobell, L. C. (1973). Individualized behavior therapy for alcoholics. *Behavior Therapy, 4,* 49–72.

Sobell, M. B., & Sobell, L. C. (1976). Second-year treatment outcome of alcoholics treated by individualized behavior therapy: Results. *Behavior Research and Therapy, 14,* 195–215.

Sobell, M. B., & Sobell, L. C. (1978). *Behavioral treatment of alcohol problems: Individualized therapy and controlled drinking.* New York: Plenum.

Sobell, M. B., & Sobell, L. C. (1982). Controlled drinking: A concept coming of age. In K. R. Blankstein & J. Polivy (Eds.), *Self-control and self-modification of emotional behavior: Vol. 7. Advances in the study of communication and affect* (pp. 143–162). New York: Plenum.

Sola, A. E., & Bonica, J. J. (1990). Myofascial pain syndromes. In J. J. Bonica (Ed.), *The management of pain* (2nd ed., pp. 352–357). Malvern, PA: Lea & Febiger.

Solomon, G. F., & Moos, R. L. (1964). Emotions, immunity, and disease: A speculative theoretical integration. *Archives of General Psychiatry, 11,* 657–674.

Sonstroem, R. J. (1984). Exercise and self-esteem. *Exercise and Sport Sciences Reviews, 12,* 123–155.

Sontag, S., Graham, D. Y., Belsito, A., Weiss, J., Farley, A., Grunt, R., Cohen, N., Kinnear, D., Davis, W., Archabault, A., Achord, J., Thayer, W., Gillies, R., Sidorov, J., Sadesin, S. M., Dyck, W., Fleshler, B., Cleator, I., Wenger, J., & Opekun, A., Jr. (1984). Cimetidine, cigarette smoking, and recurrence of duodenal ulcer. *New England Journal of Medicine, 311,* 689–693.

Sorenson, S. B., Upchurch, D. M., & Shen, H. (1996). Violence and injury in marital arguments: Risk patterns and gender differences. *American Journal of Public Health, 86,* 35–40.

Sours, J. A. (1980). *Starving to death in a sea of objects: The anorexia nervosa syndrome.* New York: Aronson.

Spanos, N. P., Perlini, A. H., & Robertson, L. A. (1989). Hypnosis, suggestion, and placebo in the reduction of experimental pain. *Journal of Abnormal Psychology, 98,* 285–293.

Spiegel, D. (1992). Effects of psychosocial support on patients with metastatic breast cancer. *Journal of Psychosocial Oncology, 10,* 113–120.

Spiegel, D. (1993). Social support: How friends, family, and groups can help. In D. Goleman & J. Gurin (Eds.), *Mind/body medicine: How to use your mind for better health* (pp. 331–349). Yonkers, NY: Consumer Reports Books.

Spiegel, D., & Bloom, J. R. (1983). Group therapy and hypnosis reduce metastatic breast cancer pain. *Psychosomatic Medicine, 45,* 333–339.

Spiegel, D., Bloom, J. R., & Yalom, I. D. (1981). Group support for patients with metastatic cancer. *Archives of General Psychiatry, 38,* 527–533.

Spiegel, D., Kraemer, H. C., Bloom, J. R., & Gottheil, E. (1989). Effect of psychosocial treatment on survival of patients with metastatic breast cancer. *Lancet, ii,* 888–891.

Spielberger, C. D., & Frank, R. G. (1992). Injury control: A promising field for psychologists. *American Psychologist, 47,* 1029–1030.

Stachnik, T. J. (1980). Priorities for psychology in medical education and health care delivery. *American Psychologist, 35,* 8–15.

Stall, R. (1986). Respondent-identified reasons for change and stability in alcohol consumption as a concomitant of the aging process. In C. R. Janes, R. Stall, & S. M. Gifford (Eds.), *Anthropology and epidemiology: Interdisciplinary approaches to the study of health and disease* (pp. 275–302). Boston: Reidel.

Stall, R., McKusick, L., Wiley, J., Coates, T. J., & Ostrow, D. G. (1986). Alcohol and drug use during sexual activity and compliance with safe sex guidelines for AIDS: The AIDS Behavioral Research Project. *Health Education Quarterly, 13,* 359–371.

Stamler, J., Wentworth, D., & Neaton, J. D. (1986). Is relationship between serum cholesterol and risk of premature death from coronary heart disease continuous and graded? Findings in 356, 222 primary screenees of the Multiple Risk Factor Intervention Trial (MRFIT). *Journal of the American Medical Association, 256,* 2823–2828.

Stamler, R., Stamler, J., Gosch, F. C., Civinelli, J., Fishman, J., McKeever, P., McDonald, A., & Dyer, A. R., (1989). Primary prevention of hypertension by nutritional-hygienic means. *Journal of the American Medical Association, 262,* 1801–1807.

Stamler, R., Stamler, J., Grimm, R., Gosch, F. C., Elmer, P., Dyer, A. R., Berman, R., Fishman, J., Van Heel, N., Civinelli, J., &

McDonald, A. (1987). Final report of a four-year randomized controlled trial—The Hypertension Control Program. *Journal of the American Medical Association, 257,* 1484–1491.

Stampfer, M. J., Colditz, G. A., Willett, W. C., Speizer, F. E., & Hennekens, C. H. (1988). A prospective study of moderate alcohol consumption and the risk of coronary heart disease and stroke in women. *New England Journal of Medicine, 319,* 267–273.

Stampfer, M. J., Hennekens, C. H., Manson, J. E., Colditz, G. A., Rosner, D., & Willett, W. C. (1993). Vitamin E consumption and the risk of coronary heart disease in women. *New England Journal of Medicine, 328,* 1444–1449.

Stanton, A. L. (1987). Determinants of adherence to medical regimens by hypertensive patients. *Journal of Behavioral Medicine, 10,* 377–394.

Stanton, W. R., Mahalski, P. A., McGee, R., & Silva, P. A. (1993). Reasons for smoking or not smoking in early adolescence. *Addictive Behaviors, 18,* 321-329.

Starr, C., & Taggart, R. (1984). *Biology: The unity and diversity of life* (3rd ed.). Belmont, CA: Wadsworth.

Stason, W., Neff, R., Miettinen, O., & Jick, H. (1976). Alcohol consumption and nonfatal myocardial infarction. *American Journal of Epidemiology, 104,* 603–608.

Steele, C. M., & Josephs, R. A. (1990). Alcohol myopia: Its prized and dangerous effects. *American Psychologist, 45,* 921–933.

Steele, C. M., Southwick, L., & Pagano, R. (1986). Drinking your troubles away: The role of activity in mediating alcohol's reduction of psychological stress. *Journal of Abnormal Psychology, 95,* 173–180.

Steenland, K. (1992). Passive smoking and the risk of heart disease. *Journal of the American Medical Association, 267,* 94–99.

Stehr, P. A., Glonginger, M. F., Kuller, L. H., Marsh, G. M., Radford, E. P., & Weinberg, G. B. (1985). Dietary vitamin A deficiencies and stomach cancer. *American Journal of Epidemiology, 121,* 65–70.

Stein, M., & Miller, A. H. (1993). Stress, the immune system, and health and illness. In L. Goldberger & S. Breznitz (Eds.), *Handbook of stress: Theoretical and clinical aspects* (2nd ed., pp. 127–141). New York: Free Press.

Stein, M., Schleifer, S. J., & Keller, S. E. (1981). Hypothalamic influences on immune response. In R. Ader (Ed.), *Psychoneuroimmunology* (pp. 429-447). New York: Academic Press.

Stein, P. N., & Motta, R. W. (1992). Effects of aerobic and nonaerobic exercise on depression and self-concept. *Perceptual and Motor Skills, 74,* 79–89.

Steinmetz, H. M., & Hobson, S. J. G. (1994). Prevention of falls among the community-dwelling elderly: An overview. *Physical and Occupational Therapy in Geriatrics, 12,* 13–29.

Steinmetz, K. A., Kushi, L. H., Bostick, R. M., Folsom, A. R., & Potter, J. D. (1994). Vegetables, fruit, and colon cancer in the Iowa Women's Health Study. *American Journal of Epidemiology, 139,* 1–15.

Stern, J. L. (1991). Cervix. In M. Dollinger, E. H. Rosenbaum, & G. Cable (Eds.), *Everyone's guide to cancer therapy* (pp. 277–284). Kansas City: Somerville.

Sternbach, R. A. (1966). *Principles of psychophysiology: An introductory text and readings.* San Diego, CA: Academic Press.

Sternbach, R. A. (1978). Clinical aspects of pain. In R. A. Sternbach (Ed.), *The psychology of pain.* New York: Raven.

Stevenson, T., & Lennie, J. (1992). Empowering school students in developing strategies to increase bicycle helmet wearing. *Health Education Research, 7,* 555–566.

Stewart, A., Greenfield, S., Hays, R. D., Wells, K., Rogers, W. H., Berry, S. D., McGlynn, E. A., & Ware, J. E., Jr. (1989). Functional status and well-being of patients with chronic conditions. *Journal of the American Medical Association, 262,* 907–913.

Stewart, W. F., Lipton, R. B., Celentano, D. D., & Reed, M. L. (1992). Prevalence of migraine headache in the United States. *Journal of the American Medical Association, 267,* 64–69.

Stillman, M. J. (1977). Women's health beliefs about cancer and breast self-examination. *Nursing Research, 26,* 121–127.

Stoddard, J. J., & Miller, T. (1995). Impact of parental smoking on the prevalence of wheezing respiratory illness in children. *American Journal of Epidemiology, 141,* 96–102.

Stokols, D. (1972). On the distinction between density and crowding: Some implications for future research. *Psychological Review, 79,* 275–277.

Stone, A. A., Bovbjerg, D. H., Neale, J. M., Napoli, A., Valdimarsdottir, H., Cox, D., Hayden, F. G., & Gwaltney, J. M., Jr. (1992). Development of the common cold symptoms following experimental rhinovirus is related to prior stressful life events. *Behavior Medicine, 18,* 115–120.

Stone, A. A., Reed, B. R., & Neale, J. M. (1987). Changes in daily event frequency precedes episodes of physical symptoms. *Journal of Human Stress, 13,* 70–74.

Stone, G. C. (1979). Health and the health system: A historical overview and conceptual framework. In G. C. Stone, F. Cohen, & N. E. Adler (Eds.), *Health psychology—A handbook* (pp. 1–17). San Francisco: Jossey-Bass.

Stone, G. C. (1982). *Health Psychology:* A new journal for a new field. *Health Psychology, 1,* 1–6.

Stone, G. C. (1984). A final word [editorial]. *Health Psychology, 3,* 585–589.

Stone, G. C. (1987). The scope of health psychology. In G. C. Stone, S. M. Weiss, J. D. Matarazzo, N. E. Miller, J. Rodin, C. D. Belar, M. J. Follick, & J. E. Singer (Eds.), *Health psychology: A discipline and a profession* (pp. 27–40). Chicago: University of Chicago Press.

Stone, G. C., Weiss, S. M., Matarazzo, J. D., Miller, N. E., Rodin, J., Belar, C. D., Follick, M. J., & Singer, J. E. (1987). Health psychology in the twenty-first century. In G. C. Stone, S. M. Weiss, J. D. Matarazzo, N. E. Miller, J. Rodin, C. D. Belar, M. J. Follick, & J. E. Singer (Eds.), *Health psychology: A discipline and a profession* (pp. 513–524). Chicago: University of Chicago Press.

Stone, R., Cafferata, G. L., & Sangl, J. (1987). Caregivers of the frail elderly: A national profile. *Gerontologist, 27,* 616–626.

Stone, S. V., Dembroski, T. M., Costa, P. T., Jr., MacDougall, J. M. (1990). Gender differences in cardiovascular reactivity. *Journal of Behavioral Medicine, 13,* 137–156.

Story, M., & Faulkner, P. (1990). The prime time diet: A content analysis of eating behavior and food messages in television program content and commercials. *American Journal of Public Health, 80,* 738–740.

Stout, N. A., Jenkins, E. L., & Pizatella, T. J. (1996). Occupational injury mortality rates in the United States: Changes from 1980 to 1989. *American Journal of Public Health, 86,* 73–77.

Strain, E. C., Mumford, G. K., Silverman, K., & Griffiths, R. R. (1994). Caffeine dependence syndrome: Evidence from case histories and experimental evaluation. *Journal of the American Medical Association, 272,* 1043–1047.

Straus, M. A., Gelles, R. J., & Steinmetz, S. K. (1980). *Behind closed doors: Violence in the American family.* Garden City, NY: Anchor.

Streingart, R. M., Packer, M., Hamm, P., Coglianese, M. E., Gersh, B., Geltman, E. M., Sollano, J., Katz, S., Moyé, L., Basta, L. L., Lewis, S. J., Gotlieb, S. S., Bernstein, V., McLwan, P., Jacobson, K., Brown, E. J., Kukin, M. L., Kantrowitz, N. E., & Pfeffer, M. A. (1991). Sex differences in the management of coronary artery disease. *New England Journal of Medicine, 325,* 226–230.

Streissguth, A. P., Barr, H. M., Sampson, P. D., Parrish-Johnson, J. C., Kirchner, G. L., & Martin, D. C. (1986). Attention, distraction, and reaction time at age 7 years and prenatal alcohol exposure. *Neurobehavioral Toxicology and Teratology, 8,* 717–725.

Striegel-Moore, R. H., Silberstein, L. R., & Rodin, J. (1986). Toward an understanding of risk factors for bulimia. *American Psychologist, 41,* 246–263.

Stroebel, C. F., & Glueck, B. C. (1976). Psychophysiological rationale for the application of biofeedback in the alleviation of pain. In M. Weisenberg & B. Tursky (Eds.), *Pain: New perspectives in therapy and research.* New York: Plenum.

Strong, C. A. (1895). The psychology of pain. *Psychological Review, 2,* 329–347.

Stuart, R. B. (1967). Behavioral control of overeating. *Behavior Research and Therapy, 5,* 357–365.

Stuart, R. B. (1974). Teaching facts about drugs: Pushing or preventing? *Journal of Educational Psychology, 66,* 189–201.

Study: Nonsmoking cancer rates increase. (1994, June 2). *The Lake Charles American Press,* p. 32.

Stunkard, A. J. (1989). Perspectives on human obesity. In A. J. Stunkard & A. Baum (Eds.), *Perspectives on behavioral medicine: Eating, sleeping, and sex* (pp. 9–30). Hillsdale, NJ: Erlbaum.

Stunkard, A. J., Harris, J. R., Pedersen, N. L., & McClean, G. E. (1990). The body-mass index of twins who have been reared apart. *New England Journal of Medicine, 322,* 1483–1487.

Stunkard, A. J., & Koch, C. (1964). The interpretation of gastric motility: I. Apparent bias in the reports of hunger by obese persons. *Archives of General Psychiatry, 11,* 74–82.

Stunkard, A. J., & Penick, S. (1979). Behavior and modification in the treatment of obesity: The problem of maintaining weight loss. *Archives of General Psychiatry, 36,* 801–806.

Stunkard, A. J., Sørensen, T. I. A., Hanis, C., Teasdale, T. W., Chakraborty, R., Schull, W. J., & Schulsinger, F. (1986). An adoption study of human obesity. *New England Journal of Medicine, 314,* 193, 198.

Suchman, E. A. (1965). Social patterns of illness and medical care. *Journal of Health and Human Behavior, 6,* 2–16.

Suls, J., & Wan, C. K. (1993). The relationship between trait hostility and cardiovascular reactivity: A quantitative review and analysis. *Psychophysiology, 30,* 615–626.

Sundstrom, E. (1978). Crowding as a sequential process: Review of research on the effects of population density on humans. In A. Baum & Y. M. Epstein (Eds.), *Human response to crowding* (pp. 31–116). Hillsdale, NJ: Erlbaum.

Susser, M. (1991). What is a cause and how do we know one? A grammar for pragmatic epidemiology. *American Journal of Epidemiology, 133,* 635–648.

Susser, M. (1995). Editorial: The tribulations of trials—Intervention in communities. *American Journal of Public Health, 85,* 156–158.

Svarstad, B. L. (1976). Physician-patient communication and patient conformity with medical advice. In D. Mechanic (Ed.), *The growth of bureaucratic medicine: An inquiry into the dynamics of patient behavior and the organization of medical care* (pp. 220–238). New York: Wiley.

Svendsen, K. H., Kuller, L. H., Martin,. M. J., & Ockene, J. K. (1987). Effects of passive smoking in the Multiple Risk Factor Intervention Trial. *American Journal of Epidemiology, 126,* 783–795.

Swain, J. F., Rouse, I. L., Curley, C. B., & Sacks, F. M. (1990). Comparison of the effects of oat bran and low-fiber wheat on serum lipoprotein levels and blood pressure. *New England Journal of Medicine, 322,* 147–152.

Swan, G. E., & Carmelli, D. (1995). Characteristics associated with excessive weight gain after smoking cessation in men. *American Journal of Public Health, 85,* 73–77.

Swan, G. E., & Denk, C. E. (1987). Dynamic models for the maintenance of smoking cessation: Event history analysis of late relapse. *Journal of Behavioral Medicine, 10,* 527–554.

Swartzman, L. C., & McDermid, A. J. (1993). The impact of contextual cues on the interpretation of and response to physical symptoms: A vignette approach. *Journal of Behavioral Medicine, 16,* 183–198.

Sweet, J. J., Rozensky, R. H., & Tovian, S. M. (1991). Clinical psychology in medical settings: Past and present. In J. J. Sweet, R. H. Rozensky, & S. M. Tovian (Eds.), *Handbook of clinical psychology in medical settings.* New York: Plenum.

Syrjala, K. L., & Chapman, C. R. (1984). Measurement of clinical pain: A review and integration of research findings. In C. Benedetti, C. R. Chapman, & G. Moricca (Eds.), *Advances in pain research and therapy: Vol. 7. Recent advances in the management of pain.* New York: Raven.

Sytkowski, P. A., Kannel, W. B., & D'Agostino, R. B., (1990). Chances in risk factors and the decline in mortality from cardiovascular disease: The Framingham Heart Study. *New England Journal of Medicine, 322,* 1635–1641.

Szmukler, G. I., Eisler, I., Russell, G. F. M., & Dare, C. (1985). Anorexia nervosa, parental "expressed emotion" and dropping out of treatment. *British Journal of Psychiatry, 147,* 265–271.

Talbott, E., Helmkamp, J., Matthews, K., Kuller, L., Cottington, E., & Redmond, G. (1985). Occupational noise exposure, noise-induced hearing loss, and the epidemiology of high blood pressure. *American Journal of Epidemiology, 121,* 501–514.

Taller, H. (1961). *Calories don't count.* New York: Simon & Schuster.

Tang, J-L., Morris, J. K., Wald, N. J., Hole, D., Shipley, M., & Tunstall-Pedoe, H. (1995). Mortality in relation to tar yield of cigarettes: A prospective study of four cohorts. *British Medical Journal, 311,* 1530–1533.

Tartaglia, L. A., Dembski, M., Weng, X., Deng, N., Culpepper, J., Devos, R., Richards, G. J., Campfield, L. A., Clark, F. T., Deeds, J., Muir, C., Sanker, S., Moriarty, A., Moore, K. J., Smutko, J. S., Mays, G. G., Woolf, E. A., Monroe, C. A., & Tepper, R. I. (1995). Identification and expression cloning of a leptin receptor, OB-R. *Cell, 83,* 1263–1271.

Tausig, M. (1982). Measuring life events. *Journal of Health and Social Behavior, 23,* 52–64.

Tavris, C. (1992). *The mismeasure of woman.* New York: Simon and Schuster.

Taylor, C. B., Fortmann, S. P., Flora, J. A., Kayman, S., Barrett, D. C., Jatulis, D. E., & Farquhar, J. W. (1991). Effect of long-term community health education on body mass index: The Stanford Five-City Project. *American Journal of Epidemiology, 134,* 235–249.

Taylor, H. L., Klepetar, E., Keys, A., Parlin, W., Blackburn, H., & Puchner, T. (1962). Death rates among physically active and sedentary employees of the railroad industry. *American Journal of Public Health, 52,* 1697–1707.

Taylor, S. E. (1979). Hospital patient behavior: Reactance, helplessness, or control? *Journal of Social Issues, 35*(1), 156–184.

Taylor, S. E. (1982). The impact of health organizations on recipients of services. In A. W. Johnson, O. Grusky, & B. H. Raven (Eds.), *Contemporary health services: Social science perspectives* (pp. 103–137). Boston: Auburn House.

Taylor, S. E. (1983). Adjustment to threatening events: A theory of cognitive adaptation. *American Psychologist, 38,* 1161–1173.

Taylor, S. E. (1990). Health psychology: The science and the field. *American Psychologist, 45,* 40–50.

Taylor, S. E., & Aspinwall, L. G. (1993). Coping with chronic illness. In L. Goldberger & S. Breznitz (Eds.), *Handbook of stress: Theoretical and clinical aspects* (2nd ed., pp. 511–531). New York: Free Press.

Taylor, S. P., Gammon, C. B., & Capasso, D. R. (1976). Aggression as a function of alcohol and threat. *Journal of Personality and Social Psychology, 34,* 938–941.

Taylor, S. P., & Leonard, K. E. (1983). Alcohol and human physical aggression. In R. G. Geen & E. I. Donnerstein (Eds.), *Aggression: Theoretical and empirical reviews* (Vol. 2, pp. 77–101). New York: Academic Press.

Tedesco, L. A., Keffer, M. A., Davis, E. L., & Christersson, L. A. (1993). Self-efficacy and reasoned action: Predicting oral health status and behaviour at one, three, and six month intervals. *Psychology and Health, 8,* 105–121.

Tedesco, L. A., Keffer, M. A., & Fleck-Kandath, C. (1991). Self-efficacy, reasoned action, and oral health behavior reports: A social cognitive approach to compliance. *Journal of Behavioral Medicine, 14,* 341–355.

Teitelbaum, P. (1955). Sensory control of hypothalamic hyperphagia. *Journal of Comparative and Physiological Psychology, 48,* 156–163.

Telch, C. F., & Telch, M. J. (1985). Psychological approaches for enhancing coping among cancer patients: A review. *Clinical Psychology Review, 5,* 325–344.

Terman, L. M., & Oden, M. H. (1947). *Genetic studies of genius: The gifted child grows up* (Vol. 4) Stanford, CA: Stanford University Press.

Thayer, R. E., Newman, J. R., & McClain, T. M. (1994). Self-regulation of mood: Strategies for changing a bad mood, raising energy, and reducing tension. *Journal of Personality and Social Psychology, 67,* 910–925.

Thistle, H. G., Hislop, H. J., Moffroid, M., & Lowman, E. W. (1967). Isokinetic contractions: A new concept of resistance exercise. *Archives of Physical Medicine and Rehabilitation, 48,* 279–282.

Thoits, P. A. (1983). Dimensions of life events that influence psychological distress: An evaluation and synthesis of the literature. In H. B. Kaplan (Ed.), *Psychosocial stress: Trends in theory and research* (pp. 33–103). New York: Academic Press.

Thomas, W., White, C. M., Mah, J., Geisser, M. S., Church, T. R., & Mandel, J. S. (1995). Longitudinal compliance with annual screening for fecal occult blood. *American Journal of Epidemiology, 142,* 176–182.

Thompson, B. W. (1994). *A hunger so wide and so deep: American women speak out on eating problems.* Minneapolis: University of Minnesota Press.

Thompson, D. R., & Meddis, R. (1990a). A prospective evaluation of in-hospital counseling for first time myocardial infarction in men. *Journal of Psychosomatic Research, 34,* 237–248.

Thompson, D. R., & Meddis, R. (1990b). Wives' responses to counseling early after myocardial infarction. *Journal of Psychosomatic Research, 34,* 249–258.

Thompson, E. L. (1978). Smoking education programs 1960–1976. *American Journal of Public Health, 68,* 250–257.

Thompson, L., & Walker, A. J. (1989). Gender in families: Women and men in marriage, work, and parenthood. *Journal of Marriage and the Family, 51,* 845–871.

Thompson, P. D. (1982). Cardiovascular hazards of physical activity. *Exercise and Sports Sciences Reviews, 10,* 208–235.

Thompson, P. D., Funk, E. J., Carleton, R. A., & Sturner, W. Q. (1982). The incidence of death during jogging in Rhode Island joggers from 1975 through 1980. *Journal of the American Medical Association, 247,* 2535–2538.

Thompson, R. A., & Sherman, R. T. (1993). *Helping athletes with eating disorders.* Champaign, IL: Human Kinetics Publishers.

Thompson, R. J., & Matarazzo, J. D. (1984). Psychology in United States medical schools: 1983. *American Psychologist, 39,* 988–995.

Thornicroft, G. (1990). Cannabis and psychosis: Is there epidemiological evidence for an association? *British Journal of Psychiatry, 157,* 25–33.

Thun, M. J., Day-Lally, C. A., Calle, E. E., Flanders, W. D., & Heath, C. W., Jr. (1995). Excess mortality among cigarette smokers: Changes in a 20-year interval. *American Journal of Public Health, 85,* 1223–1230.

Tilkian, A. G., & Daily, E. K. (1986). *Cardiovascular procedures: Diagnostic techniques and therapeutic procedures.* St. Louis: Mosby.

Tinker, J. E., & Tucker, J. A. (1994, August). *Environmental contexts surrounding natural recovery from obesity.* Paper presented at the American Psychological Association Convention, Los Angeles, CA.

Tischenkel, N. J., Saab, P. G., Schneiderman, N., Nelesen, R. A., Pasin, R. D., Goldstein, D. A., Spitzer, S. B., Woo-Ming, R., & Weidler, D. J. (1989). Cardiovascular and neurohumoral responses to behavioral challenge as a function of race and sex. *Health Psychology, 8,* 503–524.

Tobler, N. S. (1986). Meta-analysis of 143 adolescent drug prevention programs: Quantitative outcome results of program participants compared to a control or comparison group. *Journal of Drug Issues, 16,* 537–567.

Tomkins, S. S. (1966). Psychological model for smoking behavior. *American Journal of Public Health, 56* (Suppl. 12), 17–20.

Tomkins, S. S. (1968). A modified model of smoking behavior. In E. F. Borgatta & R. R. Evans (Eds.), *Smoking, health and behavior* (pp. 165–188). Chicago: Aldine.

Toniolo, P., Riboli, E., Protta, F., Charrel, M., & Coppa, A. P. (1989). Calorie-providing nutrients and risk of breast cancer. *Journal of the National Cancer Institute, 81,* 278–286.

Tønnesen, P., Nørregaard, J., Mikkelsen, D., Jørgensen, S., & Nillson, F. (1993). A double-blind trial of a nicotine inhaler for smoking cessation. *Journal of the American Medical Association, 269,* 1208–1271.

Tønnesen, P., Nørregaard, J., Simonsen, K., & Säwe, U. (1991). A double-blind trial of a 16-hour transdermal nicotine patch in smoking cessation. *New England Journal of Medicine, 325,* 311–315.

Toobert, D. J., & Glasgow, R. E. (1991). Problem solving and diabetes self-care. *Journal of Behavioral Medicine, 14,* 71–86.

Tortu, S., Beardsley, M., Deren, S., & Davis, W. R. (1994). The risk of HIV infection in a national sample of women with injection drug-using partners. *American Journal of Public Health, 84,* 1243–1249.

Travell, J. (1976). Myofascial trigger points: A clinical view. In J. J. Bonica & D. Albe-Fessard (Eds.), *Advances in pain research and therapy* (Vol. 1). New York: Raven.

Traven, N. D., Kuller, L. H., Ives, D. G., Rutan, G. H., & Perper, J. (1995). Coronary heart disease mortality and sudden death: Trends and patterns in 35- to 44-year-old white males, 1970–1990. *American Journal of Epidemiology, 142,* 45–52.

Travis, J. (1995, August 19). One Alzheimer's gene leads to another. *Science News, 148,* 118.

Treiber, F. A., Davis, H., Musante, L., Raunikar, R. A., Strong, W. G., McCaffrey, F., Meeks, M. C., & Vandernoord, R. (1993). Ethnicity, gender, family history of myocardial infarction, and menodynamic responses to laboratory stressors in children. *Health Psychology, 12,* 6–15.

Tremblay, A., Plourde, G., Després, J-P., & Bouchard, C. (1989). Impact of dietary fat content and fat oxidation on energy intake in humans. *American Journal of Clinical Nutrition, 49,* 799–805.

Treviño, F. M., Moyer, E., Valdez, B., & Stroup-Benham, C. A. (1991). Health insurance coverage and utilization of health services by Mexican Americans, mainland Puerto Ricans, and Cuban Americans. *Journal of the American Medical Association, 265,* 233–237.

Trevisan, M., Krogh, V., Freudanheim, J., Blake, A., Muti, P., Panico, S., Farinaro, E., Mancini, M., Menotti, A., Ricci, G., & Research Group ATS-RF 2 of the Italian National Research Council. (1990). Consumption of olive oil, butter, and vegetable oils and coronary heart disease risk factors. *Journal of the American Medical Association, 263,* 688–692.

Tucker, L. A. (1989). Use of smokeless tobacco, cigarette smoking, and hypercholesterolemia. *American Journal of Public Health, 79,* 1048–1050.

Tucker, L. A., & Friedman, G. M. (1989). Television viewing and obesity in adult males. *American Journal of Public Health, 79,* 516–518.

Tulkin, S. R. (1987). Health care services. In G. C. Stone, S. M. Weiss, J. D. Matarazzo, N. E. Miller, J. Rodin, C. D. Belar, M. J. Follick, & J. E. Singer (Eds.), *Health psychology: A discipline and a profession* (pp. 121–135). Chicago: University of Chicago Press.

Turk, D. C. (1978). Cognitive behavioral techniques in the management of pain. In J. P. Foreyt & D. P. Rathjen (Eds.), *Cognitive behavior therapy.* New York: Plenum.

Turk, D. C., & Meichenbaum, D. (1991). Adherence to self-care regimens: The patient's perspective. In J. J. Sweet, R. H. Rozensky, & S. M. Tovian (Eds.), *Handbook of clinical psychology in medical settings* (pp. 249–266). New York: Plenum.

Turk, D. C., Meichenbaum, D., & Genest, M. (1983). *Pain and behavioral medicine: A cognitive behavioral perspective.* New York: Guilford Press.

Turk, D. C., & Nash, J. M. (1993). Chronic pain: New ways to cope. In D. Goleman & J. Gurin (Eds.), *Mind/body medicine: How to use your mind for better health* (pp. 111–130). Yonkers, NY: Consumer Reports Books.

Turk, D. C., & Rudy, T. E. (1988). Toward an empirically derived taxonomy of chronic pain patients: Integration of psychological assessment data. *Journal of Consulting and Counseling Psychology, 56,* 233–238.

Turk, D. C., & Rudy, T. E. (1992). Classification logic and strategies in chronic pain. In D. C. Turk & R. Melzack (Eds.), *Handbook of pain assessment* (pp. 409–428). New York: Guilford Press.

Turk, D. C., Wack, J. T., & Kerns, R. D. (1985). An empirical examination of the "pain-behavior" construct. *Journal of Behavior Medicine, 8,* 119–130.

Turner, J. A., & Chapman, C. R. (1982a). Psychological interventions for chronic pain: A critical review. I: Relaxation training and biofeedback. *Pain, 12,* 1–21.

Turner, J. A., & Chapman, C. R. (1982b). Psychological interventions for chronic pain: A critical review. II: Operant conditioning, hypnosis, and cognitive-behavior therapy. *Pain, 12,* 23–46.

Turner, J. A., & Clancy, S. (1988). Comparison of operant behavioral and cognitive-behavioral group treatment for chronic low back pain. *Journal of Consulting and Clinical Psychology, 56,* 261–266.

Turner, J. A., Deyo, R. A., Loeser, J. D., Von Korff, M., & Fordyce, W. E. (1994). The importance of placebo effects in pain treatment and research. *Journal of the American Medical Association, 271,* 1609–1614.

Turner, J. A., & Jensen, M. P. (1993). Efficacy of cognitive therapy for chronic low back pain. *Pain, 52,* 169–177.

Turner, J. A., Herron, L. D., & Pheasant, H. C. (1981). MMPI prediction of outcome following back surgery. *Pain Supplement, 1,* S244 (Abstract).

Turner, J. A., & Romano, J. M. (1984). Evaluating psychologic interventions for chronic pain: Issues and recent developments. In C. Benedetti, C. R. Chapman, & G. Moricca (Eds.), *Advances in pain research and therapy: Vol. 7. Recent advances in the management of pain.* New York: Raven.

Turner, J. A., & Romano, J. M. (1990). Physiologic and psychological evaluation. In J. J. Bonica (Ed.), *The management of pain* (2nd ed., pp. 595–609). Malvern, PA: Lea & Febiger.

Twycross, R. G. (1978). Relief of pain. In C. M. Saunders (Ed.), *The management of terminal disease.* Chicago: Yearbook Publishers.

U.S. Bureau of the Census (USBC). (1973). *Statistical abstracts of the United States, 1973* (94th ed.). Washington, DC: U.S. Government Printing Office.

U.S. Bureau of the Census (USBC). (1974) *Statistical abstracts of the United States, 1974* (95th ed.). Washington, DC: U.S. Government Printing Office.

U.S. Bureau of the Census (USBC). (1975). *Historical statistics of the United States: Colonial times to 1970, Part 1.* Washington, DC: U.S. Government Printing Office.

U.S. Bureau of the Census (USBC). (1985). *Statistical abstracts of the United States: 1984,* Washington, DC: U.S. Government Printing Office.

U.S. Bureau of the Census (USBC). (1994). *Statistical abstracts of the United States: 1994* (114th ed.). Washington, DC: U.S. Government Printing Office.

U.S. Bureau of the Census. (1995). *Statistical abstracts of the United States, 1995* (115th ed.). Washington, DC: U.S. Government Printing Office.

U.S. Department of Health, Education, and Welfare (USDHEW). (1979). *Smoking and health: A report of the Surgeon General* (DHEW Publication No. 79-50066). Washington, DC: U.S. Government Printing Office.

U.S. Department of Health and Human Services (USDHHS). (1984a). *The health consequences of smoking: Chronic obstructive lung disease. A report of the Surgeon General* (DHHS Publication No. PHS-50205). Washington DC: U.S. Government Printing Office.

U.S. Department of Health and Human Services (USDHHS). (1984b). *The 1984 report of the Joint National Committee on Detection, Evaluation, and Treatment of High Blood Pressure.* Washington, DC: U.S. Government Printing Office.

U.S. Department of Health and Human Services (USDHHS). (1987). *Sixth special report to the U.S. Congress on alcohol and health.* (DHHS Publication No. ADM 87-1519). Washington, DC: U.S. Government Printing Office.

U.S. Department of Health and Human Services (USDHHS). (1988). *The health consequences of smoking: Nicotine addiction. A report of the Surgeon General, 1988* (DHHS Publication No. DC 88-8406). Washington, DC: U.S. Government Printing Office.

U.S. Department of Health and Human Services (USDHHS). (1989). *Reducing the health consequences of smoking: 25 years of progress. A report of the Surgeon General* (DHHS Publication No. CDC 89-8411). Rockville, MD: U.S. Government Printing Office.

U.S. Department of Health and Human Services (USDHHS). (1990a). *Alcohol and health: Seventh special report to the U.S. Congress* (DHHS Publication No. ADM 90-1656. Washington, DC: U.S. Government Printing Office.

U.S. Department of Health and Human Services (USDHHS). (1990b). *The health benefits of smoking cessation: A report of* the Surgeon General (DHHS Publication No. CDC 90-8416). Washington, DC: U.S. Government Printing Office.

U.S. Department of Health and Human Services [USDHHS]. (1990c). Healthy people 2000: National health promotion and disease prevention objectives. (PHS Publication No. 91-50212). Washington, DC: Author.

U.S. Department of Health and Human Services (USDHHS). (1993a). Eighth Special Report to the U.S. Congress on Alcohol and Health. Washington, DC: National Institution of Alcohol Abuse and Alcoholism. Washington, DC: U.S. Government Printing Office.

U.S. Department of Health and Human Services (USDHHS). (1993b). National Institutes of Health fact book. Washington, DC: U.S. Government Printing Office.

U.S. Department of Health and Human Services (USDHHS). (1994a). Cigarette smoking among adults—United States, 1993. Washington, DC: U.S. Government Printing Office.

U.S. Department of Health and Human Services (USDHHS). (1994b). Healthy people 2000 review 1993. (DHHS Publication No. PHS 94-1232-1). Washington, DC: U.S. Government Printing Office.

U.S. Department of Health and Human Services (USDHHS). (1994c). National household survey on drug abuse: Population estimates 1993. DHHS Publication No. (SMA) 94-3017. Rockville, MD: Substance Abuse and Mental Health Services Administration.

U.S. Department of Health and Human Services (USDHHS). (1994d). Surveillance for selected tobacco use behavior—United States, 1900–1994. Washington, DC: U.S. Government Printing Office.

U. S. Department of Health and Human Services (USDHHS). (1995). Healthy people 2000 review, 1994 (DHHS Publication No. PHS 95-1256-1). Washington, DC: U.S. Government Printing Office.

U.S. Public Health Service (USPHS). (1964). Smoking and health: Public Health Service report of the Advisory Committee to the Surgeon General of the Public Health Service (PHS Publication No. 1103). Washington, DC: U.S. Government Printing Office.

Vaillant, G. E. (1983). The natural history of alcoholism: Causes, patterns, and paths to recovery. Cambridge, MA: Harvard University Press.

van Assema, P., Pieterse, M., Kok, G., Eriksen, M., & de Vries, H. (1993). The determinants of four cancer-related risk behaviours. Health Education Research, 8, 461–472.

van den Brandt, P. A., Goldbohn, A., & van 't Veer, P. (1995). Alcohol and breast cancer: Results from the Netherlands Cohort Study. American Journal of Epidemiology, 141, 907–915.

Van der Does, A. J., & Van Dyck, R. (1989). Does hypnosis contribute to the care of burn patients? Review of evidence. General Hospital Psychiatry, 11, 119–124.

Van der Ploeg, H. M., & Vetter, H. (1993). Two for the price of one: The empirical basis of the Grossarth-Maticek interviews. Psychological Inquiry, 4, 65–66.

Van Hasselt, V. B., Morrison, R. L., Bellack, A. S., & Hersen, M. (1988). Handbook of family violence. New York: Plenum.

Vartianen, E., Fallonen, U., McAlister, A. L., & Puska, P. (1990). Eight-year follow-up results of an adolescent smoking prevention program: The North Karelia Youth Project. American Journal of Public Health, 80, 78–79.

Vega, G. L., & Grundy, S. M. (1989). Comparison of lovastatin and gemfibrozil in normolipidemic patients with hypoalphalipoprotienemia. Journal of the American Medical Association, 262, 3148–3153.

Veil, H. O. F., & Baumann, R. (1992). Comments on concepts and methods. In H. O. E. Veiel & U. Baumann (Eds.), The meaning and measurement of social support (pp. 313–319). New York: Hemisphere.

Vena, J. E., Graham, S., Zielezny, M., Brasure, J., & Swanson, M. K. (1987). Occupational exercise and risk of cancer. American Journal of Clinical Nutrition, 45, 318–327.

Vena, J. E., Graham, S., Zielezny, M., Swanson, M. K., Barnes, R. E., & Nolan, J. (1985). Lifetime occupational exercise and colon cancer. American Journal of Epidemiology, 122, 357–365.

Verbrugge, L. M. (1983). Multiple roles and physical health of women and men. Journal of Health and Social Behavior, 24, 16–30.

Verbrugge, L. M. (1989. The twain meet: Empirical expalantion of sex differences in health and mortality. Journal of Health and Social Behavior, 30, 282–304.

Verreault, R., Brisson, J., Deschénes, L., Naud, F., Meyer, F., & Belanger, L. (1988). Dietary fat in relation to prognostic indicators in breast cancer. Journal of the National Cancer Institute, 80, 819–825.

Verschuren, W. M. M., & Kromhout, D. (1995). Total cholesterol concentration and mortality at a relatively young age: Do men and women differ? British Medical Journal, 311, 779–783.

Vetter, H. (1993). Further dubious configurations in Grossarth-Maticek's psychosomatic data. Psychological Inquiry, 4, 66–67

Vincent, P. (1971). Factors influencing patient noncompliance: A theoretical approach. Nursing Research, 20, 509–516.

Von Korff, M., Barlow, W., Cherkin, D., & Deyo, R. A. (1994). Effects of practice style in managing back pain. Annals of Internal Medicine, 121, 187–195.

Vitaliano, P. P., Maiuro, R. D., Russo, J., Mitchell, E. S., Carr, J. E., & Van Citters, R. L. (1988). A biopsychosocial model of medical student distress. Journal of Behavioral Medicine, 11, 311–331.

Wadden, T. A., Stunkard, A. J., Brownell, K. D., & Day, S. C. (1984). Treatment of obesity by behavior therapy and very low calorie diet: A pilot investigation. Journal of Consulting and Clinical Psychology, 52, 692–694.

Wagenaar, A. C., Maybee, R. G., & Sullivan, K. P. (1988). Mandatory seat belt laws in eight states. A time-series evaluation. Journal of Safety Research, 19, 51–70.

Waldron, I. (1988). Gender and health-related behavior. In D. S. Gochman (Ed.), Health behavior: Emerging research perspectives (pp. 193–208). New York: Plenum.

Walker, B., Goodwin, N. J., & Warren, R. C. (1992). Violence: A challenge to the public health community. Health Watch National Symposium: Impact of violence on African-American children and adolescents: A public health challenge (1990, New York). Journal of the National Medical Association, 84, 490–496.

Wall, P. D. (1980). The role of the substantia gelatinosa as a gate control. In J. J. Bonica (Ed.), Pain. New York: Raven.

Wall, P. D., & Jones, M. (1991). Defeating pain: The war against a silent epidemic. New York: Plenum.

Wallace, J. (1985). Behavior modification methods as adjuncts to psychotherapy. In S. Zimberg, J. Wallace, & S. B. Blume (Eds.), Practical approaches to alcoholism psychotherapy (2nd ed.). New York: Plenum.

Wallston, B. S., Alagna, S. W., DeVellis, B. M., & DeVellis, R. F. (1983). Social support and physical health. Health Psychology, 2, 367–391.

Walsh, J. M. E., & Grady, D. (1995). Treatment of hyperlipidemia in women. Journal of the American Medical Association, 274, 1152–1158.

Walsh, T. D., & Leber, B. (1983). Measurement of chronic pain: Visual Analog Scales and McGill Pain Questionnaire compared. In J. J. Bonica, U. Lindblom, & A. Iggo (Eds.), Advances in pain research and therapy (Vol. 5). New York: Raven.

Walter, L., & Brannon, L. (1991). A cluster analysis of the Multi-dimensional Pain Inventory. *Headache, 31,* 476–479.

Wannamethee, G., & Shaper, A. G. (1992). Physical activity and stroke in British middle-aged men. *British Medical Journal, 304,* 597–601.

Wannamethee, G., Shaper, A. G., & Macfarlane, P. W. (1993). Heart rate, physical activity, and mortality from cancer and other noncardiovascular diseases. *American Journal of Epidemiology, 137,* 735–748.

Ward, A., & Morgan, W. (1984). Adherence patterns of healthy men and women enrolled in an adult exercise program. *Journal of Cardiac Rehabilitation, 4,* 143–152.

Watson, D., & Pennebaker, J. W. (1989). Health complaints, stress, and distress: Exploring the central role of negative affectivity. *Psychological Review, 96,* 234–254.

Watson, D., & Pennebaker, J. W. (1991). Situational, dispositional, and genetic bases of symptom reporting. In J. A. Skelton & R. T. Croyle (Eds.), *Mental representation in health and illness* (pp. 60–84). New York: Springer-Verlag.

Webster, D. W., Gainer, P. S., & Champion, H. P. (1993). Weapon carrying among inner-city junior high school students: Defensive behavior vs. aggressive delinquency. *American Journal of Public Health, 83,* 1604–1608.

Weiner, H. H. (1977). *Psychobiology and human disease.* Hillsdale, NJ: Erlbaum.

Weinstein, N. D. (1980). Unrealistic optimism about future life events. *Journal of Personality and Social Psychology, 39,* 806–820.

Weinstein, N. D. (1983). Reducing unrealistic optimism about illness susceptibility. *Health Psychology, 2,* 11–20.

Weinstein, N. D. (1984). Why it won't happen to me: Perceptions of risk factors and susceptibility. *Health Psychology, 3,* 431–457.

Weinstein, N. D. (1988). The precaution adoption process. *Health Psychology, 7,* 355–386.

Weinstein, N. D., & Klein, W. M. (1995). Resistance of personal risk perceptions to debiasing interventions. *Health Psychology, 14,* 132–140.

Weinstein, N. D., & Nicolich, M. (1993). Correct and incorrect interpretations of correlations between risk perceptions and risk behaviors. *Health Psychology, 12,* 235–245.

Weinstein, N. D., & Sandman, P. M. (1992). A model of the precaution adoption process: Evidence from home radon testing. *Health Psychology, 11,* 170–180.

Weisner, C., Greenfield, T., & Room, R. (1995). Trends in the treatment of alcohol problems in the US general population, 1979 through 1990. *American Journal of Public Health, 85,* 55–60.

Weisner, C., & Schmidt, L. (1992). Gender disparities in treatment for alcohol problems. *Journal of the American Medical Association, 228,* 1872–1876.

Weiss, S. M. (1984). Community health promotion demonstration programs: Introduction. In J. D. Matarazzo, S. M. Weiss, J. A. Herd, N. E. Miller, & S. M. Weiss (Eds.), *Behavioral health: A handbook of health enhancement and disease prevention* (pp. 1137–1139). New York: Wiley.

Weiss, S. M. (1987). Health psychology and other health professions. In G. C. Stone, S. M. Weiss, J. D. Matarazzo, N. E. Miller, J. Rodin, C. D. Belar, M. J. Follick, & J. E. Singer (Eds.), *Health psychology: A discipline and a profession* (pp. 61–73). Chicago: University of Chicago Press.

Welch, H. G., & Fisher, E. S. (1992). Let's make a deal: Negotiating a settlement between physicians and society. *New England Journal of Medicine, 327,* 1312–1315.

Wellisch, D. K. (1981). Intervention with the cancer patient. In C. K. Prokop & L. A. Bradley (Eds.), *Medical psychology: Con-tributions to behavioral medicine* (pp. 230–240). New York: Academic Press.

Wellness Management. (1995). Passport To Health reaches kids at risk. *Wellness Management: Newsletter of the National Wellness Association, 11* (2), 1, 5–6.

Wertlieb, D. L., Jacobson, A., & Hauser, S. (1990). The child with diabetes: A developmental stress and coping perspective. In *Psychological aspects of serious illness: Chronic conditions, fatal diseases, and clinical care* (pp. 61–101). Washington, DC: American Psychological Association.

Wesch, D., Lutzker, J. R., Frisch, L., & Dillon, M. M. (1987). Evaluating the impact of a service fee on patient compliance. *Journal of Behavioral Medicine, 10,* 91–101.

Whalen, C. K., Henker, B., O'Neil, R., Hollingshead, J., Holman, A., & Moore, B. (1994). Optimism in children's judgments of health and environmental risks. *Health Psychology, 13,* 319–323.

Whelan, E. (1978). *Preventing cancer.* New York: Norton.

Whitaker, A., Davis, M., Shaffer, D., Johnson, J., Abrams, S., Walsh, B. T., & Kalikow, K. (1989). The struggle to be thin: A survey of anorexic and bulimic symptoms in a non-referred adolescent population. *Psychological Medicine, 19,* 143–163.

White, D. R., & White, N. M. (1988). Causes and effects of obesity: Implications for behavioral treatment. In W. Linden (Ed.), *Biological barriers in behavioral medicine* (pp. 35–62). New York: Plenum.

White, J. H., & Schnaulty, N. L. (1977). Successful treatment of anorexia nervosa with imipramine. *Diseases of the Nervous System, 38,* 567–568.

Whitehead, W. E., Crowell, M. D., Heller, B. H., Robinson, J. C., Schuster, M. M., & Horn, S. (1994). Modeling and reinforcement of the sick role during childhood predicts adult illness behavior. *Psychosomatic Medicine, 56,* 541–550.

Whitemore, A. S., Perlin, S. A., & DiCiccio, Y. (1995). Chronic obstructive pulmonary disease in lifetime nonsmokers: Results from NHANES. *American Journal of Public Health, 85,* 702–706.

Whitlock, F. A., & Siskind, M. (1979). Depression and cancer: A follow-up study. *Psychological Medicine, 9,* 747–752.

Wiebe, D. J., & Williams, P. G. (1992). Hardiness and health: A social psychlophysiological perspective on stress and adaptation. *Journal of Social and Clinical Psychology, 11,* 238–262.

Wiens, A. N., & Menustik, C. E. (1983). Treatment outcome and patient characteristics in an aversion therapy program for alcoholism. *American Psychologist, 38,* 1089–1096.

Wikler, D. (1987). Who should be blamed for being sick? *Health Education Quarterly, 14,* 17–25.

Wilcox, D., & Dowrick, P. W. (1992). Anger management with adolescents. *Residential Treatment for Children and Youth, 9,* 29–39.

Wiley, J. A., & Camacho, T. C. (1980). Life-style and future health: Evidence from the Alameda County Study. *Preventive Medicine, 9,* 1–21.

Willett, W. C., Green, A., Stampfer, M. J., Speizer, F. E., Colditz, G. A., Rosner, B., Monson, R. R., Stason, W., & Hennekens, C. H. (1987). Relative and absolute excess risks of coronary heart disease among women who smoke cigarettes. *New England Journal of Medicine, 317,* 1303–1309.

Willett, W. C., Hunter, D. J., Stampfer, M. J., Colditz, G., Manson, J. E., Spiegelman, D., Rosner, B., Hennekens, C. H., & Speizer, F. E., (1992). Dietary fat and fiber in relation to risk of breast cancer. *Journal of the American Medical Association, 268,* 2037–2044.

Willett, W. C., Manson, J. E., Stampfer, M. J., Colditz, G. A., Rosner, B., Speizer, F. E., & Hennekens, C. H. (1995). Weight, weight change, and coronary heart disease in women: Risk within the "normal" weight range. *Journal of the American Medical Association, 273,* 461–465.

Willett, W. C., Stampfer, M. J., Colditz, G. A., Rosner, B. A., Hennekens, C. H., & Speizer, F. E. (1987a). Dietary fat and the risk of breast cancer. *New England Journal of Medicine, 316,* 22–28.

Willett, W. C., Stampfer, M. J., Colditz, G. A., Rosner, B. A., Hennekens, C. H., & Speizer, F. E. (1987b). Moderate alcohol consumption and the risk of breast cancer. *New England Journal of Medicine, 316,* 1174–1180.

Williams, A. F., & Lund, A. K. (1992). Injury control: What psychologists can contribute. *American Psychologist, 47,* 1036–1039.

Williams, A. F., & Wells, J. K. (1993). Factors associated with high blood alcohol concentrations among fatally injured drivers in the United States, 1991. *Alcohol, Drugs and Driving, 9,* 87–96.

Williams, B. K., & Knight, S. M. (1994). *Healthy for life: Wellness and the art of living.* Pacific Grove, CA: Brooks/Cole.

Williams, G. C., Grow, U. M., Freedman, Z. R., Ryan, R. M., & Deci, E. L. (1996). Motivational predictors of weight loss and weight-loss maintenance. *Journal of Personality and Social Psychology, 70,* 115–126.

Williams, M. V., Parker, R. M., Baker, D. W., Parikh, N. S., Pitkin, K., Coates, W. C., Nurss, J. R. (1995). Inadequate functional health literacy among patients at two public hospitals. *Journal of the American Medical Association, 274,* 1677–1682.

Williams, P., & Dickinson, J. (1993). Fear of crime: Read all about it? The relationship between newspaper crime reporting and fear of crime. *British Journal of Criminology, 33,* 33–56.

Williams, P. G., Wiebe, D. J., & Smith, T. W. (1992). Coping processes as mediators of the relationship between hardiness and health. *Journal of Behavior Medicine, 15,* 237–255.

Williams, R. B., Jr. (1989). *The trusting heart: Great news about Type A behavior.* New York: Times Books.

Williams, R. B., Jr. (1993). Hostility and the heart. In D. Goleman & J. Gurin (Eds.), *Mind/body medicine: How to use your mind for better health* (pp. 65–83). Yonkers, NY: Consumer Reports Books.

Williams, R. B., Barefoot, J. C., Califf, R. M., Haney, T. L., Saunders, W. B., Pryor, D. B., Hlatky, M. A., Siegler, I. C., & Mark, D. B. (1992). Prognostic importance of social and economic resources among medically treated patients with angiographically documented coronary artery disease. *Journal of the American Medical Association, 267,* 520–524.

Williams, R. B., Jr., Haney, T. L., Lee, K. L., Kong, Y., Blumenthal, J. A., & Whalen, R. E. (1980). Type A behavior hostility and coronary atherosclerosis. *Psychosomatic Medicine, 42,* 539–549.

Williamson, D. F. (1993). Descriptive epidemiology of body-weight and weight change in U.S. adults. *Annals of Internal Medicine, 119,* 646–649.

Williamson, D. F., Madans, J., Anda, R. F., Kleinman, J. C., Giovino, G. A., & Byers, T. (1991). Smoking cessation and severity of weight gain in a national cohort. *New England Journal of Medicine, 324,* 739–745.

Williamson, D. F., & Pamuk, E. R. (1993). The association between weight loss and increased longevity: A review of the evidence. *Annals of Internal Medicine, 119,* 731–736.

Williamson, D. F., Pamuk, E., Thun, M., Flanders, D., Byers, T., & Heath, C. (1995). Prospective study of intentional weight loss and mortality in never-smoking overweight US white women aged 40–64 years. *American Journal of Epidemiology, 141,* 1128–1141.

Williamson, D. F., Serdula, M. K., Anda, R. F., Levy, A., & Byers, T. (1992). Weight loss attempts in adults: Goals, duration, and rate of weight loss. *American Journal of Public Health, 82,* 1251–1257.

Willich, S. N., Lewis, M., Lowell, H., Arntz, H., Schubert, F., & Schröder, R. (1993). Physical exertion as a trigger of acute myocardial infarction. *New England Journal of Medicine, 329,* 1684–1690.

Wilson, C. P. (Ed.). (1983). *Fear of being fat: The treatment of anorexia nervosa and bulimia.* New York: Aronson.

Wilson, G. T. (1980). Behavior modification and the treatment of obesity. In A. J. Stunkard (Ed.), *Obesity* (pp. 325–344). Philadelphia: Saunders.

Wilson, G. T. (1987). Cognitive studies in alcoholism. *Journal of Consulting and Clinical Psychology, 55,* 325–331.

Wilson, G. T. (1989). The treatment of bulimia nervosa: A cognitive-social learning analysis. In A. J. Stunkard & A. Baum (Eds.), *Perspectives in behavioral medicine: Eating, sleeping, and sex* (pp. 73–98). Hillsdale, NJ: Erlbaum.

Wilson, G. T. (1993). Binge eating and addictive disorders. In C. G Fairburn & G. T. Wilson (Eds.), *Binge eating: Nature,assessment, and treatment* (pp. 97–120). New York: Guilford Press.

Wilson, P. W. F., Christiansen, J. C., Anderson, K. M., & Kannel, W. B. (1989). Impact of national guidelines for cholesterol risk factor screening. *Journal of the American Medical Association, 262,* 41–44.

Wilson, V. E., Morley, N. C., & Bird, E. I. (1980). Mood profiles of marathon runners, joggers, and non-exercisers. *Perceptual and Motor Skills, 50,* 117–118.

Windsor, R. A., Lowe, J. B., & Bartlett, E. E. (1988). The effectiveness of a worksite self-help smoking cessation program: A randomized trial. *Journal of Behavioral Medicine, 11,* 407–421.

Winett, R. A. (1995). A framework for health promotion and disease prevention programs. *American Psychologist, 50,* 341–350.

Wing, R. R. (1992). Behavioral treatment of severe obesity. *American Journal of Clinical Nutrition, 55,* 545S–551S.

Wingard, D. L., Berkman, L. F., & Brand, R. J. (1982). A multivariate analysis of health-related practices: A nine-year mortality follow-up of the Alameda County study. *American Journal of Epidemiology, 116,* 765–775.

Winkleby, M. A., Flora, J. A., & Kraemer, H. C. (1994). A community-based heart disease intervention: Predictors of change. *American Journal of Public Health, 84,* 767–772.

Winkleby, M. A., Jatulis, D. E., Frank, E., & Fortmann, S. P. (1992). Socioeconomic status and health: How education, income, and occupation contribute to risk factors for cardiovascular disease. *American Journal of Public Health, 82,* 816–820.

Winter, R. (1994, September–October). Which pain relievers work best? *Consumers Digest, 33,* 76–79.

Wise, E. H., & Barnes, D. R. (1986). The relationship among life events, dysfunctional attitudes, and depression. *Cognitive Therapy and Research, 10,* 257–266.

Wiseman, C. V., Gray, J. J., Mosimann, J. E., & Ahrens, A. H. (1992). Cultural expectations of thinness in women: An update. *International Journal of Eating Disorders, 11,* 85–89.

Wolf, S. (1950). Effects of suggestion and conditioning on the action of chemical agents in human subjects—The pharmacology of placebos. *Journal of Clinical Investigation, 29,* 100–109.

Wolf, S. L., Nacht, M., & Kelly, J. L. (1982). EMG feedback training during dynamic movement for low back pain patients. *Behavior Therapy, 13,* 395–406.

Wolfgang, M. E. (1957). Victim precipitated criminal homicide. *Journal of Criminal Law and Criminology, 48,* 1–11.

Wolters, P. L., Brouwers, P., Moss, H. A., & Pizzo, P. A. (1994). Adaptive behavior of children with symptomatic HIV infection before and after ziovudine therapy: Special Section: Pediatric AIDS. *Journal of Pediatric Psychology, 19,* 47–61.

Wong, M., & Kaloupek, D. G. (1986). Coping with dental treatment: The potential impact of situational demands. *Journal of Behavioral Medicine, 9,* 579–597.

Wood, P. D., Stefanick, M. L., Dreon, D. M., Frey-Hewitt, B., Garay, S. C., Williams, P. T., Superko, H. R., Fortmann, S. P., Albers, J. J., Vranizan, K. M., Ellsworth, N. M., Terry, R. B., & Haskell, W. L. (1988). Changes in plasma lipids and lipoproteins in overweight men during weight loss through dieting compared with exercise. *New England Journal of Medicine, 319,* 1173–1179.

Woodforde, J. M., & Fielding, J. R. (1975). Pain and cancer. In M. Weisenberg (Ed.), *Pain, clinical and experimental perspectives.* St. Louis: Mosby.

Woodside, D. B., Garner, D. M., Rockert, W., & Garfinkel, P. E. (1990). Eating disorders in males: Insights from a clinical and psychometric comparison with female patients. In A. E. Andersen (Ed.), *Males with eating disorders* (pp. 100–115). New York: Brunner/Mazel.

Wooley, S. C., & Garner, D. M. (1991). Obesity treatment: The high cost of false hope. *Journal of the American Dietetic Association, 91,* 1248–1251.

Worden, J. K., Flynn, B. S., Merrill, D. E., Waller, J. A., & Haugh, L. D. (1989). Preventing alcohol-impaired driving through community self-regulation training. *American Journal of Public Health, 79,* 287–290.

Worksite Wellness Works. (1995a, May). Corporate leaders laud benefits of wellness. *Worksite Wellness Works, 11* (2), 1, 4.

Worksite Wellness Works. (1995b, May). Medical claims-based study shows $4.75 savings for every $1. *Worksite Wellness Works, 11* (2), 8.

Wu, J. M. (1990). Summary and concluding remarks. In J. M. Wu (Ed.), *Environmental tobacco smoke: Proceedings of the international symposium at McGill University 1989* (pp. 367–375). Lexington, MA: Heath.

Wyden, P. (1965). *The overweight society.* New York: Morrow.

Wynder, E. L., Goodman, M. T., & Hoffmann, D. (1984). Demographic aspects of the low yield cigarette: Considerations in the evaluation of health risks. *Journal of the National Cancer Institute, 72,* 817–822.

Wysocki, T. (1989). Impact of blood glucose monitoring on diabetic control: Obstacles and interventions. *Journal of Behavioral Medicine, 12,* 183–205.

Wysocki, T., Green, L., & Huxtable, K. (1989). Blood glucose monitoring by diabetic adolescents: Compliance and metabolic control. *Health Psychology, 8,* 267–284.

Yager, J., Grant, I., Sweetwood, H. L., & Gerst, M. (1981). Life event reports by psychiatric patients, nonpatients, and their partners. *Archives of General Psychiatry, 38,* 343–347.

Yano, K., Rhoads, G. G., Kagan, A., & Tillotson, J. (1978). Dietary intake and risk of coronary heart disease in Japanese men living in Hawaii. *American Journal of Clinical Nutrition, 31,* 1270–1279.

Yates, A., Leehey, K., & Shisslak, C. M. (1983). Running—an analogue of anorexia? *New England Journal of Medicine, 308,* 251–255.

Yeaton, W. H., Smith, D., & Rogers, K. (1990). Evaluating understanding of popular press reports of health research. *Health Education Quarterly, 17,* 223–234.

Yep, G. A. (1993). HIV prevention among Asian-American college students: Does the health belief model work? *Journal of American College Health, 41,* 199–205.

Young, D. R., Haskell, W. L., Jatulis, D. E., & Fortmann, S. P. (1993). Associations between changes in physical activity and risk factors for coronary heart disease in a community-based sample of men and women: The Stanford Five-City Project, *American Journal of Epidemiology, 138,* 205–216.

Young, L. D. (1993). Rheumatoid arthritis. In R. J. Gatchel & E. B. Blanchard (Eds.), *Psychophysiological disorders: Research and clinical applications* (pp. 269–298). Washington, DC: American Psychological Association.

Zador, P. L., & Ciccone, M. A. (1993). Automobile driver fatalities in frontal impacts: Air bags compared with manual belts. *American Journal of Public Health, 83,* 661–666.

Zastowny, T. R., Kirschenbaum, D. S., & Meng. A. L. (1986). Coping skills training for children: Effects on distress before, during, and after hospitalization for surgery. *Health Psychology, 5,* 231–247.

Zavela, K. J., Davis, L. G., Cottrell, R. R., & Smith, W. E. (1988). Do only the healthy intend to participate in worksite health promotion? *Health Education Quarterly, 15,* 259–267.

Zhang, J., Feldblum, P. J., & Fortney, J. A. (1992). Moderate physical activity and bone density among perimenopausal women. *American Journal of Public Health, 82,* 736–738.

Zimbardo, P. G. (1969). The human choice: Individuation, reason, and order versus deindividuation, impulse, and chaos. In W. J. Arnold & D. Levine (Eds.), *Nebraska symposium on motivation.* Lincoln: University of Nebraska Press.

Zimberg, S. (1985a). Principles of alcoholism psychotherapy. In S. Zimberg, J. Wallace, & S. B. Blume (Eds.), *Practical approaches to alcoholism psychotherapy* (2nd ed.). New York: Plenum.

Zimberg, S. (1985b). Psychiatric office treatment of alcoholism. In S. Zimberg, J. Wallace, & S. B. Blume (Eds.), *Practical approaches to alcoholism psychotherapy* (2nd ed.). New York: Plenum.

Zimmerman, M. (1983). Methodological issues in the assessment of life events: A review of issues and research. *Clinical Psychology Review, 3,* 339–370.

Zimmerman, R. S., & Olson, K. (1994). AIDS-related risk behavior and behavior change in a sexually active heterosexual sample: A test of three models of prevention. *AIDS Education and Prevention, 6,* 189–204.

Zinberg, N. E. (1981). Social interactions, drug use, and drug research. In J. H. Lowinson & P. Ruiz (Eds.), *Substance abuse: Clinical problems and perspectives* (pp. 91–108). Baltimore: Williams & Wilkins.

Zinberg, N. E. (1984). *Drug, set, and setting: The basis for controlled intoxicant use.* New Haven, CT: Yale University Press.

Zonderman, A. B., Costa, P. T., & McCrae, R. R. (1989). Depression as a risk for cancer morbidity and mortality in a nationally representative sample. *Journal of the American Medical Association, 262,* 1191–1195.

Zubin, J., & Spring, B. (1977). Vulnerability—a new view of schizophrenia. *Journal of Abnormal Psychology, 86,* 103–127.

Zuckerman, M., Ball, S., & Black, J. (1990). Influences of sensation seeking, gender, risk appraisal, and situational motivation on smoking. *Addictive Behaviors, 15,* 209–220.

Zyazema, N. Z. (1984). Toward better patient drug compliance and comprehension: A challenge to medical and pharmaceutical services in Zimbabwe. *Social Science and Medicine, 18,* 551–554.

Name Index

Subject Index

Photo Credits